Rabbi Edward Reichman, MD

THE
ANATOMY
OF
JEWISH
LAW

A Fresh Dissection
of the Relationship
Between Medicine,
Medical History,
& Rabbinic Literature

OU Press
Yeshiva University Press
Maggid Books

The Anatomy of Jewish Law:
A Fresh Dissection of the Relationship Between
Medicine, Medical History, and Rabbinic Literature

OU Press
An imprint of the Orthodox Union
11 Broadway, New York, NY 10004
www.oupress.org

Maggid Books
An imprint of Koren Publishers Jerusalem Ltd.
POB 8531 New Milford, CT 06776-8531, USA
& POB 4044, Jerusalem 9104001, Israel
www.maggidbooks.com

Yeshiva University Press
500 West 185th Street, New York, NY 10033

The publication of this book was made possible
through the generous support of *The Jewish Book Trust.*

ISBN 978-1-59264-579-4

Printed and bound in the United States

ספר זה מוקדש
לעילוי נשמות הורי היקרים

This book is dedicated in loving memory of
my dear parents, *aleihem hashalom*

Rabbi Baruch Reichman
Rebbetzin Shoshana Reichman

הרב ברוך בן יצחק אייזיק
רייזל שושנה בת אהרן יוסף

The love and guidance that flowed from my wonderful
parents shepherded me to this milestone in my life. They
completely embodied and exemplified the ideals of a
true Torah life in all its manifestations. My parents both
descended from prominent *Yerushalmi* families. My father
was a descendant of the Hakham Tzvi, and my mother's
grandfather, Rabbi David Weingarten, founded the General
Israel Orphanage Home in Yerushalayim. My father was one
of the few to personally receive *semikha* from Rav Yitzchak
Hutner *zt"l*, of Yeshivas Rabbeinu Chaim Berlin. He served
as a rabbi in Wisconsin for fifty years. His care and concern
for his congregants was legendary. My mother was the
consummate *rebbetzin* and teacher par excellence. Yet, they
were most proud of the family they raised. Their love and
devotion have been a constant source of inspiration for me.
They will be forever missed! May their holy נשמות continue
to have an עליה and may they be מליצי יושר for our family.

ת.נ.צ.ב.ה.

ספר זה מוקדש
לעילוי נשמות מחותני היקרים

This book is dedicated in loving memory of
my dear parents-in-law, *aleihem hashalom*

Professor Louis H. Feldman
Mrs. Miriam Feldman

אליעזר צבי בן שמואל
מרים בת משה יעקב

My father-in-law was Professor of Classics at Yeshiva
University for over fifty years. A world-renowned expert
on Josephus, his dedication to scholarship and academia
was legendary. He was a proud, *frum* Jew and wore his
yarmulka to conferences all over the world, long before
that was the norm. My mother-in-law was a survivor
of the Holocaust, whose escape with her two sisters
saved all their lives. Their love for family, combined
with hard work and dedication to an ideal, have been
a constant source of inspiration for me. They will be
forever missed! May their holy נשמות continue to have
an עליה and may they be מליצי יושר for our family.

ת.נ.צ.ב.ה.

Contents

Foreword by Rabbi Professor Avraham Steinberg, MD   xi
Preface   xiii
Acknowledgements   xvii
Introduction: The Impact of Medical History on Medical Halakha   xxi

FERTILITY AND REPRODUCTION

The Rabbinic Conception of Conception:
An Exercise in Fertility   3

The Doctrine of the Seven-Chamber Uterus   38

Parashat Tazria and Childbirth: An Open and Shut Case   58

Is There Life After Life? Superfetation in Medical,
Historical and Rabbinic Literature   70

Midrash, Miracles, and Motherhood: The Birth of Dinah and
the Definition of Maternity—*Tzarikh Iyun LeDina*   85

The First Halakhic Discussion of Ovarian Transplantation   111

Uterine Transplantation and the Case of
the Mistaken Question   153

Shared Biological Paternity in Rabbinic Literature: From Goliath
to Mitochondrial DNA and the Three-Parent Embryo   175

ANATOMY AND PHYSIOLOGY

The Anatomy of the Human Body in Rabbinic
Literature: The 248 "*Evarim*"   199

The Anatomy of Halakha   209

The Anatomy of Prayer   231

The Illusive and Elusive *Luz* Bone   245

Are Two Heads Really Better Than One? Halakhic Issues
Relating to Conjoined Twins and a Two-Headed Person   272

The Incorporation of Pre-Modern Scientific Theories into
Rabbinic Literature: The Case of Innate Heat   296

DISEASES AND THERAPEUTICS

The Impact of Medieval Medicine on Medical
Halakha: The Case of Mumia   321

A Tale of Two Stones in the Eighteenth Century   344

The Use of Anesthesia in Circumcision: A
Reevaluation of the Halakhic Sources   351

Lessons from the First Halakhic Analysis of Vaccination   374

Ebola: A New Disease with an Ancient Tradition   385

Lehitra'ot Ebola, Goodbye Rubella, Hello Zika   393

Precedented Times: The Rabbinic Response to
COVID-19 and Pandemics Throughout the Ages   403

DEATH AND RESUSCITATION

The Halakhic Definition of Death in Light of Medical History   431

The Resuscitation of Halakha: An Animated Discussion   464

A Matter of Life "in" Death: Postmortem
Caesarean Section in Jewish Law   477

MEDICINE AND RABBINIC LITERATURE

Biblical and Talmudic Medicine: A Bibliographical Essay   511

A Letter from a Torah Sage of the Eighteenth Century to
the Faculty of a Medical School: The Selective Deference of
Rabbi Yonatan Eybeschuetz to Medical Expertise   522

Glossary   543

Index   553

Foreword

Many sources in the Bible and even many more examples in the Talmud relate to diseases, treatments, medical advice, and other medical-related issues. Several experts in the past have attempted to interpret these matters based on the medical knowledge in the relevant periods. They based their remarks on their vast knowledge of the biblical and the talmudic literature combined with their knowledge of the history of medicine.

The previous experts in the field of Jewish medical history have covered almost exclusively appropriate passages in the Bible and the Talmud only. There has been hardly any effort in discussing and studying medical-historical issues in the halakhic literature of Codes and Responsa.

The knowledge of medical history is very important in understanding the reality according to which a particular *posek* reached his medical-halakhic conclusions. There has been a paucity of studies in medical history related to the halakhic literature. This book is, therefore, a unique and important addition to the field of medicine and halakha enabling one to apply halakhic precedence to current questions and dilemmas.

Rabbi Professor Edward Reichman, MD is one of less than a handful of experts who utilize their vast knowledge of the Codes and Responsa literature combined with his wide-range knowledge of medical history in order to shed light on numerous issues with halakhic relevance discussed in the halakhic literature.

I have been privileged to know Rabbi Dr. Reichman for many years and to participate with him in numerous conferences on medicine and halakha. It has always been an outstanding learning experience to listen to the eloquent and in-depth lectures by Rabbi Dr. Reichman.

Now everyone has the opportunity to learn Rabbi Dr. Reichman's unique contribution to medicine and halakha through his excellent book, *The Anatomy of Jewish Law: A Fresh Dissection of the Relationship Between Medicine, Medical History, and Rabbinic Literature.* This book is replete with many examples from the halakhic literature where Rabbi Dr. Reichman discovers in a masterful way the underlying medical-historical reality through which the *posek* discusses and concludes his position. The book covers all fields of medicine and halakha, by *poskim* throughout the generations and geographic locations.

It is indeed an in-depth treatise of a unique field, written by a unique individual and expert, both in halakha and in medical history.

I highly recommend to everyone in the fields of medicine and halakha that they acquire and study this exceptional work.

Rabbi Professor Avraham Steinberg, MD

Preface

I f you deem this book worthy of purchase, you will need to decide where on the shelves of your precious library it should be placed. In its broadest sense, it clearly belongs in the class of Judaism and science; yet, as our generation has witnessed a massive expansion in this domain, we need to further sub-classify this literature into genus and species.

This book deals primarily with medicine, the understanding of the human body, and the treatment of human disease, as opposed to other scientific endeavors. As such, you will find no discussion of evolution, creation, astronomy and the heliocentric theory, or physics. To be sure, there are significant areas of intersection.[1] Within the genus of Judaism and medicine, further subdivision is needed.

There are two major species within this genus, each with its own subdivisions.

---

1. Chief amongst them is the so-called topic of *nishtaneh hateva*, addressing scientific passages in Ḥazal that seemingly conflict with our modern understanding. This is not the primary purpose of this book, though any work on the frontier of science is invariably swept into the proverbial tide of *nishtaneh hateva*. We do refer to this topic periodically and reference the relevant literature.

- Medical halakha (Jewish medical ethics or Jewish bioethics)
- Jewish medical history

Medical Halakha

Rabbinic authorities have been addressing medical issues since the giving of the Torah. While great Torah sages have continued to address medical issues in the modern era,[2] the founder or grandfather of the academic field of contemporary Jewish medical ethics in the modern era is considered to be Rabbi Immanuel Jakobovits, *zt"l*, whose Ph.D. dissertation from University College of London was published as *Jewish Medical Ethics* in 1959. Since then, the field has blossomed.[3]

Jewish Medical History

There is another species in the genus of Judaism and medicine which focuses on Jewish medical history and its relationship to general medical history. Studies range from the biblical and talmudic period to Maimonides and up to the modern era.[4]

Rarely, if ever, do we find crosspollination between these two species. In the writings of medical halakha, you will scarcely find mention of medical history; likewise, the authors of Jewish medical history rarely invoke halakhic literature. The present work attempts to interface

---

2. See Fred Rosner, ed., *Pioneers in Jewish Medical Ethics* (Jason Aronson, 1997). The great rabbinic authorities include Rabbi Shlomo Zalman Auerbach, *zt"l*, Rabbi Shalom Yosef Elyashiv, *zt"l*, Rabbi Moshe Feinstein, *zt"l*, Rabbi Eliezer Waldenberg, *zt"l*, Rabbi Asher Weiss, *shlit"a* and Rabbi Yitzhak Zilberstein, *shlit"a*.

3. The additional foundational pillars of the field who followed shortly thereafter include Rabbi J. David Bleich, Rabbi David Feldman, Dr. Fred Rosner, and Rabbi Dr. Moshe Tendler. They were in turn followed by the second generation of scholars who continued to expand the field, including Dr. Abraham Abraham, Rabbi Dr. Mordechai Halperin, Rabbi Yigal Shafran, Rabbi Dr. Avraham Steinberg, and Rabbi Dr. Akiva Tatz. There are now third and fourth generations continuing to expand the field.

4. Authors who have contributed to this field include Zohar Amar, Ron Barkai, Gerrit Bos, Kenneth Collins, John Efron, Ronald Eisenberg, Gad Freudenthal, Harry Friedenwald, Frank Heynick, Maoz Kahana, Yehudah Leib Katznelsen, Samuel Kottek, Tzvi Langerman, Joshua Leibowitz, David Margalit, Suessman Muntner, Michael Nevins, Moshe Perlman, Julius Preuss, Fred Rosner, David Ruderman, Eliezer Sariel, Joseph Shatzmiller, Avraham Ofir Shemesh, H. J. Zimmels, and Nimrod Zinger.

these largely disparate, dissociated disciplines in hopes of demonstrating that the Jewish and general history of medicine can shed light on, and provide context for, the world of medical halakha.

In the essays before you, we trace medical notions of anatomy, physiology, and therapeutics across time and genres of rabbinic literature. Oft times, our analysis is enlightened or enhanced by a study of the contemporaneous medical history. A few authors, such as Preuss, Zimmels, and Jakobovits, invoked medical theories contemporaneous with the sources they discussed. Their approach, in varying degrees, was performed on a macro, or horizontal, level, and they generally did not plumb the depths of specific topics.

In a sense, this book is an attempt to expand this approach and to apply it vertically. We pick up where they left off, following their lead to its logical extension. This work is by no means comprehensive or encyclopedic, nor is it systematic. The topics chosen to illustrate this approach merely represent the particular interests of the author.

These essays have previously appeared in a wide variety of publications over a span of years. They have been extensively revised, updated and integrated for this publication. The chapters of this book need not be read in sequence and are largely independent. As a result, there will be some limited repetition and overlap between chapters, including footnotes. They do however interrelate with each other, and when viewed in totality, will hopefully reflect a common theme of the value of placing medical halakhic sources into their historical context. It is the hope that this work will spark more research in this area where few have trodden.

Does this endeavor necessitate the creation of a new species or simply the new interrelationship of existing species? I will leave this to the reader to decide. Could this type of research impact the field of contemporary medical halakha? I will leave this to the *poskim* to decide.

As to where this book should sit on your bookshelf, I would suggest placement right between the sections on medical halakha and Jewish medical history, perhaps closer to the former, and serving as a bridge between them. It can serve as a supplement or complement to enhance your appreciation of the vast pre-modern rabbinic literature dealing with medical matters. This literature is the foundation upon which contemporary halakhic discussions are based.

Acknowledgements

It is with profound gratitude to *Hakadosh Barukh Hu* that I offer this humble contribution in partial fulfillment of my obligation of "*kitvu lakhem et hashira hazot,*" to write my own Torah scroll, as it were. The gifts Hashem has bestowed upon my family and me are wholly undeserved, and I hope that this effort will serve as a small attempt *lihagdil Torah uleha'adira,* to enhance the glory and greatness of Torah.

I feel blessed to have been born into such a wonderful family, stemming from many generations of *Yerushalmim.* To my knowledge, I am the first physician in a long line of rabbis, scholars, and *gomlei ḥasadim* on both my paternal and maternal sides. My parents, Rabbi Barukh, *z"l* and Shoshana, *a"h* were ideal role models in every sense, encouraging and inspiring me throughout my life. This book is dedicated to their memory.

I feel blessed to have such an amazing wife, Sara, who not only was a superb editor for this book but is my life EDitor (not a typo) as well. My children, Shmulie and Rivka, Ari, Shoshana, and Elana, are the joys of my life. I pray that Sara and I, *b'ezrat Hashem,* continue to have much *naḥas* from our beautiful family. I thank Howard and Elkie, Leah and Brad, and Moshe and Ellen for their love and support and for being such wonderful siblings.

I feel privileged to have been born at a time when scientific advances have progressed more rapidly than any other time in history. I have had the *zechus* of being exposed to the great personalities in the field of medical halakha, who have all influenced me in varying degrees, both as teachers and mentors, as well as through their writings. I was a student of Rabbi Dr. Moshe Tendler, *shlit"a* and Rabbi Dr. J. David Bleich, *shlit"a* during my years of education at Yeshiva University. I also learned from the *shiurim* of Rabbi Tzvi Flaum, *shlit"a*.

I chose to do my residency training where Dr. Fred Rosner was chairman. I recall the frequent visits to his office when, without exception, there was a handwritten manuscript of the latest medical halakhic topic on his desktop. He has been a mentor to me, a staunch supporter of my research, and has had a profound effect on my life. After residency, we learned Rambam every Friday together at his home for many years until he moved to Israel. Dr. Rosner contributed sections to two of the articles in this book on the topics of the Luz Bone and anesthesia in circumcision.

Over the years, I have had the great fortune to both attend and lecture at the conferences of a number of organizations such as the Association of Orthodox Jewish Scientists, the National Institute of Judaism and Medicine, and Torah in Motion. It is during these conferences that I was exposed to many great personalities in the field, including Rabbi Dr. Avraham Steinberg, *shlit"a*, from whom I have learned immeasurably and whose relationship I deeply cherish. I am profoundly appreciative of his contributing the Foreword to this book.

Aside from the classic works of rabbinic literature, the works that were most influential in the early years of my research for this book were those of Julius Preuss, H. J. Zimmels, and Rabbi Lord Immanuel Jakobovits, *zt"l*, as well as the Jewish medical history journal *Koroth*. A significant portion of my medical historical research was done at the Wellcome Institute for the History of Medicine in London. I recall the librarian mentioning that I was the first Orthodox Jew they had seen in the library since Rabbi Jakobovits, who conducted the research for his dissertation there. Dr. Nigel Allen, past curator of the Wellcome Institute's Oriental Collection, was instrumental in exposing me to the field of Jewish medical history.

On one trip to London, I attempted to visit the House of Commons to hear Margaret Thatcher during her weekly appearance. Unfortunately, the House of Commons gallery was full, so we were shunted to the House of Lords instead. As it turned out, the topic of debate on the floor of the House of Lords was the status of the human embryo. Rabbi Lord Jakobovits was one of the first speakers of the day. His impassioned and articulate speech had a profound impact on me. I would later have the pleasure of visiting him at his home in London over the years. I also spent time in Jerusalem with Professor Joshua Leibowitz, z"l, and Professor Samuel Kottek (current editor of Koroth), two of the leaders in the field of Jewish medical history, who both inspired my passion for Jewish medical history.

I thank those who have provided me an opportunity to share some of these topics in a public lecture forum, which assisted in the development and refinement of the research. These include Sam Lasko of Lasko Tours; Rabbi Moshe and Corrine Fuchs; Robert Frucher and Matty Klein of Leisure Time Tours; Joel Mael and the *Hashkama Minyan* at Young Israel of Lawrence-Cedarhurst; the Edward Avenue *Ḥabura*; Rabbi Ephraim Mintz and Rabbi Mordechai Dinerman of the Jewish Learning Institute and National Jewish Retreat, and Rabbi Jay Kelman and Dr. Lazer Friedman of Torah in Motion.

This book would not have been possible without the aid of countless librarians, archivists and colleagues who were instrumental in recommending or acquiring oftentimes rare references. Tzvi Erenyi and Zalman Alpert of the Yeshiva University Library were always available for consultation, as were many others at institutions throughout the world mentioned by name in the footnotes. The ubiquitous Menachem Butler could always be counted on to obtain the unobtainable or to send an unsolicited rare reference.

A number of the chapters of this book have previously appeared in the following journals and books: *Tradition; Hakirah; Journal of the History of Medicine and Allied Sciences; Jewish Action; Torah U'Madda Journal; Verapo Yerapei: Journal of Torah and Medicine of the Albert Einstein College of Medicine Synagogue; BDD Journal of Torah and Scholarship; Mitoch HaOhel series* (Yeshiva University Press); F. Rosner, ed., *Pioneers in Jewish Medical Ethics* (Jason Aronson, 1997); F. Rosner, *Encyclopedia of Biblical and Talmudic Medicine* (Jason Aronson, 2000); F. Rosner, H. Goldstein, E. Reichman, eds., *Studies in Jewish Medical Ethics* (Hojers Forlag, 2008); Y. Steinberg, ed., *Berakha Le'Avraham*: Tribute volume in honor of Rabbi Dr. Avraham Steinberg's sixtieth birthday (Jerusalem, 2008); K. Collins, E. Reichman and

Acknowledgements

A. Steinberg, eds., *In the Pathways of Maimonides: Studies in Maimonides, Medical Ethics, and Jewish Law—A Tribute to Dr. Fred Rosner* (Maimonides Research Institute, 2015). They have been extensively revised, updated and integrated for this publication. I thank all the publishers for permission to republish the material here.

OU PRESS, under the leadership of Rabbi Menachem Genack, has been involved with this project since the outset. I thank Rabbi Simon Posner at OU Press for his tremendous support, dedication, and persistent efforts in seeing this publication to fruition. I cannot thank Yocheved Goldberg enough for her countless hours of excellent editing and her dedication to this project. I also thank Rabbi Daniel Feldman and Rabbi Dr. Stuart Halpern at YU Press for facilitating a joint publication with OU PRESS. Thanks as well are due to Matthew Miller and his staff at Maggid Books, with a special note of gratitude to managing editor Caryn Meltz, for their professionalism.

The Atran Foundation provided a generous donation towards the publication of the book, for which I am most grateful.

It is deeply meaningful to me and so very much appreciated that this book is generously sponsored by Isaac and Diana Corre in honor of Isaac's parents, Rabbi Dr. Alan and Mrs. Nita Corre, *aleihem hashalom*. Isaac, or Crow as I fondly call him, was my closest childhood friend in Milwaukee, and we were inseparable. I fondly recall those simpler days when the most complex decision I would have each week was whether Isaac should come to my house Shabbos afternoon, or I to his. Many of my most cherished childhood memories include Isaac and his family. Professor and Mrs. Corre were pillars of the Milwaukee Jewish community, as were my dear parents. Rabbi Dr. Corre was a towering intellectual and Professor of Hebrew Studies at the University of Wisconsin. Mrs. Corre was director of the Jewish Home and Care Center in Milwaukee. Her devotion, vision and leadership were legendary. They both served as wonderful role models for me. Furthermore, my parents, *a"h*, and the Corres, *a"h*, were the closest of friends and shared a mutual and deep admiration for each other. There is no question that our parents are smiling down from heaven knowing that they have successfully passed the mutual admiration society to the next generation.

Introduction

The Impact of Medical History on Medical Halakha

T here is a foundational idea about the creation of the world expressed by *Ḥazal*: *HaKadosh Barukh Hu histakel be'Oraita ubara alma*—God literally looked into the text of the Torah and created the world. In essence, the Torah is the divine blueprint for the world's creation. I submit that the converse is true for man. *Adam histakel be'alma ubara Oraita*—the human being examines the world around him and creates, in a figurative sense, the Torah. When one delves into the workings of the world through the study of medicine and science, he or she brings the Torah to life and gains an appreciation of God's role in the creation of the world.

The crowning glory of God's creation is the human being. To understand the creation of the human being, the process of conception and birth, human anatomy and physiology, is to understand the human being's Creator. Therefore, people in every generation have sought to gain greater insight into the workings of the human body and the world of medicine.

Regarding the very creation or birth of the human being, the Talmud informs us of the origin of a minor anatomical feature of major consequences called the philtrum—the small infra-nasal indentation. According to tradition, the fetus learns the entire corpus of Torah in utero.[1] Just prior to birth, however, the baby receives the touch of an angel, which causes the indentation of the philtrum. This afflicts the child with transient amnesia, causing the child to forget all he has learned, necessitating years of laborious effort to restore this lost knowledge. What could possibly be the benefit to the child of such a seemingly cruel act? Many have suggested that the very process of reacquiring the Torah through years of struggle and tireless effort (*yegiah*) will lead to a more meaningful and everlasting relationship with the Torah and its Creator. A person can then, theoretically, with proper devotion and effort, ultimately return to his state of knowledge in utero, when he had mastered the entire Torah.

What of the study of science, however, and the understanding of human physiology? Does the individual child learn the intricacies of medicine and science in utero, only to forget and subsequently relearn them all with proper effort? Assumedly not, at least not as an individual. In fact, while it is theoretically possible for one person to learn the entire corpus of Torah teachings, this is decidedly not the case for science and medicine. While throughout the ages we have been blessed with Torah sages who have been the repositories of all extant Torah knowledge, no such analogue exists in science. There is no one human being who possesses all knowledge of medicine and science. The greatest minds in the history of medicine and science knew only the minutia of their specific fields. Einstein knew little about human physiology.

Science, by definition, is a collaborative endeavor, advanced only through the accumulated efforts of thousands of great minds across the span of time. Perhaps, analogous to a person as an individual working to restore his lost knowledge of the Torah, all of humanity works tirelessly to restore the knowledge of the scientific workings of the world that was known at the time of creation, attempting to reverse our global amnesia. This endeavor has progressed slowly, with each generation adding

---

1. *Nidda* 30b.

incrementally to our collective knowledge of science and medicine, and thus our appreciation of *HaKadosh Barukh Hu.*

Some advances have incorporated and built on pre-existing theories, while others have rejected or supplanted previous notions. This evolution of the understanding of medicine is reflected in the rabbinic literature throughout the centuries.

Rabbinic authorities at every stage of history invariably sought medical consultation, either directly or indirectly, prior to rendering decisions on *materia medica.*[2] The accumulated literature of centuries of medical halakhic discourse serves as the foundation for contemporary medical halakhic analysis. As this literature spans the chronological gamut of scientific and medical discovery, it is essential to view each source in its proper historical context.

The objective of this book is to sensitize the reader to the historical dimension of medical halakhic research. Modern rabbinic authorities integrate the most current medical information in order to address contemporary medical halakhic issues. Rabbis of previous generations most assuredly did the same, though the state of medical knowledge and authoritative sources clearly differed from that of today. What is often neglected is the value of an understanding of medical history as a supplement or adjunct to the study of medical halakha.

This book illustrates how a medical historical approach can be informative. Below I enumerate some specific ways this methodology will be helpful to an understanding of the overall corpus of medical halakhic literature. As this field of research remains largely unexplored, this exercise is an attempt to pave the path for future exploration. It is my hope that these categories and examples will be expanded, refined, restructured, or replaced as research in this area evolves. I make no pretense to determine the halakhic relevance of this research. This lies exclusively in the domain of the great Torah sages and rabbinic authorities. At the very least, it is my hope that this approach will enhance Torah study and provide an appreciation of the ongoing and continuously evolving relationship between science, medicine, and Jewish law.

---

2. See chapter, "A Letter from a Torah Sage of the Eighteenth Century."

I. TEXTUAL INTERPRETATION

On a microcosmic level, an understanding of medical history can enhance or facilitate the interpretation of a particular text in a number of ways.

Identification of Personalities

Modern medical halakhic responsa, despite their reliance on modern medicine and their inclusion of detailed scientific information, rarely contain references to specific physicians or scientists. In contrast, pre-modern medical halakhic literature frequently contains such specific references. This is due, in large part, to the nature of medical training and tradition in the pre-modern era. Whereas today, medical students study textbooks that are a composite of multiple authors, the medical student curriculum of the Middle Ages and Renaissance consisted of selected works of a handful of authors, primarily from Greek antiquity.[3] Three of these authors, Hippocrates (c. 460 BCE–c. 368 BCE),[4] Galen (c. 130 CE–c. 200 CE)[5] and Avicenna (980 CE–1037 CE),[6] are often cited in rabbinic literature. The references may be accompanied by the title of physician,[7] but sometimes there is no indication of the secular or medical origin of the author.[8] Avicenna is called Ibn Sina in Hebrew and could easily be mistaken for a rabbinic source. The names of these physicians did not require identification by the rabbinic authors, as they were undoubtedly familiar to the contemporary reader. In fact, the works of all the aforementioned medical authors were frequently translated into Hebrew[9] and were an integral part of the Jewish physician's library.

---

3. S. D'Irsay, "Teachers and Textbooks of Medicine in the Medieval University of Paris," *Annals of Medical History* 8 (1926), 234–239; S. Cooper, "The Medical School of Montpellier in the Fourteenth Century," *Annals of Medical History: New Series* 2 (1930), 164–195, esp. 174; N. G. Siraisi, *Medieval and Early Renaissance Medicine* (University of Chicago Press, 1990), 70–77.

4. *Teshuvot Maharashdam, Ḥ.M.,* 364. Hippocrates is referred to as *Avukrat* in Hebrew.

5. Ibid.; *Teshuvot Maharshakh* 2:160; *Tzitz Eliezer,* 10:25, chap. 4.

6. *Teshuvot Darkhei No'am, Y. D.,* 26; *Noda BiYehuda, Mahadura Tinyana, Y. D.,* 21; *She'eilat Ya'avetz* 1:41 and 171.

7. *Teshuvot Maharsham, Ḥ.M.,* 364; *Noda BiYehuda, Mahadura Tinyana, Y. D.,* 21.

8. *She'eilat Ya'avetz* 1:41 and 171.

9. E. Lieber, "Galen in Hebrew: The Transmission of Galen's Works in the Medieval Islamic World," in *Galen: Problems and Prospects* (Wellcome Institute for the History

Knowing the nature of an author's reference can enhance the reader's interpretation. It is helpful to know that the author is citing a medical authority when discussing a medical matter. Such reliance on physicians could contribute to the general discussion on the reliance on medical knowledge in halakha (*ne'emanut harofim*). On a pragmatic note, knowing that the citation is not rabbinic in origin may also prevent fruitless searches for a reference.

Clarification of Concepts and Terminology

Just as medical personalities mentioned in rabbinic literature may be unfamiliar to the modern reader, the same is true for medical terminology and theories. Rabbinic literature throughout history, ranging from biblical to halakhic commentaries, is replete with allusions to medical theories. These theories are variously assimilated depending on the context and are better understood in their proper medical historical milieu. Many of the chapters in this book address such theories, such as the theory of innate heat, the doctrine of the seven-chamber uterus, and pre-modern theories of reproductive, cardiac, and respiratory physiology.

Prevention of Misapplication

Another dimension of textual interpretation enhanced by the study of medical history is an appreciation of the medical facts from which a halakhic decision is derived. For example, in the assessment of medical risk in halakha and the permissibility of undergoing potentially dangerous procedures, a passage from the works of R. Yaakov Emden is oft quoted.[10] The medical condition R. Emden discusses is the very same medical

---

of Medicine, 1981), 167–186; one need only peruse the index of H. D. Isaacs, *Medical and Para-Medical Manuscripts in the Cairo Geniza Collection* (Cambridge University Press, 1994) under Galen, Hippocrates and Avicenna to appreciate the popularity of these authors. For a list of extant Hebrew manuscripts of Avicenna's Canon, see B. Richler, "Manuscripts of Avicenna's Canon in Hebrew Translation: A Revised and Up-to-Date List," *Koroth* 8:3–4 (August, 1982), 145–68. Avicenna's Canon is the first Hebrew medical book to be printed and the only extant Hebrew medical incunable (Naples, 1491). See also J. O. Leibowitz, "Ibn Sina in Hebrew," *Koroth* 8:1–2 (June, 1981), 3–8; D. Wilk, "One Thousandth Anniversary of Ibn Sina: Notes from the Library," ibid., 91–95.

10. *Mor UKetzia, O. H.,* 328.

condition which is the basis for the classic responsum on autopsy by R. Yeḥezkel Landau. The chapter "A Tale of Two Stones" is devoted to placing these responsa in their proper medical historical context and suggesting how this might impact their extrapolation to a modern context.

II. TEXTUAL CONTEXTUALIZATION

An awareness of medical history may also enable the reader to look beyond the text itself and appreciate the particular source in its historical context. What precipitates discussion of certain issues at a certain period in history? A number of our chapters highlight this dimension.

One of the first responsa addressing the issue of autopsy and anatomical dissection is that of R. Yeḥezkel Landau of eighteenth-century Prague.[11] Our chapter "A Tale of Two Stones" explains why this important topic was not addressed previously by Rambam or the *Shulḥan Arukh*.

Another example of the importance of chronology in the interpretation of medical discussions in rabbinic literature can be found not in the halakhic literature but in the exegetical literature. In our chapter "The Doctrine of the Seven-Chamber Uterus" we discuss a curious anatomical notion which is employed by a number of medieval exegetes in their explication of certain biblical passages.[12] If this is how the uterus was thought to be constructed, why is this anatomical notion not mentioned in the Talmud? It would certainly be important for the clarification of the laws of *nidda*. Furthermore, we find no primary rabbinic source mentioning this doctrine after the seventeenth century. Here again, an appreciation of medical history sheds light on these questions.

Similar to the doctrine of the seven-chamber uterus, rabbis of the sixteenth and seventeenth centuries address the halakhic ramification of a medicine called mumia which was derivative from the human corpse. Our chapter on mumia explains why discussions of mumia are not to be found either before or after this time period.

---

11. *Noda BiYehuda, Mahadura Tinyana Y. D.*, 210.
12. On what follows, and for a comprehensive treatment of this notion, see chapter, "The Doctrine of the Seven-Chamber Uterus."

Included in this category are discussions about specific diseases in past halakhic literature which are no longer prevalent today, such as smallpox. In addition to smallpox, we have chapters on Rubella, Ebola and Zika. Even Zika, which only surfaced during the writing of this book, has already receded from our memories. As I write these words, we are still immersed in the Covid-19 pandemic, to which we also devote an entire chapter. Therein we compare the halakhic and Jewish communal responses to Covid-19 with the rabbinic responses to previous pandemics.

III. TEXTUAL UTILIZATION

Not only does the study of medical history enhance textual understanding and chronological sensitivity of rabbinic texts, in broadening our scope to view the entire system of halakha, it can also aid in finding halakhic discussions and analyses that can serve as direct or indirect precedents in modern halakhic discourse. As in the practice of medicine, where certain historical medical theories or treatments are occasionally exhumed and resuscitated for modern use, such as the case of leeches, there are many long-forgotten episodes in the history of medical halakha that might bear relevance to modern medical halakhic discourse.

Some of these narratives may have direct relevance to modern discourse, dealing with substantively similar issues, albeit from a different scientific vantage point. Examples of this type, which are developed in the chapters of this book, include the halakhic discussions on smallpox vaccination in the eighteenth century; a journal exchange in the early twentieth century about the halakhic ramifications of ovarian and uterus transplantation; discussions across the centuries of the possibility of shared paternity based on a passage in Talmud Yerushalmi; deliberations on the legal implications of resuscitation after death long before CPR was possible.

Other medical halakhic narratives, especially when viewed as part of a continuum of the interface of science and halakha, may provide theological or philosophical foundations with which to address new scientific discoveries.[13] Some contemporary halakhic issues, such as abortion or Sabbath issues and medicine, can be directly extrapolated

---

13. See, for examples, chapters, "The Resuscitation of Halakha" and "Shared Biological Paternity in Rabbinic Literature."

from the extant halakhic corpus. The same principles and precedents are simply applied to the newly evolving circumstances. Other issues, however, such as genetic engineering, cloning, and surrogate motherhood, being products entirely of modern composition, have no clear halakhic precedents and test the limits of rabbinic creativity in finding relevant material in the existing body of halakhic literature.[14] It is in the latter circumstances that analysis of earlier halakhic discussions, where rabbinic authorities were grappling with new scientific discoveries, could contribute to modern dialogue and discourse.[15]

Viewing a collection of rabbinic responses to a particular category of scientific discovery may yield theological or halakhic patterns and themes that would not be discernible from viewing one historically isolated incident. The lessons and principles gleaned from this approach could be assimilated or adapted to our modern context.

Cloning and genetic engineering reflect a paradigm shift in our ability to manipulate the human body, and in the way we view the human being. The attendant halakhic issues relate not only to the pragmatic concerns of the definition of personhood and parentage, but also to the larger issues of interference in the process of procreation and the divine order. To assist in the exploration of these broader issues, it might be helpful to return to previous episodes in history where the rabbis were confronted with similar concerns. In the early responsa on artificial insemination, for example, the first form of human intervention in the process of procreation, one may find themes that could be applied equally to the issue of cloning. Concerns expressed in these responsa, such as the dissolution of the family structure, ambiguity of lineage, the generation of people with uncertain parentage, and the propriety of intervening in matters once thought to be the provenance of God exclusively, are all equally applicable to a discussion of cloning. While not always explicitly stated in this book, these ideas can be extrapolated from its pages.

A general approach to scientific theories that seemingly conflict with rabbinic tradition can likewise be gleaned from previous historical

---

14. See chapter, "Midrash, Miracles, and Motherhood: The Birth of Dinah and the Definition of Maternity—*Tzarikh Iyun LeDina.*"
15. See chapter, "The Resuscitation of Halakha."

chapters. In the sixteenth century, in a world that accepted the geocentric theory as absolute, objective fact, Copernicus dared challenge this age-old notion so invested with theological significance. With the heliocentric theory came a reevaluation of the earth's place in the universe. In the seventeenth century, Francesco Redi, with his simple yet elegant experiments, put the first nail in the coffin of the long-held notion that insects generate spontaneously. In the nineteenth century, Darwinism sparked a debate and reassessment of the evolution of the human being in relation to the earth. Each of these paradigmatic shifts in the histories of astronomy,[16] reproductive physiology,[17] and biology[18] produced a response in rabbinic literature. We explore lesser-known historical notions in anatomy and physiology throughout the book. Lessons or themes extracted from this literature contribute to the discourse on modern issues.

---

16. Andre Neher, *Jewish Thought and the Scientific Revolution of the Sixteenth Century: David Gans (1541–1613) and His Times*, trans. D. Maisel (Oxford University Press, 1986); J. Brown, *New Heavens and a New Earth: The Jewish Reception of Copernican Thought* (Oxford University Press, 2013).

17. Y. Lampronti, *Paḥad Yitzḥak*, s. v., *tzeida asura*; E. Dessler, *Mikhtav MeEliyahu*, 4, ed. A. Carmell (5748), 355, n. 4; D. B. Ruderman, "Contemporary Science and Jewish Law in the Eyes of Isaac Lampronti and Some of His Contemporaries," *Jewish History* 6:1–2 (1992), 211–224, reprinted in ibid., *Jewish Thought and Scientific Discovery in Early Modern Europe* (Yale University Press, 1995); A. Carmell and Y. Levi, "Re'ot HaEinayim BiKeviut HaHalakha," *Hama'ayan* 23:1 (*Tishrei*, 5743), 64–69; I. Herzog, *Heikhal Yitzḥak*, O. H., 29; N. Slifkin, "The Spontaneous Sweat-Louse," in his *Sacred Monsters* (Zoo Torah, 2007), 349–381; M. Meiselman, "Lice and Fleas," in his *Torah, Ḥazal and Science* (Israel Bookshop, 2013), 300–320.

18. The literature on evolution merits its own bibliography. See, for example, articles in A. Carmell and C. Domb, eds., *Challenge: Torah Views on Science and its Problems* (Feldheim Publishers, 1978); D. W. Weiss, *The Wings of the Dove: Jewish Values, Science and Halakhah* (B'nai B'rith Books, 1987); L. C. Dubin, "The Reconciliation of Darwin and Torah in 'Pe-er ha'Adam' of Vittorio Hayim Castiglioni," *Italia Judaica* 4 (1993), 273–284; essays in H. Branover and Ilana Coven Attia, eds., *Science in the Light of Torah: A B'or Ha'Torah Reader* (Jason Aronson, 1994); B. Sterman, "Judaism and Darwinian Evolution," *Tradition* 29:1 (Fall 1994), 48–75; L. Spetner, *Not by Chance: Shattering the Modern Theory of Evolution* (Judaica Press, 1996); N. Aviezer, *Fossils and Faith: Evolution, Darwin, Dinosaurs and the Bible* (Ktav, 1998); N. Slifkin, *The Challenge of Creation* (Zoo Torah, 2012).

IV. CONCLUSION

The principles distilled from the rich history of rabbinic literature, in conjunction with a knowledge and appreciation of medical history, will better equip us to confront the ever-increasing complexities of the medical discoveries that lie ahead. This exercise will hopefully give the reader not only a greater appreciation of the scope and breadth of rabbinic integration of medical knowledge throughout the ages, but will also provide a context and framework within which to address future halakhic issues.

Fertility and Reproduction

The Rabbinic Conception of Conception: An Exercise in Fertility

The extraordinary technological advances of this century have been applied with full force to the field of science and, in particular, to genetics and reproductive medicine. Humankind now has more control over its own reproduction than ever before in history, such that the old notion of the doctor playing God has taken on new meaning. In the ultimate form of *imitatio Dei*, it now appears that just as God creates, so does mankind. Scientists have the ability to manipulate almost every step in the process of procreation.

Although all acknowledge the value of this technology, it is not without its cost. Whereas the Talmud mentions only three partners in creation—the father, the mother, and God—current reproductive practices have expanded the list of potential partners to include the sperm donor, egg donor, surrogate mother, mitochondrial DNA donor, and possibly artificial reproductive seed donor. If our current experience is any measure, then introducing more partners clearly introduces more complications, be they emotional, financial, legal or ethical.

To solve these ethical dilemmas, secular ethicists utilize philosophical principles; some with historical precedent, and others, simply based on human imagination. In either case, ethicists are in no way bound to the ideas of the past. We, however, as Orthodox Jews who subscribe to the halakhic process and live by the words of Ḥazal, employ the past to solve the dilemmas of the present and future. We turn to our predecessors for both halakhic and ethical guidance.

All contemporary halakhic discussions of reproductive technology cite sources ranging from antiquity to the Renaissance to modern times. As the understanding of reproductive anatomy and physiology has changed throughout the centuries, the author of each source, depending on its historical period, assumes a unique understanding of embryology and reproductive medicine. Therefore, an awareness of the embryological theories contemporary with each author may aid our understanding of his discussion of medical or scientific ideas. Furthermore, if the context of the source is halakhic, it may enhance our appreciation of the halakhic issues with which the author is dealing. This knowledge can perhaps assist current *poskim* (rabbinic authorities) in their utilization of rabbinic source material for incorporation into medical halakhic responsa. I therefore suggest that we pause for a moment from addressing modern halakhic dilemmas of reproductive technology and look backward to consider our predecessors' conception of conception.

This chapter discusses selected passages from rabbinic literature from antiquity to modern times that explicitly address or allude to theories relating to reproduction. The sources will be discussed both in their own right, as well as in a medical historical context. Although rabbinic sources cover the gamut of issues of reproduction and heredity, I have chosen to concentrate on three topics for purposes of illustration, each highlighting a different aspect of reproductive medicine. The first topic addresses the very nature of the male and female seeds, focusing largely on embryology—in other words, who contributes what material to the fetus. The second section traces the history of artificial insemination, a matter of reproductive physiology, and contains sources that are often quoted in contemporary halakhic discussions. Therefore, the rabbinic sources in this section will receive disproportionately more in-depth study than the secular. The final section addresses a particular notion regarding reproductive anatomy. In each section, the secular sources will be discussed separately. In the first section only, as a historical introduction, the secular sources will precede the Jewish.

I. EMBRYOLOGY

1) Secular Sources

Almost all major figures in the history of science in antiquity devoted time to the study of animal and human embryology.[1] As knowledge of anatomy[2] and physiology was limited, theories were based on simple observation and philosophical intuition. Analogies were often made to agriculture, the male seed compared to the plant seed and the uterus, to the nourishing earth.[3] The male contribution to conception was readily

---

1. For an overview of the history of embryology, see J. Needham, *A History of Embryology* (New York, 1959); Howard Adelmann, "A Brief Sketch of the History of Embryology before Fabricius" in his translation of *The Embryological Treatises of Hieronymous Fabricius of Aquapendente* (Ithaca, 1967), I, 36–70. For references to embryology in Jewish sources, see Samuel Kottek, "Embryology in Talmudic and Midrashic Literature," *Journal of the History of Biology* 14:2 (Fall 1981), 299–315; David I. Macht, "Embryology and Obstetrics in Ancient Hebrew Literature," *John Hopkins Hospital Bulletin* 22: 242 (May, 1911), 1–8; W. M. Feldman, "Ancient Jewish Eugenics," *Medical Leaves* 2 (1939), 28–37; D. Shapiro *Obstetrique des Anciens Hebreus* (Paris, 1904); W. M. Feldman, *The Jewish Child* (London, 1917), 120–144; H. J. Zimmels, *Magicians, Theologians and Doctors* (Edward Goldston and Son, 1952), 62–64; Needham, op. cit., 77–82; Julius Preuss, *Biblical and Talmudic Medicine* (Hebrew Pub. Co., 1978), 41–138; Ron Barkai, *Les Infortunes De Dinah: Le Livre De La Generation—La Gynecologie Juive au Moyen Age* (Paris, 1991) (I thank Mr. Tzvi Erenyi for bringing this latter book to my attention).

2. There are no clearly documented human dissections from the time of Rashi, although scattered references to autopsies and dissections appear in the thirteenth and fourteenth centuries. Mundinus (1270–1326) is recognized to have been the first to incorporate human anatomical dissection into the medical curriculum. See, for example, C. D. O'Malley, *Andreas Vesalius Of Brussels* (Berkeley, 1964), 1–20; Ludwig Edelstein, "The History of Anatomy in Antiquity," in *Ancient Medicine* (Baltimore, 1967), 247–302; Charles Singer, *A Short History of Anatomy and Physiology from the Greek to Harvey* (New York, 1957); Mary Niven Alston, "The Attitude of the Church Towards Dissection Before 1500," *Bulletin of the History of Medicine* 16:3 (October, 1944), 221–238; Nancy Sirasi, *Taddeo Alderotti and His Pupils* (Princeton, 1981), 66–69. For further discussion on anatomy in rabbinic literature, see the section below, Anatomy and Physiology.

3. Hippocrates in his essay "The Seed and the Nature of the Child" devotes a lengthy section to agriculture. He says, "You will find that from beginning to end the process

observable, as the male seed was emitted outside the body. The nature of the female contribution, however, was a matter of intense debate.

Female Seed

Since the female seed was not visible to the naked eye and was not emitted externally, its very existence was a matter of conjecture. As a result, two competing theories evolved in antiquity which coexisted until pre-modern times.[4] Galen,[5] following in the footsteps of Hippocrates,[6] maintained that both the male and female contributed seed. The exact identity of the female seed was in question, but he conjectured it might be located in the uterus. He also claimed that the male semen provides the material for the development of the nerves and the walls of the arteries and veins in the fetus, while the menstrual fluid is the source of the blood.[7] Aristotle, on the other hand, denied the existence of a female seed, claiming that only the male possessed seed. This seed provided the "form" and the "principle of the movement" of the fetus, whereas

---

of growth in plants and humans is exactly the same." G. E. R. Lloyd, ed., *Hippocratic Writings* (New York, 1978), 341; A. J. Brock (trans.), *Galen On the Natural Faculties* (London, 1916), 19.

4. See Joseph Needham, *A History of Embryology* (New York, 1959) for extensive discussion of ancient theories of embryology. For a comprehensive account of pre-Aristotelian theories of sexual generation, see Erna Lesky in *Die Zeugungs und Vererbungslehre der Antike und ihre Nachwirkung* (Mainz, 1950). This work is widely quoted. See also the classic work by Monica Green, *The Transmission of Ancient Theories of Female Physiology and Disease Through the Early Middle Ages* (Doctoral Dissertation, Princeton University, 1985) and Sarah George, *Human Conception and Fetal Growth: A Study in the Development of Greek Thought From Presocrates through Aristotle* (Doctoral Dissertation, University of Pennsylvania, 1982).

5. Galen discusses his theories of generation in many places. See, for example, Margaret Talmadge May, trans., *Galen: On the Usefulness of the Parts of the Body* 2 (Ithaca, 1968), 620–654. See also Anthony Preus, "Galen's Criticism of Aristotle's Conception Theory," *Journal of the History of Biology* 10:1 (Spring 1977), 65–85.

6. Modern scholarship has revealed that the Hippocratic corpus is not the work of one author. For ideas of conception see, for example, G. E. R. Lloyd, ed., *Hippocratic Writings* (New York, 1978), 317–346, chapter entitled "The Seed and the Nature of the Child."

7. Preuss, op. cit., 83. See also Needham, op. cit., 78 who quotes a similar idea from Hippocrates.

the female provided the material from which the fetus was formed; i.e., the menstrual blood.[8]

It can be argued which of these theories predominated throughout the Middle Ages, but the falsehood of Aristotle's theory was decisively demonstrated by William Harvey. Harvey (1578–1657), known best for his description of the circulation of the blood, was also a pioneer in the field of embryology. While the ovum had not yet been described in his lifetime, he nonetheless postulated that all living beings must derive from eggs.[9] Aside from placing the first nail in the coffin of the theory of spontaneous generation,[10] Harvey superseded Aristotle and paved the path for Reinier de Graaf, who in 1672 first described the egg follicle.[11] The microscopic female human egg as we now know it was

---

8. See A. L. Peck, (trans.), *Aristotle: Generation of Animals* (Cambridge, 1942), 71, 100–101, note a, 109–112.

9. *Exercitationes de Generatione Animalium* (Amsterdam, 1651), later translated and annotated by Gweneth Whitteridge, *Disputations Touching the Generation of Animals* (Oxford, 1981).

10. The belief in spontaneous generation in Jewish and secular sources merits its own article. A passage in *Masekhet Shabbat* 107b seems to indicate that the rabbis believed that lice could spontaneously generate. This passage, as well as others that conflict with our current understanding of science, have been the subject of many a heated discussion. Francesco Redi (1620–1697) was the first to scientifically study spontaneous generation and he dealt the theory its first major blow in his work, *Esperienze Intorno Alla Generazione Deg'lisetti* (Florence, 1668). Louis Pasteur (1833–93) laid the theory to rest. For treatment of this topic in Jewish sources see Yitzḥak Lampronti, *Paḥad Yitḥak* (Bnei Brak, 1980), s. v., *"Tzedah HaAsura"*; Arye Carmell ed. Eliyahu Dessler, *Michtav MeEliyahu* 4 (Jerusalem, 1984), 355, note 4; Arye Carmel and Yehuda Levi, *"Re'ot HaEinayim Bek'viut HaHalakha,"* *HaMa'ayan* 23:1 (*Tishri*, 1983), 64–69; David Ruderman, "Contemporary Science and Jewish Law in the Eyes of Isaac Lampronti of Ferrara and Some of His Contemporaries," *Jewish History* 6:1–2 (1992), 211–224; N. Slifkin, "The Spontaneous Sweat-Louse," in his *Sacred Monsters* (Zoo Torah, 2007) 349–381: M. Meiselman, "Lice and Fleas," in his *Torah, Chazal and Science* (Lakewood, NJ: Israel Bookshop, 2013), 300–320; E. Reichman, "The Riddle of Samson and the Spontaneous Generation of Bees: The Bugonia Myth, the Crosspollination that Wasn't, and the *Heter* for Honey That Might Have Been," in Menachem Butler and Marian E. Frankston, eds., *Essays for a Jewish Lifetime: Burton D. Morris Jubilee Volume* (New York: Hakirah Press), in press.

11. See his *De Mulierum Organis Generationi Inservientibus Tractatus Novus* (Leyden, 1672).

not described until 1827, when Karl Ernst von Baer published his classic description of the mammalian ovum.[12]

Male Seed

There were three Greek theories regarding the origin of the sperm.[13] The encephalo-myelogenic doctrine claimed that the sperm was ultimately derived from the brain, and it traversed the spinal cord on its way to the male genital organs. The second theory, of which Hippocrates was an advocate, was called the pangenesis doctrine and contended that the sperm was derived from the entire body. The sperm extracted from each limb would yield the corresponding limb in the fetus. Aristotle supported the hematogenic doctrine, claiming that the seed originated from blood, and was in fact nothing but blood in a certain state of coagulation.

Although a male seed was always acknowledged, it was not until 1677 that Antonie van Leeuwenhoek first visualized the human spermatozoa under the microscope.[14]

Preformation and Epigenesis[15]

The discovery of the egg follicles by de Graaf and the spermatozoa by van Leeuwenhoek gave birth to two opposing theories regarding the embryological development of the fetus in utero. Some maintained that the fetus formed in a stepwise fashion with the development of one organ or limb preceding the next, i.e., epigenesis. Others believed that within the seed, either male or female, there existed a minuscule complete preformed being that simply enlarged during the course of gestation. These so-called preformationists were split into two camps, those claiming

---

12. *De Ovi Mammalium et Hominis Genesi* (Leipzig, 1827).

13. See Pieter Willem van der Horst, "Sarah's Seminal Emmission: Hebrews 11:11 in the Light of Ancient Embryology" in *Greeks, Romans and Christians: Essays in Honor of Abraham J. Malherbe,* edited by David Balch et al. (Minneapolis, 1990), 287–302. I thank Dr. Shnayer Leiman for directing me to this source, which places a number of rabbinic sources in the context of Greco-Roman theories of embryology. Horst provides a nice summary of these three theories. See also Sarah George, op. cit.

14. A. W. Meyer, "The Discovery and Earliest Representation of Spermatozoa," *Bulletin of the Institute of the History of Medicine* 6:2 (February, 1938), 89–110.

15. See, for example, Needham, op. cit., 205–211; A. Du Bois, "The Development of the Theory of Heredity," *CIBA Symposia* 1:8 (November, 1939), 235–246.

that the preformed child was within the female egg (ovists) and those claiming it was within the male sperm (animalculists).[16]

So convinced of this belief was one animalculist that he drew a diagram of a completely formed child crouched within the confines of one human sperm. This figure became known as the homunculus.[17] It is unclear exactly when the theory of preformation was disproved, but it had its supporters up to the late nineteenth century.

2) Jewish Sources[18]

Equipped with this historical background, we can approach the Jewish sources throughout the ages that address embryological theories both explicitly and implicitly. For the sake of clarity, I have separated, as above, the sections on male and female seed. Since the same sources often discuss both seeds, there will be, by necessity, limited repetition. For the repeated sources, the bibliographical information will be referenced the first time the source is mentioned.

Female Seed

The talmudic source that serves as the foundation of all subsequent rabbinic discussions on embryology, especially with regard to the female seed, is found in *Masekhet Nidda* (30a):

> Our Rabbis taught: There are three partners in the creation of man: God, the father, and the mother. The father emits (*mazria*) the white substance, from which are derived the bones, vessels (*gidim*),[19] fingernails, brain and the white of the eye. The mother

---

16. According to the theory of preformation, either Adam or Eve, depending on whether one was an ovist or animalculist, contained within them the preformed bodies of all the people that would populate the earth. Within each preformed seed must exist preformed seed of the next generation, and so on.
17. Regarding the origins of this depiction and its initial false attribution to van Leeuwenhoek, see A. W. Meyer, op. cit.
18. See David Feldman, *Marital Relations, Birth Control and Abortion in Jewish Law* (New York, 1974), esp. chaps. 6 and 7, for his excellent treatment of these topics. Some of the sources from this section derive from this book.
19. The term *gidim* is ill-defined and can possibly mean blood vessels, nerves or tendons. It has been used interchangeably in rabbinic literature. The clarification of Hebrew

emits (*mazra'at*) the red substance, from which are derived the skin, flesh, hair, and the black of the eye.[20] God provides the spirit (*ruaḥ*), the soul (*neshama*),[21] the beauty of the features, vision for the eyes, hearing for the ears, speech for the mouth... and intelligence. When the time comes for a man to depart this world, God takes back His part, leaving behind the contributions of the mother and father.

It seems clear that the rabbis, similar to Galen and in contrast to Aristotle, clearly acknowledged both a male and female seed, the female seed appearing to be identified with the menstrual blood. It is interesting to note that the list of organs that are derived from the respective seeds roughly resembles that of Galen. However, even though Galen was a contemporary of R. Yehuda HaNasi, the compiler of the Mishna, there is absolutely no mention of Galen, or Hippocrites for that matter, in the

---

medical terms, especially in the Middle Ages, has plagued many a doctor and historian throughout history. The confusion stems from differing etymologies of medical terms, ranging from Latin, to Greek and later Arabic, as well as the fact that these terms were not easily rendered into Hebrew. Some terms were transliterated, others translated, and often entirely new words were devised. This confusion led many Jewish physicians to include a glossary of medical terms in their books. On Hebrew terminology see, for example, Juan Jose Barcia Goyanes, "Medieval Hebrew Anatomical Names" *Koroth* 8:11–12 (1985), 192–201; A. S. Yahuda, "Medical and Anatomical Terms in the Pentateuch in Light of Egyptian Medical Papyri," *Journal of the History of Medicine* 2:4 (Autumn, 1947), 549–573. Multiple articles have appeared over the years in the journal *HaRofeh HaIvri* on the topic of Hebrew medical terminology. For an excellent review on this general topic, see R. Barkai, "The Rise of Hebrew Medical Literature," in his *A History of Jewish Gynaecological Texts in the Middle Ages* (Brill: Leiden, 1998), 6–37.

20. It is interesting that blood is not mentioned as one of the contributions of the female seed, especially since this seed, according to the Gemara is itself comprised of blood. For a discussion about this discrepancy see *She'iltot DeRav Aḥai Gaon, She'ilta* 56 and commentaries of R. Isaiah Berlin (*She'ilat Shalom*) and R. Naftali Tzvi Yehuda Berlin (*HaEmek She'ela*) on this passage. I thank Dr. Meyer Halberstam for directing me to this source.

21. The terms *ruaḥ, nefesh* and *neshama* are all abstract and difficult to define. They are often used interchangeably. See Samuel S. Kottek, "The Seat of the Soul: Contribution to the History of Jewish Medieval Psycho-Physiology," *Cliomedica* 13:3–4 (1978), 219–246.

entire text of the Mishna and Talmud.[22] As a result, any suggestion of cross-cultural borrowing is purely speculative.

The next source appears in the biblical commentary of R. Moses ben Naḥman. Although Naḥmanides is known for his exceptional talmudic scholarship, he was also a practicing physician, purportedly at Montpellier,[23] the major center of medicine in the Middle Ages.[24] As a matter of fact, one of the few references we have to Naḥmanides' medical practice states that he treated a non-Jew for infertility.[25] Naḥmanides comments on the phrase in Vayikra, *"isha ki tazria veyalda zakhar."*[26] The root of the word *"tazria"* is *"zera"* or seed; hence the translation could be, "when a woman emits seed." Whereas most biblical commentators interpret this phrase to mean when a woman conceives and thereby ignore the issue of the existence of the female seed, Naḥmanides takes this opportunity to address rabbinic theories of embryology:

---

22. Rabbinic sources of the Middle Ages and beyond clearly knew of Galen. In addition, Galen himself was at least peripherally familiar with Jews and Jewish medicine. For further discussion on Galen, see chapter, "The Halakhic Definition of Death."

23. We know of Naḥmanides' medical practice primarily from the responsa of his student, R. Shlomo ibn Aderet (Rashba). Responsa numbers 177, 413 and 825 discuss Naḥmanides' use of an astrological figure of a lion to cure a kidney ailment. The Rashba discusses the halakhic issues involved in using astrological figures. See also R. H. Y. D. Azulai, *Shem HaGedolim Ma'arekhet Gedolim*, s. v., *"Ramban."* Medical historians have mentioned that Naḥmanides practiced in Montpellier. See Isaac Alteras, "Jewish Physicians in Southern France during the thirteenth and fourteenth Centuries," *JQR* 68 (1977–1978), 218. No Jewish sources that I have found place Naḥmanides as a physician in Montpellier.

24. On the University at Montpellier in the Middle Ages see Sonoma Cooper, "The Medical School of Montpellier in the Fourteenth Century," *Annals of Medical History*, new series 2 (1930), 164–195; *CIBA Symposia* 2:1 (April, 1940), entire issue devoted to Montpellier. Regarding the Jewish presence at Montpellier, see E. Lehmann, "Jewish Physicians in Provence, Languedoc, and at the Medical School of Montpellier in the 11th, 12th and 13th Centuries," (Hebrew) *Koroth* 3:9–10 (August, 1965), 455–471; Luis Garcia-Ballester, "Dietetic and Pharmacological Therapy: A Dilemma Among Fourteenth Century Jewish Practitioners in the Montpellier Area," *Clio Medica* 22 (1991), 23–37; Joseph Shatzmiller, "Etudiants Juifs a la Faculte de Medicine de Montpellier Dernier Quart du XIV Siecle," *Jewish History* 6:1–2 (1992), 243–255; idem, *Jews, Medicine and Medieval Society* (University of California Press, 1994).

25. Rashba, responsum 120, also quoted in R. Yosef Karo, *Bedek HaBayit* on *Y. D.*, 154.

26. For additional discussion on this phrase, see chapter, *"Parashat Tazria* and Childbirth."

...Although it says, "when a woman emits seed..." the implication is not that the fetus is made from the female seed. For even
though a woman has ovaries (*beitzim*) analogous to those of the
male (*beitzei zakhar*) [testicles], either no seed is made there,
or the seed has nothing to do with the fetus. Rather the term
"*mazra'at*" refers to the uterine blood...that unites with male seed.
In their opinion [*Masekhet Nidda* above] the fetus is created from
the blood of the woman and the white [semen] of the man, and
both of them are called seed...and likewise is the opinion of the
doctors regarding conception. The Greek philosophers thought
that the entire body of the fetus derives from menstrual blood,
and that the man only provides...form to the material.

The mere fact that Naḥmanides mentions this embryological debate
reflects that it still was a topic of discussion in his time. Here Naḥmanides
accepts the contribution of a female seed and identifies that seed with
the uterine blood, based on the passage in the Gemara. He states that
this is also the position of the doctors. As we know that Naḥmanides
was himself a physician, we accept this statement with more authority.
Although he mentions no names of specific doctors, he may be align-
ing the talmudic position with the teachings of Galen. Naḥmanides also
clearly rejects what we know to be Aristotle's position.

R. Baḥya ben Asher (thirteenth century) follows Naḥmanides in
his interpretation of the phrase in Vayikra but adds a novel explanation of
the term "*tazria*." He suggests it means, "When a woman gives over the
zera." The *zera*, he maintains, is a deposit which is given to the woman
by the man for safekeeping as a plant seed is deposited in the ground. In
both cases the matured seed is to be returned from its repository when
the time is right.[27] As we have mentioned above, the agricultural analogy is one that has been used since antiquity.

While Naḥmanides claims that a woman may or may not have
her own seed independent of the menstrual blood, Maimonides clearly
acknowledges the existence of a female seed.

---

27. Commentary on Vayikra, 12:2.

...between the *ḥeder* and the *prozdor*[28] lie the two ovaries of the woman and the pathways [fallopian tubes] wherein her seed matures.[29]

Maimonides does not, however, address whether this seed has any role in conception. This issue is discussed in the following sources.

R. Shimon ben Tzemaḥ Duran (1361–1444), also known as Tashbetz, devotes a significant section of his philosophical work, *Magen Avot*, to the anatomy and physiology of reproduction. In this citation he confronts the issue of the female seed:

> Regarding whether the female seed has a role in conception, this has been debated by Aristotle and Galen. We have explained that *Ḥazal* say it has no role whatsoever in conception...The philosophers have concluded that the female seed has no role in conception...and they reached the same conclusion that was received by *Ḥazal* from the prophets and teachings of the Torah.[30]

R. Duran later identifies the menstrual blood as the contribution of the female.

In contradistinction to the above source which acknowledges the existence of an independent female seed but gives this seed no role in conception, the following reference grants a prominent role to this seed. This passage is excerpted from the work of R. Meir ben Isaac Aldabi (1310–1360), the grandson of R. Asher ben Yeḥiel, entitled *Shevilei Emuna*.[31]

---

28. These terms derive from the Mishna in *Nidda* 2:5 and have been the source of much discussion regarding their anatomical identification. See, for example, M. Halperin, *Realia and Medicine in Seder Nashim* (Schlesinger Institute, 2011), 3–40 (Hebrew).

29. *Hil. Isurei B'iah* 5:4.

30. 40a.

31. This book is a compilation of theories in philosophy, theology, psychology and medicine. The material was culled from the existing literature of that time, as stated by Aldabi in his introduction, but unfortunately there are no references, for

... and next to the uterus are the woman's two ovaries ... and from them the female seed flows into the cavity of the uterus. When the male seed is emitted into the uterus the female seed also is emitted from the ovaries and joins with the male seed to form the fetus.[32]

This appears to be the first Jewish source that ascribes such significance to the female ovarian seed and thus ends our discussion of Jewish sources prior to the works of Harvey and Leeuwenhoek. In summary, all the Jewish sources espouse the doctrine of the two seeds, both male and female, yet opinions differ as to the identity and contribution of the female seed. These sources are better understood in the context of the ongoing scientific debate in the secular world regarding the existence and nature of the female seed.

We now turn to some Jewish references to embryology at a time when the scientific world had recently undergone major upheaval. The sperm had been identified, the existence of a female egg was universally accepted, although the egg itself had not yet been observed, and the theories of preformation and epigenesis were being debated.

Tobias Cohn (1652–1729),[33] a graduate of the famous University of Padua,[34] was educated in this scientific milieu. His classic work, *Ma'aseh Tuvia*, covers topics including botany, cosmology, and medicine,

---

which R. Aldabi apologizes. This book was first printed in 1518 in Riva di Trento, but because of its immense popularity it has been reprinted many times over the centuries, including a recent printing in Jerusalem, 1990.

32. *Shevilei Emuna* (Jerusalem, 1990), 197–198.

33. For biographical information on Tuvia Cohn, see his introduction to *Ma'aseh Tuvia*. See also Dr. D.A. Friedman, *Tobias Cohn* (Tel Aviv, 1940); *Encyclopedia Judaica*, s. v., "Cohn, Tobias"; and see David B. Ruderman, *Jewish Thought and Scientific Discovery in Early Modern Europe* (Wayne State University Press: New Edition, August 1, 2001).

34. On the Jews of the University of Padua see, for example, Cecil Roth, "The Medieval University and the Jew," *Menora Journal* 9:2 (1930), 128–141; Jacob Shatzky, "On Jewish Medieval Students of Padua," *Journal of History of Medicine* 5 (1950), 444–447; Cecil Roth, "The Qualification of Jewish Physicians in the Middle Ages," *Speculum* 28 (1953), 834–843; David B. Ruderman, "The Impact of Science on Jewish Culture and Society in Venice (with Special Reference to Jewish Graduates of Padua's Medical School) in Gli Ebrei e Venezia (Venice, 1983), 417–448. See also, E. Reichman, "The Valmadonna

and the following passage on embryology reflects the climate of his time. As Cohn was well educated in rabbinic as well as scientific literature, his words are of particular relevance to our discussion.

> Aristotle, who rejected the Torah of Moses, brought a number of disappointing proofs that the menstrual blood is in place of the seed, and besides this, a woman has no other seed. However, recent physicians, who accept our holy Torah, have…brought other proofs which contradict his disappointing proofs…The first proof is that one cannot deny the existence of a female seed, for it was not for naught that a woman was created with *beitzim* and pathways that transmit seed similar to a man.
> …There is almost no need for the proofs brought by the great physician Harvey on the existence of a female seed…The great physicians of late maintain that the purpose of the ovaries (*beitzim*) is to give rise to tiny eggs (*beitzim*), similar to fish eggs, which have been seen with the microscope.[35]

This is possibly the first Hebrew source that uses the term *beitza* to describe the female egg as we understand it today. In all previous sources, the term *beitzim* is used to refer to the ovaries or testicles interchangeably, and the female seed is called simply her *zera*. Given an understanding of the history of embryology, this observation makes perfect sense, as it is only during this period that Harvey's theory of the existence of a female egg was developed.

A more detailed physiological description of conception is found in the anatomical work of Baruch Schick (1744–1808),[36] entitled *Tiferet*

Trust Broadside Collection and a Virtual Reunion of the Jewish Medical Students of Padua," *Verapo Yerapei: Journal of Torah and Medicine of the Albert Einstein College of Medicine Synagogue* 7 (2017).

35. (Cracow, 1908), 118. Note his mention of the microscope, which was first designed in the late seventeenth century.

36. Note that this author has been variously referred to as Baruch of Shklov, Baruch Shklover or Baruch Schick, the latter name under which he is listed in *Encyclopedia Judaica*. For biographical information see David Fishman, *Science, Enlightenment, and Rabbinic Culture in Belorussian Jewry, 1772–1804* (Ph.D. dissertation, Harvard

Adam. Schick is perhaps best known for translating Euclid's geometry into Hebrew for the Vilna Gaon.[37] In this excerpt, the author, after discussing the passage from *Masekhet Nidda*, mentions the single egg.[38]

> ...in the body of the woman are found the ovaries...the seed emitted by the man...induces the emission of a single egg from the ovaries...

The next passage alludes to another embryological theory and stems from a question entertained by R. Yaakov Emden (d.1776) regarding whether it was possible for a virgin woman to conceive in the absence of conjugal relations, e.g., bathhouse insemination. In this passage, he invokes the theory of preformation, particularly that of the animalculists, to answer the above question in the affirmative. The references to the male and female seeds are as follows:[39]

> ...such a thing is decidedly not in the realm of the impossible... as *Hazal* said "maybe she conceived in the bathhouse?" [*Hagiga* 14b]... and this is compatible with the ideas of the scientists, who describe only a limited role for the female seed in conception (...but it is now clear that the female seed provides no material contribution to the fetus whatsoever... and this does not contradict what is written in the Torah, *"isha ki tazria veyalda."* See the commentary of Nahmanides on this verse and you will

University, 1985); ibid., "A Polish Rabbi Meets the Berlin Haskalah: The Case of R. Baruch Schick," *AJS Review* 12:1 (Spring,1987), 95–121; Noach Shapiro, "R. Baruch Schick Mi-Shklov," *HaRofe HaIvri* 34:1–2 (1961), 230–235 (Hebrew); David Margalit, "Dr. Baruch Schick V'Sifro 'Tiferet Adam,'" *Koroth* 6:1–2 (August,1972), 5–7 (Hebrew). There is debate in the above sources as to whether Baruch Schick was a physician. See also Israel Zinberg, *A History of Jewish Literature: The German-Polish Cultural Center* (New York, 1975), 271–274.

37. Hague, 1780. In the introduction to this book appears the oft quoted notion, in the name of the Vilna Gaon, that scientific knowledge is needed for the study of Torah.

38. *Tiferet Adam* (Berlin, 1777), 3. This book was printed together with *Amudai Shamayim*, an astronomical work by the same author. As this latter work appears first in the combined volume, the book is often referenced by its name only.

39. This is a loose translation from *Iggeret Bikoret* (Zhitomer, 1868), 25b.

see that it is not a contradiction.)[40] They have found through the use of the glass [microscope] and other experiments that man, like birds and fish, is created from an egg in the ovary of the woman. And in the male seed they have seen... the image of a tiny human being, complete with its limbs...

R. Emden goes on to explain that the preformed fetus in the male seed receives its nourishment and sustenance, including warmth and moisture, from the female seed. It is interesting to note that he accepts the notion of the homunculus (preformation) and claims that this is in consonance with the commentary of Nahmanides. We mentioned above that Nahmanides granted no role to a female seed independent of the menstrual blood. However, Nahmanides does maintain, based on the Gemara in *Nidda*, that the menstrual blood does contribute materially to the fetus. This latter notion, I believe, would not be compatible with the theory of preformation. In any case, R. Emden incorporates the contemporary embryological theories into his halakhic discussion.

The final selection in this section comes from the work of Pinhas Eliyahu Hurwitz (1765–1821), *Sefer HaBrit*.[41] This work is a compilation of medical and scientific theories culled from sources in many languages and served as a valuable resource for its Jewish audience, to whom many of these ideas were inaccessible. This fact accounts for the book's popularity and multiple reprintings. This selection gives a balanced view of the opposing embryological theories and at the same time incorporates the teachings of *Hazal*:

> Some scholars have written that all the features of the entire human body, complete with its limbs, are found within the egg of the woman... and some scholars have written that within the seed of the man is the form of a minuscule human being, for when male seed... are viewed under the microscope small creatures can be seen

---

40. Parentheses are in original text.
41. On this work, see D. Ruderman, *A Best-Selling Hebrew Book of the Modern Era* (University of Washington Press, 2015).

within them moving to and fro...God knows the truth of this matter. However, it is known in truth that the woman also emits seed, as the verse explicitly states, *"isha ki tazria."* And her seed is not white, but red as Ḥazal have said" the mother emits the red substance."[42]

In conclusion of our discussion of the female seed, it is apparent that these sources do not reflect a consensus of opinion regarding the identity and nature of the female seed. Many of the sources, irrespective of the theories they espouse, attempt to align their positions with the words of Ḥazal; in particular, the passage from *Masekhet Nidda*.

Male Seed

We now analyze a selection of Jewish sources that address theories regarding the origin and nature of the male seed. Some of these sources have already been discussed in the above section on the female seed. We begin with a passage from the Talmud, from which we can infer the understanding of the origin of the male seed:

> Levi was sitting in a bathhouse and observed a man fall and strike his head. He said, "His brains were agitated (*nitmazmez*)"... Abaye said, "He has lost the ability to procreate."[43]

According to Rashi, the implication is that an injury to the brain somehow affects the male seed. This is an allusion to the encephalo-myelogenic theory of the origin of the sperm.[44]

In *Sefer HaBahir*, a kabbalistic work attributed to R. Neḥunia ben HaKana (a first-century *Tanna*), the reference to the encephalo-myelogenic doctrine is more explicit:[45] "The spinal cord, which comes from the brain, enters the male organ (*amma*) and from there comes the seed."

---

42. *Sefer HaBrit* (Jerusalem, 1990), vol. 1, chap. 2, 240.
43. *Ḥullin* 45b.
44. Loc. cit., s. v., *"she'eino molid."*
45. *Sefer HaBahir* has also been referred to as *Midrash R. Neḥunia ben HaKana.* Naḥmanides refers to it by this title in his biblical commentary. This citation is from chapter 51 and is quoted by Moshe Perlman in his *Midrash HaRefua* (Tel Aviv, 1926), 23.

Meir ben Isaac Aldabi (1310–1360) (see above) mentions the encephalo-myelogenic as well as the pangenesis doctrine, but does not indicate which one he advocates:

> The scientists have debated. Some say the seed comes from the brain, by way of the spinal cord, to the testicles, and there it matures and whitens. There are two proofs to this: pain in the spine will sometimes heal with emission of seed, and one whose spinal cord is severed cannot procreate. However, Hippocrates maintains that the seed is an extract from all the limbs of the body.[46]

Tashbetz refers to the pangenesis doctrine: "We must ascertain ... if the seed derives from the entire body or not. Behold, the ancients have said this ..."[47] But he ultimately rejects this in favor of the hematogenic doctrine of Aristotle, which he claims Ḥazal also espoused:

> ... and this is their intent, z"l, when they said, "The seed is intermixed" (*mebalbel zarei*). The meaning of this phrase is that from all the limbs there is a combined power, not that each limb yields its corresponding limb [pangenesis doctrine] ... this is their opinion, z"l, in agreement with the opinion of the philosopher [Aristotle].[48]

In summary, up to this point, we have seen Jewish sources referring to all three theories regarding the origin of the male seed.[49] We now shift our attention to the period following the discoveries of Leeuwenhoek

---

46. *Shevilei Emuna* (Jerusalem, 1990), *netiv* 4, 211.

47. *Magen Avot*, 38b. Tashbetz mentions some of the proofs to this doctrine. These proofs make fascinating reading and reflect the medieval understanding of heredity, particularly the inheritance of acquired characteristics. The concept of heredity in Ḥazal is another topic that merits medical/historical analysis.

48. Ibid., 39a.

49. The encephalo-myelogenic doctrine was also mentioned by R. Yeḥiel Mikhel Epstein in his halakhic work *Arukh HaShulḥan*, E. H., 23:3.

and Harvey, when the theories of epigenesis and preformation were prevalent.

In the passage cited above, Pinḥas Eliyahu Hurwitz refers to the theory of preformation and mentions the position of the animalculists as well as the ovists. In the following quote, he invokes the position of the animalculists in a novel interpretation of a talmudic passage:

> ... and they have seen with a microscope that in the seed of a man... exist tiny creatures, whose form resembles that of man, and that are alive and move within the drop.
>
> With this we see how all the words of *Ḥazal* are to be believed and how all their words are truthful and just... even regarding those matters which seem far-fetched or inconceivable... Our Talmud treats this sin [*hotza'at zera levatala*—wasteful emission of the male reproductive seed] harshly, equating it to murder, as it is written, R. Eliezer ben Yaakov said that one who emits seed wastefully is considered as if he killed a soul... and so said R. Yitzḥak and R. Ami in *Masekhet Nidda*. This statement seemed so far-fetched in the eyes of the philosophers amongst our people...who were unaware of the looking glass mentioned above [microscope]. How could it be considered murder prior to the conception of the child ... when the human being had not yet appeared? ... the seed at this time is only fluid from the brain[50] and is still substance without form... But now, after it has been seen with the aforementioned instrument that living beings in the image of man move to and fro within the seed, it is remarkable ... to hear such a thing. Every intelligent person would judge such a sin as truly equivalent to murder.[51]

While most Jewish sources accepted the theory of preformation, it is my opinion that Baruch Schick (1744–1808) (see above) stood alone in rejecting the theory of preformation in favor of epigenesis:

---

50. This is a reference to the encephalo-myelogenic doctrine.
51. *Sefer HaBrit* (Jerusalem, 1990), *ma'amar* 16, chapter 3, 232–233.

The limbs of the body are not all formed at once, rather they grow one by one like a tree… Some have said that the form of a small human being is found within the egg, and there is no place for their words. Still others have said that within the male seed is found the image of a tiny living being, their proof being that when the male seed is viewed under the microscope moving objects, like worms,[52] can be observed. They therefore say that these worms are in fact little human beings… This assertion is also baseless. First, if they are correct, why are there so many worms [sperm]. Second, the very form of the worm attests that it is not the likeness of a man.[53]

Despite Schick's refutation of the theory of preformation, it was still perpetuated by rabbinic sources, especially with reference to the prohibition of *hotza'at zera levatala*.[54] This may be due, in part, to the fact that while *Sefer HaBrit* was a popular, widely read work, *Tiferet Adam* was more obscure.

In summary, we have seen Jewish sources that cover the gamut of embryological theories regarding the origins of the male seed. As with the female seed, attempts were made to align these theories with the words of Ḥazal, including areas of halakha. An historical understanding

---

52. Many scientists of that time referred to sperm as seminal worms. See for example, William Cullen, trans., *Albrecht Haller, First Lines of Physiology* (Edinburgh, 1786), 205.

53. *Tiferet Adam* (Berlin, 1777), 3b–4a. Other arguments against the preformationists are cited in Needham, op. cit., 210. It appears from the last sentence of this quote that Schick may himself have viewed the sperm under the microscope. There is debate amongst historians whether Schick had a laboratory where he performed medical experimentation. See Shapiro, op. cit., 234–235; Israel Zinberg, op. cit., 282. It is also noteworthy that this entire passage is strikingly similar to the writings of Albrecht Haller, whose works were very popular in the scientific world at the time Schick was writing. Compare the passage below with the one by Schick:

> To the father, some have attributed everything; chiefly since the seminal worms, now so well known, were first observed in the male seed by the help of the microscope… But in these animals, there is a proportion wanting betwixt their number and that of the fetuses; they are also not to be constantly observed throughout the tribes of animals. (from Cullen, op. cit., 205–206)

A broader comparison between *Tiferet Adam* and the works of Haller may yield interesting results.

54. R. Yosef Ḥayyim ben Eliyahu, *Rav Pe'alim*, vol. 3, E. H., 2; R. Yeḥiel Mikhel Epstein, *Arukh HaShulḥan*, E. H., 23:1; R. Eliezer Waldenberg, *Tzitz Eliezer*, vol. 9, 51.

of the various embryological theories contemporary with each of these sources gives us a better appreciation of each author's context and scientific frame of reference.

II. REPRODUCTIVE PHYSIOLOGY— ARTIFICIAL INSEMINATION[55]

Artificial insemination is a commonly practiced procedure for the treatment of infertility. Although the procedure has grown tremendously in popularity and application over the last few decades, the concept of intentionally injecting sperm into a woman for the purpose of impregnation dates back to at least the mid-eighteenth-century, when John Hunter successfully inseminated a woman whose husband had a severe form of hypospadias.[56] As early as 1934, Hermann Rohleder wrote the first history of the artificial impregnation of human beings.[57] However, since the widespread application of this procedure is, as stated, only relatively recent, it is in this period that we find the proliferation of rabbinic responsa dealing with every imaginable halakhic consequence of artificial insemination.[58] But what sources could there be in the Talmud or *Rishonim* that could possibly aid in the halakhic explication of this seemingly novel procedure? To answer this question, we must mention yet another form of artificial insemination, this one more indirect in nature. There was a widely held belief, dating back to antiquity, that a woman could become pregnant in a bathhouse, for it was thought that

---

55. Numerous authors have previously written on this topic from an historical perspective. See H. J. Zimmels, *Magicians, Theologians and Doctors* (London, 1952); Immanuel Jakobovits, *Jewish Medical Ethics* (New York, 1959), 244–250. This essay treats the topic more comprehensively.

56. John Hunter (1728–1793) was a prominent scientist and comparative anatomist who is known for his self-experimentation with venereal disease. His original manuscripts detailing his application of artificial insemination are currently housed at the Hunterian Museum in London, where one can also see on display thousands of human and animal anatomical specimens which Hunter collected during his lifetime.

57. *Test Tube Babies* (New York, 1934).

58. See, for example, Fred Rosner, *Modern Medicine and Jewish Law*, 2nd ed. (New York, 1991), 85–100; Abraham Steinberg, *Entzyclopedia Hilkhatit Refuit* (Jerusalem, 1988), 148–161. For a bibliography of responsa on this topic, see R. Yaakov Weinberg and R. Maier Zichal, "*Hazra'a Melakhutit,*" *Assia* 55 (December, 1994), 75–89.

when a woman bathes in a bath into which a man had previously emitted sperm, she may become pregnant. In the following section, I will briefly trace the history of the notion of artificial insemination in both Jewish and non-Jewish sources, from antiquity to the present.

1) Jewish Sources

Two early references to so-called "bathhouse insemination" have served as the source for virtually all contemporary halakhic discussions on modern artificial insemination. The first case is mentioned in *Hagiga*[59] in the course of a discussion about whether a *Kohen Gadol* (High Priest), who is prohibited from marrying any woman who is not a virgin, may marry a pregnant woman who claims she is still a virgin.[60] How could a virgin possibly be pregnant? Shmuel attests that it is possible to have intercourse without perforating the *betulim* (hymen), but the Gemara entertains another possibility, that of impregnation in the bathhouse, in which case, the woman, still a virgin, would be permitted to marry a *Kohen Gadol*.

The second case is mentioned in the *Alphabet of Ben Sira*[61] in reference to the nature of Ben Sira's birth. This narrative work, of questionable date and authorship (some date this work from the Geonic period), details the life of Shimon ben Sira (second century BCE), the author of *Divrei Shimon Ben Sira* (The Wisdom of Ben Sira). The relevant passage appears in the first section of this work, which is a biography of Ben Sira from his conception to the age of one year. The passage, apparently omitted in many editions, describes how the prophet Jeremiah was simultaneously both the father and grandfather of Ben Sira. Ben Sira's mother was Jeremiah's daughter. Jeremiah was forced by evil men to perform

---

59. 14b–15a. Some have construed this passage to be a sarcastic allusion to the Christian doctrine of immaculate conception. See R. Yehoshua Baumel, *Emek Halakha*, 1:68; Jakobovits, op. cit., 359, n. 31. Preuss, op. cit., 477, has already pointed out that this cannot be, as the doctrine of the Immaculate Conception was not yet known at the time of Ben Zoma (first century CE).

60. See *Tosafot*, loc. cit., s. v., "*betula*." Whether it is only claimed or actually verified that the woman is a virgin is a matter of discussion.

61. I consulted the text based on an Oxford manuscript, published in A. M. Haberman, *Ḥadashim Gam Yeshanim* (Jerusalem, 1976), 125–127.

an act of onanism in a bathhouse, and his daughter conceived from his emissions when she inadvertently bathed in the same bath. Ben Sira was born seven months later,[62] the product of artificial insemination.[63] The text further mentions that it is no mere coincidence that the numerical value of the Hebrew letters (*gematria*) of "Sira" equals that of "Yirmiyahu," thereby hinting that Ben Sira was, in fact, the son of Jeremiah.

Not everyone accepted the veracity of this story of Ben Sira's birth. Solomon ibn Verga (c. 1460–1554) states in his historical narrative *Shevet Yehuda* that Ben Sira was the grandson of Yehoshua ben Yehotzadak and makes no mention of any relation to Jeremiah.[64] R. David Ganz, the seventeenth century chronicler, claims that this story is mere exaggeration, as "I have not found it anywhere in the Talmud, and I have not heard from my teachers that it is found in any Aggada or Midrash."[65]

---

62. See Pieter W. Van Der Horst, "Seven Months' Children in Jewish and Christian Literature from Antiquity," in his *Essays on the Jewish World in Early Christianity* (Gottington, 1990), 233–247. (I thank Dr. Shnayer Leiman for this reference.) Van Der Horst does not include Ben Sira in his list. There is a notion in *Ḥazal* that babies born in the seventh and ninth months are viable, whereas those born in the eighth month are not (see, for example, *Shabbat* 135a and *Yevamot* 80a). This was a prevalent notion in antiquity and the Middle Ages and is another example of a topic where a medical historical analysis may shed light on rabbinic sources. This issue has been previously addressed. See Neria Gutal, "*Ben Shemona: Pesher Shitat Ḥazal Benoge'a Lev'ladot Bnei Shemona*," *Assia* 55–56 (1989), 97–111; Dr. Rosemary Reiss and Dr. Avner Ash, "*Ben Shemona—Mekorot Klasi'im L'Emuna Amamit*," ibid., 112–17. See also Ron Barkai, "A Medieval Hebrew Treatise on Obstetrics," *Medical History* 33 (1988), 96–119, esp. 101–104. For further information on the secular sources see Ann Ellis Hanson, "The Eight Months' Child and the Etiquette of Birth: Obsit Omen!" *Bulletin of the History of Medicine* 61 (1987), 589–602; Sarah George, op. cit., 204–233.

63. The text also mentions that the *Ammoraim* Rav Zeira and Rav Pappa were also born by artificial insemination, but unlike Ben Sira, the identity of their fathers was unknown. Yeḥiel Halprein in his *Seder HaDorot* (Jerusalem, 1988), section 2, 118, quotes *Sefer Yuḥsin* by Abraham Zacuto, who, in turn, quotes this notion from *Sefer Kabbalat HaḤasid*. Halprein then cites the original source of this idea from the *Alphabet of Ben Sira* and subsequently refutes the belief that R. Zeira and R. Pappa were products of artificial insemination. He does not, however, assail the belief that Ben Sira was a product of artificial insemination.

64. (Pietrikov, 1904), introduction.

65. *Tzemaḥ David*, section 1, *eleph revi'i*, 448. See also *Tzitz Eliezer*, vol. 9, no. 51, gate 4, chap.1, letter *tet*.

Assuming for our discussion the veracity of the passage in the *Alphabet of Ben Sira*, some important halakhic points can be derived, which explains why it has been so extensively quoted by subsequent *Rishonim* and *Aharonim*. Ben Sira is clearly assumed to be the product of Jeremiah and his daughter. Whether this was known to Jeremiah by *ruah hakodesh* or whether this is because Jeremiah's daughter was trusted to have been a virgin is unclear. In either case, despite the fact that Ben Sira was the product of an halakhically illicit relationship, nowhere do we find aspersions cast on his lineage, and never is he referred to as a *mamzer* (legal bastard). The implication is that only the marital act can create the prohibition of *arayot* (illicit sexual relations) and label the resultant child a *mamzer*. The relevance of this to artificial insemination with donor sperm should be obvious. Secondly, Ben Sira was known as the son of Jeremiah. This fact implies that a child born from artificial insemination may be considered halakhically related to the sperm donor.

One of the earliest references to the case of Ben Sira is by R. Peretz ben Eliyahu of Corbeil (c. 1295) in his glosses on *Sefer Mitzvot Katan* (also referred to as *Amudei Gola*).[66] He states that a woman need not refrain from sleeping on her husband's sheets while she is a *nidda* out of the concern that she might bear a child from the remnant seed on the sheet and the child will be a *ben nidda*. However, R. Peretz does warn that a married woman should not sleep on the sheets of a strange man. Why R. Peretz differentiated between these two cases is a matter of halakhic import, but implicit in these statements is that R. Peretz

---

66. This reference is mentioned by the *Bayit Hadash* (R. Y. Sirkes 1561–1640) in Y. D., 195 (s. v., *"v'lo"*) as appearing in the *"hagahat Semak yashan"* of R. Peretz. The glosses of R. Peretz first appeared in the printed text of *Sefer Mitzvot Katan* in the mid 1500s and all subsequent editions invariably contained these glosses. I consulted the 1556 Cremona edition and could not find this particular gloss. It seems that this gloss remained in manuscript form and was never printed; hence the term *"yashan"* of the Bah likely refers to an old manuscript edition. This fact is further evidenced by the comment of R. Hayyim Y. D. Azulai (*Birkei Yosef E. H.*, 1:14) that after much effort he was finally able to locate this particular gloss of R. Peretz in an old manuscript.

A passage similar to that of R. Peretz appears in the *Shiltei HaGiborim* on the Rif (*Shavuot* 2a) attributed to an author referred to by his acronym, *HR"M*. R. Eliezer Waldenberg (*Tzitz Eliezer* vol. 9, no. 51, gate 4, chap. 1, letter *het*) has postulated that this may be a misprint, and the text should actually read *HR"P*, an acronym for HaRav Rabbenu Peretz.

acknowledged that a woman could become pregnant in this manner. He brings proof from the case of Ben Sira who, despite being the product of an halakhically illicit union, was not considered a *mamzer* as no conjugal relations (*bi'ah*) had taken place. Jacob Moelin (c. 1365–1427) also mentions the case of Ben Sira in the *Likutei Maharil*, where it appears as a statement without particular halakhic context.[67]

More elaborate treatment of this topic is found in the responsa of R. Shimon ben Tzemaḥ Duran,[68] to whom a question was posed about a woman who claimed to have had a virginal conception. R. Duran, who was also a physician, was asked to determine whether this was in fact possible, and, if so, what would be the halakhic ramifications. Whether this so-called bathhouse impregnation was actually feasible or simply contrived for the sake of halakhic analysis was a matter of intense debate amongst the *Aharonim*, as we shall soon see. Tashbetz was one of few *Rishonim* who addressed this topic. He concludes that it is feasible, marshaling evidence from the aforementioned passage in *Masekhet Ḥagiga*, as well as from the case of Ben Sira. With respect to the latter he prefaces with the disclaimer that "if we believe the Apocrypha" then we have proof from Ben Sira. What is particularly interesting is the Tashbetz's reference in a gloss to two of his contemporaries, one an unnamed non-Jew and the other named R. Abraham Israel, both of whom claimied to have been familiar with cases of virginal women who had conceived.

The next Jewish reference to artificial insemination is not rabbinic in origin, but appears in the case studies of the famous marrano physician Amatus Lusitanus (1511–1568).[69] This discussion, like the aforementioned passage of Ben Sira, is not found in all versions of Lusitanus' classic work, *Centuriæ*, as it was expurgated by the censors.[70] Here Lusitanus invokes the notion of artificial insemination (*sine concubito*) to exonerate a nun with a uterine mole who was accused of impropriety. He adduces his

---

67. *Sefer Maharil*, Shlomo Spitzer, ed. (Jerusalem, 1989), 611–612.

68. 3:263.

69. On Lusitanus, see essays in Harry Friedenwald, *The Jews and Medicine* 1 (Baltimore, 1944), 332–390. The section relevant to our discussion is on page 386. Preuss (op. cit., 464) also quotes Lusitanus in discussing the Gemara in Ḥagiga.

70. Friedenwald, op. cit., 363, n. 98.

proofs from the case of Ben Sira, as well as from other scientific sources discussed below.

Another famous Jewish physician makes mention of artificial insemination in his work,[71] but this particular work is halakhic, not medical in nature. R. Yitzḥak Lampronti (1679–1756),[72] in his magnum opus, *Paḥad Yitzḥak*, poses the following riddle: A child is the son of a woman who was impregnated by her father, yet he is not a *mamzer*. How is this possible?[73] He answers, "This is Ben Sira," and recounts the incident in the bathhouse, "as is written in '*ketubot*.'" This reference is clearly not to the talmudic tractate by the same name, as we have already mentioned that the story derives from the *Alphabet of Ben Sira*. The term "*ketubot*" can be translated as "the writings," without reference to a specific body of work.[74]

---

71. See the work of another famous Jewish physician, Tobias Cohn, who mentions artificial insemination in his *Ma'aseh Tuviah* (Cracow, 1908), section 3, 118b.

72. Although known for his halakhic expertise, Lampronti was a prominent Italian physician and a graduate of the University of Padua. See Abdelkader Modena and Edgardo Morpugo, *Medici E Chirurghi Ebrei Dottorati E Licenziati Nell Universita Di Padova dal 1617 al 1816* (Bologna, 1967), 55–57. Lampronti consulted the famous physician Morgagni for assistance with his difficult medical cases. Saul Jarcho elaborates on these consultations in his article, "Dr. Isaac Lampronti of Ferrara," *Koroth* 8:11–12 (1985), 203–206. For more on Lampronti, see D. Ruderman, "Contemporary Science and Jewish Law in the Eyes of Isaac Lampronti and Some of His Contemporaries," *Jewish History* 6:1–2 (1992), 211–224; D. Margalit, "R. Yitzḥak Lampronti: Rabbi, Physician, Lexicographer," (Hebrew) in his *Ḥakhmei Yisrael KeRofim* (Mosad Harav Kook, 5722) 152–174; H. Savitz, "Dr. Isaac Lampronti: Rabbi, Physician, Teacher, Preacher, Encyclopaedist," in his *Profiles of Erudite Jewish Physicians and Scholars* (Spertus College, 1973), 29–32. For a collection of all the medical matters in R. Lampronti's magnum opus, see D. Margalit, "Medical Articles in the Encyclopedia Paḥad Yitzḥak by R. I. Lampronti," (Hebrew) *Koroth* 2:1–2 (April, 1958), 38–60.

73. *Paḥad Yitzḥak* (Bnei Brak, 1980), s. v., "*Ben Bito*." David Margalit does not mention this passage in his essay, "*Erkhim Refui'im ShebeEntzyclopedia HaHilkhatit Paḥad Yitzḥak L'R. Y. Lampronti*," *Koroth* 2:1–2 (April, 1958), 38–61.

74. Although the *Wisdom of Ben Sira* is included in the works of the Apocrypha, the *Alphabet of Ben Sira* is not. See R. Yehoshua Baumel, *Emek Halakha*, no. 68, regarding the quotation of R. Lampronti: "…even though he did not cite his source for this, still his words are believed, and this *tzaddik* is free from iniquity." R. Baumel apparently thought the word "*ketuvim*" to be a generic reference, not a reference to a specific work or body of works.

We now turn to the scientific question of whether bathhouse impregnation is even possible. Implicit from all the above sources is that they accepted the possibility of this unique form of artificial insemination. However, few of them address the question specifically, with the exception of Tashbetz and Lusitanus, both of whom accept the possibility. One of the first to expressly deny the possibility of such an event was R. Yehuda Rosanes (d. 1727), who articulates his position in his glosses to Maimonides' *Mishneh Torah*, entitled *Mishneh LeMelekh*.[75] R. Rosanes maintains that a woman can only become pregnant through the completion of the natural marital act (i.e., *gemar bi'ah*). He brings support for this notion from talmudic sources, and also discusses the talmudic teaching that a woman cannot become pregnant from the first intercourse (*bi'ah rishona*). Based on these as well as other sources, he concludes that bathhouse impregnation as impossible.

This passage from the *Mishneh LeMelekh* is cited widely by subsequent authorities, some with approbation,[76] others with condemnation, as we will soon see. Although a number of *Aharonim* mention the *Mishneh LeMelekh* approvingly, including R. Moses Schick, perhaps his most enthusiastic advocate was R. Solomon Schick. In a responsum to R. Yosef Edinger, coincidentally a student of R. Moses Schick, R. Solomon Schick states assuredly, with no ambiguity, that bathhouse impregnation could never happen. In addition to quoting R. Rosanes and R. Moses Schick as concurring, he interprets the passage in *Hagiga* in a novel fashion. As the aforementioned passage follows the story of the four rabbis who entered "*pardes*" (however it is to be defined), and one of those rabbis is the same Ben Zoma of our relevant passage, and this Ben Zoma was harmed by his journey into "*pardes*," R. Solomon Schick maintains that the Gemara is possibly mocking him. Never, according

---

75. *Hil. Ishut*, 15:4. See also *Mishneh LeMelekh* on *Hil. Isurei Bi'ah* 17:15 where R. Rosanes discusses these matters in great detail and states that the passage of Ben Zoma in *Hagiga* is not considered halakhic.

76. See, for example, Malakhi ben Yakov HaKohen (d.1785–1790), *Yad Malakhi* (Berlin, 1857), *klalei hadinim* no. 247; R. Moshe Schick, known as Maharam Schick, *Taryag Mitzvot* no.1.

to R. Solomon Schick, did the Gemara actually believe that bathhouse insemination could occur.[77]

Other authorities subsequent to R. Rosanes have independently questioned the possibility of bathhouse impregnation. R. Ḥayyim (1835–1909), author of *Ben Ish Ḥai,* espouses a novel position in his work, *Torah Lishma.*[78] R. Ḥayyim was asked whether he would allow sperm procurement from an ill man to facilitate a proper medical diagnosis. The questioner maintained that since the sperm could subsequently be used to impregnate a woman, this should mitigate the prohibition of *hashhatat zera.* R. Ḥayyim's contention is that "nature has changed" (*nishtaneh hateva*)[79] with respect to artificial insemination. Whereas insemination through an intermediary medium (e.g., bathhouse impregnation) was possible in the times of the *Tannaim* due to their greater bodily strength and potency of their seed, such was not the case from the time of the *Ammoraim* and onward. He maintains that if it were at all possible, it would be an extremely rare occurrence as was the case mentioned by the Tashbetz. Therefore, as the likelihood of impregnating a woman with the remaining seed was so remote, sperm procurement would not be allowed.[80] Around the time this responsum was written, John Hunter performed the first successful artificial impregnation of a human being. However, this success was not widely publicized.[81]

Along a similar vein, a number of *Aharonim* also maintained that bathhouse impregnation was not possible in their time due to the changed nature. However, it was the changed nature of the baths, they maintained, not that of the seed, that explained why insemination was

---

77. *Teshuvot Rashban,* E. H., no. 8.
78. (Jerusalem, 1976), no. 481. R. Ḥayyim wrote these responsa under a pseudonym.
79. The concept of "*nishtaneh hateva*" has been invoked many times in rabbinic literature. See, for example, *Tosafot in Avoda Zara* 24b, s. v., "*Para*"; *Tosafot in Ḥullin* 47a, s. v., "*kol*"; E. H. 156:4 in the Rema. Two areas where authorities often discuss this principle are *Hil. Treifot* and *metzitza* in *mila.* See also later in this article regarding the two pathways of the male genital organ.
80. R. Ḥayyim cites other reasons for forbidding sperm procurement in this case, such as, some seed might spill in the process of collection, or, even if they collect all the seed, it might not all be used for the purpose of insemination. These concerns have been voiced by current *poskim* in their discussions on artificial insemination.
81. See Rohleder, op. cit.

Fertility and Reproduction

no longer possible.[82] According to this opinion, since the baths in talmudic times were heated from below,[83] it was theoretically possible for insemination to occur, either because a man was more likely to emit seed in this kind of bath, or because this particular heat source was more conducive to the survival of the seed.[84]

While others questioned the possibility of bathhouse impregnation, as we have seen, it was R. Rosanes who was always hailed as the main opponent to this notion. His position did not remain unopposed, as a number of *Aharonim* reject his contention.[85] There were three different approaches in response to R. Rosanes. R. Yehonatan Eybeschuetz (1690–1764) argued against R. Rosanes based on a re-analysis of the *talmudic* passages that R. Rosanes cites, concluding that the latter's interpretations were incorrect, hence, artificial insemination is possible.[86] R. Hayyim Yosef David Azulai (1724–1806) mentioned on three separate occasions in his writings that bathhouse impregnation was possible because it was accepted as fact by the Gemara, as well as by

---

82. R. Yaakov Reischer, *Iyun Yaakov* (Wilhelmsdorf, 1725), on *Masekhet Hagiga* 14b. See also R. Pinchas Horowitz, *Pitha Zuta al Hil. Nidda UTevilla* (London, 1958), 195:7, who explains the position of R. Reischer. Both of these sources question why Maimonides omits the case of Ben Zoma from his code.

83. See *O. H.* 230:3 and *Mishna Berura*, loc. cit.

84. R. Yekutiel Greenwald, in his *Kol Bo Al Aveilut* (New York, 1947), 305–330, n. 8, states that the majority of *poskim* hold that bathhouse insemination could never happen. However, if it were ascertainable that such an event had occurred, the parents and children would be obligated to mourn for each other. Another halakhic question unique to a child born from bathhouse insemination is whether such a child could have his *mila* performed on Shabbat. See R. Moshe Bunim Pirutinsky, *Sefer HaBrit* (New York, 1973), 9, who states, based on the interpretation of R. Hananel to the Gemara in *Hagiga*, that since such a birth is considered miraculous, and not by natural methods of conception, the *mila* could not be performed on shabbat. See also J. David Bleich, "Circumcision of a Child *Sine Concubito*," in his *Bioethical Dilemmas* 2 (Targum Press, 2006), 93–97; Y. Kohn and G. Weitzman, "Shabbat Brit of a Child Conceived Through Medical Intervention," *Journal of Halacha and Contemporary Society* 61 (Spring 2011), 56–81.

85. Many *Aharonim* still maintained the possibility of bathhouse impregnation without specifically addressing the *Mishneh LeMelekh*. See R. Yaakov Emden *Iggeret Bikkoret* (Zhitomer, 1868) and *She'ilat Yaavetz*, vol. 2, no. 97.

86. *Bnei Ahuva* (Jerusalem, 1965), on Maimonides, *Hil. Ishut* chap. 15.

a number of prominent *Rishonim*.[87] The third approach of refutation is scientific in nature and was taken by R. Baruch Mordechai ben Yaakov Libschitz (1810–1885). R. Rosanes had stated that conception could only be accomplished with *gemar bi'ah*. R. Libschutz responded that with respect to bathhouse impregnation, the waters of the bath could transport the seed to the internal organs of the woman, thereby effectively accomplishing the same result as *gemar bi'ah*.[88]

Contemporary *poskim*, in their discussions on modern therapeutic artificial insemination, refer to some of the aforementioned sources. However, as the possibility of such an occurrence, at least in the modern medical context, is an accepted fact, little space is devoted to the scientific question of feasibility.[89] More time is apportioned for the resolution of attendant halakhic dilemmas.

2) Secular Sources[90]

The notion of virginal or non-natural conception dates back to antiquity and antedates Christianity.[91] Explicit reference to the phenomenon of artificial insemination, however, is found in sources from the Middle Ages. Avicenna in his *Canon* on medicine and Averroes (d. 1198) in his *Colliget* acknowledge the possibility of artificial

---

87. *Birkei Yosef*, E. H., 1:14; *Yair Ozen, ma'arekhet* 1 no. 93; *P'tach Einayim* on Ḥagiga 14b. See also R. Y. S. Nathanson, *Shai LeMoreh*, Glosses on E. H., 1;6; ibid., *Responsum Shoel UMeshiv*, Vol. 3, section 3, nos. 34 and 132 (end); R. Eliezer Fleckles, *Teshuva MeAhava*, Y. D., no. 195.

88. *Brit Yaakov* (Warsaw, 1876), E. H., no. 4. The author employs the same logic with respect to R. Peretz's pronouncement about a woman becoming pregnant from seed remaining on the sheets. Here, too, he maintains that a woman may use the sheets for internally cleaning herself, thereby bringing the seed into close proximity with the uterus.

89. See R. Shalom Mordechai Schwadron (1835–1911), *She'elot UTeshuvot Maharsham* (New York, 1962), vol. 3, no. 268, who was asked whether it was permissible to undergo artificial insemination.

90. For the material on artificial insemination in medieval times, I have relied on secondary sources, primarily Preuss. The primary sources are in Arabic and Latin and, for the most part, remain untranslated into English.

91. See Robert Graves, *The Greek Myths* (Baltimore, 1955), 51 for descriptions of non-natural methods of conception. I thank Dr. Louis Feldman for this reference.

impregnation.[92] Thomas Aquinas (d. 1274) relates that a woman became pregnant from lying in a bed into which sperm was previously discharged.[93] As discussed above, R. Peretz of Corbeil, a contemporary of Aquinas accepted this possibility and therefore dealt with the halakhic ramifications. Amatus Lusitanus quotes Avicenna and Al-Jazzar (tenth century)[94] as authorities who accept artificial insemination.[95]

In 1750, a pamphlet entitled *Lucina Sine Concubito* by Dr. Abraham Johnson was published in London.[96] It was submitted by Johnson to the Royal Society, the pre-eminent scientific body in England, and is comprised of a personal account of a patient of Johnson's, whom the latter believed had conceived by artificial insemination. In this fantastical essay, Johnson postulates the means by which this insemination was achieved. He believed, based on classical sources, that the reproductive seed derived from the western winds and was accidentally ingested by his female patient. He further claimed that he tested his theory experimentally on his housemaid, without her consent, and achieved positive results (i.e., the maid became pregnant). He therefore submitted his results to the Royal Society with suggestions for wider applications of his technique.

While the belief in bathhouse insemination persisted into the twentieth century,[97] similar to the Jewish sources above, it was not without its detractors. Paolo Zacchias (1584–1659), physician to Pope

---

92. Preuss, 464.

93. Ibid. Preuss provides no reference for this statement.

94. On this author see Gerrit Bos, "Ibn Al-Jazzar on Women's Diseases and Their Treatment," *Medical History* 37 (1993), 296–312. In personal communication Dr. Bos says he is unaware of any reference to artificial insemination in the extant works of Al-Jazzar.

95. Preuss, 464.

96. This work was reprinted and appended to Hermann Rohleder, *Test Tube Babies* (New York, 1934).

97. Preuss, 464, cites Stern, who stated that the belief in bathhouse insemination was still prevalent in Turkey at that time, i.e., early twentieth century. See also George Gould and Walter Pyle, *Medical Curiosities* (New York, 1896), 42–45, who state that the possibility of bathhouse insemination was still being debated. They also relate an extraordinary, if not fantastical, story from the Civil War of how a woman, struck in the abdomen with a bullet that previously hit the testicle of a soldier, gave birth, after 278 days, to an eight-pound boy.

Innocent X and prominent medical legal writer,[98] rejects the possibility, as did the great scientist Albrecht Haller (1708–1777).[99]

In conclusion, since the possibility of bathhouse insemination would be difficult to disprove, whether it has or can actually occur remains a mystery.[100]

III. REPRODUCTIVE ANATOMY—THE TWO PATHWAYS (*SHNEI SHVILIN*)

1) Jewish Sources

Rabbinic sources throughout the ages have discussed the intricate details of male reproductive anatomy, as it directly relates to the laws governing the definition of an halakhically infertile man (i.e., *petzua daka* and *kerut shafkha*).[101] In the context of one such discussion, the Gemara in *Bekhorot* (44b) makes a statement that seems somewhat puzzling today. The Gemara states that there are two pathways in the male genital organ, one for urine and one for seed,[102] and that these two pathways are separated by a fine membrane the width of a garlic peel whose integrity is necessary for fertility. Should this membrane rupture and allow communication between the two channels, the man may be rendered halakhically infertile *(petzua daka)* and consequently may be forbidden to marry.

The existence of these two pathways in the male organ was an accepted fact amongst *Rishonim* and early *Aḥaronim*, and many halakhic discussions revolved around cases where one or the other pathway was perforated, especially in cases of hypospadias (i.e., when the opening of the urethra is not at the tip of the *ever*, but at varying points along the

---

98. On Zacchias and other medical legal writers see Bernard Ficarro, "History of Legal Medicine," *Legal Medicine Annual* (1979).

99. Both Zacchias and Haller are mentioned in Preuss, op. cit., 464.

100. Although I have been unable to find any contemporary medical references to bathhouse insemination, I have found an interesting case which attests to the viability of the human sperm. See Douwe A.A. Verkuyl, "Oral Conception: Impregnation Via the Proximal Gastrointestinal Tract in a Patient with an Aplastic Vagina," *British Journal of Obstetrics and Gynaecology* 95 (September, 1988), 933–934.

101. See E. H., 5.

102. See also Rashi on *Yevamot* 75b, s. v., "*guvta.*"

shaft).[103] In the latter case, it was unclear whether the existing opening was only for the urine, which could easily be ascertained, or whether it was also for the seed, which was halakhically difficult to determine given the prohibition of *hotza'at zera levatala*. The following section highlights some of the sources, both Jewish and secular, that have addressed this unique anatomical notion.

R. Shimon ben Tzemaḥ Duran mentions the notion of the two pathways in his philosophical work, *Magen Avot*.[104]

> ...for the organs of reproduction in the man are two, the *ever* and the *beitzim* [testicles]...and *Ḥazal* added the *ḥutei beitzim*[105] ...should any of these three organs be damaged a man will be rendered infertile...and *Ḥazal* have written extensively on these topics, based on their *kabbala*, and have understood matters that scientists have not...and in the Canon [of Avicenna][106] it states that there are three pathways, one for urine, one for seed and one for [other] fluids...but this does not appear to be so according

---

103. See *Otzar HaPoskim* (Jerusalem, 1962), E. H., 5, no.25 and Abraham Tzvi Hirsch Eisenstadt, *Pitḥei Teshuva*, E. H., 5, no. 5 for a series of halakhic queries regarding both acquired and congenital variants of the male genitalia.

104. 37b. A loose translation of the passage follows.

105. It is a matter of debate as to the halakhic definition of *ḥutei habeitzim*. For our purposes we can assume it refers to the vas deferens.

106. Avicenna (980–1037), known in Hebrew sources as Ibn Sina, was a Persian physician of great renown. His main work, *The Canon*, was considered the authoritative work on medicine for many centuries, and is quoted extensively by rabbinic sources. The only extant Hebrew medical incunabula is a copy of Avicenna's *Canon* (Naples, 1491). Many Hebrew manuscripts of Avicenna were found in the Cairo Geniza. See Haskell D. Isaacs, *Medical and Para-Medical Manuscripts in the Cambridge Genizah Collections* (Cambridge, 1994).

It appears that the printer of *She'elot UTeshuvot Ḥavot Yair* (reprinted, Jerusalem, 1973) by R. Yair Bacharach was not familiar with the work of Avicenna, as I believe there is a misprint in responsum no. 234. In this responsum, addressing the permissibility of using talmudic remedies for medical treatment, R. Bacharch discusses a particular theory of medical therapeutics. R. Bacharach claims that he found support for this theory in "*Sefer HaKinyan Le'even Pinah.*" I have found no bibliographical reference to such a work, and, given the medical context of the statement, believe the proper reading should be "*Sefer HaKanon le'Ibn Sina.*"

> to *Ḥazal* [who say there are two] ... all this is based on the true
> *kabbala*, which the scientists have not acquired ... and since the
> wisdom of our sages has been lost through the exiles we must
> labor [to restore it] ... and one should not err and say that *Ḥazal*
> were not expert in the sciences ...

Most *poskim* have understood the passage in *Bekhorot* to mean that
there are two pathways extending all the way to the tip of the *ever*, and
such was clearly the opinion of R. Moses Sofer in considering the suggestion of physicians to repair a hypospadias.[107] R. Yisroel Yehoshua
Trunk (1820–1893), however, interpreted the Gemara differently. He
understood the two pathways for urine and seed to refer to the internal anatomy, but not that they extended into the *ever*. It is a mistake
to think this, he maintained, as both the urine and seed traverse one
path in the *ever*.

Ḥazon Ish, R. Avraham Yeshayahu Karclitz (1878–1953), apparently agreed with the anatomical observation of R. Trunk, but did not
accept his interpretation of the Gemara:

> In the Gemara, it states that there were two pathways, one for
> the urine and one for the seed ... in this matter, the nature has
> changed (*nishtanu hativ'im*),[108] as today there is only one path-
> way in the *ever*.[109]

Ḥazon Ish also claimed, based on his discussion with physicians, that the
particular part of male anatomy under discussion is subject to variation,
be it a function of time or of geographical location.[110] R. Yosef Ḥayyim

---

107. R. Moshe Sofer, *Teshuvot Ḥatam Sofer* (Vienna, 1882) vol. 6, no. 64, s. v., *"akh ma."*
108. See the position of R. Yosef Ḥayyim above in section on artificial insemination.
109. *Ḥazon Ish* (Bnei Brak, 1991) *E. H.*, 12, no. 7.
110. Ibid. See *Tzitz Eliezer*, vol.10. no. 25, chap. 24. These two sources deal with the
     halakhic aspects of prostate surgery, which can involve intentional ligation of the
     vas deferens. The issue discussed is whether such a procedure renders the patient
     a *kerut shafkha* (one who is castrated and therefore prohibited from marrying into
     the people of Israel). On this topic, see the important responsum of R. Moses
     Feinstein, *E. H.*, vol. 4, nos. 28 and 29.

mentions a number of such anatomical variants that were found in the city of Bagdad.[111]

2) Secular Sources

The notion of there being more than one pathway in the *ever* was prevalent in the Middle Ages, especially in the Arab world,[112] but does not appear to have clear roots in antiquity. Galen, a contemporary of R. Yehuda HaNasi, states unequivocally that there is one path for both urine and semen,[113] though Hippocrates appears to have supported the two-path theory.[114] Avicenna, as quoted by R. Duran above, claimed there were three canals in the *ever*, and Mondino (d.1326), the Italian anatomist, described a separate canal for the sperm.[115] These ideas permeated the works of the Renaissance artist and anatomist Leonardo da Vinci (1452–1519), who drew two distinct passages in his anatomical drawings.[116]

Andreas Vesalius (1514–1564) is credited with rectifying the Arab belief and clarifying, by anatomical dissection, that there is only one

---

On the effect and importance of geographical location in the *Talmud* as compared to classical sources see Stephen Newmyer, "The Concept of Climate and National Superiority in the Talmud and its Classical Parallels," *Transactions and Studies of the College of Physicians of Philadelphia*, series 5, vol. 5, no. 1 (March, 1983), 1–12. On the concept of climatology in general, see Genevieve Miller, "'Airs, Waters and Places' in History," *Journal of the History of Medicine* 17 (January, 1962), 129–140. The notion of climatic changes in time and place has been employed to explain the concept of *"nishtaneh hateva."*

111. *Rav Pe'alim*, vol. 3, *E. H.*, no. 12.

112. Preuss, op. cit., 110; *Magen Avot*, cited in the text above; Cecil Roth, ed., *Encyclopedia Judaica*, 2 (Jerusalem), 932.

113. Margaret Talmadge May, ed., *Galen: On the Usefulness of the Parts of the Body* (Ithaca, 1968), 660.

114. See *Hippocrates: Generation. Nature of the Child*, Volume X of the Loeb Classical Library (Harvard University Press, 2010), 9: "…the seed passes through the middle of the testicles to the penis, not running where the urine does, but contained in another passage which exists for it." I thank Dr. Moshe Pinchuk for this reference.

115. J. Playfair McMurrich, *Leonardo da Vinci, the Anatomist* (Baltimore, 1930), 202.

116. Ibid., 180; Charles D. O'Malley and J. B. de C. M. Saunders, *Leonardo on the Human Body* (New York, 1983), 460–463.

pathway in the *ever*.[117] He also postulates how the Arabs arrived at their conclusion.[118] Interestingly, by way of discussion, he cites an actual case of a young man from Padua who had two passages at the tip of the *ever*, one for semen and one for urine.[119]

The susceptibility of the urethra to anatomical variation, and in particular to duplication, has been recorded in medical case records.[120] Frank Netter, in his contemporary classic, *The CIBA Collection of Medical Illustrations*, draws accessory urethral channels as an example of congenital variations.[121]

IV. CONCLUSION

The understanding of embryology, as well as reproductive anatomy and physiology, has changed significantly over the centuries. The sources in rabbinic literature that address these issues, whether directly or indirectly, reflect these changes. It is essential for the modern reader to appreciate the historical dimension when learning or extrapolating from these sources.

---

117. See C. D. O'Malley, *Andreas Vesalius of Brussels* (Berkeley, 1964), 358. The appendix contains a selection of translations from Vesalius' famous work, *De Humani Corporis Fabrica* (Basel, 1543).

118. Preuss, op. cit., 110.

119. C. D. O'Malley, et al., trans., *William Harvey: Lectures on the Whole of Anatomy* (Berkeley, 1961), 142, n. 509. Harvey followed Vesalius and confirmed that there was only one path in the *ever*.

120. See George Gould and Walter Pyle, *Anomalies and Curiosities of Medicine* (New York, 1896), 317. They also quote the case studies of Fabricius Hildanus (1560–1624), Marcellus Donatus (1538–1602) and others, including Vesalius.

121. *Reproductive System*, vol. 2 (New York, 1988), 31. Here, however, the accessory urethra ends in a blind pouch and does not carry either sperm or urine.

The Doctrine of the Seven-Chamber Uterus

INTRODUCTION[1]

Rabbinic Literature is replete with references to medical and scientific theories from previous centuries. In particular, in the area of anatomy, we find a number of notions that confound the modern reader.[2] For example, the Mishna in *Ohalot* (1:8) enumerates 248 limbs,[3] the Talmud[4] states that there are two passages in the male reproductive organ,[5] and the Mishna in *Nidda* (2:5) uses a metaphor for female reproductive anatomy that to this day eludes clarification.[6] Contrary to the popular

---

1. The author wishes to thank Dr. Shlomo Sprecher, *a"h* for his valuable contributions to this article.
2. On the general history of anatomy and anatomical dissection in rabbinic literature, see chapter, "The Anatomy of Halakha."
3. On the 248 limbs, see chapter, "The Anatomy of the Human Body in Rabbinic Literature."
4. *Bekhorot* 44b.
5. See chapter, "The Rabbinic Conception of Conception."
6. R. Moses Sofer, in his commentary to *Nidda* 18a, concludes that Rashi and *Tosafot* were mistaken in their anatomical interpretation of the metaphor mentioned in the Mishna, while Maimonides' position is more consistent with known anatomical teachings. For more on this topic, see Abraham. S. Abraham, "Introduction to *Hilkhot Nidda*" in his *Nishmat Avraham* (Hebrew) Y. D., 66–69; M. Halperin, "On

belief that these notions are unique and exclusive to rabbinic literature, many of these notions are based on contemporaneous medical or scientific doctrine. Appreciating the historical context of these statements better enables the reader to analyze these sources. The larger issue—how to deal with passages in rabbinic literature that seemingly conflict with our modern understanding of medicine—has received extensive treatment over the last few years and will not be addressed herein.[7] Moreover, the present topic does not have halakhic ramifications and is therefore less theologically problematic. In this chapter, I focus on the history of a curious anatomical notion found in rabbinic literature. This notion, known as the doctrine of the seven-chamber uterus, has been previously explored by medical historians. The rabbinic sources that incorporate this doctrine, which span roughly eight centuries and many areas of

---

the Meaning of the Term '*Rechem*' in *Chazal*," *Assia* 61–62 (*Nisan*, 5758), 105–109 (Hebrew); M. Halperin, "The Terms *Lul* and *Aliyah* of *Chazal*," letter in *Assia* 65–66 (*Elul*, 5759), 181–183 (Hebrew); Y. Levi, "The Terms of Female Reproductive Anatomy According to Rashi in the Talmud," *Assia* 63–64 (*Kislev*, 5759), 169–176 (Hebrew); I. M. Levinger, "The Structure of the Female Reproductive System in the Human and in Cattle," *Koroth* 4:8–10 (June, 1968), 611–615 (Hebrew); D. Malach, "More on the Meaning of the Term '*Rehem*' in *Hazal*," letter to the editor in *Assia* 67–68 (*Shevat*, 5761), 206–208 (Hebrew); T. Meachum, "Critical Edition of *Masekhet Nidda*" (Ph.D. Dissertation, Hebrew University, 5749), 224–230; J. Preuss, "Female Reproductive Anatomy," in his *Biblical and Talmudic Medicine*, trans. F. Rosner (Jason Aronson, 1993), 113–121; M. Halperin, *Realia and Medicine in Seder Nashim* (Schlesinger Institute, 2011), 3–40 (Hebrew).

7. For treatment of this fascinating and complex topic see D. Frimer, "*Kevi'at Avhut al yedei Bedukat Dam beMishpat haYisraeli ubemishpat haIvri*," in M. Halperin, ed., *Sefer Assia* 5 (Jerusalem, 1986), 185–209; D. Cohen, "*Shinuy Hateva*: An Analysis of the Halachic Process," *Journal of Halacha and Contemporary Society* 31 (Spring 1996); S. Sprecher, "*Divrei Hazal VeYedi'ot Mada'iyot*," B.D.D. 2 (Winter 1996), 2–39; S. Z. Leiman, "R. Israel Lipshutz and the Mouse that is Half Flesh and Half Earth: A Note on Torah U-Madda in the Nineteenth Century," in *Hazon Nachum* (Yeshiva University Press, 1997), 449–458; N. Gutal, *Sefer Hishtanut HaTeva'im BeHalakha* (Makhon Yahdav, 5758); A. Steinberg, *Encyclopedia of Jewish Medical Ethics*, trans. F. Rosner (Feldheim, 2003), s. v., "change in nature"; N. Slifkin, *Mysterious Creatures* (Targum Press, 2003), 17–41; M. Halperin, "Science and Medicine in the Talmud: *Kabbalah o Actualia*," *Assia* 71–72 (January, 2003), 90–102 (Hebrew); Yehuda Levi, *The Science in Torah: The Scientific Knowledge of the Sages* (Feldheim, 2004); M. Meiselman, *Torah, Chazal and Science* (Israel Bookshop, 2013).

rabbinic literature, will constitute the core of this chapter. This exercise serves as another example of how an understanding of medical history can enhance our study of rabbinic literature.[8]

I. THE DOCTRINE OF THE SEVEN-CHAMBER UTERUS[9] IN MEDICAL HISTORY

The anatomical composition and function of the uterus was a matter of debate in antiquity.[10] One of the debated issues was the number of compartments that the uterus possessed. Hippocrates discussed the possibility of multiple chambers or compartments to the uterus, and this notion was adopted by many writers in antiquity. In the Middle Ages, a number of physicians espoused a specific belief that the human uterus comprised seven chambers or cells: three on the right, three on the left, and one in the middle. Furthermore, the location of the fetus within the uterus was thought to affect the sex determination of the offspring. The male embryos were believed to develop on the right, the female ones on the left. The embryos developing in the center would be hermaphrodites.

This doctrine of the seven-chamber uterus, which finds its expression in anatomical illustrations of this period,[11] is virtually non-existent

---

8. This is particulary relevant for notions that are not in consonance with contemporary understanding of medicine.
9. On this doctrine, see Fridolf Kudlien, "The Seven Cells of the Uterus: The Doctrine and its Roots," *Bulletin of the History of Medicine* 39:5 (1965), 415–423; idem, "The Legal Aspect of the Doctrine of the Seven Uterine Cells," *Bulletin of the History of Medicine* 40:6 (1966), 544–546; Robert Reisert, "Der Siebenkammerige Uterus," *Wurzburger Medizinhistorische Forschungen* 39 (1986); Christine Boot, "Neufunde Zum, Siebenkammerigen Uterus," *Sudhoffs Archiv Zeitschrift Für Wissenschaftsgeschichte* 71:2 (1987), 233–235. For a review and comments on Reisert's work, see Monica Green in Speculum 66:2 (April, 1991), 468–469.
10. For an overview of the historical notions of the uterus, see L. Dean-Jones, *Women's Bodies in Classical Greek Science* (Clarendon Press, 1994); H. King, *Hippocrates' Woman* (Rutledge, 1998); E. M. Ramsey, "Concepts of the Uterus: A Historical Perspective," in T. Chard, Jurgis Gediminas Grudzinkas, *The Uterus* (Cambridge University Press, 1993).
11. See Christoph Ferckel, "Diagramme der Sexualorgane in Mittelalter- lichen Hand- schriften," *Archiv für Geschichte der Medizin* (1917), 255–264; Alfred Plaut, "Historical and Cultural Aspects of the Uterus," *Annals of the New York Academy of Science* 75:2 (January, 1959), 389–411. For later illustrations of the uterus, see K. Petrucelli,

prior to the Middle Ages.[12] The obvious question is how such a doctrine could develop when simple visual inspection of the human uterus clearly contradicts it. The short answer to this question lies in understanding the history of anatomical dissection. While human dissection was performed briefly in antiquity, systematic dissection of the human body was not routinely performed until the early Renaissance. Anatomical teaching was primarily based on theory and philosophy, with only occasional limited correlation with anatomical dissection.

Although the exact origins of the doctrine in the aforementioned form remain unclear, it is believed to have historical roots in antiquity, representing a synthesis of the right-left theory[13] of sex determination[14]

"The Misrepresented Uterus: The Progression of Uterine Depictions in Anatomical Atlases Between the Sixteenth and Eighteenth Centuries," *Journal of Biocommunication* 25:4 (1998), 10–13. Some attribute the doctrine to Leonardo da Vinci as well, based on one of his illustrations of the uterus. See C. D. O'Malley and J. B. de C. M. Saunders, *Leonardo on the Human Body* (Dover Publications, 1952), 464. Da Vinci's more elaborate illustrations of the uterus do not seem consistent with the seven-chamber doctrine. See J. Playfair McMurrich, *Leonardo da Vinci, the Anatomist* (Williams and Wilkins, 1930), 200–201.

12. On the transmission of gynecological theories from antiquity, see M. Green, *The Transmission of Ancient Theories of Female Physiology and Disease through the Early Middle Ages* (Ph.D. Dissertation, Princeton University, 1985).

13. The right-left theory was adopted in different variations by Hippocrates and Galen, as well as many other Greek authors. See, for example, A. L. Peck, trans., *Aristotle: Generation of Animals* (Harvard University Press, 1942), 371–374; Owsei Temkin, trans., *Soranus' Gynecology* (Johns Hopkins University Press, 1956), 44–45; Margaret T. May, *Galen on the Usefulness of the Parts of the Body* (Cornell University Press, 1968), 635–638; Sarah George, *Human Conception and Fetal Growth: A Study of Greek Thought from the Presocratics Through Aristotle* (unpublished dissertation, University of Pennsylvania, 1982), 69–96, 109–110; Joan Cadden, *Meanings of Sex Differences in the Middle Ages* (Cambridge University Press, 1993), 195–201. The theory was also partially adopted by William Harvey. See C. D. O'Malley, et al., *William Harvey: Lectures on the Whole of Anatomy* (University of California Press, 1961), 70 and 138.

14. On sex determination, see, for example, G. E. R. Lloyd, ed., *Hippocratic Writings* (Penguin Books, 1950), 317–346; May, op. cit., *Galen on the Usefulness of the Parts of the Body*, 634–638; George, *Human Conception and Fetal Growth: A Study of Greek Thought from the Presocratics Through Aristotle*, op. cit., 109–119; Lars L. Cederqvuist

with the theories of the mathematical significance of the number seven.[15] The source of the seven-cell theory probably lies in the influence of *De Spermate*, a pseudo-Galenic treatise used from the twelfth century that asserted that parts of the body were divided into sevens.[16] The doctrine of the seven-cell uterus in its completed form was adopted by anatomists at Salerno, as well as by the prominent anatomist of Bologna, Mondino de Luzzi (c. 1270–1326).[17] Singer claims that Mondino must have culled the doctrine from the writings of Michael Scot (1180–1250),[18] astrologer in the court of Emperor Frederick II,[19] although recent historians have advanced different theories. I focus on Michael Scot because of his documented Jewish connections and the likelihood that one of his works was cited by rabbinic sources. The doctrine of the seven-cell uterus is found in the third of Scot's major works, entitled *Liber Physionomiae*,[20] which was also variously called *De Secretis Naturae* and *De Procreatione*.[21] The roughly twenty editions of this work that were published before 1500 are testimony to its popularity in the Middle Ages,[22] and Scot is

---

and Fritz Fuchs, "Antenatal Sex Determination: A Historical Review," *Clinical Obstetrics and Gynecology* 13:1 (1970), 159–177; Ursula Mittwoch, "Erroneous Theories of Sex Determination," *Journal of Medical Genetics* 22:3 (1985), 164–170.

15. See Kudlien, op. cit. On the importance of numerology in gynecology in antiquity, see George, op. cit., *Conception and Fetal Growth: A Study of Greek Thought from the Presocratics Through Aristotle*, 204–226.

16. Danielle Jacquart and Claude Thomasset, *Sexuality and Medicine in the Middle Ages*, trans. Matthew Adamson (Princeton University Press, 1988), 34.

17. Kudlien, op. cit., and Reisert, op. cit.

18. On Scot, see Lynn Thorndyke, *Michael Scot* (Nelson Publishers, 1965). Thorndyke also devotes a chapter to Scot in his *History of Magic and Experimental Science* 2 (Columbia University Press, 1923), 307–337; According to J. D. Galinsky and J. T. Robinson, "Rabbi Jeruham b. Meshullam, Michael Scot, and the Development of Jewish Law in Fourteenth-Century Spain," *Harvard Theological Review* 4 (2007), 489–504, the best up-to-date biography and bibliography on Michael Scot is Charles Burnett's entry on Scot in *Grundriss der Geschichte der Philosophie* (ed. Ruedi Imbach and Peter Schulthess).

19. Charles Singer, *A Short History of Anatomy and Physiology from the Greeks to Harvey* (Dover Publications, 1957), 81.

20. Michael Scot, *De Secretis Naturae* (Lugduni, 1580), 264.

21. Thorndyke, op. cit., 4–8.

22. Ibid.

likely to be at least partially responsible for the wide dissemination of the seven-cell doctrine.

Scot is known to have collaborated with the Jewish philosopher and physician Jacob Anatoli, the son-in-law of Samuel ibn Tibbon, at the Sicilian court of Emperor Frederick II, where they were engaged in translating and disseminating Arabic science and philosophy. During Anatoli's tenure at court, he had close contact with Michael Scot. In fact, Scot mentions a formula in his *Alchemy* that was taught to him by "Rabbi Jacob the Jew," identified as Anatoli.[23] Could Scot have been responsible for transmitting his theory of the seven-chamber uterus to the Jewish community through these connections?

Similar to its hazy origins, the doctrine's disappearance cannot be traced to a specific date. Berengario de Carpi (1470–1530) wrote in his *Isogogae* that it is a sheer lie to say that the uterus has seven chambers.[24] In an accompanying illustration, a woman is shown pointing a finger at her non-septated uterus while symbolically placing her foot on books that have perpetuated the erroneous notion of the seven-cell uterus.[25] Vesalius (1514–1564) likewise rejects the seven-cell doctrine in his *De Humani Corporis Fabrica*, mentioning Michael Scot by name.[26] Parenthetically, this also supports the notion that Scot is responsible for the proliferation of the doctrine. Although two prominent anatomists

---

23. C. Sirat, *A History of Jewish Philosophy in the Middle Ages* (Cambridge University Press, 1990), 226–228, details the relationship of Anatoli and Scot and identifies "Rabbi Jacob the Jew" to be Anatoli. On how citations from the works of Michael Scot indirectly found their way into the halakhic literature of the Middle Ages through the mediation of Jacob Anatoli, see J. D. Galinsky and J. T. Robinson, "Rabbi Jeruham b. Meshullam, Michael Scot, and the Development of Jewish Law in Fourteenth-Century Spain," *Harvard Theological Review* 4 (2007), 489–504.

24. Plaut, "Historical and Cultural Aspects of the Uterus," *Annals of the New York Academy of Science* 75:2 (January, 1959), 389, quotes Carpi's words verbatim and discusses the famous illustration. He does not mention that the illustration is found in the *Isogogae*.

25. Carpi himself believed the uterus to be bilocular. See James P. McMurrich, *Leonardo da Vinci, the Anatomist* (Williams and Wilkins Co., 1930), 200–201.

26. See Lynn Thorndyke, *History of Magic and Experimental Science* 5 (Columbia University Press, 1941), 526; C. D. O'Malley, *Andreas Vesalius of Brussels* (University of California Press, 1964), 32 and 279. Thorndyke, op. cit., 523, points out that Vesalius makes no reference to Carpi's earlier rejection of the seven-cell doctrine.

explicitly rejected the doctrine in the early sixteenth century, it was still being quoted in the seventeenth century.[27]

II. THE SEVEN-CHAMBER UTERUS IN RABBINIC SOURCES[28]

The doctrine of the seven-chamber uterus is not found anywhere in the Talmud. It is, however, found repeatedly in rabbinic literature spanning from the Middle Ages to pre-modern times. Given that the doctrine was a product of the Middle Ages (see above), its absence from talmudic literature is understood. The doctrine's first appearance in rabbinic literature follows shortly after its introduction in medieval medical science. The mention of this distinctly medical doctrine is not restricted to the medically related rabbinic literature. In fact, it can be found in many diverse areas. I specifically present the sources categorized by type of rabbinic literature to illustrate that an appreciation of the medical historical context is not limited to the study of medical halakha and can be of use to all students of rabbinic literature.

---

27. Kudlien, "The Seven Cells of the Uterus: The Doctrine and its Roots," op. cit., 416; idem, "The Legal Aspect of the Doctrine of the Seven Uterine Cells," op. cit., 545–546.
28. This topic of the seven-chamber uterus doctrine has received scarce treatment in Jewish scholarship. There is no mention of it in H. J. Zimmels, *Magicians, Theologians and Doctors* (Edward Goldston and Son, 1952), which covers medicine in rabbinic responsa from the twelfth to nineteenth centuries. This glaring omission is likely attributable to the fact that the seven-chamber doctrine has no halakhic ramifications, and Zimmels' work encompasses primarily halakhic responsa. The present essay likewise includes no references to the doctrine in halakhic responsa. The doctrine merits brief mention in J. Trachtenberg, *Jewish Magic and Superstition* (Meridian Books: Cleveland, 1961), 188 and 303 (n. 13); M. Brayer, *The Jewish Woman in Rabbinic Literature: A Psychological Perspective* (Ktav, 1986), 304–305. See also R. Margaliyot's *Mekor Chesed*, notes on *Sefer Chasidim* (Mosad HaRav Kook, 5717), no. 515, p. 443, and the superb article of Sharon Faye Koren, "Kabbalistic Physiology: Isaac the Blind, Nahmanides, and Moses de Leon on Menstruation," *AJS Review* 28:2 (2004), 317–339, where she discusses the doctrine at n. 34, in addition to addressing the right-left theory, the anatomy of the uterus, and theories of reproductive physiology in rabbinic sources. For a general discussion of notions of female anatomy in the secular and rabbinic literature of the Middle Ages, including brief mention of the seven- chamber doctrine, see R. Barkai, *Les Infortunes De Dinah: Le Livre de la Generation: La Gynecologie Juive au Moyen Age* (Paris, 1991), 35–58. I thank Professor Barkai for his research suggestions.

Biblical Commentaries

The doctrine of the seven-chamber uterus is first explicitly mentioned in rabbinic literature in the early thirteenth century, where it appears in a number of biblical commentaries to Vayikra (12:2): "If a woman has conceived seed, and borne a male child, then she shall be unclean seven days." As the verse speaks of a woman giving birth to a male child, the commentaries take the opportunity to address both female anatomy and sex determination.[29] A number of medieval Biblical commentators, known collectively as the *Ba'alei HaTosafot,* invoke a version of the doctrine of the seven-chamber uterus in their commentaries to this verse. While there are slight variations amongst them, each describes three chambers on the right, from which a male fetus forms, three on the left, from which a female fetus forms, and one in the center, from which either an *androginos* (hermaphrodite) or *tumtum* (fetus with ambiguous genitalia) develops.

The original doctrine of the seven-chamber uterus mentions that a hermaphrodite is formed from the center chamber, but, to my knowledge, does not mention a *tumtum* as a possible product from this chamber. Although some of the rabbinic commentators cite this doctrine from a medical source, it is possible that the rabbinic sources, on their own initiative, added the notion of the birth of a *tumtum.* As many Jewish laws and obligations are gender specific, the rabbis are concerned with determining the legal gender of every individual. As a result, there are

---

29. This verse also served as a springboard for discussion of reproductive physiology throughout the ages. See chapter, "The Rabbinic Conception of Conception: An Exercise in Fertility." For Jewish references to sex selection and sex determination, see Joshua Trachtenberg, *Jewish Magic and Superstition* (Meridian Books, 1961), 188–189 and 303; Fred Rosner, "The Biblical Secret for Choosing One's Baby's Sex," *Israel Journal of Medical Sciences* 15 (September, 1979), 784–787; N. Kass, "Sex Determination—Medically and in the Talmud," *Koroth* 7:11–12 (June, 1980), CCLXLIII-CCCI; J. Preuss, *Biblical and Talmudic Medicine,* trans. F. Rosner (Hebrew Publishing Company, 1978), 389–391; Yosef BaGad, *Nahalei Ha'Eshkolot* 2 (self-publication), 440–449. No one has yet thoroughly studied the right-left theory as found in Jewish sources, but it is noteworthy that Maimonides (1135–1204) was skeptical of the doctrine in his commentary to Hippocrates. See Suessman Muntner, Maimonides, *Kitvei Refuah* 3 (Mosad HaRav Kook, 1961), 105 and 109.

numerous discussions in rabbinic sources about individuals whose gender status is ambiguous. As both the hermaphrodite and the *tumtum* are in this category, they are often discussed together.[30] It, therefore, follows that whenever the rabbis discuss the topic of hermaphrodites, *tumtum* is likely to be included.

Four of the commentaries, *Sefer HaGan* (thirteenth century),[31] *Tosafot* (twelfth-thirteenth centuries),[32] the commentary of R. Asher ben Yeḥiel (c. 1250–1327),[33] and the commentary of R. Isaac ben Judah Halevi,[34] cite as the source of this doctrine Abraham ibn Ezra (1089–1164), quoting *Sefer Toldot*, the *Book of Procreation*.

30. See, for example, *Mishna Bikurim* 4:5 and Tractate *Yevamot* 81a. On the hermaphrodite and *tumtum* in rabbinic literature see W. M. Feldman, *The Jewish Child* (London, 1917), 130; Zimmels, *Magicians, Theologians and Doctors*, op. cit., 214, n. 112; David Margalit, "*Tumtum v'Androgenus*," *Koroth* 6:11–12 (August, 1975), 777–780; Zvi J. Hacohen Kook, "*Dinei Androgenus*," *Koroth* 7:1–2 (April, 1976), 79–80; Shlomo Y. Zevin, *Entzyclopedia Talmudit* 2 (Encyclopedia Publishers: Jerusalem,1990), 55–60; ibid., 19 (Encyclopedia Publishers: Jerusalem, 1991), 182–246; J. Preuss, *Biblical and Talmudic Medicine*, trans. F. Rosner (Hebrew Publishing Company, 1978), 226–228.

31. Little biographical information exists about the author of this work, who is known simply as R. Aharon. Dr. J. Mitchell Orlian, based on internal evidence from *Sefer haGan*, concludes that R. Aharon lived in northern France in the first half of the thirteenth century and wrote *Sefer HaGan* about the year 1240. See his *Sefer HaGan: Text and Analysis of the Biblical Commentary* (doctoral dissertation, Bernard Revel Graduate School, Yeshiva University, New York, 1973), now issued by Mosad HaRav Kook (Jeusalem, 2009). I thank Dr. Orlian for allowing me to view the manuscript prior to its publication. The relevant passage appears on folio 158R (Vienna National Library, Hebrew Codex II, 28, Swartz Catalogue, II, 19:5).

32. See *Otzar Perushim* (Shulsinger Brothers, 1950), 48. This commentary is not the work of a single hand, but is ascribed to a group of medieval bliblical and talmudic commentators from France and Germany, known as the Tosafists. See Cecil Roth, ed., *Encyclopedia Judaica* 15 (Keter Publishing House, 1972), 1278–1285.

33. See *Otzar Perushim* (n. 27), 48. This commentary is ascribed to R. Asher ben Yeḥiel (1259–1327), known as *Rosh*, but the authorship has been debated. See Menachem M. Kasher, *Sarei HaEleph* (Torah Sheleimah Publications, 1984), 67–68.

34. See his biblical commentary *Paneaḥ Raza* (Jerusalem, 1965), 298. The author actually quotes from *Sefer HaGan*, who in turn cites Ibn Ezra. *Paneaḥ Raza* is replete with references to *Sefer HaGan*. See Orlian, *Sefer HaGan: Text and Analysis of the Biblical Commentary*, op. cit.; Ḥayyim Y. D. Azulai, *Shem HaGedolim*, section 2, s. v., "*Paneaḥ Raza*."

In fact, no mention of *Sefer Toldot*, nor any explicit reference to the seven-chamber doctrine, can be found in the extant published writings of Ibn Ezra, although it should be noted that not all of his writings have survived. There is, however, an indirect allusion to the seven-chamber doctrine in Ibn Ezra's Biblical commentary (see below).

Although the identification of *Sefer Toldot*, apparently mentioned by Ibn Ezra as the source of the doctrine, is uncertain, there are a number of possible contenders. There is a *Sefer HaToledet*, which is a Hebrew adaptation of Muscio's Latin version (sixth century) of the *Gynaecia* written by Soranus (second century).[35] This could not be the *Sefer Toldot* of Ibn Ezra for two reasons. First and foremost, Soranus, upon whose book this work is ultimately based, did not espouse the seven-chamber doctrine, so Ibn Ezra cannot be referring to this work. In addition, while the exact date of composition of this manuscript is still a matter of debate, it most likely appeared after the era of Ibn Ezra.[36]

As mentioned above, Michael Scot appears to be responsible for popularizing the doctrine of the seven-chamber uterus. One of the titles used for Scot's work is *de Procreatione*, which could be translated into Hebrew as *Sefer Toldot*. However, as Ibn Ezra died before Michael Scot's birth, he cannot be referring to this version of *Liber Physionomiae*. A possible, though improbable, scenario would be that these medieval commentators are referring to Scot's work, and the attribution to Ibn Ezra is erroneous. Perhaps one author attributed the reference to Ibn Ezra, and the other commentators simply perpetuated his error. However,

---

35. For Soranus' description of the anatomy of the uterus see, for example, Owsei Temkin, *Soranus' Gynecology* (Johns Hopkins University Press, 1956), 8–14. Soranus' work on gynecology was translated and abbreviated by Muscio (sixth century) and translated into Hebrew as *Sefer Toledet*. See Ron Barkai, "Jewish Medical Treatises in the Middle Ages," in Berger, ed., *Jews and Medicine* (Beit Hatefutsoth, 1995), 45–88, esp., 68–71, and idem, *A History of Jewish Gynaecological Texts in the Middle Ages*, Brill's Series in Jewish Studies 20 (1998). This is an excellent reference for the history of gynecology in Jewish sources in the Middle Ages. See also the excellent review essay of this book by Gerrit Bos in *Jewish Quarterly Review, New Series* 89:1–2 (July-October, 1998), 101–122. Bos has translated and annotated many medieval medical texts from the Jewish and Arabic tradition, including the works of Maimonides.

36. Ibid.

Sefer HaGan is one of the commentaries that cites Ibn Ezra, and his other references to Ibn Ezra are reliably found in the latter's extant works. In addition, as discussed below, we find allusion to the doctrine of the seven-chamber uterus in the existing works of Ibn Ezra.

R. Hezekiah ben Manoah (mid-thirteenth century) omits the reference to Ibn Ezra in his biblical commentary, *Hizkuni*, and cites the doctrine in the name of *Sefer Toldot*.[37] As R. Hezekiah made use of the commentaries of both Ibn Ezra and *Ba'alei HaTosafot* for his work,[38] it is likely that he copied the doctrine from one of these two sources and accidentally omitted the attribution to Ibn Ezra. C. D. Chavel, in his edition of *Hizkuni*, postulates that R. Hezekiah was likely aware that his predecessors, including the *Ba'alei HaTosafot*, quoted this notion in the name of Ibn Ezra, but since R. Hezekiah did not find it explicitly in the works of Ibn Ezra, he intentionally omitted the attribution out of concern for its veracity, and simply cited the source as *Sefer Toldot*.[39]

R. Dr. Abraham Lifschutz devotes an article to the references to Ibn Ezra in the *Ba'alei HaTosafot* (including the commentaries discussed above) on the Torah that are not found in the published editions of the Ibn Ezra.[40] He discusses our passage, and while he was unable to find any explicit reference to the seven-chamber doctrine in the works of Ibn Ezra, he did discover reference to a related or parallel passage in a journal article by Shmuel David Luzzatto (1800–1865), the renowned Italian philologist, poet and biblical exegete, about an unpublished Ibn Ezra manuscript. In an article in 1839, Shmuel David Luzzatto states that

---

37. Hayyim D. Chavel, ed., *Hizkuni* (Mosad HaRav Kook, 1988), 362–363.
38. Ibid., 7.
39. Ibid., 362. Chavel also mentions that *Paneah Raza* cites the doctrine of the seven-cell uterus in the name of *Sefer HaGan*. Chavel, however, is unfamiliar with this work, as it was never published in his lifetime. See also A. Leibowitz, "Doctors and Medical Knowledge in the Tosafist Circles," *Tradition* 42:2 (2009), 19–34, n. 37, who discusses this passage from *Hizkuni*. I thank David Guttman and Shlomo Sprecher for this reference.
40. A. Lifschutz, "The Ibn Ezra in the Commentaries of Ba'alei HaTosafot," *HaDarom* 28 (*Tishrei*, 5729), 202–221 (Hebrew). The author of this article was a high school *Tanakh* teacher of mine. This article, which I came across only recently, was published prior to the time I attended his class. Had I only then appreciated the extent and breadth of his scholarship!

he found mention of a work of Ibn Ezra not previously mentioned in any Ibn Ezra bibliography.[41] In a manuscript of Ibn Ezra, arranged or compiled by Daniel ben Shlomo HaRofeh in 1448, on the Torah portion of *Tazria*,[42] Daniel HaRofeh cites a comment of Ibn Ezra from his *Sefer Moladot* discussing the difference in days of impurity observed postpartum by a woman for the birth of a boy (seven) versus that of a girl (fourteen). The quote from *Sefer Moladot* reads as follows:

> If a woman lies on her right side, it (the seed) will enter on the right and she will give birth to a male. The impurity will rapidly exit. Therefore, she is impure for seven days and pure for thirty-three days. If she lies on the left, she will give birth to a girl and the impurity will not rapidly exit. Therefore, she is impure for fourteen days.[43]

Although unknown previously to Luzzatto, *Sefer HaMoladot*, an astrological treatise of Ibn Ezra, has been well studied in the modern era. The only resemblance this passage bears to the seven-chamber doctrine is the mention of the right-left theory of conception. There are no anatomical details of the womb, or the possibility of the birth of a hermaphrodite as specifically mentioned in the name of Ibn Ezra by the *Ba'alei HaTosafot*. Therefore, this cannot be our source of the doctrine from Ibn Ezra.

However, much to my astonishment, when I consulted a copy of the original manuscript of Daniel HaRofeh, I found something quite

---

41. See S. D. Luzzatto in *Kerem Ḥemed* 4 (1839), 137–138. I thank Zalman Alpert of the Yeshiva University Gottesman Library for helping me locate this volume.

42. This manuscript is described in H. Hirschfeld, *Descriptive Catalogue of the Hebrew Mss. of the Montefiore Library* (Macmillan and Co.: London, 1904), 4 (manuscript no. 15).

43. In a footnote to Luzzatto's article of 1839, S. Y. Rapoport claims that he was in possession of a manuscript of Ibn Ezra entitled *Sefer Molad HaAdam*, also called *Sefer HaMoladot*, and that after reading through the entire work, he found no reference to this passage. I consulted Professors Shlomo Sela and Tzvi Langermann, as well as Meira Epstein, author of an English translation of *Sefer HaMoladot*, and all confirmed that there is no mention of this notion or passage in the extant versions of Ibn Ezra's *Sefer Moladot*.

unexpected—a detailed description of the seven-chamber doctrine.[44] This passage, found in the marginalia, simply states the doctrine with no attribution either to *Sefer Toldot, Sefer Moladot,* or to Ibn Ezra. In addition, the phraseology and additional details of the doctrine in this manuscript are at slight variance with the statement of the doctrine attributed to Ibn Ezra by the *Ba'alei HaTosafot.* Is this marginal note to be attributed to Ibn Ezra, or is it an interpolation by Daniel HaRofeh, commenting on the text? Could this be the source of the attribution of the seven-chamber doctrine to Ibn Ezra? This is the only known detailed mention of the doctrine in any extant work of Ibn Ezra.

There remain a number of unresolved questions regarding the attribution of the seven-chamber doctrine to Ibn Ezra and the apparent citation by Ibn Ezra of *Sefer Toldot* as the source of this doctrine. While we now know of a manuscript of the biblical commentary of Ibn Ezra that mentions the doctrine, it is not at all clear that this mention is from Ibn Ezra (eleventh century), as opposed to the manscript's compiler (fifteenth century). Furthermore, the detailed mention of the seven-chamber doctrine in this manuscript contains no attribution to *Sefer Toldot,* or to any other source. In addition, the exact identity of the *Sefer Toldot* still remains a mystery.

If the reference to the seven-chamber doctrine in the manuscript of Daniel HaRofeh is indeed a citation from Ibn Ezra, and if Ibn Ezra, perhaps elsewhere, quotes *Sefer Toldot* as the source of the doctrine, this would clearly eliminate Michael Scot as the author of *Sefer Toldot,* since Scot was born some years after Ibn Ezra's death. But as we still have no documented evidence that Ibn Ezra himself quoted the doctrine in the name of *Sefer Toldot,* this possibility cannot be completely excluded.

---

44. Jewish National Library manuscript collection, manuscript number F4538, p. 196v. I greatly thank Yael Okun of the JNL for her assistance in locating the manuscript. This manuscript was part of the Montefiore Library manuscript collection in England, which contained many of Shmuel David Luzzatto's personal manuscripts, as well as those of Leopold Zunz (1794–1886), the German historian and founder of the modern 'science of Judaism.' Many of the manuscripts from this collection were recently sold at auction by Sotheby's Auction House. Parenthetically, the passage from *Sefer Moladot* described by Luzzatto appears in full on the next page of the manuscript (p. 196r) as a separate note in the margin.

Another biblical commentary contemporary with the Tosafists, known as the *Da'at Zekenim MiBa'alei HaTosafot* (unknown authorship), cites the doctrine of the seven-chamber uterus in the name of *Sefer HaTeva*,[45] and mentions neither Ibn Ezra, nor *Sefer Toldot*. As the citation of the doctrine itself is nearly verbatim as that cited in the aforementioned commentaries, *Sefer HaGan*, *Tosafot*, and the work of R. Asher ben Yeḥiel, all of whom attribute the doctrine to Ibn Ezra in the name of *Sefer Toldot*, this likely represents an unintentional error in transmission. Alternatively, *Sefer HaTeva* may be a generic name for a work of medicine and science. However, there is an alternative possibility. Scot's work, as mentioned above, had more than one title. The most popular title was *De Secretis Naturae*. As the Hebrew word *"teva"* means nature, it is theoretically possible that the *Da'at Zekenim MiBa'alei HaTosafot* refers to Scot's work, independent of any previous rabbinic tradition. This is, of course, pure conjecture, as we have no other evidence that *Ba'alei HaTosafot* had the language skills or cultural orientation to absorb "gentile" wisdom. In addition, Scot's work was entitled "The Secrets of Nature," a translation of which would be something akin to *Sefer Sitrei HaTeva*. It is an interesting coincidence, however, that the books named by the *Ba'alei HaTosafot* as the sources of the doctrine—*Sefer HaTeva* and *Sefer HaToldot*—are the very two names for Michael Scot's work wherein the doctrine appears, *De Secretis Naturae* and *De Procreatione*.

Although there are differences between the aforementioned medieval commentaries on the verse in Vayikra, and I have suggested possible explanations for the discrepancies, it is more likely that they all derive the version of the seven-chamber doctrine from a common tradition or source.

While the aforementioned biblical commentators bring up the doctrine of the seven-chamber uterus as part of discussions on female physiology, some biblical commentators use the doctrine in the explication of biblical passages. Based on the verse in Shemot 1:7: "And the children of Israel were fruitful, and increased abundantly, and multiplied, and grew exceedingly mighty; and the land was filled with them,"

---

45. Vayikra 12:2.

a number of rabbinic commentaries state that the Jews in Egypt had multiple gestational pregnancies, sextuplets according to Rashi.[46] In this vein, Ibn Ezra makes the following comment: "I have seen a woman who gave birth to quadruplets, and physicians explain how a woman could give birth to seven children."[47] Although detailing neither the female anatomy nor the right-left theory, Ibn Ezra could possibly be alluding here to the doctrine of the seven-chamber uterus, which explains anatomically how a woman could theoretically give birth to seven children. This clearly is not the exact passage in Ibn Ezra referenced by the aforementioned medieval commentators, as neither the language nor the content correlates.

Other commentaries on this verse are more explicit in their reference to the seven-chamber doctrine. R. Issachar Eilenburg (1570–1623) invokes the seven-chamber doctrine in explaining why specifically six children were born to the women in Egypt, neither more nor less.[48] Based on the doctrine, as a woman had seven uterine chambers, she could potentially give birth to seven children at a time, three males, three females, and one *androgenus* or *tumtum*. The women of Egypt were blessed in that they gave birth to *only* six children at a time, being spared the curse of bearing an *androgenus* or *tumtum*. The Maharal (R. Judah Loew ben Bezalel c. 1525–1609) echoes the same approach in his commentary to the verse in Shemot, invoking the seven-chamber doctrine in identical fashion.[49] R. Yisrael Yaakov Algazi (Jerusalem, eighteenth century) cites the doctrine in the interpretation to this verse in his *Haggadah, Magid Devarav L'Yaakov,*[50] and further expands upon it with linguistic analysis, claiming that one of the miracles in Egypt was that all the Jewish children born in Egypt were themselves fertile, and none was conceived from the center uterine chamber. Such a child would be an *androgenus* or *tumtum* and, consequently, infertile.

---

46. Ad loc.

47. Commentary to Shemot 1:7.

48. *Tzeda L'Derekh* (Prague, 1623), on Shemot 1:7.

49. Joshua D. Hartman, ed., *Gur Aryeh* vol. 3 (Makhon Yerushalayim, 1991), 6–7.

50. (Izmir, 1767), 167.

Compendia of Prayers and Customs

In the thirteenth and fourteenth centuries, there was a genre of rabbinic literature consisting of compilations of laws on prayers and customs of the Jewish calendar year.[51] In one such work, there is a reference to the seven-chamber doctrine. R. David ben Joseph Abudraham (fourteenth century), in his commentary on the prayer recited daily after the performance of normal bodily excretory functions, launches into a discussion of human physiology, including reproduction.[52] It is in the context of a discourse on sex determination that R. Abudraham cites the seven-chamber doctrine as one theory explaining how women conceive a female fetus versus a male. If a woman lies on her left side, he explains, the woman will conceive from one of the three uterine cells on the left, thereby producing a female child.

Philosophical Works

In 1360, Meir ben Isaac Aldabi (c. 1310–c. 1360),[53] grandson of R. Asher ben Yeḥiel (*Rosh*), completed a philosophical work entitled *Shevilei Emuna* (Paths of Faith). This work, although philosophical in focus, contains a wealth of medical and scientific information, with chapters on anatomy, embryology and physiology.[54] The author devotes a chapter to each organ of the body, and the following quote appears in the chapter on the uterus: "…it has seven chambers, three on the right and four on the left. If the woman leans slightly to her right after intercourse she will conceive a female child, and if to her left, a male child."[55]

---

51. Examples of these works include *Sefer HaManhig* by R. Abraham ben Nathan HaYarḥi of Lunel, *Shibolei HaLeket* by R. Zedekiah ben Abraham, and *Kol Bo*, of unknown authorship.

52. *Abudraham HaShalem* (Hathiya Press, 1963), 35–37.

53. See Cecil Roth, ed., *Encyclopedia Judaica* 2 (Keter Publishing House, 1972), 551–552.

54. See, D. Schwartz, "Towards the Study of the Sources of R. Meir Aldabi's Shevilei Emunah," *Sinai* 114 (1994), 72–77. Schwartz focuses mainly on the philosophical sources, noting that R. Aldabi borrowed from Gershon ben Shlomo's *Sha'ar HaShamayim*, as well as from Arabic sources. He does not discuss the origin of R. Aldabi's medical information.

55. *Shevilei Emuna* (Riva Di Trento, 1559), *netiv* 4. This passage is found in the Jerusalem (5750) edition at page 198.

Although Aldabi does not cite a source for the seven-chamber doctrine, it is clearly not his rabbinic predecessors. It is remarkable that he does not cite the doctrine as cited in the commentary attributed to his own grandfather, R. Asher ben Yeḥiel, who mentions the classic version of the doctrine. First, Aldabi counts four chambers on the left instead of three on the left and one in the center, thereby eliminating the possibility of the birth of a hermaphrodite. Second, he deviates from the classic right-left theory, linking female children to the right side of the uterus instead of the left. Some have claimed that Aldabi derived much of his material from the encyclopedic *Sha'ar HaShamayim* of Gershon ben Shlomo of Arles.[56] He clearly did not borrow this interpretation of the doctrine from this work, as another version of the doctrine appears therein.[57] As this theory likely did not originate with Aldabi, perhaps it is testimony to a variation of the seven-chamber doctrine in the Arabic literature.

Hebrew Medical Works

Although most Hebrew medical works are not classically considered part of the corpus of post-rabbinic literature, there are some such works that may deserve this distinction. While the majority of Hebrew medical works throughout history are devoid of religious content, a few medical treatises were composed by physicians who were also scholars and who incorporated Jewish legal discourse into

---

56. This theory was advanced by Moritz Steinschneider in his *Die Hebräischen Übersetzungen des Mittelalters und die Juden als Dolmetscher: Ein Beitrag zur Literaturgeschichte des Mittelalters; meistenteils nach Handschriftlichen Quellen* (Berlin, 1893), 9–27. On Gershon ben Shlomo of Arles, see F. S. Bodenheimer, trans., *The Gate of Heaven* (Jerusalem, 1953) and J. T. Robinson, "Gershom ben Solomon's *Sha'ar Ha-Shamayim*: Its Sources and Use of Sources," in S. Harvey, ed., *The Medieval Hebrew Encyclopedias of Science and Philosophy* (Amsterdam Studies in Jewish Thought, volume 7, 2000).

57. See *Sha'ar HaShamayim* (Rodelheim, 1801), 47–48, which seems to maintain that there were 3 chambers in the uterus. The one on the right would yield a male child, the one on the left a female, and the one in the center a hermaphrodite. This is a variant of the right-left theory, a precursor to the seven-chamber doctrine, but does not resemble the variant of the doctrine as mentioned by R. Aldabi.

their works. One such example is the medical volume of Jacob Zahalon (1630–1693),[58] *Otzar HaHayyim*. Zahalon was not only a physician trained at the University of Rome, but also the rabbi of the Italian community of Ferrara, where he was known for his homiletic prowess.[59] The introduction to *Otzar HaHayyim* begins with a Jewish legal discussion of the permissibility of practicing medicine and tampering with the divine order.

The penultimate chapter of Zahalon's work is devoted to women's diseases and is introduced with a brief note on female anatomy. Here Zahalon states, "… some say the uterus comprises seven chambers, yet others refute this notion." Despite his medical training at an Italian university, where he undoubtedly read Vesalius' rejection of the seven-chamber doctrine in the *Fabrica*, Zahalon still mentions the doctrine as an acceptable, although disputed, anatomical notion. It is noteworthy that Tobias Cohen,[60] another Italian-trained physician with rabbinic schooling, makes no mention of the seven-chamber doctrine in his classic treatise *Ma'asei Tuvia*,[61] which was published roughly twenty-five years after *Otzar HaHayyim*.

---

58. On Zahalon and his work see, for example, Harry A. Savitz, "Jacob Zahalon, and His Book, 'The Treasure of Life,'" *New England Journal of Medicine* 213:4 (July, 1935), 167–176; Harry Friedenwald, "Jacob Zahalon of Rome: Rabbi, Physician, Author and Moralist," in *The Jews and Medicine* 1 (Ktav, 1967), 268–279; Jonathan Jarashow, "Yakov Zahalon and the Jewish Attitude Towards Medicine," *Koroth* 9:9–10 (1989), 725–736.

59. See Henry A. Sosland, *A Guide for Preachers: The Or HaDarshan of Jacob Zahalon—A Seventeenth Century Italian Preacher's Manual* (Jewish Theological Seminary, 1987).

60. On Cohen see, for example, David A. Friedman, *Tuvia HaRofeh* (Palestine Jewish Medical Association, 1940); Nigel Allan, "Illustrations From the Wellcome Institute Library: A Jewish Physician of the Seventeenth Century," *Medical History* 28:3 (July, 1984), 324–328; David Ruderman, *Jewish Thought and Scientific Discovery in Early Modern Europe* (Yale University Press, 1995), 229–255; E. Lepicard, "An Alternative to the Cosmic and Mechanic Metaphors of the Human Body? The House Illustration in *Ma'aseh Tuviya* (1708)" *Medical History* 52 (2008), 93–105.

61. (Bragadin, Venice, 1707–1708). For a comparison of the works of Zahalon and Cohen, see David Ruderman, op. cit., 232–239.

Talmudic Commentaries

In the book of *Shmuel*,[62] it is recounted that for a short period during the reign of King David, the Ark of the Covenant was kept in the house of Oved-edom HaGitti. Oved-edom was rewarded for his efforts, as the verse states, "and the Lord blessed Oved-edom, and his entire household." The Talmud[63] elaborates on the nature of this blessing, stating that Oved-edom's wife, and each of his eight daughters-in-law, gave birth to sextuplets.[64] R. Akiva Eiger (1761–1837), in his *Gilyon HaShas*, cites R. Eilenburg's biblical commentary to Shemot, which explains, based on the seven-chamber doctrine that the Jewish women in Egypt gave birth to sextuplets, having been spared the curse of conceiving a hermaphrodite or tumtum. R. Eiger, as is usual for his notes, makes no personal comment, and leaves the reader to apply the citation to the current context. Assumedly, the women of Oved-edom's family were also blessed with sextuplets and spared the curse of a child conceived from the central uterine chamber.

However, R. Zekharia Yeshayahu HaKohen Yolles, in his *Sefer HaTorah V'HaHokhma* written in the late nineteenth century,[65] questions R. Akiva Eiger's application of the seven-chamber doctrine to the Talmud's discussion of Oved-edom's progeny. The talmudic passage states that the sixty-two children of Oved-edom were all male (*anshei*

---

62. II Shmuel 6:10–12.
63. *Berakhot* 63b–64a.
64. The calculation is based on a passage in I Divrei HaYamim 26:8 that states that Oved-edom had 62 children. To obtain this total, it is suggested that Oved-edom's wife and eight daughters-in-law each had sextuplets, equaling 54 children. To this, we add Oved-edom's own eight sons to achieve a total of 62. It should be noted that the Midrash in *Bamidbar Rabba*, chap. 4 and in *Shir HaShirim Rabba*, chap. 2, as well as the Jerusalem Talmud in Tractate *Yevamot* 22b, offer a different calculation, without requiring each woman to have had sextuplets. This theory, based on a different textual analysis, suggests that each woman was able to conceive two children every month for three successive months, thus also equaling a total of 54 children. R. Aryeh Loeb Jellin (1820–1886), in his commentary *Yefeh Einayim* to the passage in Tractate *Berakhot*, considers this latter theory to be more outside the realm of nature than that described in Tractate *Berakhot*.
65. (Vilna, 5673), 381.

ḥayil), whereas according to the seven-chamber doctrine, half, or thirty-one, should have been female.[66]

III. CONCLUSION

In this section, we have discussed a curious anatomical notion found in the history of medicine known as the doctrine of the seven-chamber uterus, which is expressed in rabbinic literature from the twelfth through the late nineteenth centuries. The *Ba'alei HaTosafot* attributed this doctrine to Abraham ibn Ezra, although it has previously not been found in any of Ibn Ezra's extant works. In this essay, we identified a previously unknown reference to the seven-chamber doctrine in a fifteenth-century manuscript of Ibn Ezra, although it is unclear if the mention of the doctrine is to be attributed to Ibn Ezra himself, or to the manuscript's copyist. The exact source quoted in the early rabbinic literature as the origin of this doctrine—*Sefer Toldot* quoted in the name of Ibn Ezra by numerous *Ba'alei HaTosafot*; or the *Sefer HaTeva*, as cited by the *Da'at Zekenim MiBa'alei HaTosafot*—remains a mystery. It is possible, though speculative, that Michael Scot, through his Jewish connections, contributed to the dissemination of the doctrine in Jewish circles, especially since the names *Sefer Toldot* and *Sefer HaTeva* correspond to the Latin names for Scot's work, which cites the seven-chamber doctrine. In sum, the appreciation of the medical historical context of the doctrine of the seven-chamber uterus enhances our understanding of the rabbinic literature wherein this doctrine appears.

---

66. See also R. M. Efrati, "The Case of Edom HaGiti," *Nezer HaTorah* (*Tevet*, 5768), 324–325.

Parashat Tazria and Childbirth: An Open and Shut Case

I. INTRODUCTION: MEDICINE IN RABBINIC LITERATURE[1]

Throughout the centuries, rabbinic commentators have often used their works as a vehicle or springboard for medical and scientific discussion, sometimes in the service of textual biblical interpretation; other times, simply as narrative tangent. The Torah portion of *Tazria*, where human childbirth and its associated laws are addressed, is the biblical source of many medical discussions in rabbinic writings throughout the centuries. Appreciating the diversity and historical context of these writings is our objective.

Biblical commentaries of past centuries can often be challenging to interpret. However, persistence coupled with consultation of additional *seforim* (works of rabbinic literature) is often rewarded with a

---

1. The definitive work on biblical and talmudic medicine remains Julius Preuss, *Biblical and Talmudic Medicine*, trans. Fred Rosner (Hebrew Publishing Company, 1978). See also the many works of Dr. Fred Rosner on this topic, including his *Encyclopedia of Biblical and Talmudic Medicine* (Jason Aronson, 2000).

better understanding of the difficult passages. There are, however, certain medically related passages for which the conventional approach will not yield fruits. A cursory review of the major commentaries on the first few verses of the portion of *Tazria*, for example, will leave the twenty-first century reader utterly bewildered. Search as one may in standard *seforim*, one is unlikely to reach any clearer perceptions or achieve any greater wisdom. One will encounter in pre-modern rabbinic commentaries a number of notions on reproductive physiology and anatomy that simply defy or elude modern understanding. Some of these notions are a product of their historical period and reflect the evolution of science, while others are uniquely Jewish in nature. This chapter discusses some of the medically related passages in rabbinic literature on the portion of *Tazria*.

II. MEDICAL PASSAGES IN THE RABBINIC DISCUSSIONS ON *PARASHAT TAZRIA*

On the first section of the *parasha*, we find a number of rabbinic discussions relating to human reproduction. The discussions cover a number of topics, including anatomy, physiology, and embryology, each of which will be treated separately. We will cite representative primary sources for each section, though the same medical notion, or variation thereof, may be expressed in other sources.

Anatomy

Human anatomy, in all its gloriously detailed intricacies, is well understood today. There are no debates about the configuration or structure of the parts of the human body. All the parts have been identified and labeled, and the occasional anatomical variants have been categorized. The human uterus is of course amongst them. There are indeed some variations of this pear-shaped, single chamber structure, and sometimes the chamber can even be partially divided in two. However, the description found in the *Da'at Zekenim MiBa'alei HaTosafot* does not seem to correspond to any known anatomical variant:[2]

---

2. Vayikra 12:2.

And some say it is found in the *Book of Nature* that the womb of a woman has seven chambers—three on the right, three on the left, and one in the center. If the seed enters the right chambers, she will beget a male child; if it enters the left chambers, she will beget a female child, and if it enters the center chamber, it will result in the birth of a *tumtum* (ambiguous genitalia) or androgynous (hermaphrodite).

Here, the *Da'at Zekenim MiBa'alei HaTosafot* is not referencing an idea of his own, or of specifically rabbinic origin for that matter, but one he explicitly cites from contemporaneous medical literature. Was the uterus of this historical period indeed comprised of seven chambers? If not, how could such a notion gain currency when even the most cursory inspection of the body would dispel it? A comprehensive discussion of this unique anatomical doctrine is found in the previous chapter.

Embryology[3]

Human embryology is the branch of biology that deals with the formation, early growth and development of the human being. The *Midrash Rabba* on this portion contains a magnificently detailed embryological description of the fetus in utero.

How is the fetus positioned in its mother's womb? Folded and resting like a notebook (*pinkas*). Its head is positioned between its knees; its hands on the sides of the head … the mouth is sealed and the navel (umbilicus) is open. It receives nourishment from

---

3. For references to embryology in Jewish sources, see David I. Macht, "Embryology and Obstetrics in Ancient Hebrew Literature," *John Hopkins Hospital Bulletin* 22:242 (May, 1911), 1–8; W. M. Feldman, *The Jewish Child* (London, 1917), 120–144; W. M. Feldman, "Ancient Jewish Eugenics," *Medical Leaves* 2 (1939), 28–37; Samuel Kottek, "Embryology in talmudic and Midrashic Literature," *Journal of the History of Biology* 14:2 (Fall, 1981), 299–315; H. J. Zimmels, *Magicians, Theologians and Doctors* (London, 1952), 62–64; Julius Preuss, *Biblical and Talmudic Medicine* (Hebrew Publishing Co., 1978), 41–138; Pieter Willem Van Der Horst, "Sarah's Seminal Emission: Hebrews 11:11 in the Light of Ancient Embryology" in *Greeks, Romans and Christians: Essays in Honor of Abraham J. Malherbe*, edited by David Balch et al. (Minneapolis, 1990), 287–302.

what its mother eats, and drinks from what she drinks. It does not excrete waste lest it kill its mother. When it exits ... the closed passages open and the open passages close.[4]

This description is as accurate today as it was then. There is, however, an embryological passage in the Talmud, related to this portion, which requires further discussion. The beginning of *Tazria* details the periods of purity and impurity that a woman is required to observe upon the birth of a child. The total combined periods of purity and impurity for the birth of a female child, eighty days, are double that for the male child, forty days. While this difference has spawned many homiletic interpretations, R. Yishmael posits an embryological basis for this differentiation.

> R. Yishmael says if she miscarried on the forty-first day following conception, she must observe the *tum'ah* [impurity] laws of a male birth ... And if she miscarried on the eighty-first day following conception, she must observe the *tum'ah* laws of a female birth, for the basic form of a male embryo is completed by the forty-first day and the basic form of a female embryo is completed by the eighty-first day.[5]

The sages attempt to refute R. Yishmael by citing an experiment performed by Cleopatra on her maidservants who were condemned to death. She sacrificed them forty days after they had conceived in order to examine the anatomical composition of the fetuses. Inspection revealed that both the male and female fetuses were formed by forty days. R. Yishmael's response to the results of this experiment is instructive:[6]

---

4. *Vayikra Rabba* 14:7.
5. *Nidda* 30a.
6. The talmudic exchange about the validity and possible shortcomings of the experiment is remarkable and reflects sensitivity to the experimental method we utilize today. It should be noted that the Talmud records another version of the experiment with different results. For more on the experiment of Cleopatra, see J. Needham, *A History of Embryology* (New York, 1959), 65–66, and Samuel Kottek, 299–315.

> I bring you a proof from the Torah, and you bring me a proof from imbeciles?[7]

While the sages marshal support from sources external to the rabbinic tradition, R. Yishmael maintains that his embryological approach has "proof from the Torah." While some medical and scientific traditions may be co-opted from contemporaneous medicine, this may not always be the case. It should be noted that the notion of the disparate growth and formation rates for the male and female fetus was espoused in antiquity by a number of writers, with the formation of the female fetus believed to take longer than that of the male.[8] However, the exact numbers forty and eighty for the embryological formation of the two genders is not mentioned in external sources.

The period of forty days appears in another related passage in the Talmud that cites our Torah portion. It discusses the propriety of praying for the gender of a child after the woman has already conceived.

> If his wife is pregnant and he said, "May it be Your will that my wife give birth to a male," this is a prayer in vain.[9]

The Talmud challenges the assumption that prayer will not help by citing the story of the birth of Dinah. As the Talmud records, Leah was pregnant with a male child, and based on her concern for the role of her sister Rachel in the birth of the twelve tribes, she prayed to God that her child should not be male. The Talmud relates that her prayers were answered and a male child was converted to a female child in utero.[10]

---

7. *Nidda* 30b.
8. These authors include Empedocles, Asclepiades, and Hippocrates. See Preuss and Kottek. While the exact numbers of forty and eighty do not appear in known sources from talmudic times, Thomas Aquinas later claimed that male embryos were "ensouled" at about forty days, while female embryos were not "ensouled" until about eighty days in the womb.
9. *Berakhot* 60a.
10. On the many versions of the story of the birth of Dinah, including an analysis of the contemporary halakhic ramifications of this story in cases of surrogate motherhood, see chapter, "Midrash, Miracles, and Motherhood: The Birth of Dinah and the Definition of Maternity—*Tzarikh Iyun LeDina.*"

The Talmud considers whether the case of Leah was a miraculous or natural event and posits that perhaps Leah's prayer took place within the first forty days of gestation, when the gender of the fetus is not yet determined.

While some have attempted to interpret this passage in light of contemporaneous medical history, others have attempted to explain it in light of modern science. I cite two examples of the latter, the first being one of the earliest examples from the modern era, and the second being one of the most recent contributions.

The following passage, referring to the talmudic discussion on the ability to pray for the gender of a child within forty days after conception has occurred, appeared in *Medical Leaves*, a journal dedicated to the study of Jewish medical history and contemporary Jewish medical problems, in 1939.[11]

> This utterly fantastic speculation assumes considerable interest in the light of the very recent researches… which shows that even such an apparent absurdity is not altogether outside the realm of scientific possibility. As is well known, every early embryo is primarily bisexual, in that it possesses both Wolffian and Mullerian ducts, which are the precursors of the male and female genital organs, respectively. The chromosomal influence of the particular fertilizing spermatozoon determines which of these pairs of ducts shall ultimately atrophy. Atrophy of the Mullerian ducts results in a male child, and atrophy of the Wolffian ducts produces a female child… Hence, although sex is normally determined at the moment of conception by the chromosome constitution of the fertilizing spermatozoon, this gametic influence may, in certain cases, and under not understood and uncontrollable circumstances, as well as in varying degrees, be overcome.

---

11. W. M. Feldman, "Ancient Jewish Eugenics." Between 1937 and 1943, five volumes of the journal *Medical Leaves* were published. W. M. Feldman himself wrote about this very passage earlier in his *The Jewish Child* (London, 1917), 140.

The next citation appeared in the 2009 issue of the journal *B'Or Ha'Torah* on science and Judaism,[12] and is, in essence, a scientifically updated version of the above passage.

> A well-known passage in the Talmud states that parents can pray for the gender of their unborn child only during the first forty days of pregnancy. Another passage states that the female identity of an embryo takes eighty days to be formed.
>
> At first blush, this appears to be contradictory to the basic facts of reproductive biology. Isn't the gender of the embryo determined at the moment of conception? A more careful analysis reveals that the chromosomal makeup of the fertilized egg, XX or XY, is not the only factor determining the embryo's gender. The successful expression of the SRY gene located on the short arm of the Y chromosome is another crucial factor.
>
> In fact, it takes approximately forty days from the time of conception for male gender to become irreversibly determined and about eighty days for female gender to be determined.
>
> One can only wonder at the prophetic insight of the Talmud sages, who pinpointed the precise time frame for the formation of gender long before the science of genetics was developed.

Physiology

Another aspect of biology that is found in the biblical commentaries of this portion is the physiology of conception, in particular, the respective contributions of the man and woman to the fetus. While a more expansive analysis of the rabbinic understanding of reproductive physiology throughout the ages is contained in the first chapter of this section, a brief discussion of this topic is appropriate here because of its appearance in *Parashat Tazria*. Naḥmanides, for example, himself a physician, comments on the physiology of conception on the verse "if a woman is *tazria* and gives birth to a male child." The root of the word *tazria*, *zera*,

---

12. L. Poltorak, "On the Embryological Foresight of the Talmud," *B'Or Ha'Torah* 19 (2009), 19–24. I thank Dr. Poltorak for sending me a copy of her article.

implies the presence of a reproductive seed of the woman. It is this very issue that Naḥmanides addresses in his comments.[13]

> ... although it says, "when a woman emits seed" ... the implication is not that the fetus is made from the female seed. For even though a woman has *"beitzim"* [ovaries] analogous to those of the male *"beitzei zachar"* [testicles], either no seed is made there, or the seed has nothing to do with the fetus. Rather the term *"mazra'at"* refers to the uterine blood ... that unites with the male seed. In their opinion (*Nidda* 31a) the fetus is created from the blood of the woman and the white [semen] of the man, and both of them are called seed ...[14] and likewise is the opinion of the physicians regarding conception. The Greek philosophers believed that the entire body of the fetus is formed from the menstrual blood and the [seed of the] man gives form to the matter.

As Naḥmanides explicitly mentions medical theories from external sources, appreciation of these sources in their historical context is warranted. Naḥmanides alludes to a major debate that raged since antiquity. Since the female seed was not visible to the naked eye, and was not emitted externally, its very existence was a matter of conjecture until modern times. As a result, two competing theories evolved in antiquity which coexisted until pre-modern times. Aristotle, the Greek philosopher to whom Naḥmanides refers, denied the existence of a female

---

13. For an analysis of this Ramban and discussion of the rabbinic understanding of the female contribution to conception, see David Feldman, *Marital Relations, Birth Control and Abortion in Jewish Law* (New York, 1974), especially chapters 6 and 7; chapter, "The Rabbinic Conception of Conception: An Exercise in Fertility"; Kottek, op. cit.; Van Der Horst, op. cit.; S. F. Koren, "Kabbalistic Physiology: Isaac the Blind, Naḥmanides and Moses De Leon on Menstruation," *AJS Review* 28:2 (2004), 317–339.

14. This refers to the passage in *Nidda* (31a) that there are three partners in the formation of man—God, the father and the mother. On this passage, see Marvin Gold, "Genetic Imprinting and Gene Silencing," *B'Or Ha'Torah* 16 (2006), 19–31, as an example how modern science is used to reinterpret rabbinic passages on medicine. See also R. Kiperwasser, "Three Partners in a Person: The Bereishit and Development of Embryological Theory in Biblical and Rabbinic Judaism," *Lectio Difficilior* 2 (2009). See also chapter, "Rabbinic Conception of Conception."

seed, claiming that only the male possessed seed. This seed provided the "form" and the "principle of movement" to the fetus, whereas the female provided the material from which the fetus was formed, i.e., the menstrual blood. Galen, on the other hand, following in the footsteps of Hippocrates, maintained that both the male and female contributed seed. The exact identity of the female seed was in question, but he conjectured it may be located in the uterus. He also claimed that the male semen provides the material for the development of the nerves and the walls of the arteries and veins, whereas the menstrual fluid is the source of the blood. Naḥmanides, citing the talmudic passage (*Nidda* 31a), aligns the rabbinic tradition with the two-seed theory.

Gender Determination

Our final section addresses the issue of gender determination as reflected in a passage from the Talmud.

> R. Yitzḥak said in the name of R. Ami, if the woman emits seed (*mazra'at*) first, she bears a male; if the man emits seed first, she bears a female, as it is stated: *isha ki tazria veyalda zakhar* (When a woman emits seed and bears a male).[15]

As discussed briefly above, the very word *mazra'at* for the woman is a matter of debate. While the word *mazria* for the male unequivocally refers to the emission of male seed, the analogous term for the female was not traditionally interpreted in a parallel fashion.[16]

This notion of gender determination associated with the precedential emission of reproductive seed appears to be uniquely rabbinic. While scientists since antiquity struggled to solve the mystery of gender

---

15. *Nidda* 31a.
16. In pre-modern times, when the identity and function of the woman's contribution to the fetus was in question, *mazra'at* was understood by many to refer to the female climax. On this passage, see D. Feldman; Fred Rosner, "Sex Preselection and Predetermination," in his *Biomedical Ethics and Jewish Law* (Ktav, 2001), 165–173; A. Korman, *HaAdam VeTivo BeMada UVeYahadut* (Tel Aviv, 5763), 112–118; Preuss, 390–391; N. Kass, "Sex Determination: Medically and in the Talmud," *Koroth* 7:11–12 (June, 1980), 293–301; Yaakov Levi, "*Isha Ki Tazria*," *Koroth* 5:9–10 (July, 1971), 716–717.

determination, a study of contemporaneous medical theories of antiquity does not reveal this specific notion. Furthermore, the notion appears to be driven by the linguistic phrasing of the biblical verse. The Maharal elaborates upon this in his *Gur Aryeh*.[17] In explaining why the verse, *"isha ki tazria veyalda zachar"* is used as a source for the notion that if a woman emits seed first, a male child will result, the Maharal asserts that the Torah could have written, "When a woman emits seed, if it is a male child, then certain laws apply; if it is a female child, then certain laws apply." The fact that the Torah writes, "When a woman emits seed and begets a male child," it means that if she emits seed first, she will, with certainty, beget a male child.[18]

Commentators over the centuries have posited explanations for the talmudic principle based on the medical knowledge of their time. Examples include the commentaries of Sforno (sixteenth century),[19] *Keli Yakar* (seventeenth century),[20] *Sefer HaBrit* (nineteenth century)[21] and the *Torah Temimah* (early twentieth century).[22]

The modern era is no exception. In light of advances in the understanding of reproductive physiology in the modern era, this passage has been reinterpreted. Dr. L. B. Shettles observed that the Y chromosome travels faster than the X chromosome, so that if a woman ovulates prior to marital relations, there is a greater likelihood that the Y chromosome will reach the egg first, resulting in a male child.[23] This observation led

---

17. Vayikra 12:2.

18. The talmudic principle that a woman's emitting seed first is associated with the birth of a male child has a corollary principle in biblical interpretation that male children mentioned in the Torah are associated with their mothers, while female children are associated with their fathers. See *Nidda* 31a, Rashi on Bereshit 34:1 and 46:15. For an analysis of these passages in Rashi and their relationship to the nature of Dinah's birth discussed in the talmudic passage above, see chapter, " Midrash, Miracles, and Motherhood: The Birth of Dinah and the Definition of Maternity—*Tzarikh Iyun LeDina*."

19. Vayikra 12:2.

20. Ibid.

21. (Warsaw, 5629), Part 1, Section 17, Ch. 2. I thank Dr. Abe Lipshitz for this reference.

22. Vayikra 12:2.

23. L. B. Shettles and D. M. Rorvik, *Your Baby's Sex* (New York, 1970), 56. He also takes into account the nature of the acidity of the secretions of the reproductive tract during climax and around the time of ovulation.

to the reinterpretation of the talmudic passage. The word *mazra'at* could refer to ovulation, the emission of the female seed, analogous to the emission of the male seed. Thus, if a woman emits seed first (i.e., ovulates), she will beget a male child. This reinterpretation of the rabbinic passage was known even to Shettles himself and is found repeatedly in works of Jewish medical ethics.

Whether the Shettles method has scientific merit remains a matter of debate. The opinion that the timing of ovulation bears on the subsequent gender of the progeny cannot be easily proved or disproved. While it seems anachronistic to interpolate this understanding into the talmudic passage, written some 1,500 years prior to the identification and visualization of the egg and the physiological understanding of ovulation, one cannot discount the possibility of a *mesora* for this notion which is only now better understood in light of modern medicine. Just as one learns the Torah forgotten in utero only later in life, perhaps humanity, over generations, is gradually learning the forgotten secrets of medicine and human reproduction.

III. CONCLUSION

In this chapter, we have discussed some selections from rabbinic literature on the portion of *Tazria* that relate to medicine; in particular, human reproduction. We have interpreted some passages in light of contemporaneous medical history. This approach can be applied to other medically related passages in rabbinic literature, but it must be applied judiciously. Clearly when the rabbinic authorities of earlier centuries themselves refer to external medical sources, as is the case for the seven-chamber uterus and the theories about the contributions of the male and female to the fetus, a review of those sources and their context is beneficial in understanding the interpretations. However, there are some areas where the rabbinic medical discussions are not in consonance with known contemporaneous medical doctrines. In these areas, one cannot simply attribute these notions to ancient doctrines. In addition, there may be an element of *mesora* at play in these cases, as is perhaps the case with the position of R. Yishmael cited above and the talmudic approach to gender determination. In some instances, modern advances have led to fresh interpretations and perhaps vindication of the pre-modern rabbinic sources. Some of these interpretations are convincing. Others, less so. Nevertheless, those who consider all pre-modern rabbinic passages on medicine as erroneous and antiquated relics of the past are mistaken, as are those who vigorously defend all such passages as medically correct. Each passage requires independent analysis. But we must always exercise humility, awe and respect for the words of Hazal as we continue to search and explore these areas.

In the aforementioned description of the fetus in utero from the *Midrash Rabba*, it states that when the baby exits the womb and enters the outside world, the previously closed passages open, and the open passages shut. The same expression is applied to the study of Torah in general. Sometimes opening one avenue of analysis closes another and vice versa. Navigating the maze of the openings and closings of the medical passages in rabbinic literature is a challenging and oft-times rewarding task. Satisfactory resolution of some of these challenges, however, may not be forthcoming until we exit this world and enter the world to come.

Is There Life After Life? Superfetation in Medical, Historical and Rabbinic Literature

I. CASE REPORT

On January 18, 2008, a unique medical case was reported in the British newspaper, the *Daily Mail*. Two babies were carried in the same womb, born only one minute apart, yet Thomas and Harriet Mullineux are not twins. They were conceived three weeks apart thanks to an extraordinary twist of nature. Their mother Charlotte had been pregnant with twins when at seven weeks she miscarried one of them. But two weeks later, she discovered, after undergoing a follow-up ultrasound, that she was carrying another fetus, conceived separately and still growing in her womb. The surviving twin and the new baby were born in May of 2007.

This case, which may represent an extraordinarily rare, and not well documented, phenomenon, is the substance of this chapter. We shall address the medical, historical, and halakhic aspects of this case.

II. SUPERFETATION IN HISTORICAL
AND MEDICAL LITERATURE

The process whereby a woman becomes pregnant and then subsequently conceives again during another ovulatory cycle is called superfetation. Superfetation has been discussed for centuries, and the possibility of conception during an existing pregnancy has been debated since antiquity. It was assumed to be possible by Hippocrates, Aristotle and Pliny. William Harvey reports that in order to hide her knavery, a certain maid who was pregnant from her master went to London for the duration of her pregnancy, where she delivered a child in September. She then returned home. In December of the same year, she was unexpectedly delivered of another child, assumedly a product of superfetation, which proclaimed the crime that she had so cunningly concealed before.[1] Modern medicine, however, remains skeptical of the possibility of superfetation.

One must distinguish between superfetation, when a woman already pregnant conceives again from a later ovulation, from what is termed superfecundation, when a woman ovulates two eggs during one cycle, yet there are two separate instances of fertilization, perhaps even days apart. The possibility of superfecundation has been accepted since antiquity and clearly proven scientifically in the DNA age in cases when twins have been identified genetically as having two different fathers.[2]

---

1. For an extensive review of the premodern sources discussing superfetation, see G. M. Gould and W. L. Pyle, *Anomolies and Curiosities of Medicine* (W. B. Saunders, 1896), 46–48. See also Y. V. O'Neill, "Michele Savonarola and the *Fera* or Blighted Twin Phenomenon," *Medical History* 18 (1974), 222–239. Our discussion is about the possibility of natural superfetation. With the advent of assisted reproductive technologies, and the intentional introduction of reproductive seed or fertilized embryos at both different times and locations, the possibility of superfetation increases significantly. Hormonal manipulation further increases the possibility by reversing the body's normal mechanisms for preventing a second simultaneous pregnancy.
2. The first scientifically proven case of superfecundation was recorded by G. K. Doring, 1960 (cited in O'Neill, op. cit., at note 67), but there have been a number of others subsequently. See, for example, E. Girela, et al., "Indisputable Double Paternity in Dizygous Twins," *Fertility and Sterility* 67:6 (June, 1997), 1159–1161. On superfecundation, see F. Rosner, "Superfecundation in Mythology, History and Poetry," *New England Journal of Medicine* 300(1979), 49; D. Rabinerson, et al., "Superfecundation and Superfetation--The Forgotten Entities," (Hebrew) *Harefuah* 147:2 (February, 2008), 155–8. The most curious and convincing examples of superfecundation are

Proving superfetation beyond reasonable doubt, however, has remained elusive. Even in the modern age of ultrasound and DNA testing, it has not been unanimously accepted as possible. Modern reproductive physiology teaches that once pregnancy is achieved, it is generally not possible for a woman to conceive again subsequently until after the completion of the pregnancy. Once a first pregnancy is achieved, progesterone, secreted first by the corpus luteum and then subsequently by the placenta, supresses further ovulation and additionally makes the female reproductive tract much less receptive to male reproductive seed. It has been observed that twins are occasionally of significantly different sizes or weights, and some consider this proof that they were conceived at different times. The size or weight disparity, however, is not sufficient proof, as there are a number of other medical conditions to which this can be attributed. Several articles have appeared over the last few decades claiming to have confirmed superfetation with differing levels of confidence.[3] However, an article from 2003 denies any possibility of superfetation and attributes all such cases to other phenomena.[4] Despite the logical and scientific conclusion that superfetation is not possible, many such cases have been recorded throughout history. There are two approaches to these cases. Either they are all attributable to some other phenomenon and indeed superfetation is impossible, or alternatively, despite scientific evidence to the contrary, superfetation is possible, although admittedly exceedingly rare.

---

those in which children of different colors, either twins or near the same age, are born to the same woman. Depending on the race of the parents, however, this phenomenon can be explained without resorting to the rare case of superfecundation.

3. For example, N. Baijal, et al., "Discordant Twins with the Smaller Baby Appropriate for Gestational Age—Unusual Manifestation of Superfoetation: A Case Report," *BMC Pediatrics* 7:2 (January 19, 2007); A. Harrison, et al., "Superfetation as a Cause of Growth Discordance in a Multiple Pregnancy," *Journal of Pediatrics* 147:2 (August, 2005), 254–255; T. Steck and S. Bussen, "Conception During Pregnancy (superfetation)," *Human Reproduction* 12:8 (August, 1997), 1835–1836; J. Bertrams and H. Preuss, "A Case of Twins with Probable Superfetation," (German) *Zeitschrift fur Rechtsmedizi Journal of Legal Medicine* 84:4 (1980), 319–321.

4. I. Blickstein "Superfecundation and Superfetation: Lessons From the Past on Early Human Development," *Fetal and Neonatal Medicine* 14:4 (October, 2003), 217–219.

III. SUPERFETATION IN RABBINIC LITERATURE

The notion of superfetation is found in rabbinic literature and is first discussed in the Talmud.[5]

> Rav Bivi taught the following Baraisa before Rav Nachman: Three women may use a wad inserted in their bodies to prevent conception. These are a minor, a pregnant woman, and a nursing woman. A minor may do this because of the concern that she may become pregnant and she may then die. A pregnant woman may do it because of the concern that she may render her fetus a *sandal*. A nursing woman may do it because of the concern that she may be forced to wean her child and he will consequently die.[6]

The Gemara in *Yevamot* discusses three cases for which the use of a *mokh*, a form of contraceptive, is permitted.[7] The common denominator of these cases is the concern that some medical harm may result from a pregnancy. One of the three women permitted to use a *mokh* is one who is pregnant, lest her fetus become a *sandal*. Rashi *ad loc* describes a *sandal* as a malformed, non-viable fetus with no recognizable human

---

5. For previous discussions on this topic, see I. Jakobovits, *Jewish Medical Ethics. A Comparative and Historical Study of the Jewish Religious Attitude to Medicine and its Practice* (Bloch Publishers, 1959), 325, n. 132; J. Preuss, *Biblical and Talmudic Medicine*, trans. F. Rosner (Hebrew Publishing Company, 1978), 386–387; D. M. Feldman, *Birth Control in Jewish Law: Marital Relations, Contraception and Abortion as Set Forth in the Classic Texts of Jewish Law* (New York University Press, 1968), 180–187; A. Steinberg, "Twins: Medical and Halakhic Perspectives," (Hebrew) in A. Steinberg, ed., *Sefer Assia* 2 (Schlesinger Institute, 5741), 232–239; S. Kottek, "Twins in Jewish and Historical Sources," (Hebrew) in A. Steinberg, ed., *Sefer Assia* 2 (Schlesinger Institute, 5741), 240–245.

6. *Yevamot* 12b.

7. The identity of a *mokh*, whether used before or after relations, and the nature of its contraceptive effect are a matter of rabbinic debate. This *sugya* is the main source of contemporary discussions on the permissibility of contraception in general. See D. M. Feldman, *Birth Control in Jewish Law: Marital Relations, Contraception and Abortion as set forth in the classic texts of Jewish Law* (New York University Press, 1968); M. D. Tendler, "Contraception and Abortion," in F. Rosner, ed., *Medicine and Jewish Law* (Jason Aronson, 1993); J. D. Bleich, "*Besugya deshalosh nashim*," in his *BeNetivot HaHalakha* 3 (New York, 5761), 1–4.

facial features.[8] The simple explanation of this passage is that when a pregnant woman becomes pregnant subsequently with another child, one fetus will physically restrict the growth of the other, whose development will be retarded, resulting in a malformed fetus appearing like a *sandal*. This seems to accept the possibility of superfetation. Rashi indeed explains that the second pregnancy impedes the development of one of the fetuses, resulting in a gross malformation resembling a *sandal*, and a resultant miscarriage. *Tosafot*,[9] however, argue against Rashi's position and point out that the *Talmud Bavli* explicitly rejects the possibility of superfetation. The relevant passage is found in *Nidda* 27a.

> R. Avin bar Rav Adda said in the name of Rav Menaḥem of Kefar Shearim, and some say of Beit Shearim: There was an incident in which a child was delayed in being born three months after its twin. And if you have any doubts as to the veracity of this report, behold, [those twins] sit before us in the house of study! And who are they? Yehuda and Ḥizkiya, the sons of R. Ḥiyya.
>
> But the master said that a woman cannot conceive and conceive again while she is still pregnant with the first child! Abaye said: There was one drop of semen which divided into two and developed into separate children. One's formation was completed at the beginning of the seventh month, and one's formation was completed at the beginning of the ninth month.

In this passage, the Gemara recounts a story of two brothers who were born three months apart and subsequently survived, as evidenced by the fact that they were both students in the yeshiva together at that time. In

---

8. Most identify the *sandal* with the fetus compressus (compressed) or fetus papyraceous (flattened remarkably through loss of fluid and most of the soft tissue) described in the medical literature. See Preuss, 386 and Feldman, 183. See O'Neill, op. cit., 229 for a discussion of all the possible consequences of the death in utero of a twin fetus, including a description that would fit well with the Talmud's term *sandal*. For an expansive analysis of the term *sandal*, see Federico Dal Bo, "A Foetus Shaped Like a Sandal: Birth Anomalies in Talmudic Tractate *Nidda*," in Lennart Lehmhaus, ed., *Defining Jewish Medicine* (Harrassowitz Verlag, 2021), 93–118.

9. *Yevamot* 12b, s. v., "*shema*."

fact, these siblings were none other than the children of R. Ḥiyya, Yehuda and Ḥizkiya. The Gemara then queries: How could this be possible, when Mar states that a woman cannot become pregnant again if she is already pregnant (i.e., superfetation is *not* possible)? The Gemara responds that this was *not* a case of superfetation, rather, conception occured at one time and the reproductive seed divided into two. One child was born at seven months gestation, while the other was born at nine months.[10]

If the *Talmud Bavli* explicitly rejects the possibility of superfetation, *Tosafot* ask, how could Rashi use this idea to explain why a pregnant woman may use a *mokh*? *Tosafot* answer that according to Rashi, the phrase "*Ein isha mit'aberet veḥozeret umit'aberet*" does not mean that a woman cannot *conceive* subsequently if she is pregnant, rather, it means that even though she can conceive, the product of such a conception

---

10. This explanation itself requires further elaboration. The word used is "*tipa*," which usually refers to the male reproductive seed prior to fertilization. Splitting of the male seed is not physiologically possible, nor would it, by itself, produce two embryos. If "*tipa*" refers to the embryo, which was split, then the brothers would have to be identical twins. Excluding superfetation, the simplest explanation is that two eggs were ovulated and fertilized, yet they were born at different times. This is a known, though uncommon, occurrence termed interval delivery in modern scientific terminology. This however would not explain the phrase, "*tipa aḥat hayta v'neḥlika l'shtayim*."

There is a notion in Ḥazal that babies born in the seventh and ninth months are viable whereas those born in the eighth month are not (see, for example, *Shabbat* 135a and *Yevamot* 80a). This was a prevalent notion in antiquity and the Middle Ages. On the Jewish sources on this notion, see *Ḥazon Ish Y. D.*, 155; Abraham. S. Abraham, *Nishmat Avraham* (English) (Mesorah/Artscroll), vol. 1, 185, 228 and vol. 3, 244; Pieter W. Van Der Horst, "Seven Months' Children in Jewish and Christian Literature from Antiquity," in his *Essays on the Jewish World in Early Christianity* (Gottington, 1990), 233–47; Neria Gutal, "*Ben Shemona: Pesher Shitat Ḥazal B'noge'a Livladot Bnei Shemona*," *Assia* 55–56 (1989), 97–111; Ron Barkai, "A Medieval Hebrew Treatise on Obstetrics," *Medical History* 33 (1988), 96–119, esp. 101–104. For further information on the secular sources see Ann Ellis Hanson, "The Eight Months' Child and the Etiquette of Birth: Obsit Omen!" *Bulletin of the History of Medicine* 61 (1987), 589–602; Sarah George, *Human Conception and Fetal Growth: A Study in the Development of Greek Thought From Presocrates through Aristotle* (Doctoral Dissertation, University of Pennsylvania, 1982), 204–233; C. R. King, "The Eight Month Fetus: Classical Sources for a Modern Superstition," *Obstetrics and Gynecology* 72:2 (August, 1988), 286–287; R. Reiss and A. Ash, "The Eight Month Fetus: Classical Sources for a Modern Superstition," *Obstetrics and Gynecology* 71:2 (February, 1988), 270–273.

will not survive to viability, but will invariably be miscarried as a mal-formed *sandal*. Therefore, according to Rashi, it would appear that while superfetation is technically possible for conception, it is not possible for viability. Thus, the production of two healthy, viable children from superfetation, such as the sons of R. Chiya, is not possible.

Rabbenu Tam, however, maintains that even conception after existing pregnancy is not possible (i.e., even superfetation for conception is not possible). He therefore posits an entirely different explanation as to why a pregnant woman may use a *mokh*. According to Rabbenu Tam, if a woman is pregnant with twins, and has relations with her husband, it is possible the male reproductive seed alone may interpose between the two fetuses and cause one to be malformed in the shape of a *sandal*.

While the *Talmud Bavli* clearly maintains that "*Ein isha mit'aberet vehozeret umit'aberet*," which is variously interpreted by Rashi and Rab-benu Tam as either superfetation is not possible at all, or it is possible only for conception, but not to viability, the position of the *Talmud Yerushalmi* appears to be otherwise.

A passage in the *Talmud Yerushalmi* seems to explicitly affirm the possibility of superfetation.[11] The passage attempts to identify a scenario in a case of *yibum* where a woman cohabits with both her husband, who subsequently dies, and the *yavam* (levir) within a certain period of time such that there will be uncertainty as to the father of the child. At the conclusion of the passage, it states that you learn from this that a preg-nant woman can become pregnant again at a later time.

However, this reading is not accepted by all. The *Korban HaEda* on the *Yerushalmi* amends the text to read that a pregnant woman can-not again become pregnant, in consonance with the *Talmud Bavli*.[12] R. Hayyim Yosef David Azulai, while not amending the text of the *Yerush-almi*, nonetheless concludes that the statement, "*at shema mina sheha'isha mit'aberet vehozeret umit'aberet*" means that a woman may indeed be able to conceive during pregnancy, but only a non-viable fetus would result,

---

11. *Yevamot* 22b (chapter 4, halakha 2). Jakobovits, op. cit., n. 132, p. 325; Preuss, op. cit., 387. Both interpret the *Yerushalmi* as limiting the possibility of superfetation to coitions that occur within forty days of each other.

12. The Artscroll *Yerushalmi* adopts this version based on the *Korban HaEdah*.

similar to the position of Rashi. Based on his reading of other passages in the *Yerushalmi*,[13] he maintains that the *Yerushalmi* does not accept the possibility of superfetation with the birth of a healthy, living viable second child.

In *Sefer Ḥasidim* by R. Yehuda HaḤasid (twelfth century), it is written that within forty days, a woman can become pregnant from two men. This appears to be referring to a case of superfetation, where a woman can become pregnant from one man, then subsequently become pregnant from another man.[14]

In the fifteenth century, R. Shimon b. Tzemaḥ Duran mentions a case of superfetation in the course of answering a query on the laws of *nidda*:

> A sage testified that he saw [the case of] a woman in Rome who gave birth to a child and, after four months, went into labor and gave birth to another child. When they brought her before the Great Church for an explanation, she declared that when she was in her fifth month of pregnancy, she cohabited with another and became pregnant by him; the first child, she said, is her husband's and the second another's. They accordingly "stoned" her. This case was listed in the medical books to show that the retentive power of the womb [can be very strong] and that there are women who, however, are inordinately weak and miscarry.[15]

In the early eighteenth century, R. Yitzḥak Lampronti, rabbi/physician and graduate of the University of Padua, writes in his encyclopedia *Paḥad Yitzḥak*[16] that occasionally a pregnant woman may again conceive and

---

13. Especially *Nidda* chapter 3, p. 51, halakha 4.
14. Alternatively, it may be referring to another case discussed in the Gemara about the possibility of a woman conceiving one child who is the product of two fathers. See chapter, "Shared Biological Paternity."
15. Translation by Feldman, op. cit.
16. S. v., "*me'uberet.*" On R. Lampronti, see D. Ruderman, "Contemporary Science and Jewish Law in the Eyes of Isaac Lampronti and Some of His Contemporaries," *Jewish History* 6:1–2 (1992), 211–224; D. Margalit, "R. Yitzḥak Lampronti: Rabbi, Physician, Lexicographer," (Hebrew) in his *Ḥakhmei Yisrael KeRofim* (Mosad Harav Kook, 5722)

achieve a second pregnancy. This seems to go against the conclusion of the *Talmud Bavli*. However, a closer reading reveals that R. Lampronti is referring here to superfecundation, as opposed to superfetation. He brings proof to his comment by citing a case from America of a woman who bore twins one after another, but the twins were of different colors, assumedly from different fathers. This more likely refers to a case where the woman engaged in relations with two different men within a short period after she ovulated two eggs, each egg being fertilized by a different man. As discussed above, superfecundation, as this is called, has been accepted since antiquity and scientifically proven in modern medical literature.

Abraham b. Mordekhai Halevi (Cairo, seventeenth century) ponders the halakhic implications of the talmudic statement, "a woman cannot conceive if already pregnant," and assumes it is not an absolute statement, but rather a reflection that superfetation is an extremely rare occurrence. Thus, he is willing to invoke its possibility in selective halakhic circumstances.[17] For example, with respect to *tum'at leida* (the impurity associated with childbirth), if a woman gives birth to a second child shortly after the first, he would assume the more common circumstance that the two pregnancies were conceived at the same time. Therefore, a woman need not begin a new counting of days of impurity. However, regarding possible danger to a pregnant woman, he would be concerned about the small possibility of superfetation and its impact on the existing fetus and would allow use of a contraceptive *mokh*. It is R. Halevi's third case that spawned a lengthy response by R. Hayyim Yosef David Azulai (known as the Hida).[18] In this theoretical test case, R. Halevi states that if a woman gives birth very shortly after her husband leaves for a long journey, and then gives birth again some months later (seven or nine), we may exonerate the wife of any possible wrongdoing

152–174; H. Savitz, "Dr. Isaac Lampronti: Rabbi, Physician, Teacher, Preacher, Encyclopaedist," in his *Profiles of Erudite Jewish Physicians and Scholars* (Spertus College: Chicago, 1973), 29–32. For a collection of all the medical matters in R. Lampronti's magnum opus, see D. Margalit, "Medical Articles in the Encyclopedia Paḥad Yitzḥak by R. I. Lampronti," (Hebrew) *Koroth* 2:1–2 (April, 1958), 38–60.

17. *Gan HaMelekh*, 130, in *Ginat Veradim*.
18. *Birkei Yosef, E. H.*, 4:8

by assuming that she conceived again while pregnant. Consequently, the second child, as the first, is a product of her husband. This presupposes not only that a woman can conceive while pregnant but assumes superfetation with a subsequent live birth.[19]

It is this last presupposition with which R. Azulai takes issue. He engages in a lengthy review of the halakhic literature relating to the notion about whether a pregnant woman can again become pregnant and concludes that although there are debates about the possibility of conceiving while pregnant (see the foregoing), none of the rabbinic authorities accepts the possibility of superfetation with subsequent live birth of both fetuses, an assumption made by R. Halevi in his third case.

R. Azulai mentions two major areas where the issue of superfetation is discussed in rabbinic literature. One is the passage in *Yevamot* above. He notes that even though Rabbenu Tam maintains that conception after pregnancy is not possible, he acknowledges that according to Rashi conception is indeed a possibility. However, even according to Rashi, if superfetation did occur, one of the fetuses would certainly become a *sandal* and be severely malformed and non-viable. Even Rashi would concur that the birth of two healthy children through superfetation is impossible. Rather, the talmudic phrase "*Ein isha mit'aberet vehozeret umit'aberet*" is to be interpreted to mean that a pregnant woman cannot have a viable second child from superfetation.

The other area that R. Azulai discusses in order to prove that superfetation with the birth of viable children is rejected by all *Rishonim* is a case of twins where one dies prior to thirty days, and the other survives. In general, a child who dies prior to thirty days after birth is considered a *nefel*, a non-viable child, and no mourning practices are observed. However, if there is strong evidence that it was a viable child, mourning may be required. In a case of twins, if one child survives, it may reflect upon the status of the other twin, who may likewise be considered viable, even though death occurred prior to thirty days. As such,

---

19. R. Halevi's case asssumes the wife conceived while in her later stages of pregnancy and gave birth to the second child seven or nine months after the delivery of the first. Even modern science does not record or acknowledge this extreme case of superfetation.

mourning for the deceased twin may be required. This is indeed the position of the *Rashbatz*, as cited by R. Azulai, that mourning for the deceased twin is required despite the occurrence of death prior to thirty days.[20] This argument presupposes that the twins were conceived at the same time. In fact, the *Rashbatz* cites the passage in the *Bavli* that "*Ein isha mit'aberet vehozeret umit'aberet*" as proof to his position. If, however, one assumes that a pregnant woman can again conceive at a later time, it is possible that the child that died prior to thirty days was indeed of an earlier gestational age and was in fact not viable. Mourning would thus not be required.

R. Yosef Karo codified a variation of this case in his *Shulḥan Arukh*, but the questionable integrity of our printed text has led to much debate about its interpretation.[21] The printed text reads: "There are some who say in a case of twins, if one dies within thirty days, and the second twin lives—*and dies*—after thirty days, we do not mourn for him [the second twin]."

According to this version, if the first twin died before thirty days, and the second died after thirty days, we do not mourn even for the second twin, who lived beyond thirty days. The *Levush* (as cited in the *Taz*) explains that if the second twin is ill at the time of the first twin's death, since they both derive from the same conception, both are considered non-viable, and mourning is not required even for the older twin. The *Taz* is in wonderment of this decision, as how could one refrain from mourning for a child who survived more than thirty days, whatever the circumstances may be? He maintains that the original source of this halakha was not a case of neonatal death of the second twin, rather, the second twin survived. He maintains that the word "*vamet*" (and dies) should be removed from the text. In this case, the halakha states that even though the second twin survived, mourning is not required for the *first* twin who died before thirty days. While the *Taz* argues convincingly that this is clearly a more logical alternative than that of the *Levush*, this decision is not consistent with the logic and decision of the *Rashbatz*

---

20. See Y. Baumel, *Emek Halakha* 1:5 for further discussion of the case of mourning for twins.

21. *Y. D.*, 374:9 and commentaries, ad loc.

cited above, who would require mourning for the first twin, even if he died within thirty days, based on the notion that *"Ein isha mit'aberet vehozeret umit'aberet."*

While R. Azulai railed against R. Halevi for accepting the possibility of superfetation (with the birth of two healthy children), one of his close friends and colleagues, R. Yom Tov Algazi, seems to have accepted the possibility as well. In R. Algazi's commentary on Naḥmanides' work on *Hilkhot Bekhorot*,[22] he questions the pronouncement of *Talmud Yerushalmi* that one can fulfill the mitzva of *peru urevu* through the birth of a *mamzer*.[23] As the mitzva could only be accomplished through illicit, biblically forbidden relations, the mitzva should be nullified under the rule of *mitzva haba'a be'aveira* (a mitzva performed through the violation of a Torah prohibition). R. Algazi offers a novel case that would allow the fulfillment of the mitzva despite the production of a *mamzer*. If a man's brother dies childless, he is required to perform *yibum*. However, one must wait three months after his death (the time frame defined in the Talmud by which it would be physically apparent that a woman is pregnant) lest his wife be pregnant, in which case *yibum* may not be required.[24] In this case, the surviving brother waited the requisite three months, but, despite physical appearance to the contrary, the wife turned out to be pregnant. The resultant child of their union would be a *mamzer*, but the brother's act, which was an *ones* (purely accidental and unforseen), was not in violation of any prohibition. Therefore, this would not fall under the umbrella of *mitzva haba'a be'aveira*.

In the 1910 edition of the journal *Vayelaket Yosef*, R. Yisrael Klein questions the solution of R. Algazi on the grounds that the Talmud clearly states in *Nidda* 27 that a pregnant woman cannot conceive again. How is it possible then for a woman three plus months pregnant to conceive a second child that will be born as a *mamzer*? R. Klein was unable to find a satisfactory answer to his question and left the issue unresolved.

---

22. R. Y. T. Algazi on chapter 8 of Maimonides' *Hil. Bekhorot*, published in the back of the Vilna Shas *Bekhorot*, p. 56, column 4, s. v., *"ulam."* See *Yerushalmi Yevamot*, chapter 2.

23. R. Algazi addresses the debate as to whether the statement of the *Yerushalmi* that one can fulfill the mitzva of *peru urevu* is definitive or left unanswered.

24. The child would have to be born alive to preclude *yibum*. Pregnancy alone is not sufficient, as the Torah states *"uben ein lo."*

Some years later, R. Ephraim Billitzer recounted R. Klein's question and provided a creative solution.[25] According to R. Billitzer, in the case discussed by R. Algazi, the man who died had two wives. The surviving brother performed *yibum* with one wife after three months, but the other wife was subsequently found to be pregnant, obviating the need for *yibum*. Thus, there would be no concern about superfetation, no case of *mitzva haba'a be'aveira*, as it was an *ones*, the resultant child would be a *mamzer*, and the mitzva of *peru urevu* would be fulfilled.[26] R. Billitzer acknowleges that this key fact that the man had two wives, is not specifically mentioned in the text by R. Algazi. While this is indeed a clever solution, it appears to be a case of *ikar haser min hasefer* (i.e., it is not clearly mentioned in the text).

I would humbly suggest a different possible solution to the question posed by R. Klein. While it is true by all accounts that the *Talmud Bavli* rejects the possibility of superfetation (with the birth of two healthy children), as R. Algazi's close friend, R. Azulai, convincingly proves, however, R. Algazi's entire discussion revolves around a passage in the *Yerushalmi* (that one can fulfill the mitzva of *peru urevu* through the birth of a *mamzer*). The *Yerushalmi* appears to explicitly reject the opinion of the *Talmud Bavli*,[27] and accepts the possibility of superfetation. Therefore, the original question of R. Klein in *Vayelaket Yosef* does not apply.

The notion of superfetation also arose in another context in the eighteenth century. It was not always clear throughout history how twins were formed embryologically. For example, some maintained that twins could not be formed from one marital act, while others believed that one act could create multiple births. This issue finds its expression in a homily of R. Yonatan Eybeschuetz and serves as the basis of a question of suspicion of infidelity posed to R. Yeḥezkel Landau.

In discussing the lineage of David HaMelekh, R. Eybeschuetz queries why the progeny of the union of Yehuda and Tamar should

---

25. *She'elot UTeshuvot Yad Ephraim E. H.*, 1.

26. R. Billitzer does find a possible allusion to it based on a turn of phrase of the R. Y. T. Algazi.

27. R. Azulai, op. cit., is of the opinion that even the *Yerushalmi* rejects the possibility of superfetation with the birth of two healthy children.

be considered tainted.[28] After all, prior to *matan Torah*, the obligation of *yibum* devolved upon the father as well as on the brother. Therefore, Yehuda was fulfilling a mitzva through his union with Tamar and the resulting progeny should not only be free of stain, they should be considered superior. To answer this question, R. Eybeschuetz posits that only the first coition fulfills the mitzva of *yibum*, and furthermore, twins cannot be born of one coition, but rather require two. As a result, only the first of the twins, who was conceived through the process of a mitzva, is associated with royalty. The second twin however, would be susceptible to stain.

It is this notion of the requirement of two coitions to produce twins that was read and integrated by an eighteenth-century European businessman. Prior to his departure on a long journey, this man engaged in marital relations with his wife. Upon his return some months later, his wife gave birth to twins. Remembering the homily of R. Eybeschuetz, he assumed his wife must have been unfaithful and approached R. Yehezkel Landau for rabbinic advice.[29]

R. Landau roundly criticizes the questioner and dismisses out of hand the scientific ideas discussed in R. Eybeschuetz's essay. He further adds that not only are two coitions not required to produce twins, rather, based on talmudic passages (cited above), sequential coitions could not produce two viable twins, as one would invariably become a *sandal*. Here, R. Landau invokes the talmudic dictum that superfetation (with the subsequent birth of two viable children) is not possible. In fact, as discussed above, while superfetation is debated, the possibility of superfecundation is universally accepted. Twins could indeed be produced through sequential coitions in a case of superfecundation.

IV. CONCLUSION

For centuries, the rabbis have debated the possibility of superfetation, and while some have accepted it as a possibility, the *Talmud Bavli*, by most accounts, clearly rejects the possibility of superfetation with viable progeny. There are a number of passages in the Talmud that seemingly

---

28. *Ya'arot Devash* (Lvov, 5623), 100a.
29. *Noda BiYehuda Tinyana E. H.*, 81.

conflict with our modern understanding of science, and numerous approaches have been developed to address them.[30] The passages discussing superfetation, until now, have not been numbered amongst them. It has not been possible to determine with absolute scientific certainty that superfetation is possible. How are we to view the current case report from England? Will this current case cause us to add the talmudic discussions on superfetation to the list of passages that seemingly conflict with our modern understanding of medicine, or, like its predecessors in recent medical literature, will the gestational disparity be attributed to another medical phenomenon?[31] We reserve judgment while we await the final scientific analysis of this case. While advances in DNA testing and ultrasound have significantly enhanced our ability to assess the phenomenon of superfetation, the definitive study of this phenomenon remains a desideratum.

---

30. The phrase that has been used to resolve these apparent conflicts is *nishtaneh hateva* (nature has changed). For treatment of this topic see D. Frimer, "*Kevi'at Avhut al yedei Bedukat Dam beMishpat haYisraeli ubemishpat haIvri*," in M. Halperin, ed., *Sefer Assia* 5 (Jerusalem, 1986), 185–209; D. Cohen, "*Shinuy Hateva*: An Analysis of the Halachic Process," *Journal of Halacha and Contemporary Society* 31 (Spring 1996); S. Sprecher, "*Divrei Ḥazal VeYedi'ot Mada'iyot*," B.D.D. 2 (Winter 1996), 2–39; S. Z. Leiman, "R. Israel Lipshutz and the Mouse that is Half Flesh and Half Earth: A Note on Torah U-Madda in the Nineteenth Century," in *Ḥazon Nachum* (Yeshiva University Press, 1997), 449–458; N. Gutal, *Sefer Hishtanut HaTeva'im BeHalakha* (Makhon Yaḥdav, 5758); A. Steinberg, *Encyclopedia of Jewish Medical Ethics*, trans. F. Rosner (Feldheim, 2003), s. v., "change in nature"; N. Slifkin, *Mysterious Creatures* (Targum Press, 2003), 17–41; M. Halperin, "Science and Medicine in the Talmud: *Kabbalah o Actualia*," *Assia* 71–72 (January, 2003), 90–102 (Hebrew); Yehuda Levi, *The Science in Torah: The Scientific Knowledge of the Sages* (Feldheim, 2004); M. Meiselman, *Torah, Chazal and Science* (Israel Bookshop, 2013).

31. There are features of this case that make it more convincingly a case of superfetation as, according to reports, an ultrasound was performed when the younger twin was at a very early gestational age. This precludes the possibility of confusing this with, for example, a twin-twin transfusion or severely size-discordant twins from other causes.

Midrash, Miracles, and Motherhood: The Birth of Dinah and the Definition of Maternity— *Tzarikh Iyun LeDina*

I. INTRODUCTION

In the present age of medical discovery, with developments completely unforeseen by our predecessors, it is challenging to find legal precedent in both American law and halakha to address the attendant legal ramifications of these new technologies. The field that perhaps best typifies this trend is the specialty of reproductive medicine and the treatment of infertility. Physicians now have the ability to manipulate the process of procreation in ways previously assumed to be relegated to God alone.

For the last few decades, rabbinic authorities have searched for legal precedent to address issues such as donor insemination, surrogacy, pre-implantation genetic diagnosis, stem cell research, and the production of artificial reproductive seed. As there is rarely clear and direct precedent in the Torah, Talmud, or legal codes for such historically novel innovations, rabbinic authorities must expand their search to unconventional areas of rabbinic literature, such as the midrashic, aggadic, or other non-legal, texts. For example, early discussions on artificial insemination focused on the story of Ben Sira, a story that, while cited tangentially in halakhic sources, ultimately derives from a non-halakhic and non-midrashic source.[1]

One area in which a non-halakhic source has featured prominently in the halakhic discussions is the definition of maternity in the case of surrogate motherhood.[2] The halakhic solution to the definition of maternity in such cases remains one of the most complex issues in contemporary medical halakha. There is no consensus on this matter, and all possible legal positions have been espoused by contemporary authorities.

Of the few sources that have been found to be relevant to the halakhic discussion of maternity, we find the biblical story of the birth of Dinah. In this essay, we analyze the rabbinic approaches to this story, as well as the incorporation of this story into the exegetical literature. We then review the uses of this story in halakhic discussions on the definition of maternity. While this story has received brief, sporadic treatment in the past, this chapter provides an extensive review of the rabbinic literature on this topic.

II. THE STORY OF THE BIRTH OF DINAH

In Bereshit,[3] we read of the births of the children of Yaakov. Leah gives birth to six of the twelve tribes. For the birth of Leah's first six children, the Torah states that she conceived (*vatahar*) and she bore (*vateled*) a child. However, for the description of the birth of Dinah, the Torah deviates from the typical phrasing, stating, "And afterwards, she bore a daughter and named her Dinah." It is the use of the word "afterwards" (*ve'ahar*), as well as the change from the previous literary pattern of "she

---

1. See chapter, "The Rabbinic Conception of Conception: An Exercise in Fertility."
2. Technically, a surrogate mother provides both the egg, as well as the gestation. Mary Beth Whitehead was the first American surrogate mother. A gestational host is the term for a woman who carries an embryo created from another egg donor. This chapter refers to the case of a gestational host, though I use the commonly accepted colloquial term surrogate mother instead.
3. Chapter 30:23.

conceived and she bore" (*vatahar vateled*), that draws the attention of the *midrashim*. The multitude of interpretations and versions of the events that flow from this deviation comprise the substance of this chapter.

Version 1A—Gender Change through the Prayers of Rachel

We begin our analysis with *Bereshit Rabba*:

> And afterwards, she bore a child, etc. We learn, if one's wife is pregnant, and he prays, "May it be Your will that my wife bear a male child," behold this is a prayer in vain... R. Yehuda bar Pazi says even if the woman is sitting on the birthing stool, the gender of the child can change... as it is written, "And afterwards, she bore a daughter." Dina was originally created as a male, and through the prayers of Rachel, who said, "may Hashem add for me an additional son," the child became a female.[4]

The Midrash adds that the Matriarchs, including Rachel, were prophetesses and that Rachel asked God for only "one" additional son, in the singular, since she knew that after the birth of Yosef, only one of the total of twelve tribes was yet to be born. A number of key points can be gleaned from this Midrash. 1) Rachel is the one who prays; 2) The substance of the miracle was a gender change of the fetus in Leah's womb from male to female; 3) The event transpired *after* the birth of Yosef.[5]

The *Talmud Yerushalmi*'s approach is consistent with that of the Midrash and addresses the reason for the Torah's use of different phrasing for the birth of Dinah.

> In the name of Beit Yannai, the initial conception of Dinah was as a male, but after Rachel prayed, the fetus was changed to female,

---

4. Albeck, 72.
5. For further elaboration of this version, see R. Menachem Kasher, *Torah Shelema*, *Vayetzei*, 67; *Pardes Yosef, Parashat Vayetzei*, n. 21. *Pardes Yosef* attempts to align the commentary of Ibn Ezra, who claims that Zevulun and Dinah were twins, with the version that Rachel is the one who prayed for the gender change. *Hizkuni* and Radak also claim that Dinah was Zevulun's twin.

as it says, "And *afterwards*, she bore a daughter and named her Dinah." *After* Rachel prayed, the fetus became female.[6]

Version 1B—Gender Change through the Prayers of Leah

The *Midrash Tanḥuma*[7] has a slightly different variation of the events that led up to Dinah's birth. Similar to the *Midrash Rabba*, the discussion begins with the question of whether one can pray for the gender of a child when one's wife is already pregnant. As proof that one indeed can change the gender of the fetus through prayer, the Midrash brings the story of Leah. According to the Midrash, after she bore six sons, Leah saw through prophecy that twelve tribes would be born to Yaakov. She had already given birth to six of them and was now pregnant with another male child. According to her calculations, the two maidservants had each given birth to two, for a combined total, with her six, of ten. If she would deliver another male child, this will leave only one male child left to be born to Rachel. Rachel would then be inferior to even the maidservants who each bore two of the tribes. Leah, therefore, prayed to God:

> Master of the World, if my child is a male, Rachel will then be of even lesser status than the maidservants (who each bore two of the tribes).

The Midrash then continues:

> Immediately God heard her prayer, and the male fetus in her womb was changed to a female.

The Midrash also explains why Leah chose to call the child by the name of Dinah:

> And why did Leah call the child Dinah? Because the righteous Leah stood in judgment [*bedin*] before God. God responded to her,

---

6. *Yerushalmi Berakhot*, chap. 9, halakha 3.
7. *Vayetzei*, n. 8

> "Just as you are merciful, I will also have mercy on her [Rachel],"
> as it says immediately thereafter, "And God remembered Rachel."

While the nature of the birth described by the *Tanḥuma*, a gender change
of the fetus in utero, is identical to that of the *Midrash Rabba*, there is
one fundamental difference. In the *Tanḥuma*, it is Leah who prays, as
opposed to Rachel. Dinah's name conveys this fact. It also appears clear
from the *Tanḥuma* that Yosef was not yet born at the time of Leah's
prayer, as Leah enumerates all the existing male children, and a child
from Rachel is not amongst them.

The Talmud appears to follow the tradition of the *Tanḥuma*[8] and,
like the other sources, begins with a discussion of the effectiveness of
praying for a specific gender child once a woman is already pregnant.
As proof that prayer can effectuate gender change, the story of Leah is
mentioned. Like the *Tanḥuma*, the Talmud maintains that Leah prayed
after making the calculations of how many of the tribes would be born
by Rachel. Her prayers were answered, and the male child in her womb
converted to a female. The Talmud concludes, however, that one cannot
learn the effectiveness of prayer for gender from this case, as this case
was miraculous and an exception to the natural order.

The continuation of the passage is also relevant to our discussion. The Talmud states that perhaps the case where Leah prayed was
within forty days gestation, when one can, according to the Talmud,
change the gender with prayer. Moreover, the Talmud queries, can
one indeed change the gender with prayer even within forty days?
R. Yitzḥak, son of R. Ami, states that if a man is *mazria* (emits seed)
first it will be a female child, while if a woman is *mazra'at* (emits seed)
first, it will be a male child.[9] Thus, it is reproductive physiology, the
seed emission, which determines gender immediately, and irrevocably,

---

8. *Berakhot* 60a.

9. The words *mazria* and *mazra'at* are the masculine and feminine forms of the verb
to give forth, or emit, seed. What exactly did Ḥazal mean by the term *mazria*? For
the male, it is clearly interpreted as the emission of reproductive seed, but for the
female, it is not at all clear. Ḥazal were not aware of the woman's parallel seed emission, ovulation, although they do acknowledge a contribution of the female. For
further discussion of this passage, see chapter, "*Parashat Tazria* and Childbirth."

upon conception. Prayer could not possibly alter this. The Talmud responds by claiming that in a case of simultaneous seed emission (*hazra'a*), the gender is not immediately determined, and prayer can still have an effect for forty days. This notion of gender determination associated with precedential seed emission is a key to the explication of a number of biblical passages discussed below.

Like the *Tanḥuma*, The Talmud maintains that Leah is the one who prayed, and the nature of the miracle was an in utero gender change of the fetus from male to female.

Version 2A—Inter-Uterine Exchange of Dinah and Yosef

There is yet another variation on the birth of Dinah that is found in the *Targum Yonatan ben Uziel*.[10] It is this quite different version of the miraculous birth of Dinah that features in contemporary halakhic discussions of surrogate motherhood. According to the *Targum Yonatan* it is Leah who prayed, based on the same calculations of the total number of tribes, but the nature of the miracle was radically different:

> And God heeded the prayers of Leah and exchanged the fetus in her womb; and Yosef was placed in the womb of Rachel, while Dinah was placed in the womb of Leah.

Instead of a gender change in utero, the *Targum Yonatan* describes an inter-uterine transfer or exchange. Leah and Rachel were pregnant simultaneously, with Leah carrying a male fetus and Rachel a female fetus. After Leah's prayers, the two fetuses exchanged places, with Leah giving birth to Dinah and Rachel to Yosef. [11]

The *piyyut* (liturgical poem) "*Even Ḥug*" recited on Rosh Hashana also corroborates this version of the story.[12] The author,

---

10. Bereshit 30:21.

11. This version is often quoted from the *Maharsha* (*Nidda* 31a), who cites the *Paneaḥ Raza* as also espousing the inter-uterine transfer version and uses this version to solve a textual difficulty in the Torah raised by the account of Dinah's birth as told in *Berakhot*.

12. *Complete Artscroll Machzor for Rosh Hashanah* (Mesorah Publications, 1985), 312.

assumed to be R. Eliezer HaKalir, in talking about the travails of the infertile Rachel and her ultimate blessing of fecundity, states "to appease her by exchanging Dinah for Yosef."[13] This is generally accepted as referring to the inter-uterine exchange.

In the premier Hungarian halakha journal *Vayelaket Yosef*,[14] in an article devoted to the analysis of the story of Dinah's birth, R. Shlomo Fisher posits a novel thesis in claiming that the passage in *Berakhot* 60a actually refers to an inter-uterine exchange, consistent with the approach of the *Targum Yonatan*, and *not* to a gender change, as is conventionally thought.[15] R. Fisher bases this, in part, on two linguistic observations. 1) After recounting the incident of Dinah's birth, the Gemara discounts it as a proof to its question by claiming, "*ein mazkirin ma'aseh nissim*, we do not bring proof from miracles." R. Fisher points out that the word "miracles" is in the plural, implying that there was more than one miracle in this case. He considers this an allusion to the fact that there was an inter-uterine exchange, and thus two miracles that transpired; one for Leah and one for Rachel.[16] 2) When the Gemara recounts the nature of the miracle it states, "*miyad nehefkha lebat*," the fetus immediately converted to a female. R. Fisher notes that the word *nehefkha* is in the feminine. Had the miracle been that the male fetus converted to a female, the phrase should have been in the masculine, *nehefach*, as it

---

13. Regarding the value and perception of the *piyyutim* in the eyes of rabbinic authorities, R. Eliezer Fleckeles writes in the very first responsum of his *Teshuva MeAhava*: "Come and see how precious were the *piyyutim* in the eyes of the holy *Rishonim* to the extent that all their writings and language were well known to them (*shegura befihem*), as I will show you many examples." One example R. Fleckeles cites is the case of Dinah and the use by the *Maharsha* of the language of the *piyyut* to support his thesis.

14. *Vayelaket Yosef* 6:9 (Adar, 5664) [February-March, 1904], n. 82.

15. He does not mention that his predecessor, R. Moshe Margalit, espoused the same thesis in his *Mareh HaPanim* on the *Talmud Yerushalmi*, although the latter's analysis is not as fully developed (see further in this chapter for approach to variant versions). The *Maharsha* cited above appears to maintain this approach as well.

16. One could ask why in fact there had to be two miracles. Transferring Yosef to the womb of Rachel was necessary to accomplish the main objective of Rachel giving birth to two of the *Shevatim*. Why was it necessary for Dinah to be transferred to the womb of Leah? What did this accomplish? See *Pardes Yosef, Parashat Vayetzei*, n. 21 who cites the *Livyat Ḥen*'s answer to this question.

was the male fetus that converted. Rather, the meaning of the phrase is that the fetus was converted for *her* (Leah) into a female, after the inter-uterine exchange.[17]

R. Fisher also claims that the inter-uterine exchange can even be inferred from the Torah's language. The word that serves as the basis for the notion that Dinah's birth was unique is *"ve'aḥar,"* and "afterwards" Leah bore a daughter. The rabbis interpret the word "afterwards" to indicate after Leah made a judgment about her child. R. Fisher queries where this is alluded to in the word *"ve'aḥar?"* All this word means is that the following transcribed events happened "afterwards." R. Fisher therefore offers a novel interpretation of the use of the word as a means of alluding to the miracle of the inter-uterine exchange. After recounting the birth of Zevulun, the Torah recounts the births of Dinah and Yosef. One would obviously think that these events occurred in sequential order. However, the introduction of the word *"ve'aḥar,"* according to R. Fisher, indicates otherwise. It means that "after" the following *group* of events transpired, namely the simultaneous pregnancies of Leah and Rachel and subsequent inter-uterine exchange of Dinah and Yosef, *then* Leah gave birth to a daughter. The word *"aḥar"* implies "after" all the events recounted below, including the birth of Yosef. This is not to be understood as a standard description of consecutive events; rather the whole section needs to be considered together.

Version 2B—Inter-Uterine Exchange of Dinah and Binyamin

There is one version according to which Rachel prayed after Yosef was born, and at that stage there was an inter-uterine transfer between Leah and Rachel. However, according to this version, it was Binyamin, not Yosef, who was switched with Dinah.[18] This version is not cited extensively in the exegetical or later halakhic literature.

---

17. One could argue that the phrase should then have read *"miyad nehefkha **la** lebat,"* that the child was converted **for her** into a female.
18. This is cited in the name of *Sekhel Tov* by R. Menachem Kasher, *Torah Shelema, Vayetzei,* 67–69. R. Kasher details a number of textual variants in the *midrashim* and *Yerushalmi* about the story of Dinah's birth and raises a series of questions created by the textual inconsistencies.

Version 2C—Combination of Inter-Uterine Exchange and Gender Change

R. Avraham Yaakov HaLevi Horowitz, in his *Tzur Yaakov*,[19] offers a truly unique interpretation of the inter-uterine exchange mentioned in the *Targum Yonatan*. He claims that the physical bodies did not switch between the wombs of Leah and Rachel; rather, the male child within Leah changed to a female, and the female child within Rachel became a male. Only the souls switched after the gender changes took effect. This version contains both a gender change and an inter-uterine transfer, though the transfer was not of the physical bodies, but of the metaphysical souls. This is a synthesis of the two major versions of the birth of Dinah.[20]

Approach to the Variant Versions

R. Moshe Margalit, in his commentary *Mareh HaPanim* on the *Talmud Yerushalmi*[21] was well aware of the conflicting versions of the birth of Dinah and asserts that, for each approach, the originator of the prayer determined the nature of the subsequent miracle. According to those who maintain that Rachel is the one who prayed,[22] the prayer occurred after the birth of Yosef, and the miracle was a gender change of Leah's fetus. An inter-uterine transfer could not have been possible if Yosef was already born. According to those who maintain that Leah is the one who

---

19. N. 28. See below, section on ovarian transplantation, for further treatment of this source. See also, R. Meir Brandsdorfer, "Egg Donation and the *Yiḥus* of the Child," (Hebrew) *Yeshurun* 21 (*Nisan*, 5769) [April, 2009], 557–564, who incorporates this source into his halakhic discussions.

20. R. Tzvi Ryzman in his *Ratz KaTzvi* (E. H., chapter on *hashtalat shaḥlot* [ovarian transplants]) assumes that the simple meaning of the passage in *Berakhot* regarding the gender change is that there was a gender change for the fetuses of *both* Leah and Rachel. Perhaps he derived this from R. Horowitz (*Tzur Yaakov*, n. 28), whom he cites and who seems to imply this as well. I have not come across this approach to the passage in *Berakhot* elsewhere, and the accepted meaning of the passage is that there was only a gender change of the fetus within Leah. According to this accepted version, Rachel was not necessarily pregnant simultaneously with a female child, and there was no need for the event to involve Rachel.

21. *Yerushalmi Berakhot,* chapter 9, halakha 3, s. v., "*al shem.*"

22. *Midrash Rabba* and *Yerushalmi Berakhot.*

prayed, Rachel was pregnant, but Yosef was not yet born. The miracle was the inter-uterine exchange of Yosef for Dinah.[23]

The *Mareh HaPanim* uses this approach to interpret the conclusion in *Berakhot* that we do not learn from miracles. The conclusion of the Talmud is *not* that one cannot, in general, learn from miraculous incidents, but rather, in this case, as Leah is the one who prayed, the miracle was an inter-uterine exchange. Since there was no gender change in this miracle, one of course cannot learn about the power of prayer to change gender from this incident.

The problem with this interpretation is that the passage in *Berakhot* states explicitly that upon Leah's prayer, the fetus immediately converted to a female. It does not imply or state explicitly that there was an inter-uterine exchange. The *Tanḥuma* also maintains that Leah prayed, yet the miracle was a gender change, not an inter-uterine exchange. The *Mareh HaPanim* was not the only one to maintain that the passage in *Berakhot* in fact assumes that there was an inter-uterine exchange.[24]

III. THE STORY OF THE BIRTH OF DINAH IN BIBLICAL COMMENTARIES

The story of the birth of Dinah, especially the version of the inter-uterine exchange, has been mentioned by biblical commentators throughout the centuries to either interpret cryptic phrases or to solve seeming interpretive contradictions. The following section draws on a wide array of sources that have invoked the story of Dinah's birth in their commentaries. While the focus of these sources is purely exegetical, we can nonetheless infer from a number of them the author's position on the definition of maternity in halakha.

---

23. For another approach to the differences between the versions of the *Bavli* and the *Yerushalmi* of the birth of Dinah, and how this relates to whether Leah or Rachel prayed, see R. Yoel b. David Dispeck (1715–1793), *Pardes Dovid* (Warsaw, 1900), 47. R. Dispeck also discusses the gestational period up to which one can pray, whether up to forty days or to the time a woman sits on the birthing stool, and how this relates to the differences between the two Talmuds.

24. See position of R. Fisher, in *Vayelaket Yosef*, discussed above.

The Change of Language by the Birth of Dinah

As discussed above, the Torah's deviation from the phrase "and she conceived and she bore" (*vatahar vateled*) serves as a springboard for the discussions of Dinah's unique birth. The *Da'at Zekenim MiBa'alei HaTosafot*[25] follows the approach of the *Targum Yonatan* that the miracle was an inter-uterine transfer, and adds an additional textual interpretation. As mentioned above, in the case of Dinah's birth, the Torah deviates from the typical phrasing of "she conceived and she bore," stating instead, "and afterwards, she bore a daughter and named her Dinah." While other sources focus on the use of the word "afterwards," the *Da'at Zekenim* addresses the absence of the phrase "she conceived and she bore." By the other births, Leah both conceived and bore the same child. In this case, while she conceived one child, Yosef, she gave birth to another, Dinah, as an inter-uterine exchange occurred. That is why the Torah could not say that "she conceived and she bore" a child. This was simply not true for the birth of Dinah.[26]

The Naming of Yosef by Rachel

In his *Pardes Yosef*, R. Yosef Patsanovski employs the inter-uterine exchange to interpret the statements of Rachel after Yosef's birth.[27] In naming Yosef, Rachel says, "*asaf Hashem et ḥerpati,*" God has brought in my disgrace.[28] According to the *Pardes Yosef*, Rachel meant that her disgrace was mitigated in front of the world, as now a child was born to her. She however knew that this was not truly her child, but one conceived

---

25. Bereshit 30:21.

26. R. Ḥezkiya Manoaḥ offers the same interpretation of this verse in the *Ḥizkuni*. This interpretation would work equally well for the other version of the miracle, that there was an in utero gender change. In this case as well, it would be inaccurate to state that Leah both conceived and bore a female child, as she initially conceived a male child. A challenge to the interpretations of the *Da'at Zekenim* and *Ḥizkuni*, however, is the use of the phrase "*vatahar vateled*" for the birth of Yosef. If indeed the deviation from the phrase "*vatahar vateled*" is because there was an inter-uterine exchange, this should have applied equally to the Rachel's birth of Yosef. Yosef also was not both conceived and born by Rachel, and this phrase should have been omitted there as well. See also *HaTur HeArukh*, Bereshit 30:21.

27. *Pardes Yosef*, Parashat Vayetzei, n. 21.

28. Bereshit 30:23–24.

in the womb of Leah. She therefore says, "*Yosef Hashem li ben aḥer*," may God add on for *me* another child, a child that I will conceive and will truly be mine.[29] This assumes that Rachel was aware of the exchange. This also assumes that the "genetic" mother is the halakhic mother.

The Prelude to the Rape of Dinah

R. Eliezer Friedman, in an article in the halakha journal *Tel Talpiyot*,[30] questions the motivation behind Rashi's comment on the verse that introduces the story of the rape of Dinah, "and Dinah the daughter of Leah went out" ("*vatetzei Dinah bat Leah*").[31] Rashi compares Dinah's going out to Leah's going out. What bothered Rashi about the fact that Dinah was here referred to as the daughter of Leah, and not the daughter of Yaakov, to the extent that he needed to justify it by creating a comparison between Leah and Dinah? He answers that Rashi was compelled to address the fact that Dinah was called the daughter of Leah, and not Yaakov, in order to be consistent with his approach elsewhere. On the verse "in addition to Dinah *his* daughter,"[32] Rashi specifically notes that Dinah, a female, is associated with her father, based on the talmudic principle regarding gender determination and the timing of seed emission (see above). Therefore, when the Torah writes "and Dinah the daughter of

---

29. See similar idea in M. Carlbach, *Ḥavatzelet HaSharon, Bereshit, Vayigash* p. 658; S. Y. Freshwater, *Siftei Shlomo* on Bereshit (Beit HaMidrash Sassov, 5770), 152–155. I thank R. Daniel Feldman for drawing my attention to the latter source. R. Freshwater raises an intriguing idea that would actually yield different maternal definitions for Yosef and Dinah. He points out that Rabbenu Baḥya states that Dinah was seven months older than Yosef. If so, then at the time of the inter-uterine exchange, Dinah was seven months older as well. Perhaps, he ponders, there would be a difference in the assignment of maternity if the fetus remained in the womb longer. Thus, it is possible that Dinah, who remained in her conception-mother's womb for a prolonged period of time, might still be considered the daughter of Leah, while Yosef, having been transferred at an earlier embryological stage, might not be considered the son of Rachel. This would have potential halakhic ramifications for surrogate motherhood, where the embryo is transferred at a very early embryological stage.

30. *Tel Talpiyot* 19:7 (*Tevet*, 5671) [January, 1911], n. 58, p. 55–56. R. Friedman addresses the position of Rashi and arrives at the identical conclusion as R. Fisher, though he was clearly unaware of R. Fisher's earlier lengthy contribution.

31. Bereshit 34:1.

32. Bereshit 46:15.

Leah went out," and deviates from this pattern, Rashi is compelled to find a specific reason for the change.

However, R. Friedman questions the very position of Rashi that Dinah, a female, should be associated with her father, based on *Berakhot*, which states that Dinah was conceived originally as a male, only later to be converted to a female. Therefore, Dinah should not be called the daughter of Yaakov. R. Friedman therefore posits that Rashi did not accept the notion of a gender change; he accepted the version of the *Maharsha*, the *Targum Yonatan* and the *piyyut* that there was an inter-uterine exchange. Therefore, Dinah was conceived and born as a female and should rightfully be identified as the daughter of Yaakov. Therefore, when she is identified as "*Dinah bat Leah*," Dinah the daughter of Leah, this is a deviation from the accepted norm and begs interpretation. This is what led Rashi to provide the commentary that the goings out were parallel between Leah and Dinah.[33]

The Age of Yosef When He Descended to Egypt[34]

In the context of his lengthy essay on Rashi's approach to the birth of Dinah, R. Shlomo Fisher utilizes the story of the inter-uterine exchange to interpret a biblical passage.[35] He comments on the necessity of the Torah to mention the age of Yosef when he was sold by his brothers—seventeen years of age.[36] He mentions the tradition that all the *Shevatim* were born with a female twin.[37] Since maternal siblings are forbidden to marry according to the Noachide laws, each *shevet* married a daughter

---

33. R. Friedman offers a proof that Rashi held of the inter-uterine exchange theory based on Rashi's alternate version of the text of the passage in *Berakhot*.

34. See R. Yehoshua Yaakov Rabinowitz (1801–1901), Ein Yaakov (Pietrikov, 5655 [1895]), 17–19, for an explanation of the dreams of Yosef based on the different versions of the birth of Dinah.

35. *Vayelaket Yosef* 6:9 (*Adar*, 5664) [February-March, 1904], n. 82, p. 82. More on this essay below.

36. Bereshit 37:2.

37. See R. Fisher's article for further elaboration of this idea. He addresses whether Yosef and Dinah, who were born through unusual means, also had twins. For a review of the literature on the notion that twins were born with each *shevet*, including specific discussion about Dinah and Yosef, see M. Greenbaum, "On the Twins Born with the *Shevatim*," (Hebrew) *Nezer HaTorah* (*Nisan*, 5768), 117–121. See also *Pardes Yosef*,

from another mother. R. Fisher claims that Yosef would naturally have married Dinah, as Yosef assumed that they were from different mothers. He was unaware of the miraculous inter-uterine exchange that led to his birth. In fact, however, as both Yosef and Dinah were created from the womb of Leah, they were not only paternal siblings, they were, according to R. Fisher, maternal siblings as well. In order to prevent Yosef from the sin of illicit sexual relations (*arayot*), God arranged for him to descend to Egypt at the age of seventeen, shortly before the typical age of marriage, eighteen. This seems to imply that both conception and gestation can determine maternity, as Leah conceived Yosef, but only gestated Dinah, yet R. Fisher considers Leah to be the halakhic mother of both.

Yehuda's Appeal to his Brothers Not to Kill Yosef

R. Meir Simḥa of Dvinsk invokes the inter-uterine exchange in at least two places in his biblical commentary, *Meshekh Ḥokhma*. In the first case, he uses it to explain an extraneous phrase in the story of Yosef and his brothers.[38] In appealing to his brothers not to kill Yosef, Yehuda says of Yosef, "he is our brother, our flesh."[39] The *Meshekh Ḥokhma* explains the addition of the phrase "our flesh," in the following manner. According to *Masekhet Nidda*, there are three partners in creation. The man contributes the white substance from which are derived the bones, etc., and the woman contributes the red material from which are derived the skin and the flesh.[40] If there was an inter-uterine exchange when Yosef was born, then he was originally conceived by Leah. It was Leah, then, the woman, who contributed his flesh. Yehudah was alluding to the fact that that Yosef was both their paternal sibling, "our brother," as

---

Parashat Vayetzei, n. 21, who incorporates the twinning tradition into his commentary on the story, and also explains the Ibn Ezra's interpretation that Zevulun and Dinah were twins.

38. See second example below.

39. Bereshit 37:27.

40. For further analysis of this passage, and of the rabbinic literature that deals with the male and female contributions to the child, see chapter, "The Rabbinic Conception of Conception: An Exercise in Fertility." See also, R. Kiperwasser, "'Three Partners in a Person': The Genesis and Development of Embryological Theory in Biblical and Rabbinic Judaism," *Lectio Difficilior* 2 (2009), 1–37.

well as their maternal sibling, "our flesh," as the flesh is derived from the mother, and they shared a common mother, Leah. This assumes that the "genetic" mother is the mother. It also assumes that Yehudah was aware of the inter-uterine transfer.[41]

The Daughters of Yaakov Comfort Him

Ḥatam Sofer (R. Moshe Sofer) uses the story of the inter-uterine exchange to explain a very perplexing *Midrash*. When Yaakov mourns upon hearing of Yosef's disappearance, the Torah informs us that "all his sons and all his daughters arose to comfort him."[42] Many commentators focus on the use of the plural form for daughters. As only one daughter of Yaakov, Dinah, is listed in the Torah, what could the plural term "daughters" be referring to?[43] Some introduce here the notion that each son (*shevet*) was born with a twin, therefore Yaakov actually did have many daughters.[44] Ḥatam Sofer, however, addresses a different midrashic statement. The *Midrash* asks: "How many daughters did Yaakov have? He only had one, and even this one he would have preferred to bury." Ḥatam Sofer posits that Yaakov associated the (supposed) death of Yosef with the bad *mazal* of Rachel. He quotes Rashi as subscribing to the story of the inter-uterine exchange that Yosef was originally conceived by Leah, only to later be transferred to the womb of Rachel. Yaakov imagined that if the transfer had not occurred, Yosef would have been born to Leah and would still be alive. The twelve tribes would then still be complete. Furthermore, even the sight of Dinah was not a comfort for Yaakov in his mourning, but rather a painful reminder of these events. In some sense, he would have preferred to have buried Dinah rather than Yosef. This is the meaning of the *Midrash*, "He only had one [daughter], and even this one he would have preferred to bury." Note that Ḥatam Sofer also assumes that Rashi accepted the story of the inter-uterine exchange. He also assumes that Yaakov was aware of the exchange.

---

41. See *Teshuvot HaRabaz*, E. H. 5, who gives the identical interpretation of the phrase "our brother, our flesh."
42. Bereshit 37:35.
43. See Rashi, Bereshit 37:35.
44. See M. Greenbaum, "On the Twins Born with the *Shevatim*," (Hebrew) *Nezer HaTorah* (*Nisan*, 5768) [April, 2008], 117–121.

Shaul ben HaKena'anit and the Marriage of Dinah to Shimon

The nature of Dinah's birth also receives attention regarding the tradition that Dinah married Shimon. Among the list of Shimon's children, we find the name *Shaul ben HaKena'anit*. Ḥazal identify this child as the product of Shimon and Dinah. After being raped and kidnapped by Shekhem, Dinah would only agree to leave the city of Shekhem on the condition that Shimon marry her.[45] The nature of the prohibition against incest prior to the giving of the Torah is a matter of some debate, but the accepted opinion is that paternal siblings were permitted, while maternal siblings were forbidden.[46] How could Shimon then marry Dinah if they were maternal siblings?

The *Paneah Raza* (R. Yitzhak b. Yehuda Halevi) solves this problem by stating that Dinah was conceived in the womb of Rachel. This implies that he accepts the notion that there was an inter-uterine exchange. Since Dinah was conceived by Rachel, she was therefore the daughter of Rachel. As such, she was not a maternal sibling to Shimon, just a paternal sibling. This implies that it is conception (or genetics) that determines maternity. As this exegetical interpretation has halakhic implications, since it allowed an otherwise illicit marriage to take place, it is one of the most frequently cited sources in the halakhic literature on the definition of maternity.[47]

---

45. See, for example, Rashi, Bereshit 46:10 and *Bereshit Rabba* 80:11.

46. See, for example, Rashi, Bereshit 20:12.

47. It is this *Paneah Raza* that is cited by the *Maharsha* as the source of the belief that Dinah was born through an inter-uterine exchange. See also *Da'at Zekenim MiBa'alei HaTosafot, Tosafot Hashalem, Kotnot Or* and *Peirush HaTur HeArukh* on Bereshit 46:10.

    R. Eliyahu Mizrahi suggests a different reason why Shimon was able to marry Dinah, citing opinions that marriage according to Noachide laws is permitted for even maternal siblings. R. Meir Brandsdorfer claims that Rashi was of the same opinion. According to R. Brandsdorfer, Rashi maintained that Dinah was born through a gender change, in accordance with the conventional understanding of the passage in *Berakhot*. As such, Shimon and Dinah were both paternal and maternal siblings. The only way they could have married is if even maternal siblings were allowed to marry according to Noachide laws. See R. Meir Brandsdorfer, "Egg Donation and the *Yihus* of the Child," (Hebrew) *Yeshurun* 21 (*Nisan*, 5769) [April, 2009], 557–564.

    See R. Shimon Oshenberg's (sixteenth century) commentary on Rashi, *Devek Tov*, with notes of R. Aharon Walden (5674 edition), on Bereshit 46:10. The *Devek Tov* is quoted by R. Friedman (*Tel Talpiyot* 19:7 [*Tevet*, 5671/January, 1911], n. 58,

The List of Leah's Descendants and the Position of Rashi

In the Torah journal *Vayelaket Yosef*,[48] R. Yitzḥak Maier HaCohen Schwartz poses a question for the reader. In the enumeration of the names of the people that descended to Egypt, the Torah lists the descendants of Leah in the following fashion: "These are the sons of Leah whom she bore to Jacob... in addition to Dinah his daughter."[49] Rashi comments on the fact that the sons are called the "sons of Leah," associated with their mother, while the daughter, Dinah is identified as "Dinah *his* daughter," associated with her father. Rashi assimilates these associations with the talmudic passage on the physiology of gender determination and comments that the females are associated with Yaakov to teach you that if a man emits seed first, a female child will result, while if a woman emits seed first, a male child will result.

R. Schwartz queries how Rashi could infer the gender determination principle from this verse specifically. Rashi himself writes earlier[50] that after Leah's prayer, the child within her was changed to a female. If so, then at the time of conception, Dinah was a male. Only after Leah prayed did the male become a female. How then can we derive from here that if a man emits first, a female child will result? This child was originally a male and should thus have been associated with the mother? R. Schwartz reports that he asked this immensely challenging question to many and had never received a satisfactory response. He beckoned any reader to respond.

Some months later, R. Schwartz received a response to his vexing question. I suspect he could not have anticipated the expansiveness

---

p. 55–56) as proof that Rashi accepted the version of the inter-uterine exchange. I assume his inference is from the notes on the text by R. Walden. R. Walden implies that indeed Rashi accepted the version of the inter-uterine exchange. This very passage from the *Devek Tov* was also referenced in an earlier edition of *Tel Talpiyot* by R. Moshe Yosef Roth in his halakhic discussion on the definition of maternity in a case of ovarian transplantation. (*Tel Talpiyot*, Year 17, vol. 21 [*Tammuz*, 5668/ July, 1908], n. 176, p. 192.) See below. See also R. Mordechai Carlbach, *Ḥavatzelet HaSharon, Bereshit, Parashat Vayigash.*

48. *Vayelaket Yosef* 6:5 (*Tevet*, 5664/December, 1903), n. 49.

49. Bereshit 46:15.

50. Bereshit 30:21.

of the response provided by R. Shlomo Fisher,[51] which spans fourteen double column small print pages, and presents a thesis on the resolution of this seeming internal contradiction within Rashi, as well as an explication of the *midrashim* dealing with the miracle of the birth of Dinah.[52]

R. Fisher maintains that Rashi, as well as the passage in *Berakhot*, (see above) held that there was an inter-uterine exchange. In addition to other involved proofs to this thesis, he notes that remarkably, Rashi on the very next verse after the birth of Dinah cites a *piyyut* to aid his interpretation. The *piyyut* he cites is "*Even Ḥug*," the very same *piyyut* that details the birth of Dinah and maintains that she was born through an inter-uterine exchange (see above). Clearly, Rashi, who cited this very *piyyut* in the next verse, was familiar with the version of Dinah's birth elaborated therein, and concurred that it was an inter-uterine exchange. This answers R. Schwartz's question, for Dinah, according to the inter-uterine exchange, was always a female, from conception, and was correctly associated with her father.

The List of Rachel's Descendants

As discussed above, in enumerating the descendants of Leah amongst the seventy people who descended to Egypt, the Torah says, "These are the sons of Jacob whom she bore (*yalda*) to Jacob." It is on this verse that Rashi cites the doctrine of gender determination based on the talmudic passage, that males are conceived when the female emits seed first, and vice versa. This is inferred by the Torah's association of the woman with the male children—"These are the *sons* of Jacob whom *she* bore (*yalda*)."

When the Torah enumerates the descendants of Rachel, however, the language is different: "These are the *sons* of Rachel who were born (*yulad*) to Jacob."[53] The male children are here associated with the man. While Rashi does not comment on this deviation, the *Meshekh Ḥokhma* questions why regarding the sons of Rachel it does not say whom *she* bore (*asher yalda*), as by Leah. He answers here as well by invoking the story of the inter-uterine exchange. Rachel initially conceived a female

---

51. *Vayelaket Yosef* 6:9 (*Adar*, 5664) [February-March, 1904], n. 82.
52. A full explication of his thesis is beyond the scope of this article.
53. *Bereshit* 46:22.

child, though she gave birth to a male child. The male children listed here, while all descendants of the children *born* to Rachel, were not all descendants of children *conceived* by Rachel. Yosef was the product of an inter-uterine exchange and was not the product of Rachel's seed. He was the product of Leah's seed and was only later transferred to the womb of Rachel. The Torah could therefore not use the phrase "whom *she* bore (*asher yalda*)," associating Rachel with the birth of all these male children, as this was not in fact the case.

IV. THE USE OF THE STORY OF DINAH'S BIRTH IN HALAKHIC DISCUSSIONS ON THE DEFINITION OF MATERNITY

For centuries, the story of Dinah's birth remained confined to the exegetical literature. This was to change when technological advances facilitated the possibility of surrogate motherhood. With this new treatment for infertility it was now possible for the first time to have two possible mothers—an egg donor, or genetic mother, and a birth mother. With two candidates now vying for motherhood, the very definition of maternity in halakha was challenged. These new challenges led to the exhumation of the story of Dinah, and in particular, the version of the inter-uterine exchange.[54] Based on the story of the inter-uterine exchange, Dinah also had two possible mothers—the "genetic" mother (Rachel, who conceived her), and the birth mother (Leah, who bore her). According to this version, who was the legal mother of Dinah? Both Leah and Rachel contributed to Dinah's birth, but which carried the halakhic seal of maternity?

Contrary to popular belief, the use of the story of Dinah for halakhic purposes did not begin with the development of surrogate

---

54. The story of the inter-uterine exchange was also used for halakhic purposes to determine paternity in artificial insemination. See. R. Y. Z. Mintzberg, "Artificial Insemination," *Noam* 1 (5718) [1958], 159. To my knowledge he is the only authority to use the source in this way. This source is mentioned by R. Bick in his "Ovum Donations: A Rabbinic Conceptual Model of Maternity," *Tradition* 28:1 (Fall 1993), 28–45. See comments on R. Mintzberg's analysis by R. Y. Ben-Maier, "In Vitro Fertilization: The Relationship of the Child to the Gestational or Biological Mother," (Hebrew) *Assia* 41 (*Nisan*, 5746) [April, 1986], 25–40, at n. 8.

motherhood in the late twentieth century. The halakhic exhumation of this story began in the early twentieth century with a little-known halakhic episode whose reverberations are still felt in the halakhic literature to this very day. In 1907, in the halakhic journal *Vayelaket Yosef*, a question was posed by R. Yaakov Gordon for forum discussion:

> Physicians have developed a new procedure to treat infertility through the transplantation of reproductive organs from one woman to another. Who is the halakhic mother in this case? Would it be the donor or the recipient?

This question was not fictional but was based on a case of ovarian transplantation that had been performed successfully on an infertile woman a year earlier, with the resulting birth of a healthy child. This remarkable case—and its medical, ethical, and halakhic ramifications—is discussed elsewhere in this book,[55] but for our present purposes, it is the first time in medical history that the definition of maternity became subject to debate.

In the case of ovarian transplantation, one woman's ovarian tissue, containing the genetic material, was transplanted into the abdominal cavity of another woman. This woman then conceived and delivered a child with the donor's eggs. Who would be the halakhic mother in this case? This was one of the questions considered by the rabbis of that generation. In this historical narrative, we find, for the first time, the mention of the story of Dinah in a practical halakhic context.[56] The story was then revisited in the late twentieth century with the development of surrogate motherhood for the treatment of infertility. This section treats these two periods separately. In the more recent discussions of surrogate motherhood, the story of Dinah is frequently mentioned,

---

55. See chapter, "The First Halakhic Discussion of Ovarian Transplantation."
56. R. Bleich writes that the first to use the aggadic discussion of Dinah's birth in a halakhic discussion was R. Menasheh Grossberg in an article dated 5684 [1923]. See his "Maternal Identity Revisited," *Tradition* 28:2 (Winter 1994). R. Grossberg, like the others cited here, is addressing the case of ovarian transplantation. The literature cited here predates 5684.

though significantly downplayed, as more primary halakhic sources have superseded the non-halakhic material.

The Halakhic Discussion of Ovarian Transplantation

In providing halakhic responses to the new procedure for the treatment of infertility, ovarian transplantation, a number of authorities in the early twentieth century invoked the story of Dinah to solve the maternity riddle. However, despite utilizing the same story of the inter-uterine exchange, divergent conclusions were drawn.

Some used the inter-uterine exchange to assert that the birth mother is the halakhic mother. For example, R. Eliyahu Posek, author of *Mor Ve'Ahalot*, cites the *Targum Yonatan* and the *piyyut "Even Ḥug"* of R. Eliezer HaKalir confirming the inter-uterine exchange.[57] He further notes that Dinah is called the daughter of Leah and Yosef the son of Rachel. He interprets this to mean that the birth mother is the halakhic mother.[58]

R. Betzalel Zev Shafran (1866–1930)[59] arrives at a similar conclusion that the birth mother is the halakhic mother based on the inter-uterine exchange of Dinah and Yosef. The Torah clearly states, "and it was that Rachel gave birth to Yosef," and also, "Dinah the daughter of Leah." The Torah teaches us thereby that the birth mother is the true halakhic mother. He adds that there is nothing that is not hinted to in the Torah.

---

57. *Ohel Yitzḥak*, Year 5, Vol. 4 (*Tevet*, 5667) [December, 1906], p. 4. This was a response to the question posed by R. Yaakov Gordon in the previous issue of *Ohel Yitzḥak*, Year 5, Vol. 3 (*Kislev*, 5667) [November, 1906], p. 4. R. Gordon apparently sent this question to multiple journals. When I initially wrote on the halakhic chapter of ovarian transplantation, I was unaware of the articles in *Ohel Yitzḥak* and thought the halakhic exchange in *Vayelaket Yosef*, initiated by R. Gordon's question as well, to be the first on the topic. The question of R. Gordon in *Ohel Yitzḥak* (December, 1906) predates that printed in *Vayelaket Yosef* by almost a year and appeared some seven months after the case report of a successful ovarian transplantation by Dr. R. T. Morris was published.

58. The *pesak* of R. Posek is cited approvingly by R. Tzvi Hirsch Friedling in *HaBe'er*, Year 6, vol. 3 (5691) [1931].

59. *Teshuvot HaRabaz E. H.*, 5. He also cites R. Ḥ. Y. D. Azulai as utilizing the inter-uterine exchange to interpret a talmudic passage in his *Devash l'fi*, s. v., *"ayin hara."*

R. Moshe Yosef Roth[60] brings the inter-uterine exchange discussion from the *Paneaḥ Raza*, who comments on the identity of *Shaul ben HaKena'anit* and the question of how Shimon could marry Dinah. The *Paneaḥ Raza's* conclusion is that Dinah is halakhically the daughter of Rachel, the "genetic" mother. R. Roth therefore concludes that the ovarian donor would be the halakhic mother.[61] The same conclusion is echoed by R. Menashe Grossberg.[62]

There is one authority that discounts the use of the inter-uterine exchange, but not on halakhic grounds; rather, on purely technical grounds based on his novel interpretation of the exchange. R. Avraham Yaakov HaLevi Horowitz, in his *Tzur Yaakov*,[63] suggests a variation on the inter-uterine exchange. He claims that the physical bodies did not switch between the wombs of Leah and Rachel; rather, the male child within Leah changed to a female, and the female child within Rachel became a male. Only the souls switched after the gender changes took effect. Therefore, this story cannot be used to ascertain maternity in the case of ovarian transplantation. He bases this, in part, on the time of ensoulment. The soul of a child is bestowed upon conception. Therefore, the soul of Yosef was bestowed when he was conceived by Leah. The soul was later transferred to the male child carried by Rachel.

Contemporary Discussions of Surrogate Motherhood and the Definition of Maternity

The story of the inter-uterine exchange has also been incorporated into the contemporary halakhic discussions about the definition of maternity

---

60. *Tel Talpiyot*, Year 17, vol. 21 (*Tammuz*, 5668) [July, 1908], n. 176, p. 192.

61. See R. Menashe Klein, a contemporary *posek*, *Mishneh Halakhot Mahadura Tinyana Y. D.*, 436, who discusses uterus transplantation and uses the inter-uterine exchange in his analysis.

62. See *Sha'arei Torah, Sha'ar Menashe* 15 (5684) [1924], n. 3. R. Bleich mentions this source in his *Contemporary Halakhic Problems* 2 (Ktav, 1983), 91–93, but does not mention the context of this halakhic discussion and the entire discussion of ovarian transplantation. See also R. Yehonatan Halevi Eyebeshutz in *HaB'er*, Year 8, v. 3 (*Sivan* 5693) [June, 1933], 80, who cites R. Grossberg. In a response to R. Grossberg, R. Joshua Feigenbaum (*Sha'arei Torah* 15:4) rejects the proof of R. Grossberg, claiming that one cannot derive halakha from aggadic sources. This is also cited by R. Bleich.

63. N. 28.

in cases of surrogate motherhood.[64] Here, too, varying conclusions are drawn from the same sources. The story, however, has generally received less halakhic weight in this second, later halakhic discussion and has been largely supplanted by more purely halakhically oriented sources, with some exceptions.

R. Moshe Hershler[65] and R. Moshe HaLevi Soloveitchik[66] utilize the story for halakhic purposes and claim that based on the inter-uterine exchange, it is the birth mother who is the halakhic mother. As the Torah says, "and afterwards she bore a daughter," this implies, R. Hershler asserts, that only after the birth of the child was Dinah halakhically called Leah's daughter. Furthermore, R. Hershler adds, we have no proof whatsoever to consider the genetic mother (or egg donor) to be the mother. R. Hershler maintains that while we generally do not derive halakha from aggadic sources, we can use aggadic sources to support a logically derived conclusion (*sevara*), as is the case here. The issue of deriving halakha from aggadic sources pervades the discussions regarding the extrapolation from the story of the birth of Dinah to modern medical halakha.[67]

R. Avraham Yitzhak HaLevi Kilav[68] cites the inter-uterine exchange briefly, and while acknowledging that we do not derive halakha from aggadic sources, he nonetheless derives one principle from the story—that one can only have one halakhic mother. R. Yaakov Ariel[69] likewise minimizes the utility of the inter-uterine exchange story due to its non-halakhic nature, as well as the disparate versions of the events.

---

64. There are dozens of articles in the halakhic literature on the definition of maternity in cases of surrogate motherhood. For reviews of the major positions, see A. Steinberg, *Entzyclopedia Hilkhatit Refuit* 2 (Schlesinger Institute, 1991), s. v., "*hafraya hutz gufit*"; Abraham S. Abraham, *Nishmat Avraham* 3 (Schlesinger Institute, 2007), 30–40.

65. *Halakha URefua* 1 (Jerusalem, 5740 [1980]), 319–320.

66. "Test Tube Babies," (Hebrew) *Or HaMizrah* 100 (5741) [1981], 122–128.

67. On this topic, see A. Steinberg, *Entzyclopedia Hilkhatit Refuit* 2 (Schlesinger Institute, 1991), 135, at n. 63; Abraham. S. Abraham, *Nishmat Avraham* 3 (Schlesinger Institute, 2007), 36; I. Bernstein, "Learning Halacha from Aggadah," *Journal of Halacha and Contemporary Society* 70 (Fall 2015), 47–79.

68. *Tehumin* 5, 260–267.

69. *Tehumin* 16, 171–180.

R. Moshe Sternbuch rejects the application of the inter-uterine exchange to contemporary halakha, but not due to concern about deriving halakha from aggadic sources. He claims that we cannot derive halakha from miraculous events. R. Sternbuch maintains that logic dictates that the egg donor should be the halakhic mother. The miraculous uprooting of Dinah from Rachel's womb severed that natural maternal connection. We therefore cannot learn from this case.

More attention is given to the story of the inter-uterine exchange by R. Yisrael Meir Lau.[70] Citing the issue of Dinah's marriage to Shimon, R. Lau marshals the inter-uterine exchange in support of identifying the genetic mother as the halakhic mother. He notes that this contradicts the conclusion derived from a talmudic source[71] that the birth mother is the halakhic mother but posits that this latter ruling applies only when the original maternal-fetal connection was abrogated, as in the talmudic case of conversion.

R. Lau also raises a question that challenges the veracity of the inter-uterine exchange. If, as discussed above, Shimon was able to marry Dinah because Dinah was really the child of Rachel, then Yosef should likewise be considered the legal child of Leah, in whose womb he was conceived. The Torah seems to reject both assertions. First, Dinah is referred to explicitly as *"bat Leah,"* (daughter of Leah) and furthermore, the Torah refers to Binyamin as Yosef's maternal brother—*"Vayar et Binyamin aḥiv ben imo"* (and he saw his brother, Binyamin, his mother's son). R. Ben-Maier[72] adds another verse clearly indicating that Yosef was the child of Rachel and casting doubt on the inter-uterine exchange, "and the children of Rachel were Yosef and Binyamin."[73]

---

70. *Yaḥel Yisrael* 3:89.

71. *Yevamot* 97b.

72. R. Y. Ben-Maier, "In Vitro Fertilization: The Relationship of the Child to the Gestational or Biological Mother," (Hebrew) *Assia* 41 (*Nisan,* 5746) [April, 1986], 25–40, at n. 8. R. Ben-Maier brings an opinion from R. Shlomo Min HaHar that all these proofs are fruitless, as the terms *"ben," "bat,"* and *"yalda"* do not specifically refer to a biological relationship and are used in the Torah also to refer to simply raising a child.

73. Bereshit 35:24.

In 1981, in an early discussion on maternity in surrogate motherhood, R. Bleich mentions the inter-uterine exchange to support the position that maternal identity is determined by conception, but concludes that halakha cannot be derived from aggadic sources.[74] A decade later,[75] he cites the use of the inter-uterine exchange to support the halakhic opinion in favor of the birth mother, but does not consider the aggadic source dispositive. R. Ezra Bick addresses the story in his legal analysis and response to R. Bleich's 1991 article,[76] and brings the Tur's explanation as to how Shimon could have married Dinah as proof that maternity is derived by genetics/conception (see above section on *Shaul ben HaKena'anit*). While R. Bick states that "this is, to the best of my knowledge, the only classical halakhic source relevant to this question," he does not believe it sufficient to adjudicate the matter. He also accepts the principle that halakha cannot be based on aggadic sources, but limits this to directly applying halakha from a specific aggadic statement. He does believe and advocate that aggadic principles in general be used to guide or inform halakhic decisions in cases where no other relevant halakhic material exists, as he believes to be the case for the definition of maternity.

Additionally, R. Meir Brandsdorfer,[77] despite reaffirming the principle that halakha cannot be derived from aggadic sources, devotes a lengthy discussion to the story of Dinah and its implications for the determination of maternity. He concludes that while some erroneously infer from the story of the inter-uterine exchange that the birth mother is the halakhic mother, the story actually confirms, though cannot be used to prove, that the genetic mother, or egg donor, is the halakhic mother.

---

74. *Tradition* 19:4 (Winter 1981), 359–360.
75. R. J. David Bleich, "In Vitro Fertilization: Questions of Maternal Identity and Conversion," *Tradition* 25:4 (Summer 1991), 82–102. This article was a rebuttal to R. Bick's article in *Tradition* cited above. R. Bleich devotes little attention to the aggadic story of Dinah's birth in his extensive writings on the definition of maternity in halakha and focuses primarily on halakhic material.
76. E. Bick, "Ovum Donations: A Rabbinic Conceptual Model of Maternity," *Tradition* 28:1 (Fall 1993), 28–45.
77. R. Meir Brandsdorfer, "Egg Donation and the *Yiḥus* of the Child," (Hebrew) *Yeshurun* 21 (*Nisan*, 5769) [April, 2009], 557–564.

V. CONCLUSION

In this chapter, we have explored the different aggadic versions of the birth of Dinah and have discussed the use of this story both in the exegetical and halakhic literatures. With new and unforeseen advances in medicine, finding halakhic precedent is challenging. Contemporary rabbinic authorities, in the absence of other clear precedent, often turn to aggadic, non-halakhic material. The use of this material can shed light on the issues and possibly, with limitations, may be used for halakhic purposes. However, its use is also fraught with potential difficulty. Each instance must be analyzed independently. With regard to the use of the story of Dinah for the determination of maternity in halakha, the consensus amongst rabbinic authorities is that we do not place great weight upon this aggadic source. This is because of the general principle of not deriving halakha from aggadic sources, coupled with the conflicting conclusions drawn from this particular source by earlier scholars. This essay clearly illustrates the latter point. Herein, we have shown that there are not only many aggadic versions of the birth of Dinah, but even those who accept the inter-uterine exchange version derive different halakhic conclusions from the story. In sum, *tzarikh iyun ledina*, with its intended double entendre. Clarification is required for the law (*dina*) of maternity in surrogate motherhood; and clarification is also required for the aggadic story of Dinah's birth.

The First Halakhic Discussion of Ovarian Transplantation

I. INTRODUCTION

In contemporary discussions on issues relating to reproductive technology and infertility, a number of rabbinic authorities refer to a previous series of exchanges in the history of medical halakha. This narrative, consisting of both medical and halakhic literature, may be unfamiliar to the modern reader. But unlike other narratives in the history of medical halakha, such as the use of mummies for medicinal purposes in the sixteenth and seventeenth centuries,[1] or the treatment of smallpox in the eighteenth and nineteenth centuries,[2] which recount the use of now obsolete medical practices, this narrative is directly applicable to contemporary halakhic discussions of current and future issues in reproductive technology. Reviewing the halakhic literature of this narrative and placing it in its rightful historical context, as well as appreciating the

---

1. See chapter, "The Impact of Medieval Medicine on Medical Halakha: The Case of Mumia."
2. See chapter, "Lessons from the First Halakhic Analysis of Vaccination."

specifc medical understanding of each author, will hopefully facilitate the proper use of this material for modern medical halakhic discourse.

II. THE HALAKHIC DISCUSSION OF
OVARIAN TRANSPLANTATION

R. Eliezer Waldenberg,[3] in a series of responsa written in the 1960s on marital issues, questions whether a woman who had undergone a uterine transplant is obligated to inform her potential suitors of her operation. He cites earlier authorities who address the halakhic ramifications of such a surgery and address the definition of maternity for the resulting offspring. In 1971, R. Yitzḥak Isaac Liebes, in the context of his expansive essay on the halakhic issues of organ transplantation,[4] discusses the issues unique to ovarian transplantation, citing earlier halakhic literature on this topic. R. Azriel Rosenfeld, in a number of articles in the 1970s,[5] uses the literature on ovarian transplantation to explore the issues of gene design and human identity. Also in the 1970s, R. J. David Bleich, addressing the then new advances in assisted reproduction, draws on the literature of this little known halakhic narrative to solve the issue of maternal identity in surrogate motherhood.[6] More recently, R. Waldenberg relies on this literature in deciding the halakhic maternal identity in a case of surrogate motherhood,[7] Dr. Fred Rosner incorporates it into his discussion of sex organ transplants,[8] and R. Dr. Mordechai Halperin cites it in an article discussing the use of donated genetic material in assisted reproduction.[9]

---

3. *Tzitz Eliezer* v. 7, sect. 48, chap. 5, n. 16.
4. Y. I. Liebes, *"Be'Inyan Hashtalat Evarim,"* *Noam* 14 (Jerusalem, 5731), 28–111, esp. 86–109.
5. A. Rosenfeld, "Judaism and Gene Design," *Tradition* 13:2 (Fall 1972), 71–80; idem, "Human Identity: Halakhic Issues," *Tradition* 16:3 (Spring 1977), 58–72. I thank Dr. Joel Wolowelsky for directing me to these sources.
6. J. D. Bleich, *Contemporary Halakhic Problems* 1 (Ktav, 1977), 106–109.
7. *Tzitz Eliezer*, v. 20, sect. 49. The responsum is dated 5753.
8. F. Rosner, *Modern Medicine and Jewish Ethics*, 2nd ed. (Ktav, 1991), 115–118.
9. M. Halperin, *"Trumat Ḥomer Geneti BeTipulei Poriyut,"* in the *HaKinus HaBenleumi HaSheni: Refua, Etika VeHalakha* (Schlesinger Institute, 1996), 321–327.

As neither uterine nor ovarian transplants were performed at the time that the aforementioned rabbis were writing (in the 1970's), to what could these authorities have been referring? Are these simply hypothetical discussions for the sake of halakhic clarification, or do they have a basis in medical reality? All the aforementioned sources refer to an earlier halakhic discussion. When was this earlier body of halakhic literature written, and why? Was it composed as a halakhic intellectual exercise, or was it perhaps a response to medical and scientific advances?

Unbeknownst to many a modern reader, physicians and scientists of the late nineteenth and early twentieth centuries experimented with human ovarian transplantation, with variable success. Already from the earliest stages of experimentation, rabbinic authorities began to address the attendant halakhic ramifications. It is to this halakhic narrative, which spans roughly twenty-five years and comprises the core of this chapter, to which the aforementioned authorities refer. While the focus of this book is to highlight the importance of a medical historical approach, due to the potential value of this literature for contemporary discussions, the entire corpus of halakhic literature on ovarian transplantation is discussed in great detail.

The core section is preceded by an historical overview of ovarian transplantation, thus facilitating an appreciation of the medical context of the halakhic discussions,[10] and is followed by a discussion of the application of the early halakhic sources on ovarian transplantation to modern dilemmas. This chapter concludes with a brief look at the current state of ovarian transplantation, pondering the potential application of the aforementioned halakhic literature to future halakhic dilemmas.

III. MEDICAL HISTORY OF OVARIAN TRANSPLANTATION

Before beginning a focused discussion on the history of ovarian transplantation in the late nineteenth and early twentieth centuries, I should like to preface with a few remarks on the status of reproductive physiology and genetics during this time period. Despite the microscopic visualization of

---

10. Only the historical aspects of ovarian transplantation relevant to the halakhic discussions will be presented. The footnotes will refer the reader to sources for further study.

the human spermatozoa and ovarian follicle in the late seventeenth century, confusion still persisted regarding the respective roles of the male and female seeds in conception and heredity.[11] It was not until 1827 that the human female egg was directly visualized for the first time by Ernst von Baer, and it was only in the late nineteenth and early twentieth centuries that the process of reproduction was understood on a cellular level. Simultaneous with the research in reproductive physiology evolved the field of genetics and research into the heredity of human characteristics.[12] Although Gregor Mendel's classic study on plant hybridization was published in 1866, it lay unnoticed until 1900, the year that marks the beginning of the modern period of the study of heredity.[13] Already in the early twentieth century chromosomes were understood to be the material responsible for heredity, but it was only in 1953 that Watson and Crick first described the molecular structure of DNA.[14] Concurrent with the basic science research in the fields of reproductive physiology and genetics, clinicians during this period were also experimenting in the field of clinical reproductive medicine.

In the late nineteenth century, physicians were grappling with ways to overcome the ravages of gynecological disease. In cases of diseased ovaries or Fallopian tubes, the affected organs were usually surgically removed, not only rendering the patient infertile, but also subjecting her to early menopause. In 1895, Dr. Robert Tuttle Morris (1857–1945)[15]

---

11. See J. Needham, *A History of Embryology* (Abelard Shuman, 1959). On the Jewish sources on embryology and the contributions of the male and female seeds see chapter, "The Rabbinic Conception of Conception: An Exercise in Fertility."

12. See J. A. Peters, ed., *Classic Papers in Genetics* (Prentice-Hall, 1959) and C. Stern and E. R. Sherwood, eds., *The Origin of Genetics: A Mendel Sourcebook* (W. H. Freeman, 1966).

13. See R. A. Fisher, "Has Mendel's Work Been Rediscovered," in Stern and Sherwood, op. cit., 139–171.

14. J. D. Watson and F. H. C. Crick, "Molecular Structure of Nucleic Acids: A Structure for Deoxyribose Nucleic Acid," *Nature* 171 (1953), 737–738. Later that year, the authors proposed the chemical mechanism by which cells passed on their character accurately. See idem, "Genetic Implications of the Structure of Deoxyribonucleic Acid," *Nature* 171 (1953), 964–967.

15. For more information on Morris, see his autobiography, *Fifty Years a Surgeon* (E. P. Dutton, 1935). In chapter 15, entitled "Gland Grafting," Morris recalls his experiences with ovarian transplantation. On Morris and the general history of ovarian

postulated that transplanting a small piece of functioning ovary into a patient who had undergone bilateral ovary removal would alleviate the untoward symptoms of menopause, and possibly restore menstruation and fertility.[16] The donor tissue, he theorized, could either derive from the residual functioning ovarian tissue of the patient herself (i.e., auto-transplant), or from a functioning ovary of another patient (i.e., hetero-transplant). Regarding the reestablishment of fertility in these patients, the theory was that eggs would be spontaneously ovulated from these graft sites and would encounter the sperm in either the Fallopian tubes or uterus, as in a normal case of spontaneous conception.

Later that year, Morris reported the results of two successful ovar-ian transplants: one autotransplant, after which the patient subsequently became pregnant and aborted in the third month, and one heterotransplant,[17] after which the patient resumed menstruation but did not conceive.[18]

Two aspects of Morris' technique are important for our discus-sion, the size and location of the transplant. Only a pea-sized section of ovary was removed from the donor, with apparently no residual effect

---

transplantation, see H. H. Simmer, "Robert Tuttle Morris (1857–1945): A Pioneer in Ovarian Transplants," *Obstetrics and Gynecology* 35:2 (February, 1970), 314–328; V. C. Medvei, *The History of Clinical Endocrinology* (Carnforth, 1993), 203–206.

16. Morris first reported this novel idea in his *Lectures on Appendicitis and Notes on Other Subjects* (G. R. Putnam's Sons, 1895), before he had actually performed any such procedures.

17. A note on clarification of terminology is in order. Two forms of ovarian transplant were performed by Morris and his peers. One procedure involved the removal and replantation of a piece of the patient's own ovary, referred to in the literature interchangeably as auto- or homotransplant; the other procedure, of concern for our discussion, involved the transplantation of a donor ovary, or part thereof, into the patient, referred to interchangeably as homo- or heterotransplant. In this article, I will use the terms autotransplant and heterotransplant exclusively. In addition, throughout the medical literature on this topic, the terms grafting, implantation and transplantation are used interchangeably to refer to either auto- or heterotransplant. Articles bearing the words "ovarian transplant" in the title may deal exclusively with autotransplant. See, for example, W. S. Bainbridge, "Transplantation of Human Ovaries: Present Status and Future Possibilities," *American Journal of Obstetrics and Gynecology* 5:5 (May, 1923), 493–498.

18. R. T. Morris, "The Ovarian Graft," *New York Medical Journal* 62 (1895), 436.

on her fertility.[19] This small section was surgically implanted into one of three possible locations: the uterus, Fallopian tubes or peritoneum.[20] No other organs were transplanted, and the transplanted piece of ovary was placed deep within the pelvic organs.

In the subsequent years, a number of physicians performed research in the field of heterotransplantion, some reporting cases where the woman regained menstruation,[21] but in 1906, Morris reported a case that sent shock waves throughout the medical community. In 1902, Morris had treated a woman with polycystic ovary disease.[22] After completely removing both of the patient's ovaries with a surgical instrument designed specifically for this procedure,[23] Morris then transplanted a small piece of another woman's ovary into the peritoneum of the patient.[24] Four months later, the patient resumed menstruation, in 1905, she became pregnant, and on March 15, 1906, she delivered a baby girl weighing seven and one half pounds. In addition to Morris' personal account of this case,[25] extensive reports appeared in the French and English literature.[26]

---

19. As one ovary was entirely untouched, and the other, from which the small section was removed, remained structurally intact, there is no reason to assume that the fertility of the donor would be affected. However, as the physicians were not concerned about the donors' subsequent history, they did not comment on their subsequent fertility.

20. R. T. Morris, "Notes on Ovarian Grafting," *Medical Record* 57 (January, 1901), 83–87, esp. 85.

21. See F. H. Martin, "Transplantation of Ovaries," *Surgery, Gynecology and Obstetrics* 7 (1908), 7–21, for a report on Martin's personal cases as well as a review of the literature until that time. F. H. Martin was a pioneer in the field of ovarian transplantation and wrote extensively on the topic.

22. I do not refer here to the disease known today as polycystic ovaries (PCO), as that would be anachronistic. Rather, I simply refer to the pathological description of the ovaries by Morris.

23. The instrument was called Truffier's angiotribe, after Theodore Truffier (1857–1929), a French surgeon who pioneered the field of ovarian autotransplantation.

24. Hermann Boldt operated on the donor for uterine prolapse, and a small wedge of ovary was removed at that time in order to alleviate what was believed in those days to be ovarian congestion. See Morris' autobiography, op. cit., 217.

25. R. T. Morris, "A Case of Heteroplastic Ovarian Grafting Followed by Pregnancy and the Birth of a Living Child," *Medical Record* 69:18 (May 5, 1906), 697.

26. See Simmer, op. cit., 320, for references.

Many physicians doubted the veracity of the case, and even Morris himself was skeptical about the conclusions that could be drawn from it. Morris, as well as others, wondered whether some of the patient's own ovarian tissue had remained after the initial surgery.[27] In fact, pregnancy had been observed in cases where allegedly both ovaries were removed, and no transplant was performed.[28] Morris further speculated that a heterotransplant might stimulate activity of previously latent ovarian cells in the patient.[29]

Aside from the scientific critique of the case, it spawned numerous discussions on the ethical and legal ramifications of transplanting an ovary from one woman to another. One article in an English journal presented a discussion addressing the question of who is considered the mother of the child.[30] Dr. Freeland Barbour opined that from a medicolegal point of view, the lawyer would require an exploratory incision in order to satisfy himself that all the recipient's ovarian tissue had been removed before giving an opinion. Mr. Scott Carmichael concurred, claiming, "the crux of the whole matter was whether the ovaries had been completely excised."[31]

One group of respondents believed the donor of the ovary to be the mother. Dr. Paterson likened the organ recipient to an incubator,

---

27. See Morris' autobiography, op. cit., 215–216. Morris, however, was fairly certain that he had removed both ovaries, especially since he had used Truffier's angiotribe. In addition, Dr. Boldt, who was present at the operation, later testified that he had seen Morris remove both ovaries completely. See Simmer, op. cit., 321.

28. J. A. Robertson, "A Renewal of Menstruation and Subsequent Pregnancy After Removal of Both Ovaries," *British Medical Journal* 2 (1890), 722 (cited by Simmer). In 1901 Morris addressed this issue extensively, in his "Notes on Ovarian Grafting," *Medical Record* 57 (January, 1901), 83–87, esp. 83–84.

29. These thoughts were later published in his autobiography, *Fifty Years a Surgeon* (E. P. Dutton, 1935), 220.

30. J. H. Croom, "A Case of Heteroplastic Ovarian Grafting, Followed by Pregnancy and a Living Child: Query—Who Is the Mother?" *Transactions of the Edinburgh Obstetrical Society* 31 (1906), 194–200. The article begins by reviewing the facts of the case, then opens the question of maternity for forum discussion. The case is clearly that of Morris, but all the participants are referred to by initials only. The surgeon who removed the ovarian tissue from the donor is called Dr. B., likely referring to Dr. Hermann, but, interestingly, there is no mention of a Dr. M (i.e., Morris).

31. Croom, op. cit., 196–197.

claiming that since the life of the ovum was given to it by the donor, the donor should be considered the mother of the child.[32] Dr. Dewar also considered the ovary donor to be the mother, rendering the child (offspring of the father and another woman, not his wife) illegitimate and possibly unable to collect inheritance. Professor Croom concurred, adding, "that when a man married a woman her ovaries belonged to him; and even after they were transferred to another woman they were still his. So the offspring of the second woman must be a bastard."[33]

Others contended that the recipient, or gestational mother, was the mother, since once the ovary was removed, "it no longer belonged to the woman who supplied the graft, but had become an integral part of the woman who bore the child."[34] Dr. Taylor added that since the law does not recognize a child until after the occurrence of quickening, the only possible legal mother is the one who gave birth to the child. [35]

Some suggested observing the child as she grows, to see which mother's characteristics she develops.[36] Dr. Darling remarked that it would be easier to determine maternity if one of the mothers was white, and the other black.[37]

Morris himself mentioned some of the concerns that were voiced by others regarding ovarian heterotransplantation.[38] One of his patients wanted to know whether the ovary donor was a Methodist or Episcopalian,[39] and others objected to the procedure because the child would have "treble parentage."[40] Lawyers were concerned that such interventions would confuse the laws of entitlement of property.[41]

While work in the field of ovarian transplantation continued for a number of decades after the publication of Morris' case report, the

---

32. However, he added, if the recipient had purchased the ovary, the response might be different.
33. Croom, op. cit., 199.
34. Ibid., 198.
35. Ibid., 199.
36. Ibid., 198–200.
37. Ibid., 198.
38. See his autobiography, op. cit., 211–224.
39. Ibid., 215.
40. Ibid., 217. The phrase "treble parentage" was used by Simmer, op. cit., 321.
41. Ibid., 216.

research was largely restricted to autotransplantation.[42] A number of authors mention, *inter alia*, that conception had been known to occur in cases of heterotransplantation, but they provide no documentation.[43] It is possible that these references all refer to Morris' one case report.

Despite the immense popularity this case enjoyed shortly after its publication, it seems to have been quickly forgotten. Even Fielding Garrison, whose classic work on the history of medicine was first published in 1913, does not mention Morris' case report, let alone his general contribution to the field of ovarian transplantation.[44] In 1934, Dr. Edward Richardson, in his comments on an article on ovarian transplantation, states that "so far as I know, pregnancy following actual transplantation of ovarian tissue has not been achieved."[45]

In 1970, Hans Simmer wrote, in reference to Morris' case report, that "doubts remain about the validity of this case, especially, since as far as can be determined, in no other instance of human ovarian homo-transplant (i.e., heterotransplant) has pregnancy ensued."[46]

In conclusion, it appears that despite the intense medical research in the field of ovarian transplantation in the late nineteenth and early twentieth centuries, there is only one recorded case in the entire medical literature, albeit of questionable veracity, of pregnancy and live birth following an ovarian transplant (i.e., heterotransplant).[47] This case, which

---

42. See, for example, W. S. Bainbridge, "Transplantation of Human Ovaries: Present Status and Future Possibilities," *American Journal of Obstetrics and Gynecology* 5:5 (May 1923), 493–498; W. L. Estes Jr. and P. L. Heitmeyer, "Pregnancy Following Ovarian Implantation," *American Journal of Surgery* 24:3 (June, 1934), 563–581. See also Simmer, op. cit., 324.

43. F. H. Martin does make specific mention of Morris' case in his "Transplantation of Ovaries," *Surgery, Gynecology and Obstetrics* 7 (1908), 14. See also F. H. Martin, "Ovarian Transplantation in Lower Animals and Women: Review of the Literature and Bibliography," *Surgery, Gynecology and Obstetrics* 13 (1911), 53–63, where he quotes Mauclaire as stating that conception had occurred after auto- and heterotransplantation in animals as well as human beings. The same unsupported statement was made twelve years later by Bainbridge, op. cit., 498.

44. Simmer, op. cit., 316.

45. Richardson's note is appended to the 1934 article of Estes, op. cit.

46. Simmer, op. cit., 321.

47. There have been a number of recorded cases of pregnancy associated with autotransplant. See, for example, Estes, op. cit.

briefly sparked intense scientific debate and ethical discussion, was soon forgotten.[48] Research in the field of human ovarian heterotransplantation continued for some years after Morris' case report, with only limited success, and was essentially abandoned after the 1920s.[49]

IV. THE HALAKHA OF OVARIAN TRANSPLANTATION

The halakhic sources on ovarian transplantation deal exclusively with heterotransplantation, and are not a product of rabbinic imagination, but a response to a new medical development. The earliest halakhic responses to this new procedure appeared in a series of articles in two European journals spanning from 1907–1908. As the practice of ovarian transplant was in its infancy at this time, the authors are uniformly skeptical of the success, not to mention reality, of the procedure. In addition, their unfamiliarity with the medical facts is betrayed by the nature of their halakhic concerns.

The issue of ovarian transplantation resurfaced again in halakhic literature in the late 1920s to early 1930s, with two rabbinic scholars independently addressing the topic, followed by a series of articles in another European journal. As there was only one reported case, in 1906, of human ovarian transplantation followed by a live birth, it is unclear what precipitated the renewed interest in the topic at this time. Either the rabbinic authorities were addressing the continued research in heterotransplantation, or they were only then informed of the earlier discussions of Morris' case report. Some sources, such as R. Kamelhar's response below, confirm the latter possibility. With some exceptions, the discussants in this later stage fail to mention the existence of the earlier halakhic literature. Yet, these authors address the identical halakhic issues, even utilizing some of the same proof texts. In addition, since by this time the understanding of reproductive physiology had progressed, the rabbinic authorities of this period are significantly more familiar with

---

48. Hans Simmer is responsible for rescuing these early accounts from oblivion and granting Morris the rightful title as the first surgeon to successfully transplant human ovarian tissue. See Medvei, op. cit.

49. E. S. Taylor, *The History of the American Gynecological Society 1876–1981 and American Association of Obstetricians and Gynecologists 1888–1981* (Mosby Publishers, 1985), 94.

the medical facts. Although some medical ambiguities are scattered throughout their remarks, on the whole, they are less skeptical and more knowledgeable about ovarian transplantation than their predecessors. It will be evident that the rabbinic authorities shared many of the same factual, legal and ethical concerns as their medical counterparts.

Exchange in Vayelaket Yosef

It appears that the earliest halakhic reference to ovarian transplantation is found in the pages of *Vayelaket Yosef,* a Hungarian journal edited by Yosef Schwartz.[50] In an article published in 1907,[51] roughly one year after Morris' famous case report, R. Yaakov Gordon of England informs the readers of a new medical procedure involving the transplantation of reproductive organs from one female to another infertile female, enabling the latter to conceive.[52] Without elaborating on the details of the procedure, he ponders its halakhic implications: can one perform a transplant from mother to daughter? Is the resulting progeny considered a halakhic *bekhor* (first born)? Who is the halakhic mother, the donor or the recipient? After cursorily alluding to his own theories on the topic, R. Gordon invites a forum discussion.

The first respondent, R. Eliezer Deutch, head of the Bonyhád rabbinical court, assumes that the entire set of female reproductive organs, including the external genitalia, is transplanted in the procedure. As discussed above, only the ovary, or a part thereof, was actually transplanted. This misconception likely resulted from the ambiguity of R. Gordon's initial question. The question posed to the rabbinic authorities states that the "female reproductive organs" were transplanted, and raises the issue of *bekhor,* since in this case the "uterus belongs to another woman." As the medical literature on ovarian transplantation was unavailable to the rabbis of Eastern Europe, and the details

---

50. On the history of this journal, see I. Lewin, *Otzar Kitvei Et Torani'im* (New York, 5740), 88–95.

51. Year 10, vol. 3 (15 Ḥeshvan, 5668–October 23, 1907), 9a–9b.

52. R. Gordon states that ovarian transplantation with subsequent live birth had occurred in his country. In fact, there are no such recorded cases from England. R. Gordon is probably referring to the reports of Morris' case which appeared in the British literature. See, for example, the above discussion on Croom's article.

of the procedure were unknown to them, each simply responded to the question as it was presented, or as he understood it. The modern reader must realize that R. Deutch operates with this misconception in order to appreciate his halakhic concerns and analyses. For example, since R. Deutch believed that the external genitalia were included in the transplant, he is concerned with the issue of *erva*, as the husband would be having direct sexual contact with the reproductive organs of an *eshet ish* (another married woman).[53] R. Deutch considers this case to be halakhically comparable to having relations with a corpse; an act, although reprehensible and perhaps rabbinically prohibited, nonetheless does not constitute a biblical violation of *erva*.[54] The organs, once removed from the donor, are simply inanimate limbs of a corpse, rendering the prohibition of *erva* inapplicable to them.[55] Had R. Deutch known that only the ovary was transplanted, and that there would be no direct contact with it during marital relations, he may not have been concerned with the issue of *erva*.[56] He further concludes that, without question, and in all respects, the transplanted organs halakhically

---

53. Of course, we don't know for sure that the donor is married, but as the prohibition is biblical in nature, it is assumed so until proven otherwise. In addition, since the donor presumably had children, it is a reasonable assumption that she is married. There is no discussion about how halakha would view a circumstance where the donor was non-Jewish. See comments of R. Weinreb below in section from the journal *HaBe'er*.

54. *Yevamot* 55b and Maimonides, *Hil. Issurei Bi'ah* 1:12.

55. The respondent acknowledges that in the case of a man having relations with a complete corpse, there is a rabbinic prohibition which was instituted to prevent one from extrapolating that, amongst other things, relations with a *treifa* would be permitted. However, once the body is no longer whole, as in this case, the decree would not apply. In addition, he argues that it must be the living body that generates *erva*, and not simply the reproductive organs. For if it were the latter, one could envision a scenario whereby one could circumvent the prohibition of *erva* with a woman by replacing her reproductive organs with those of a non-*erva*. Furthermore, he argues, that if the reproductive organs were the determinant for *erva*, doubt would be cast on all legal cases of *erva*. It would impossible for witnesses to ever verify whether the reproductive organs of the female were in fact her own, or those of a non-*erva*.

56. R. Deutch might still have been concerned with the issue of *erva*, as others in the discussion address the issue of *ervah* even while acknowledging that the transplanted organs are far from sexual contact.

become part of the recipient's body. This conclusion would likely not be affected by the aforementioned misconception.

In the next issue of *Vayelaket Yosef*[57] R. Deutch addresses the issue of *bekhor*. *Ḥullin* 70a brings a hypothetical case where the birth canal is so wide that the fetus can exit without direct physical contact with the uterine (or vaginal) walls. Is the air space of the uterus sufficient to generate the status of *bekhor*, the Gemara queries, or is direct physical contact with the uterine walls required? Maimonides maintains that the fetus in this case would be a *safek bekhor* (doubtful firstborn).[58] In our case, according to R. Deutch, the uterine walls belong to the donor, while the air space belongs to the recipient. Therefore, a child born to the organ recipient would be the first to pass through the air space of her birth canal, and, according to this logic, would likewise be considered a *safek bekhor*.[59] Here, too, R. Deutch's misconception regarding the nature of the procedure impacts on his halakhic analysis. Had he understood that only a piece of ovarian tissue was transplanted, and that the uterus and external genitalia of the recipient remained intact, then the issue of *bekhor* would not be in doubt. As both the air space and the uterine walls would belong to the recipient, she would clearly determine the *bekhor* status of the child. This would not be a *safek bekhor*, but a *vaday bekhor* (certain firstborn).

Despite his reasoned response, R. Deutch still doubts the medical reality of such a transplant, advancing a rabbinic proof for this position. According to the Gemara, Sarah the Matriarch was infertile due to congenital absence of her uterus.[60] Had transplantation of reproductive organs been possible, he argues, there would have been no need for

---

57. Year 10, vol. 4 (1 *Kislev* 5668–November 7, 1907), 12a–12b.
58. *Hil. Bekhorot* 4:19.
59. Since the procedure is done for infertility, it is assumed that the recipient had no previous children. In fact, ovarian transplant was sometimes performed exclusively to preserve normal female hormonal production in previously fertile women.

R. Deutch does not consider the transplanted organs to be a halakhic barrier to the uterine air space of the recipient. He bases this on the principle that *min bemino aino hotzetz* (i.e., like substances do not constitute a halakhic barrier).
60. *Yevamot* 64b bases this on the extraneous phrase *"ein la valad."* in *Bereshit* 11:30.

God to perform a miracle to reverse Sarah's infertility.[61] He concludes by saying that would it not have been for his respect for the questioner, he would not have answered such a ridiculous query. As mentioned above, many physicians at that time also questioned the veracity of the case report of human ovarian heterotransplantation.

The discussion continues in the journal in two subsequent issues. Citing a passage from *Ḥullin*,[62] R. Sheftel Weiss believed that he had found a remarkable talmudic analogue to our case of reproductive organ transplantation.[63] In the talmudic hypothetical, the uteri of two animals are adjacent to each other and the fetus moves from one uterus to the second before being born.[64] The Gemara ponders for which animal would this fetus be considered a *bekhor*. R. S. Weiss does not elaborate, however, as to how this passage would be practically applied to our case.[65]

---

61. This reasoning seems to negate the notion of advancement in medicine and science. If such a procedure can be done today, the author argues, it must have been able to be done in the time of Sarah. While God's powers are infinite and eternal, one must acknowledge that man's ability to cure disease has undergone an evolutionary process. During the historical period of Sarah, the contemporary medical treatments would have been ineffective for congenital absence of the uterus. It was therefore necessary for God to intervene with the performance of a miracle. If God wished to bestow the gift of fertility on someone today, it might be done through a physician specializing in reproductive medicine.

62. 70a. This passage immediately follows the passage mentioned above by R. Deutch. It is interesting that R. Deutch chose not to cite it.

63. Year 10, vol. 6 (Ḥanukka 5668–December, 1907), 21b.

64. It is unclear from the passage where the exact point of contact is. *Tosafot* s. v., "*ad*" in *Ketubot* 4b considers this case to be purely hypothetical ("*davar shelo ba le'olam*").

65. The Gemara considers this a case of *teiku* (i.e., no clear solution) and Maimonides, *Hil. Bekhorot* 4:18 considers it a *safek bekhor* to the second animal (and presumably for the first as well). Applying the logic of R. Deutch above, we might consider the offspring in our case to be a *safek bekhor* to both mothers, therefore requiring a *pidyon haben* from both husbands. One could argue, however, how comparable this case is to ours. In the case of the Gemara, the fetus exits two separate uteri, each of independent halakhic status. It is, therefore, theoretically possible for both animals to have produced a *bekhor*. In our case, there is only one uterus, the status of which is in question. If the status of the uterus were clarified, there would only be one possible candidate for the *bekhor*. However, it is even possible in our case, I believe, to envision a dual *bekhor* status. The status would not be conveyed sequentially, as in the case of the Gemara, but simultaneously. The Gemara debates whether the walls of the uterus or the air space of the uterus generates the status of *bekhor*, and

Two additional concerns are briefly raised by R. S. Weiss, the prohibition of deriving benefit from a corpse,[66] and the issue of submitting to a procedure involving halakhically questionable risk.[67]

The final note on this topic in the journal was authored by R. Binyamin Arye Weiss.[68] According to R. Weiss, if this procedure would be medically possible, which he doubts, it would be halakhically forbidden to undergo, for even if there were no danger to the patients involved, the donor would be undergoing sterilization (*sirus*), a prohibition which, at the very least, is of rabbinic origin.[69] R. Weiss, like the other respondents in the journal, apparently believed that the entire set

---

Maimonides, as discussed above, considers this a *safek*. In our case, according to the conception of R. Deutch, the walls of the uterus belong to the donor, while the air space of the uterus belong to the recipient. When the fetus exits, it may therefore be simultaneously considered a *bekhor* to both women.

66. It is unclear whether the respondents believe the donation to be postmortem or from a living donor. Assumedly, R. Weiss believes it to be postmortem.

67. Regarding the permissibility of undergoing risky or unproved therapy see J. D. Bleich, "Experimental Procedures: The Concept of *Refu'ah Bedukah*," in his *Contemporary Halakhic Problems* 4 (Ktav, 1995), 203–217.

68. Year 10, vol. 9, no. 77 (*Shevat*, 5668; January, 1908), 29a. This response to R. Schwartz was subsequently published in R. Weiss' *Even Yekara*, n. 29.

69. The biblical origin for the prohibition of sterilization, or *sirus*, is Vayikra 22:24–25. The context of the biblical discussion is the prohibition of using castrated or sterilized male animals for temple sacrifice. The *Midrash Sifra*, chapter 7, extends the prohibition to all animals, both kosher and non-kosher, and the Gemara, in *Shabbat* 110b, extends the prohibition to human beings as well. To what extent this prohibition applies to females of the human species is a matter of debate. Maimonides in *Hil. Issurei Bi'ah* 16:10–11 implies that sterilization for women is only rabbinically prohibited, while *Turei Zahav, Even HaEzer* 5:6, claims that the prohibition of sterilization does not apply to women at all. For further discussion, see Joseph Ozarowski, "Tubal Ligation and Jewish Law," *Journal of Halacha and Contemporary Society* 7 (Spring 1984), 42; J. David Bleich, "Sterilization of Women," in his *Contemporary Halakhic Problems* 1 (Ktav, 1977), 96–99; Shaul Weinreb, "Tubal Ligation and the Prohibition of *Sirus*," *Journal of Halacha and Contemporary Society* 40 (Fall 2000), 5; R. Moshe Feinstein, "Women Whose Health is Endangered by Pregnancy and the Halakhah of *Sirus* for Women," in R. Moshe Hershler, ed., *Halakha URefua*, 1 (Regensberg Institute, 1980), 328–331 (Hebrew); R. Moshe Hershler, "Removing a Woman's Reproductive Organs (hysterectomy)," in R. Moshe Hershler, ed., *Halakha URefua*, 1 (Regensberg Institute, 1980), 332–335 (Hebrew); R. Yehuda Leib Gordon, "Sirus (sterilization) of a Woman," in R. Moshe Hershler, ed., *Halakha URefua* 4 (Regensberg Institute,

of reproductive organs, including both of the ovaries, was removed from the donor for transplantation. Consequently, the issue of *sirus* is without question applicable to the donor. However, had R. Weiss known that only a small piece of ovarian tissue was removed from the donor, and that the donor likely retained her fertility, he may have questioned the applicability of the laws of *sirus* to this case.[70]

If, however, one already underwent the procedure, R. Weiss adds, the halakhic mother of the offspring would be the organ recipient. R. Weiss brings proof for this position from the case in *Sota* 43b, where a branch of an *orla* tree, which is less than three years old and forbidden to eat, is grafted onto an older tree, whose fruit is permitted. The Gemara concludes that for halakhic purposes the branch becomes an integral part of the receiving tree and loses its original identity. Here, too, the transplanted organs would lose their identity and become an integral part of the recipient's body. The recipient would therefore be considered the sole halakhic mother. This argument, that once the organs are removed, they no longer belong to the donor, but become an integral part of the recipient, was advanced by physicians in their discussions on this topic as well.[71]

R. Weiss' comments are brief, and he does not elaborate exactly how the case of *orla* is applied to the case of ovarian transplantation. He makes no mention as to how he understands the nature of the donor's contribution to the subsequent offspring,[72] a point which is crucial to whether or how one can extrapolate from R. Weiss' responsum to contemporary discussions, as will be discussed below.

1985), 34–35 (Hebrew); R. Moshe Feinstein, "Hysterectomy and Oophorectomy and Sirus," in R. Moshe Hershler, ed., *Halakha URefua* 4 (Regensberg Institute, 1985), 112–113 (Hebrew).

70. While one can argue that any manipulation of the reproductive organs constitutes a violation of *sirus*, some authorities invoke *sirus* only in the presence of infertility. In any case, as many authorities consider *sirus* for a woman to be only rabbinically prohibited, this added fact that the woman in this case retains her fertility would at least have caused R. Weiss to entertain some doubt about the applicability of *sirus* to the donor in an ovarian transplant.

71. See above discussion on the history of ovarian transplantation.

72. See section below on R. Kamelhar, who also applies the analogy from *orla*, but is more explicit regarding his understanding of the donor's contribution.

Exchange in Tel Talpiyot[73]

A similar exchange of ideas on the topic of transplantation of the repro-ductive organs appeared in another Hungarian journal, *Tel Talpiyot,*[74] just a few months later. The discussion is introduced by the identical question of R. Gordon, and is followed by the response of R. Eliezer Deutch, verbatim as they appeared in *Vayelaket Yosef.*[75] In a footnote to R. Deutch's remarks, the editor argues against the latter's conclusion that the recipient is considered the sole mother, claiming that both the donor and the recipient have significant contributory roles (i.e., *zeh v'zeh gorem*). In addition, he rejects the halakhic comparison of the transplanted limbs to the limb of a corpse, for while the latter is cold and lifeless; the transplanted organs are rejuvenated in the recipient and restored to life. Sexual contact with such organs would be prohibited. He therefore considers the recipient to be a *safek erva*, in which case she would be forbidden to her husband.

The second respondent, R. Yeshaya Silverstein, head of the rabbinical court in Veitzen, likewise concludes that the transplanted organs, for halakhic purposes, become part of the recipient's body. He adduces proof from a passage in *Bekhorot* 28b regarding the *treifa* status of an animal whose uterus has been removed. In support of the position that such an animal is not a *treifa*, the Gemara mentions the practice in Alexandria, Egypt of removing the uteri of the cattle that were sold or exported.[76] Since these animals obviously lived for prolonged periods of time after the procedure (longer than twelve months), this is proof that the absence of a uterus does not consti-tute a *treifa*. R. Silverstein questions the Gemara's proof. If, by defi-nition, the absence of a particular organ constitutes a *treifa*, then the

---

73. For information on this journal see I. Lewin, op. cit., 305–306.

74. Year 17, no. 19 (*Sivan*, 5668–June, 1908), 169–171.

75. The response of R. Deutch spanned two issues in *Vayelaket Yosef.* Only the first part or R. Deutch's response is published in *Tel Talpiot.* It is possible that the editor of the latter journal read the initial discussion in *Vayelaket Yosef* and published the query and first response in his journal in order to generate further discourse.

76. The cattle from this region were considered of superior quality. Removing the uterus would prevent the buyer from using the animal for breeding, thereby insuring the seller's control of the market.

animal's subsequent lifespan is irrelevant. Even should such an animal live longer than twelve months, it would still be considered a *treifa*.[77] R. Silverstein therefore understands the proof of the Gemara that the reason absence of the uterus is not a *treifa* is because the condition can be reversed with the transplantation of a uterus from another animal. *Treifa*, by definition, only applies to an irreversible ailment. If the removed organ can be effectively replaced, then its absence does not constitute a *treifa*.[78] After transplantation the animal could return to complete health and fertility. Furthermore, the transplanted organs must be considered part of the recipient in order to sustain this proof; otherwise, the recipient would still be halakhically considered to have missing organs.

If one believed, as R. Silverstein and R. Deutch did, that the uterus was transplanted, then this proof is particularly salient. However, despite the fact that this was not the case, this analysis is still applicable to ovarian, or any organ transplant.

R. Silverstein brings further proof from the laws of *nidda*. One of the requirements for generating the *tum'ah* (impurity) of *nidda* is for the woman to actually sense the menstrual flow "*bivsara*" (in her flesh) as it exits her body.[79] In a case of transplantation of the reproductive organs, one might argue that the menstrual flow of the recipient would not be felt "in her flesh," as the organs are not hers, but those of the donor. This cannot be, contends R. Silverstein, as this would effectively circumvent all the laws of *nidda*. Rather, the organs become part of the recipient's

---

77. This is the position of R. Yeḥezkel Landau in his commentary *Dagul MeR'vava*, Y. D., 29.
78. This proof is perplexing since the entire purpose for removing the uterus was to prevent subsequent fertility of the animal. It seems clear that in Alexandria they assumed the effects of uterine removal to be irreversible. Of note, Alexandria was the major center of anatomical studies in antiquity. See, for example, essay of Ludwig Edelstein entitled "The History of Anatomy in Antiquity" in his *Ancient Medicine* (Johns Hopkins University Press, 1967), 247–301; H. Von Staden, *Herophilus: The Art of Medicine in Early Alexandria* (Cambridge University Press, 1993).
79. This halakha is derived from the term "*bivsara*" (her flesh) in Vayikra 15:19. See *Nidda* 57b and Y. D., 183:1.

body such that any flow would be considered "in her flesh."[80] This latter proof confirms that R. Silverstein believed, as R. Deutch, that the entire set of reproductive organs would be included in the transplant. Had he understood that the uterus and outflow tract of the menstrual blood remained intact in the recipient, this analysis would have been irrelevant.

The final response, by R. David Tzvi Katzburg, the journal's editor, is introduced with three prefatory comments. He first asserts that the progeny should be considered that of the birth mother (i.e., the one in whose body the fetus gestated), and not that of the organ donor, because the offspring is a composite of material from the entire body, and not just the reproductive organs. The seed, originating from the brain, travels via the spinal cord to the genital area. This notion (that the seed is a composite of material from the entire body) explains why children resemble their parents. Consequently, as the transplanted reproductive organs play only a minor role in the process of conception, the organ donor is eliminated as a candidate for maternity. The recipient, from whose entire body the seed is derived, is the only logical halakhic (and physiological) mother.

This discourse on reproductive physiology may seem enigmatic to the modern reader, as we currently understand that the embryo is formed from an equal contribution of genetic material (DNA) from a man and a woman. The parental resemblance is explained by the transmission of one's genes to one's offspring. This understanding, however, is a product of the mid-twentieth century. Prior to this period, there were a number of co-existing theories, dating back to antiquity, regarding the composition and contribution of the male and female seeds. The author actually combines two of these theories in his comment. The encephalo-myelogenic doctrine claimed that the seed originated in the brain and traveled via the spinal cord to the genital organs. Hippocrates advanced the so-called pangenesis doctrine, claiming that the seed was derivative

---

80. Today, we understand sensation to be dependent on innervation. Even if uterine transplant were possible, the severed sensory nerves could not regain their function in the recipient. Even if the transplanted organs were halakhically considered an integral part of the recipient's body, the recipient would still be unable to actually sense the menstrual flow.

from material from the entire body. Part of his logic for advancing this theory was based on the observation that offspring can resemble their parents in all bodily aspects. He, therefore, postulated that the parent must in fact be transferring material from each part of their body to their offspring. The author here alludes to this reasoning.[81]

R. Katzburg's second preface addresses the veracity of the scientific information of the query. Doubting that any successful transplant of the reproductive organs could have occurred, especially since such a revolutionary procedure would surely have been more widely publicized, he postulates that it was likely an unsuccessful experiment about which R. Gordon had heard. Nonetheless, unable to verify the facts, he hazards an educated guess as to what form of transplant would have been done.[82] He categorically dismisses the notion that the external genitalia were included in the transplant for two reasons. First, as these structures are unlikely to contribute to infertility, there would be no need to replace them. Second, it is unlikely that a woman would willingly suffer the pain of such a radical surgical procedure. He therefore postulates that the organ which was transplanted was the uterus. It is the uterus, he contends, that can prolapse outside the body and can therefore be easily excised

---

81. For more comprehensive treatment on the history of reproductive physiology as found in rabbinic sources see chapter, "The Rabbinic Conception of Conception: An Exercise in Fertility."

82. In the ensuing discussion the editor employs the rabbinic terms for the female reproductive anatomy: *prozdor, aliya,* and *mekor (ḥeder).* These terms are derived from the Mishna in *Nidda* 2:5. While the *mekor* clearly refers to the uterus, there has been much debate regarding the exact anatomical definitions of the former two terms. I shall avoid the use of these terms to prevent ambiguity, as the nuances of the definitions are not relevant to our discussion. For further discussion about the identification of these terms see, for example, Julius Preuss, *Biblical and Talmudic Medicine,* trans. F. Rosner (Hebrew Publishing Company, 1978), 115–19; Abraham S. Abraham, *Nishmat Avraham, Yoreh Deʾah* (Jerusalem, 1985), 76–79; I. M. Levinger, "*HaMivneh HaʾAnatomi shel Evarei HaMin Beʾisha UVeBaʾalei Ḥayyim,*" *Koroth* 4: 8–10 (June 1968): 611–15; Tirzah Z. Meachum, "Mishna Tractate Nidda with Introduction: A Critical Edition with Notes on Variants, Commentary, Redaction and Chapters in Legal History and Realia," (unpublished doctoral dissertation: Hebrew University, 1989), 224–231; M. Halperin, *Realia and Medicine in Seder Nashim* (Schlesinger Institute, 2011), 3–40 (Hebrew).

and replaced.[83] In addition, as the uterus houses the fetus and is adjacent to the ovaries and Fallopian tubes, its malfunction can lead to infertility. It therefore follows that this is the organ that the physicians would transplant.

While the editor's logic with respect to the transplantation of the external genitalia is correct, he nonetheless erred in his assumption that the uterus would be transplanted. As is evident from our historical discussion, it is the ovary, or part thereof, that was in fact transplanted. As with R. Deutch and R. Silverstein, one cannot fault R. Katzburg for not knowing the details of the ovarian transplantation. The relevant medical literature was unavailable to him, and he simply responded to the question as he saw fit. Nonetheless, it is important to be aware of this misconception when extrapolating from these sources.

---

83. He cites *Nidda* 41b which discusses a case where a woman's uterus becomes detached. The passage describes the fate of the uterus as *venafal la'aretz*. This could mean that the uterus falls in the direction of the ground, consistent with a case of prolapse, but this seems unlikely given the context of the passage. The phrase appears to be taken literally, that the uterus actually falls to the ground. Preuss, op. cit., 378, considers this passage to be a purely theoretical discussion. In any case, the author proves from here that the uterus is easily accessible for surgical removal and replacement.

There is, however, another passage, in *Ḥullin* 70a, that, to my mind, directly refers to a case of prolapsed uterus. The context is a discussion on the requirements for generating the status of *bekhor*. Amongst a series of different cases testing the nuances of the law, the following case is brought: *"ne'ekru kotlei beit harehem, mahu?"* What would the halakha be, the Gemara asks, if the walls of the uterus were *"ne'ekar,"* the same word used in the passage in *Nidda* 41b. The Gemara then continues, "How does one define *ne'ekru*? When the uterus is detached but still hanging from its neck." How else could one define the term? Rashi (s. v., *"ne'ekru"*) clarifies that one might have thought that *"ne'ekru"* means that the uterus actually fell to the ground, therefore the Gemara has to tell us that the uterus is still connected. I believe Rashi is implicitly alluding to the aforementioned case in *Nidda*. While making it clear that the passage in *Nidda* refers to a uterus fallen to the ground, this passage is itself an excellent description of a prolapsed uterus. Prolapse of the uterus in pregnancy, although uncommon, has been documented. See, for example, J. P. Lavery, et al., "Uterine Prolapse with Pregnancy," *Obstetrics and Gynecology* 42:5 (November, 1973), 681–3; P. S. Hill, "Uterine Prolapse Complicating Pregnancy: A Case Report," *Journal of Reproductive Medicine* 29:8 (August,1984), 631–3. Whether the case of the Gemara is actual or theoretical has no bearing on the halakhic discussion.

The third prefatory remark includes a number of rabbinic references to cases where objects are severed and reconnected. The common denominator in all the cases is that the objects may again be considered halakhically whole. The editor infers from these sources that in our case of transplantation the organs would be considered an integral part of the recipient.

Having presented his conceptual framework, the editor addresses the halakhic issues of the query. Regarding the prohibition of *erva*, it is evident to him that only the recipient's status is relevant. As the uterus becomes an integral part of the recipient, the status of the donor is irrelevant.[84]

Furthermore, in addressing the permissibility of transplanting a woman's uterus into her daughter, the editor compares the case of uterine transplant to the case of bathhouse insemination.[85] In the latter case, even if the woman were a *nidda*, the status of a *ben nidda* would not be conferred upon the child, since no illicit sexual activity took place. Likewise, he claims, in the case of uterine transplant, even though the uterus originally derived from the woman's mother, a person considered an *erva* for the husband, since the uterus becomes an integral part of the daughter's body, the husband is not technically considered to be having illicit relations with his mother-in-law.[86]

---

84. Since according to this author, only the uterus, and not the external genitalia, is transplanted, he could have dismissed the problem of *erva* by claiming that there would be no direct sexual contact with the transplanted organ. We must therefore assume one of two possibilities. Either the editor thought that the cervix was also transplanted, in which case there could potentially be direct sexual contact with the transplanted organs; or, the prohibition of *erva* can theoretically apply even without direct physical contact, as long as the organs of an *erva* are somehow involved. See below, comments of R. Weinreb in section from the journal *HaBe'er*.

85. This possibility of bathhouse insemination is first mentioned in *Ḥagiga* 14b–15a. For treatment of the sources on bathhouse insemination and artificial insemination, see chapter, "Rabbinic Conception of Conception."

86. Both cases involve a theoretically illicit union that, by virtue of unique circumstances, is not considered halakhically forbidden. But the comparison ends there. The analogy may have been somewhat better had the author invoked the case of Ben Sira, who was believed to have been the product of the seeds of the prophet Jeremiah and his own daughter, a biblically forbidden union, after the latter conceived in the bathhouse. Despite the mixture of seed of those considered *erva* to each other, due to

In the final section of this article R. Katzburg discusses the issue of *bekhor*. He claims that even though this uterus, while part of the donor, had already borne fruit and previously yielded a *bekhor*, since it takes on a new identity in the recipient, the first born for the recipient with the transplanted uterus would be considered a halakhic *bekhor*. Furthermore, he contends that the reason a caesarean birth precludes *bekhor* status is because the fetus must exit naturally through the birth canal.[87] In our case, since only the uterus is transplanted, the birth canal was always part of the recipient's body. Therefore, a child born after the transplant would in fact be the first child to exit the recipient's birth canal (assuming she had no children before the procedure).

As mentioned above regarding R. Deutch's remarks on the issue of *bekhor*, this discussion is rendered superfluous with the understanding that only the ovarian tissue is transplanted.

Two additional responses to R. Gordon's query appeared in a subsequent issue of the journal.[88] R. Yeraḥmiel Katzburg, while questioning the veracity of the medical account, is in agreement with the editor's comments on the response of R. Deutch and believes this to be a case of *zeh v'zeh gorem* (two entities contributing equally). He marshals support from the biblical stories of the Matriarchs' infertility.[89] According

---

the absence of illicit sexual contact, no prohibition was considered violated. All the more so here, in a similar case of biblical *erva*, since only the uterus is transplanted, and there is no direct mixture of seed, nor direct sexual contact with the transplanted organ, no prohibition should be considered violated. For more on the case of Ben Sira see chapter, "Rabbinic Conception of Conception."

87. The Mishna in *Bekhorot* 47b excludes a child born by caesarean section from the laws of *bekhor*. The law is codified in *Y. D.*, 305:24. Regarding the history of caesarean section in Jewish sources see chapter, "A Matter of Life 'in' Death: Postmortem Caesarean Section in Jewish Law."

88. Year 17, no. 21 (*Tammuz*, 5668–July, 1908), 191–192.

89. This is an elaboration of the same proof brought by R. Deutch above. R. Deutch mentions that Sara suffered from congenital absence of her uterus. R. Yitzḥak Yaakov Weiss, in his *Teshuvot Minḥat Yitzḥak* vol. 1, no. 125 (cited in Bleich, *Contemporary Halakhic Problems* 3 [Ktav, 1989], 124) claims that Rachel suffered from the same condition. The verse in Bereshit 29:31 describes Rachel as an "*akara*," and Rashi in *Yevamot* 42b states that the term "*akara*" is used to describe a woman who is sterile due to absence of her uterus. One could therefore apply R. Deutch's argument to the case of Rachel as well.

to rabbinic tradition God reversed the normal course of nature and "opened the wombs" of the Matriarchs. If a "natural" remedy, such as transplantation of the reproductive organs, were possible then why was it necessary for God to change the course of nature? It therefore must be that even if such a procedure were possible, the offspring would not be related exclusively to the gestational, or birth, mother. Therefore, the transplanted organs retain their independent status in the recipient. As a result, there would be a prohibition of *erva* with the donor. In addition, he rejects the editor's comparison to the case of bathhouse insemination, since in our case, as opposed to bathhouse insemination, there is actual sexual contact. He goes so far as to say that the woman might require a new marriage contract (*ketuba*) with her husband.

R. Moshe Yosef Roth offers a novel support to the position that the organ donor is the sole halakhic mother. In *Sefer Paneaḥ Raza* on *Vayigash*[90] the question is raised as to how Shimon could have married his sister Dinah.[91] Marriage of maternal siblings is forbidden even according to the Noachide laws.[92] He answers that according to tradition, Leah conceived a boy, and Rachel a girl. Through the prayers of Leah, the two were switched in utero such that Leah gave birth to a girl (Dinah), and Rachel to a boy (Yosef). Rachel is analogous to the donor in our case, having donated her fetus (and possibly uterus) to Leah, and Leah is likened to the recipient, having received the female fetus from Rachel.[93] Since Dinah was conceived

---

90. See also *Paneaḥ Raza* on *Vayetzei*, s. v., "*v'aḥar yalda bat.*"
91. This discussion is based on Bereshit 46:10 which mentions one of the children of Shimon to be *Shaul ben HaKena'anit*. The commentaries note that since Avraham was so adamant that his son not marry a woman from Canaan, it would be unlikely that Shimon would have actually married a Canaanite woman. It is therefore explained that the term *hakena'anit* refers to Dinah, as Dinah had refused to leave the city of Shechem after being raped unless Shimon agreed to marry her. This child is a product of that marriage. See commentaries of R. Eliyahu Mizraḥi, *Re'em*, ad loc. and R. Yaakov ben Asher, *Ba'al HaTurim*, ad loc. For further discussion of this topic, see chapter, "Midrash, Miracles, and Motherhood: The Birth of Dinah and the Definition of Maternity."
92. Maimonides, *Hil. Issurei Bi'ah* 14:10.
93. Although the author does not detail the analogy clearly, there is actually a double transplant, each person being both the donor of a fetus (and possibly uterus) and the recipient of a fetus.

by Rachel, Rachel is considered her halakhic mother, even though Leah was the birth mother. Therefore, since Shimon's halakhic mother was Leah and Dinah's halakhic mother was Rachel, they were only paternal siblings, and consequently permitted to marry. We therefore see that with respect to *erva*, it is the donor of the organs who determines the status.[94]

It is unclear to me how this proof of R. Roth is to be applied to our case of ovarian transplantation. In the biblical case, Rachel donates a complete fetus. What does R. Roth consider the donor's contribution to be in the case of ovarian transplantation? He must assume that the donor provides at least some material contribution, although it was too early in the history of genetics for R. Roth to have understood the female's genetic contribution. Not all the rabbinic authorities accepted the notion that the donor provided a material contribution to the subsequent child.

---

94. *Berakhot* 60a, as well as the *Yerushalmi Berakhot* 9:3 and *Midrash Tanḥuma* on *Vayetzei*, n. 8, claim that the fetus of Leah underwent a sex change from male to female, but none mentions any transfer or transplant between Rachel and Leah. Rashi quotes the *Talmud Bavli* in his commentary to Bereshit 30:21. The first mention of an actual transfer is in Targum Yonatan ben Uziel on this same verse. The author here quotes *Sefer Paneaḥ Raza* as the source for this notion, as does R. Eliyahu Mizraḥi (*Re'em* on Bereshit 46:10) and *Maharsha* on *Nidda* 31a, s. v., "*v'et*." They were perhaps unfamiliar with the passage in the Targum Yonatan. The *Maharsha* adds an additional textual support that a transfer actually took place from a line in the *piyyut* "*Even Ḥug*" which is recited on the first day of Rosh Hashanah (*Complete Artscoll Machzor for Rosh Hashanah*, Mesorah Publications, 1985, p. 312). R. Moshe Margliot (d. 1781), in his commentary *Mareh HaPanim* on the aforementioned passage in the *Yerushalmi* acknowledges the conflict of sources and also mentions the support from the *piyyut* of "*Even Ḥug*." R. Meir Simcha of Dvinsk explains two difficult biblical passages based on the notion that there was an inter-uterine transfer between Rachel and Leah. See *Meshekh Ḥokhma* on *Vayeishev*, s. v., "*veyadeinu*" and on *Vayigash*, s. v., "*bnei Rachel... asher*." See also R. Yosef Patsanovski's *Pardes Yosef* on *Vayetzei*, s. v., "*uvetargum*" for similar examples of exegesis and further sources on this topic.

Some of the above sources are mentioned in the subsequent discussions on ovarian transplant (see below), as well as in contemporary discussions on maternal identity in the case of surrogate motherhood. For an expansive treatment of the different midrashic approaches to the births of Dinah and Yosef, see chapter, "Midrash, Miracles, and Motherhood: The Birth of Dinah and the Definition of Maternity."

R. Betzalel Zev Shafran (1866–1930)

The next to discuss reproductive organ transplantation in detail is R. Shafran, a noted Rumanian rabbi and talmudic scholar, whose comments were recorded posthumously by his son.[95] In contradistinction to his predecessors, R. Shafran's knowledge of the medical facts is more precise, as by this time, some twenty years after the initial halakhic discussions, the procedure of ovarian transplant had been more widely practiced and publicized. He understood that only the ovary was transplanted, and not the uterus or external genitalia. The fundamental halakhic question, however, remained the same; who is the mother of the child?

R. Shafran makes no mention of the aforementioned halakhic interchange and offers his own opinion. To answer the question, he invokes the *Targum Yonatan ben Uziel* that Dinah, conceived by Rachel, and Yosef, conceived by Leah, underwent an inter-uterine transfer such that Rachel gave birth to Yosef and Leah to Dinah.[96] Despite being conceived in the womb of Rachel, the Torah considers Dinah to be the daughter of Leah.[97] This is clear proof, he contends, that the birth mother, not the donor of the ovary, is considered the mother. Although using the same analogy to the inter-uterine exchange as R. Roth above, R. Shafran arrives at the exact opposite conclusion.

Regarding the issue of *erva*, R. Shafran is concerned that the process somehow involves an *eshet ish* (married woman) and concludes that the matter requires further thought. He beseeches the great rabbis of his generation to address this issue more fully.

---

95. *Teshuvot HaRabaz, Teshuvot Miben HaMeḥaber*, n. 5. For a contemporary discussion of the responsum of R. Betzalel Shafran by his grandson, see E. Safran, "The Power of the Womb, the Power of Prayer," https://www.ou.org/torah/parsha/parsha-from-ou/power-womb-power-prayer/ (accessed November 25, 2017).

96. R. Shafran cites a passage from *Sefer Devash L'fi* (letter *ayin*, s. v., "*ayin hara*") of R. Ḥ. Y. D. Azulai, who applies this notion to interpret a rabbinic expression. R. Shafran himself explains a phrase in Bereshit 37:27 based on this notion. R. Meir Simcha of Dvinsk explains the phrase similarly. See *Meshekh Ḥokhma*, op. cit.

97. Bereshit 34:1.

Rabbi Yekutiel Kamelhar (1871–1937)[98]

R. Kamelhar's contribution to this debate can be found in his classic work, *"HaTalmud U'Mada'ei HaTevel,"*[99] where he mentions that at a medical conference in Chicago in 5671 (1910–1911) doctors discussed a case in which a woman gave birth to a child after undergoing an ovarian transplant.[100] He then offers his halakhic opinion of this case. Like R. Shafran, he is familiar with the medical realities of ovarian transplantation yet does not reference any previous halakhic discussions on the topic.[101] In his introductory comments, however, he is unclear as to which woman has the primary impact on the fetus. While acknowledging a possible role of the donated ovary in the subsequent conception, he seriously entertains the possibility that the transplanted ovary might stimulate the natural fertility of the recipient without providing

---

98. On R. Kamelhar see C. Roth, ed., *Encyclopedia Judaica* 10 (Keter Publishing House), 724; Y. Mundshein, *HaTzofeh LeDoro: Toldot Ḥayav UPa'alo shel HaRav Yekutiel Aryeh Kamelhar* (Reuven Mass Publishers, 5747).

99. (Lvov, 1928), 44–45.

100. Dr. F. H. Martin, Professor of Gynecology at the Post Graduate Medical School of Chicago, made a presentation at the American Gynecological Association's annual meeting in Atlantic City on May 24, 1911 (correlating to 5671), on the topic of ovarian transplantation, which was subsequently published in *Surgery, Gynecology and Obstetrics* 13 (1911), 53–63, and in the *Transactions of the American Gynecological Society* 36 (1911), 337–359. (I thank Jeffrey Anderson, librarian of the American College of Physicians in Philadelphia, for the latter reference.) Dr. Shnayer Leiman has suggested that this is the presentation referred to by Kamelhar, only he confused the city of origin of the author with the location of the conference. Martin only briefly makes reference to Morris' case report in his presentation but does not report any other cases of pregnancy following ovarian heterotransplantation. In Stewart's history of the American Gynecological Society he mentions three conferences (in 1908, 1917 and 1922) where papers on ovarian transplantation were presented. His discussions of the conferences of 1910 and 1911, which correlate to the Jewish year 5671, do not mention any papers on the topic. However, Stewart merely addresses the highlights of the conferences, but does not give a comprehensive list of the presentations. See E. S. Taylor, *The History of the American Gynecological Society 1876–1981 and American Association of Obstetricians and Gynecologists 188–1981* (Mosby Publishers, 1985), 22–23, 26–27, 94.

101. R. Kamelhar was also unaware of R. Shafran's opinion. Although R. Shafran's comments preceded 1928, the publication year of R. Kamelhar's work, they were only first published in the 1930's.

any material contribution, in which case the recipient would be the sole halakhic mother. This theory is reminiscent of Dr. Morris' comment that heterotransplant might stimulate the patient's own ovarian cells.

R. Kamelhar draws on a number of rabbinic discussions which he believes are comparable to ovarian transplantation. The first is an agricultural analogy based on a passage in *Sota* 43b which discusses the impact of tree grafting on the laws of *orla*. R. Kamelhar, perhaps unaware that R. Binyamin Weiss had earlier applied the same analogy, reaches the same conclusion that just as the grafted branch loses its original status and becomes an integral part of the post-*orla* tree,[102] likewise, in our case, the transplanted ovary loses its original status and becomes an integral part of the recipient's body. The birth mother is therefore the sole halakhic mother, and no violation of *erva* is incurred.

The second relevant rabbinic discussion is found in *Ḥullin* (79a–b) regarding whether the male seed is considered to be of halakhic significance when determining the halakhic status of a hybrid animal (*im hosheshin lezera ha'av*)[103] R. Kamelhar opines that both sides of this debate would agree that in the case of ovarian transplant the recipient is the halakhic mother. Those who maintain that the male seed is insignificant would surely hold likewise for the donated ovary. If the male seed, which clearly has an independent role in conception, is not deemed significant, all the more so the donated ovary, which has no independent role in conception, and either stimulates the natural conception of the recipient, or simply serves as a receptacle for her seed, both merely peripheral contributions.

---

102. R. Kamelhar cites the *Tosafot* in *Avoda Zara* 49a, s. v., "*she'im*" that the conclusion of the Gemara is sustained even by those who would normally hold *zeh v'zeh gorem*, since in this case the original status of the grafted branch becomes completely nullified, as the term "*batla*" used by the Gemara indicates. The original *orla* tree therefore has no contributory role whatsoever in the new entity. He also cites *Menaḥot* 69b that "*hakol holekh aḥar ha'ikar*" (the status is determined by the major or predominating element of a mixture). The passage mentions a series of cases where plants of different halakhic status are grafted onto each other. The Gemara does not conclude, as R. Kamalhar indicates, that "*hakol holekh aḥar ha'ikar*," rather, the passage ends with a *teiku* and the assumption is that one should take the stringent view in all cases.

103. This debate refers to animals, but R. Kamelhar applies it to human beings as well.

Even those who grant significance to the male seed, R. Kamelhar continues, would still not necessarily bestow such significance to the donated ovary. After all, while the male seed has an active role in conception (it is *molid*), the transplanted ovary, dissociated from the donor, is merely a receptacle which could easily have been artificial. Surely an artificial organ could have no halakhic significance, nor could such an organ be considered a halakhic mother. Without the seed of the recipient, and the physiological environment of her body, the transplanted ovary would be useless. The halakha therefore must be that the woman who gave her seed and gave birth to the child is considered the halakhic mother.

From the above analysis, it is clear that R. Kamelhar adopts the position that the donor in an ovarian transplant has no material contribution to the fetus, a position likewise entertained by contemporary physicians, as discussed above. He does not seriously consider the possibility that the egg is provided by the transplanted ovary.

The third rabbinic dictum which R. Kamelhar believes bears relevance to our case is that regarding birds which grow on trees (a.k.a. barnacle goose).[104] R. Yosef Karo in *Shulḥan Arukh*[105] categorizes these creatures as crawling insects and forbids their consumption. Even though the creatures originate from the seed of birds, since the tree, which is the dominant element (*ikar*), gives forth the eggs, the creature is halakhically considered an insect. This is yet another proof that the ovary recipient, whose role predominates in the process of conception, and who gives birth to the child, would be the halakhic mother.

R. Kamelhar reports that R. Meir Arik (1855–1926) concurred with the entire aforementioned analysis.[106] Elaborating on his position

---

104. On this belief in rabbinic sources, see H. J. Zimmels, "*Ofot haGedailim beIlan*," in *Minḥat Bikurim* (Vienna, 1926), 1–9; *Jewish Encyclopedia* 2 (Ktav, 1964), 538–540; N. Slifkin, "Vegetable Men and Tree-Geese," in his *Sacred Monstors* (Zoo Torah, 2007), 305–323. For discussion of this notion in secular sources see L. Thorndyke, *History of Magic and Experimental Science* 2 (Columbia University Press, 1923), 200, 464–465. R. Kamelhar also gives tangential treatment to this topic on p. 44, op. cit.

105. Y. D., 84:15.

106. R. Arik is the author of *Imrei Yosher*. R. Kamelhar mentions some of R. Arik's comments on the topic of the barnacle goose.

regarding the relevance of *erva* to ovarian transplantation, R. Kamelhar points out that despite the fact that Ḥavah was created from one of Adam's own ribs, Adam was not guilty of cohabitation with another male. This is true, he asserts, because the organ takes on a completely new identity in the recipient. There is therefore no prohibition of *erva* for the transplanted ovary, as this ovary acquires a new identity in the recipient and is no longer associated with the donor.

In explaining the biblical incident where the sheep of Yaakov multiplied,[107] the *Midrash*[108] claims that the water ingested by the sheep turned into reproductive seed.[109] Yet, according to R. Kamelhar there is no doubt that the offspring were considered normal sheep, to which the laws of *sheḥita* and *bekhor* would apply. This is proof that only the gestation and parturition determine the offspring's status, for despite the miraculous origin of the male seed, the sheep were considered halakhically normal.[110]

R. Kamelhar also refers to a contemporary animal experiment where the offspring's coat color was found to be identical to that of the ovary donor, a finding that apparently proved that the donor of the ovary is the mother.[111] While the Gemara does address the transmission

---

107. Bereshit 30:37–39.

108. *Bereshit Rabba* 17:7 in the name of R. Hoshea.

109. The *Midrash* continues, stating that only the *"tzurat havlad"* was lacking from this seed. This may be an allusion to the Aristotelian notion that the male provides the "form" and "principle of movement" of the fetus, and the female's sole contribution is the substance or matter from which the fetus is formed. See A. L. Peck, trans., *Aristotle: Generation of Animals* (Harvard University Press, 1942), 100–101 and 109–112. Perhaps this is the meaning of the *Midrash*. The only thing lacking from the seed was the physical formation of the fetus (i.e., *"tzurat havlad"*), which would be provided, as usual, by the female. For further discussion of Aristotle's view of conception in relation to rabbinic literature, see chapter, "Rabbinic Conception of Conception."

110. This may prove that in animals the male seed is irrelevant to the determination of halakhic status, but one cannot infer anything from here regarding the role of the female seed, as both the seed, gestation and parturition were provided by the female sheep in this case. In addition, one cannot derive halakha directly or exclusively from the Midrash.

111. He identifies the scientist by the name Weisner, and I have been unable to locate the particular citation. It is unclear whether the experiments he refers to were done with rats or insects, as R. Kamelhar uses the term *"sheretz,"* which could refer to

of characteristics (*simanim*) from parent to offspring,[112] R. Kamelhar contends that this discussion is restricted to bodily features and does not include skin color. The latter can be affected by external influences, as evidenced by the story of Yaakov's sheep acquiring a different color after gazing upon the colored rods.[113] The Midrash mentions a similar story where external influences altered the color of a fetus.[114] In addition, R. Kamelhar asserts that one cannot extrapolate from experiments on animals to human beings. Even data gleaned from the study of non-Jewish

---

either; or if they were done with animals that underwent ovarian transplant; or if they were simply genetic experiments to determine which parent is responsible for color inheritance. The latter is possible. See S. Wright, "Color Inheritance in Mammals," *Journal of Heredity* 8 (1917), 224–235.Wright reviews the literature on this topic up to his time and makes no reference to anyone named Weisner. It is possible that Weisner's experiments were published between 1917 and 1928 (the year of publication of *HaTalmud UMada'ei HaTevel*). There is, however, an article published in 1907 in the *Proceedings of the American Physicians Society* in which Guthrie (cited by F. II. Martin, "Transplantation of Ovaries," *Surgery, Gynecology and Obstetrics* 7 [1908], 20) describes a series of experiments on chickens to determine the influence of the foster mother on the offspring in cases of ovarian transplantation. He exchanged the ovaries of black and white leghorn hens and found that the transplanted ovaries function in the normal manner, and that the color characteristic of the chicks is influenced by the foster mother. The experiment that Kamelhar cites, however, apparently found that the foster mother does not affect the color of the offspring. Morris, in his autobiography, op. cit., 217, mentions that Castle grafted ovarian tissue from a black guinea pig into a white guinea pig and obtained black progeny from a white mother and father. These results are consistent with the experiment mentioned by Kamelhar.

112. *Ḥullin* 79b. The discussion here is of the halakhic identity of an animal produced from two breeds (e.g., a mule), as it relates to the prohibition of slaughtering a mother and child on the same day (*oto v'et beno*). *Talmud Yerushalmi Kilayim* 8:3 mentions, in the name of R. Yonah, that the size of an animal's ears reflects its parentage. If its ears are small, then its mother is a mare and its father a donkey; if they are large, then it is vice versa, and its father is of the equine species.

113. Bereshit 30:37–39.

114. *Bamidbar Rabba* 9:43. The *Midrash* relates the story of an Arabian King who posed the following question to R. Akiva: "Both I and my wife are black, yet my wife gave birth to a white son. Should I kill her for infidelity? R. Akiva responded: Are the statues in your house white or black? The king answered white. R. Akiva then assured him that when he had intercourse with his wife, she gazed upon the white statues and bore him a child of similar color." For more on the psychic maternal influences on the fetus see Preuss, op. cit., 391–392.

bodies cannot be applied to Jews.[115] He therefore concludes that, with respect to human beings, the father is the one who provides the seed, and the mother the one who conceives and gives birth to the child.[116]

Exchange in HaBe'er[117]

In the early 1930's there appeared an exchange of ideas on the halakhic aspects of ovarian transplantation in the Eastern European journal *HaBe'er*, much like that which appeared over twenty years earlier in the journals *Vayelaket Yosef* and *Tel Talpiyot*. The topic is introduced in a section of the journal devoted to contemporary halakhic problems,[118] and the preface of the article, authored by the editor, R. Tzvi Hirsch Freidling, explains that doctors in England and America are now successfully treating infertility by transplanting ovaries from fertile to infertile women. As Morris' 1906 case is the only recorded successful treatment of infertility with ovarian transplantation, it is unclear what precipitated the discussion of this issue in the journal at this time.

R. Freidling raises four halakhic questions: Who is the halakhic mother of the resultant child? Is there a prohibition of *erva* since the donor is a married woman? Is the child blemished (*pasul*)? Is it even permitted for a woman to undergo such a surgical procedure, or to receive another woman's organs?

---

115. For this notion, he cites the commentary of *Ḥatam Sofer* to *Avodah Zara* 31 and *Tel Torah*, by R. Meir Arik, on *Nidda* 45a. It is predicated on the belief that since non-Jews ingest non-kosher foods, their bodies have a different physiological constitution. For further discussion on this topic, see *Teshuvot Ḥatam Sofer*, Y. D., 105; E. Munk, "B'Inyan Lismokh al Rofeh Y'rei Shamayim biZman sheYediyotav Hen miSifrei Nituaḥ shel Umot HaOlam," in *V'Rapo Yerapei: Zikhron Yeshayahu* (Jerusalem, 1989), 124–126; N. Gutal, *Sefer Hishtanut HaTeva'im* (Jerusalem, 1995), 134–135, note 116.

116. R. Kamelhar assumes that in ovarian transplantation the recipient provides the egg. Consequently, as she is the one who both "conceives and gives birth to the child," she is considered the halakhic mother. R. Avraham Yaakov Horowitz, after citing R. Binyamin Weiss' *Even Yekara*, independently applies the same logic to conclude that the recipient is the halakhic mother. See his *Tzur Yaakov*, n. 28.

117. For the history of this journal see I. Lewin, op. cit., 46–48.

118. Year 6, vol. 3 (*Sivan*, 5691; May/June, 1931), 110–113. The section is entitled "*Mayim Tehorim.*"

The issue of *bekhor*, which was addressed by a number of the earlier authorities, is conspicuously absent from this list. As the rabbis of this later period were aware that only the ovary was transplanted, there was no doubt for them regarding the status of *bekhor*.

To answer the questions, R. Freidling quotes the entire response of R. Kamelhar, either ignoring or unaware of the other aforementioned discussions, and offers additional support to R. Kamelhar's position. He also cites the opinion of R. Eliyahu Posek on this issue,[119] who, similar to R. Shafran above, brings the *Targum Yonatan* to Bereshit (30:21) as proof that the birth mother is the halakhic mother. The issue of *erva* is, therefore, irrelevant because the transplanted organs become an integral part of the recipient.

R. Posek further states that one dare not undergo such a procedure because it would violate the prohibition of *ḥavala* (causing unnecessary bodily harm) for both the donor and the recipient.[120] The physician's testimony regarding the success of the procedure is not to be believed, as it is possible that these women would have become pregnant even without the transplant.[121]

R. Freidling concludes by quoting the responsum of R. Binyamin Arye Weiss, as it appeared in the latter's work *Even Yekara*.[122]

---

119. This source is cited from what appears to be a printed work of R. Posek, but the citation is an acronym which does not correspond to any of R. Posek's known printed works. It is possible that the citation appears in *Piskei Eliyahu*, but I have been unable to consult this work.

120. R. Posek does not mention the prohibition of sterilization. Perhaps he holds like the *Turei Zahav, Even HaEzer* 5:6, that while the prohibition of sterilization does not apply to women, there may be a prohibition of *ḥavala* for removing the female organs. As both the donor and recipient in ovarian transplantation have their ovaries removed, this prohibition would apply equally to both of them. R. Shaul Yisraeli employs the principles of *ḥavala* to permit accepting money for organ donation. See "Rav Shaul Yisraeli—Organ Transplants: Responsa," in *Jewish Medical Ethics* 3:1, 14–17.

121. R. Posek points out that women often conceive after years of infertility.

122. See above, end of section on *Vayelaket Yosef*, for discussion of R. Weiss' comments. Of note, R. Freidling does not reference R. Weiss' responsum where it initially appeared, in *Vayelaket Yosef*.

In a subsequent issue of *HaBe'er*,[123] the editors return to the question of ovarian transplant, publishing two additional responsa. The first is by R. Ḥanokh Henekh Shafran, who merely quotes the responsum of his father, R. Bezalel Shafran, author of *Teshuvot Rabaz*.[124] He notes that his father discusses the same issues and sources as R. Kamelhar and R. Posek, whose comments were both published in the earlier issue of the journal, despite having never seen either of their works on this subject.

The final respondent, R. Ḥayyim Zev Wolf Weinreb, addresses the halakhic issues raised by R. Freidling. In referring to the articles from *Vayelaket Yosef*, R. Weinreb is the first to mention the existence of an earlier literature on this topic. However, as he was unable to obtain the journals, this literature was not incorporated into his response.

He first addresses the comments of R. Binyamin Weiss regarding the organ donor's violation of the prohibition of sterilization (*sirus*). Explaining why R. Weiss is not concerned that the recipient, whose ovaries are also removed before the transplant, would be violating the same prohibition, R. Weinreb opines that the removal of nonfunctional ovaries may not constitute *sirus*.[125] However, he hastens to add, as one cannot trust the physician's assessment that the ovaries were in fact nonfunctional, the prohibition of *sirus* may apply to the organ recipient as well.

On the other hand, he argues, since both women's role in the sterilization procedure is passive, and the prohibition of sterilization devolves upon the one who actively performs the procedure and not the one to whom it is done (i.e., the passive recipient), perhaps neither the donor nor the recipient would violate the prohibition.[126]

---

123. Year 7, vol. 2, nos. 70–71 (*Shevat*, 5692; January/February, 1932), 88–92.
124. See above section on R. Shafran.
125. See *Minḥat Ḥinukh*, mitzva 291.
126. The same *Minḥat Ḥinukh* that R. Weinreb quotes (mitzva 291) also postulates (end of letter *aleph*) that even passive sterilization might be prohibited. The classic example of a passive recipient violating a prohibition is the prohibition of cutting the hair of the corners of the head (Vayikra 19:27, "*lo takifu p'at roshkhem*"). *Makkot* 20b states that both the *makif* and the *nikaf* get lashes. Rashi s. v., "*d'amar lakh*" opines that one possible reason for this inclusion of the passive recipient in the prohibition is the plural language of the verse (*takifu*), which alludes to more than one person who is in violation of the prohibition (i.e., both the *makif* and the *nikaf*). Applying the same logic to the case of sterilization, since the verse is stated in plural ("*uv'artzekhem lo*

R. Weinreb next takes up the issue of *havala* raised by R. Posek. While agreeing that *havala* likely applies to the donor, even if only minimal danger is involved, he contends that this prohibition does not apply to the recipient for two reasons. First, the procedure would likely be performed by expert surgeons, a fact which might minimize the *havala*, and second, the prohibition might be waived for the sake of procreation and marital harmony.

Regarding the issue of *erva* with the organs donated by a married woman (*eshet ish*), R. Weinreb advances the novel suggestion that the donor either be unmarried or non-Jewish in order to circumvent the problem.[127] However, he argues, even if the donor were an *erva*, since the ovary is placed intra-abdominally, and there would be no direct physical contact with the organ during marital relations, the prohibition of *erva* would not apply.[128] Going one step further, he maintains that even

---

ta'asu"), perhaps even the passive recipient is in violation. However, since no other authorities seem to mention or concur with this analysis, the *Minḥat Hinukh* does not consider this opinion binding.

127. It is interesting that none of his predecessors makes this suggestion. In the contemporary discussions on surrogate motherhood, the issues revolving around the use of unmarried or non-Jewish surrogates have been explored. The current Israeli surrogacy laws mandate that the surrogate be unmarried, so as to bypass the problem of *eshet ish*. The Israeli laws also require the surrogate and egg donor to be of the same religion.

128. In a parenthetical note, R. Weinreb refers the reader to *Teshuvot R. Akiva Eiger* n. 172 and to *Tiferet Yisrael* on the Mishna in the sixth chapter of *Temura* for further discussion of this issue. The *Mishna Temura* 6:5 states that even though an animal is prohibited from sacrificial use, its offspring may nevertheless be permitted. The commentaries qualify this statement as referring to a case where an animal, while still *ḥullin* (i.e., prior to being designated for temple sacrifice), mates with another animal and conceives. Generally, if a female animal has sexual relations with a male, she becomes prohibited from sacrificial use (*Mishna Temura* 6:1). The offspring in this case, a product of one animal prohibited from sacrificial use (the female), and one permitted (the male), is nevertheless permitted based on the fact that this is a case of *zeh v'zeh gorem* (i.e., both parties contributed to the production of the offspring), which in these circumstances is permitted. However, the commentaries add, if the female animal would have had sexual relations with a male animal while she was already pregnant, then her offspring would not be permitted because since the fetus is part of the mother (*ubar yerekh imo*, a matter of debate elsewhere), both the mother and fetus are considered to have had intercourse, a

if theoretically the external genitalia were also transplanted,[129] which he understood was not the case here, no violation would be incurred because once the organs are removed from the donor they lose their *erva* status and are considered mere flesh.[130]

---

fact rendering both of them prohibited from sacrificial use. R. Eiger asks, based on this Mishna, why a man is not prohibited from having intercourse with his own wife while she is pregnant with their daughter; after all, since we say *ubar yerekh imo*, then it should be considered as if he is having sexual relations with his own daughter. R. Eiger answers that sexual relations with a child less than three years of age (including a fetus) is not technically considered *erva* and is only rabbinically prohibited because of *hashḥatat zera*. Since in this case, the man is having relations with his pregnant wife, and *hashḥatat zera* is not a concern, no violation at all is incurred. Both the commentaries on the Mishna and the question of R. Eiger imply that one can theoretically violate the prohibition of *erva* even if the source of *erva* itself is deep within the body. The *Tiferet Yisrael* on *Mishna Temura* (*Boaz*, letter *gimmel*) however, questions the premise of R. Eiger. R. Eiger assumes that we consider as if the act of intercourse was done with the fetus just as it was done with the mother. If this were the case, argues the *Tiferet Yisrael*, then R. Eiger's answer is insufficient to solve other potential problems. For example, if the act of slaughtering is considered equally done to the fetus, then one could not slaughter a pregnant animal because of the prohibition of slaughtering a mother and child on the same day. The *Tiferet Yisrael* therefore contends that we do not consider as if the act were done simultaneously to both the mother and the fetus. Rather, the notion of *ubar yerekh imo* means that the fetus is subordinate to the mother and does not have independent status. If the mother becomes prohibited for sacrificial use, then so too the fetus, by virtue of its association with the mother, not by virtue of any independently committed violation. Similarly, when one has intercourse with his pregnant wife, the wife is permitted to the husband. The fetus, who is subordinate to the mother, is therefore likewise permitted. It is this logic of the *Tiferet Yisrael* which I believe R. Weinreb relies upon in claiming that there is no issue of *erva* in ovarian transplantation. Since the recipient is permitted to her husband, and the transplanted ovary is subordinate to the recipient, there is no problem of *erva*.

129. See above regarding articles in *Tel Talpiyot* and *Vayelaket Yosef*, where the respondents actually believed that the external genitalia were transplanted.

130. R. Weinreb rejects the proof of R. Freidling from Adam, asserting that one cannot extrapolate from creation. In addition, as he believes the prohibition of *erva* to be inapplicable to this case, he dismisses the question of whether the child is blemished (*pasul*). He cites the *Turei Zahav* (Y. D. 195:7) in the name of the *Semak*, regarding the concern for a woman sleeping on another man's sheets lest she conceive from the residual seed, as proof that when no prohibition is violated the offspring have no blemish. For further explication of the statement of the *Semak*, see chapter, "The Rabbinic Conception of Conception: An Exercise in Fertility."

R. Weinreb considers the question of maternal identity to be the most serious halakhic issue, and his comments on this issue reflect a very detailed understanding of the physiological basis for ovarian transplantation, far beyond that of his predecessors. According to the physicians, he writes, the female's role in conception is to provide a single egg, which is emitted from the ovary and travels towards the uterus to meet the male seed. In the case of ovarian transplant, it is the donor who provides that egg. It is therefore difficult to maintain that the donor has no maternal rights whatsoever, a position held by R. Kamelhar and R. Posek. R. Weinreb does however acknowledge that it can also be argued that the recipient has maternal rights.[131]

V. CONTEMPORARY REFERENCES TO THE
DISCUSSION OF OVARIAN TRANSPLANTATION

As mentioned in the introduction to this chapter, a number of rabbinic authorities over the last few decades have incorporated the halakhic analysis of ovarian transplantation into their discussions of modern medical halakhic issues. It is my contention that in order to effectively apply this halakhic analysis to contemporary dilemmas, one must first appreciate the historical context of each source, as well as the author's knowledge of the contemporary medicine. Then, based on a comparison of the state of medicine at the time of the author as compared to our own, a rabbinic authority can decide whether, or with what limitations, a particular source can be applied to a contemporary halakhic issue.

R. Waldenberg refers to a case of uterine transplantation in his responsa.[132] This reference is clearly a perpetuation of the

---

131. R. Weinreb responds to the factual doubts of R. B. A. Weiss by pointing out that other organs, including both upper and lower extremities, have been successfully transplanted. He raises the question of whether these organs retain their status of *tum'ah* after they have been transplanted, or whether the fact that the organ is restored to life in the recipient reverses their *tum'ah* status. This latter logic was used by R. Yehuda Unterman to permit cornea transplantation (*Shevet MiYehuda*, 313–322), as well as by R. Waldenberg in his discussion on receiving money for organ transplantation. See Abraham S. Abraham, *Nishmat Avraham* 4 (Jerusalem, 1991), 222–223. For further discussion on this topic, see chapter, "The Resuscitation of Halakha: An Animated Discussion."

132. *Tzitz Eliezer* v. 7, sect. 48, chap. 5, n. 16.

misconception held by the early discussants of ovarian transplantation, such as R. Deutch, R. Silverstein and R. Katzburg, that the uterus, and perhaps even the external genitalia were transplanted. In the context of R. Waldenberg's initial mention of this halakhic literature, however, where he addresses the issue of premarital disclosure, this misconception has no halakhic ramifications. This may not be the case, however, regarding R. Waldenberg's later responsum, where he concludes, based on R. Weiss' comments on ovarian transplantation, that in the case of surrogate motherhood, the gestational mother is the halakhic mother. Here, an historical approach to R. Weiss' responsum may impact on its interpretation and application.

R. Weiss' responsum, although later published in his *Even Yekara*, was initially published in the halakhic exchange in *Vayelaket Yosef*. At this early stage of the halakhic discussions, the belief was that the entire set of reproductive organs was transplanted. R. Weiss does not refute this notion. In addition, R. Weiss states, based on the agricultural analogy from *orla* discussed above, that the birth mother is the halakhic mother.

First, in applying a contextual approach, it must be determined what R. Weiss understood about ovarian transplantation relative to his contemporaries. As R. Weiss' comments are terse, with no accompanying explanation, it is unclear whether he believed that the donor contributed materially to the offspring, as was believed by R. Roth, for example, as well as some members of the medical community; or, that the donor organs served merely as a conduit for, or stimulant to, the recipient's egg, without providing any material contribution, a position espoused by R. Kamelhar and theorized by Dr. Morris. This ambiguity alone may preclude or limit the use of this material for modern discourse.

The next step in the analysis, a comparative approach, is predicated on the accuracy of the contextual approach. For example, if R. Weiss concurs with R. Kamelhar that the donor has no material contribution, then R. Weiss' decision may not be applicable to the modern case of surrogate motherhood, where the genetic contribution of the donor is indisputable. However, if R. Weiss concurs with R. Roth, that the donor contributes materially to the fetus, then his analysis may be applied to our modern circumstance.

In the same vein, R. Dr. Mordechai Halperin mentions the halakhic literature on ovarian transplantation in an article discussing the use of donated genetic material in assisted reproduction.[133] He cites the responsum of R. Weiss, who considers the birth mother to be the halakhic mother, to conclude that the genetic contribution is not halakhically significant for the determination of maternity. It is questionable whether one can draw this conclusion from R. Weiss' comments. R. Weiss himself, as discussed above, may have thought that the egg is provided by the organ recipient, not the donor. If such is the case, one cannot conclude from his responsum that the genetic contribution is not halakhically significant. Applying this possible interpretation of R. Weiss' comment, had he acknowledged a material or genetic contribution of the donor, he may have granted the latter halakhic maternity.

While R. Waldenberg and R. Dr. Halperin rely on the responsum of R. Weiss, which is ambiguous regarding the nature of the donor's contribution, R. Bleich, in an early essay on host mothers, turns to the work of R. Kamelhar for possible application to the issue of maternal identity.[134] As R. Kamelhar explicitly denies any material contribution of the donor, a point which R. Bleich does not mention, it is debatable whether his conclusions can be applied to a case of surrogate motherhood, where the donor's substantial contribution is irrefutable.[135] R. Rosenfeld, who

---

133. M. Halperin, *"Trumat Homer Geneti BiTipulay Poriyut,"* in *HaKinus HaBenleumi HaSheni: Refua, Etika VeHalakha* (Schlesinger Institute, 1996), 321–327. R. Dr. Halperin concurs with R. Weiss' comments that successful ovarian transplant likely never took place because they would have been unable to overcome the problem of organ rejection. Even today, he says, there have been no successful ovarian transplants. In fact, those involved in ovarian transplantation observed that a heterograft was less likely to succeed than an autograft, and that an interspecies graft was even less likely to succeed. Although ignorant at that time of the immunology of organ rejection, they nonetheless made clear observations of failed transplants secondary to rejection. See articles of F. H. Martin above, for example, where he details these observations in his conclusions.

134. J. D. Bleich, *Contemporary Halakhic Problems* 1 (Ktav, 1977), 106–109.

135. R. Kamelhar's analysis of the concept of *"hosheshin l'zera ha'av,"* and his contention that both positions in this debate would concur that the donor is not the halakhic mother, is predicated on the belief that the donor provides no material contribution to the offspring.

also incorporates passages from R. Kamelhar's work, likewise does not acknowledge that R. Kamelhar expressly denies any material contribution of the ovary donor. However, he does state that our understanding of heredity and genetics may be cause to reverse the decisions of the earlier rabbinic authorities.[136]

Although the authorities above specifically mention the halakhic literature on ovarian transplantation in their contemporary halakhic discussions on issues of assisted reproduction, and in particular surrogate motherhood, it should be noted that many contemporary authorities cite source material similar to that raised in the initial halakhic discussions of ovarian transplantation, without direct reference to this previous earlier body of halakhic exchanges.[137] In particular, two sets of sources first mentioned with reference to ovarian transplantation have been cited extensively in the maternal identity debate: the sources dealing with the inter-uterine transfer of Yosef and Dinah,[138] and the agricultural sources from *Sota* 43b and *Menahot* 69b.[139] In addition, the passage from *Hullin* 70a discussing the transfer of an animal between two uteri, first mentioned by R. Sheftel Weiss, has received some attention in contemporary

136. A. Rosenfeld, "Human Identity: Halakhic Issues," *Tradition* 16:3 (Spring 1977), 65–66.
137. The issue of the halakhic definition of maternal identity has been reviewed elsewhere and will not be repeated here. See M. J. Broyde, "The Establishment of Maternity and Paternity in Jewish and American Law," *National Jewish Law Review* 3 (1988), 117–158; E. Bick, "Ovum Donations: A Rabbinic Conceptual Model of Maternity," *Tradition* 28:1 (Fall 1993), 28–45; J. D. Bleich, "In Vitro Fertilization: Questions of Maternal Identity and Conversion," in his *Contemporary Halakhic Problems* 4 (Ktav, 1995), 237–272. I wish only to point out that arguments similar to those mentioned in the halakhic literature on ovarian transplantation have been advanced in contemporary halakhic discussions.
138. See Bleich, op. cit., note 125, 247–248, and E. Bick, op. cit., 31–32. R. Bick states that these sources were introduced into the halakhic literature concerning parenthood by R. Yisrael Minzberg in 5718, and R. Bleich mentions that this aggadic source was first cited by R. Menashe Grossbart in 5684. However, the article of R. Roth mentioned above, in *Tel Talpiyot*, Year 17, no. 21 (*Tammuz*, 5668/July, 1908), 191–192, antedates both these sources. For a comprehensive discussion on the rabbinic literature addressing the births of Yosef and Dinah, see chapter, "Midrash, Miracles, and Motherhood: The Birth of Dinah and the Definition of Maternity."
139. See Bleich, op. cit., 251–257 and Bick, op. cit., 30–31.

discussions,[140] as has the passage from *Ḥullin* 79a, cited by R. Kamelhar above.[141] As these sources are incorporated independently, without reference to the earlier halakhic discussions of ovarian transplantation, an historical analysis does not affect their interpretation. One can only speculate as to whether these authors identified these sources independently, or through their perusal of the earlier halakhic literature.

VI. THE FUTURE OF OVARIAN TRANSPLANT

The fertility benefit of ovarian transplantation has recently been largely superseded by in-vitro fertilization. Now that a donated egg can be fertilized in a petrie dish and transferred directly into a woman's uterus for implantation, it no longer seems necessary to surgically transplant ovarian tissue in order to potentially restore fertility. One might therefore think that the halakhic literature on ovarian transplant, much like Morris' case report, may soon be relegated to obscurity. Recent medical advances, however, may lead to the resurrection of this halakhic narrative.

In 2008, Dr. Sherman Silber performed the first successful whole ovary transplant, In addition, ovarian tissue transplant, in a procedure not dissimilar to that of Dr. Morris is being used to preserve fertility in patients undergoing cancer treatment.[142] Although this latter procedure typically involves replanting a woman's own ovaries,[143] a variation of autotransplantation (see above section on medical history), it is possible

---

140. Ibid., 245–246. R. Bleich states that "in point of fact, no halakhic writer has cited this text as a source for the definition of maternal identity." Although R. Sheftel Weiss, in his article in *Tel Talpiyot* discussed above, invokes this source in discussing *pidyon haben* for the offspring in ovarian transplantation, he does not specifically use it for the halakhic definition of maternity.

141. Ibid., 257–258.

142. See, for example, L. Lotz, *et. al.*, "Ovarian Tissue Transplantation: Experience From Germany and Worldwide Efficacy," *Clinical Medicine Insights: Reproductive Health* 13 (2009), 1–8.

143. There is also another recent advance which allows for the freezing of the human ovum for women wishing to preserve fertility either in cases of cancer or for other purposes. This is being used in the Jewish community to preserve fertility in women of advancing age who have not yet married. The halakhic issues for this technology merit a separate halakhic treatmeat. See, for example, E. Rybak, "Aging Ovaries and Age-Old Tradition," *Journal of Halacha and Contemporary Society* 63 (Spring, 2012), 22–50.

that it may expand to include the transplantation of another woman's ovaries. This is exactly the case discussed above in the halakhic analysis of ovarian transplantation and would undoubtedly lead to a reevaluation of this literature.

Another form of ovarian transplantation, transplanting the ovaries of an aborted fetus, is also in its infancy, although ethical objections may arrest its development. This research could potentially produce a child who will inherit the genes of a woman who herself never lived. There are clearly other halakhic issues involved with the general use of fetal ovarian tissue,[144] let alone its use in assisted reproduction, but the basic issues of ovarian transplantation for the recipient, including sterilization, *erva*, and maternal identity would be similar.

Could the aforementioned sources pertaining to ovarian transplantation be equally applied to the current and future cases of ovarian transplantation? If so, to what extent? From the early literature one can glean the attendant halakhic issues involved in human ovarian transplantation, such as the risk of the procedure to both donor and recipient, the concern for violating the prohibitions of *erva* and *sirus*, and the definition of maternity. In addition, one can find potentially relevant source material and novel halakhic analyses for application to the modern dilemmas of ovarian transplantation. However, to rely on the previous decisions of the early rabbinic authorities regarding the halakhic issues of ovarian transplantation is fraught with difficulty and should be done only with extreme caution. The author to author variability in medical and physiological knowledge, and the paradigm shift in reproductive physiology and genetics since the writing of this literature are obstacles that are not easily overcome. A medical historical analysis of the sources, including both contextual and comparative approaches, may facilitate optimal use of these sources by rabbinic authorities.[145]

---

144. See J. D. Bleich, "Fetal Tissue Research: Jewish Tradition and Public Policy," in his *Contemporary Halakhic Problems* 4 (Ktav, 1995), 171–202.

145. For the most comprehensive contemporary halakhic discussion on ovarian transplantation, see Tzvi Ryzman, *Ratz KaTzvi, Asufat Ma'amarim Pirkei Meḥkar VeIyun: Poriyut, Yuḥsin Ishut* (Tzvi Ryzman, 2 Adar, 5776).

Uterine Transplantation and the Case of the Mistaken Question

I. INTRODUCTION

In April 2000, the first successful human uterine transplantation was performed on a 26-year-old female who had lost her uterus six years earlier due to post-partum bleeding. The uterus was subsequently removed 99 days later due to complications. The donor, a 46-year-old patient with ovarian cysts, underwent a modified hysterectomy. This case was first reported in the medical literature in March 2002.[1] Since this initial case, there have been a number of successful uterus transplants followed by pregnancy and live births.[2]

In the entire field of assisted reproduction, clear halakhic precedent is hard to come by. Rabbinic authorities of previous generations simply did not and could not have addressed all unforeseen technological

---

1. W. Fageeh, et al., "Transplantation of the Human Uterus," *International Journal of Gynaecology and Obstetrics* 76:3 (March, 2002), 245–51; Albert Altchek, "Uterus Transplantation," *Mount Sinai Journal of Medicine* 70:3 (May 2003), 154–162.
2. For a review of the current state of the field by one of its pioneers, see M. Brannstrom's continually updated entry on uterine transplantation at uptodate.com.

advances. The modern *posek* is therefore presented with the challenge of finding legally relevant material. This challenge has been met in addressing the topics of artificial insemination and surrogate motherhood.[3] We are now faced with another unforeseen advance—the transplantation of the female uterus. How would halakha address this novel therapy, and could there be precedent for a procedure that was only recently performed for the first time in history?

A Remarkable Medical Case

In 1906, Robert Tuttle Morris reported a spectacular case in which he had transplanted a sliver of human ovary into the abdominal cavity of a woman whose ovaries he had personally removed. The recipient of the ovarian transplant subsequently gave birth to a healthy child. This case, which would be equally astonishing today, generated a brief flurry of literature in the medical and lay press, and was soon forgotten.

Hearing of the news of this case, R. Yaakov Gordon posed a halakhic inquiry for forum discussion in the journal *Vayelaket Yosef*:[4]

> A halakhic query: Physicians have developed a procedure to transplant reproductive organs from one woman into an infertile woman to cure infertility. Can one transplant the reproductive organs from a mother into a daughter? Who is the mother of the resultant child, the first woman or the second woman?

As R. Gordon was not familiar with the details of the case, he erroneously assumed that the entire set of female reproductive organs was transplanted, including the ovaries, the uterus and the external genitalia. Since the halakhic respondents were unfamiliar with the real case, they simply responded to the question as asked.[5]

This original question has been perpetuated in the halakhic literature since that time, with subsequent authorities addressing the issues

---

3. See, for example, A. Steinberg, *Entzyclopedia Hilkhatit Refuit* 1 (Schlesinger Institute, 1988), s. v., "*hazra'a melakhutit.*"
4. *Vayelaket Yosef*, Year 10, vol. 3 (15 Ḥeshvan, 5668/October 23, 1907), 9a–9b.
5. Many did, however, express disbelief that such a transplant was possible.

of reproductive organ transplants in different contexts. We therefore have detailed halakhic discussions from previous generations on the issue of reproductive organ, and specifically uterine, transplantation, a procedure that had never been performed. This body of halakhic literature is explored in detail in the preceding chapter. At the time I wrote the essay on which that chapter is based,[6] however, uterus transplants remained in the realm of science fiction. As they have now transitioned into the realm of scientific fact, here we revisit the original halakhic sources from the early twentieth century, extracting those that relate exclusively to uterine transplantation. While there is, by necessity, limited review and repetition from the previous halakic discussion, there is much additional material here derived from the original sources. In addition, we supplement our discussion with current scientific information and updated halakhic material.[7] Our discussion is divided into two sections—issues for the donor and issues for the recipient.

II. UTERINE TRANPLANTATION—THE DONOR

The rabbis commenting on the early case of reproductive organ transplantation raised three issues with respect to the donor. In the journal

---

6. See chapter, "The First Halakhic Discussion of Ovarian Transplantation." In the introduction to this chapter, I mentioned that while the focus of the chapter was to highlight the importance of a medical historical approach, the literature on the early halakhic discussions of reproductive organ transplant has potential value for contemporary medical halakhic discourse. I did not, however, anticipate the current case of uterine transplantation.

    Natan Slifkin, in his *Mysterious Creatures* (Targum Press, 2003), 230–232, discusses the contemporary relevance of a unique case in the Talmud of the mouse that is part earth. While there does not appear to be a living animal that correlates with this talmudic description, he relates a modern case for which the talmudic analysis is instructive. This is an unforeseen application of a seemingly irrelevant halakhic discussion. In the early literature on reproductive organ transplant, the rabbis similarly discussed issues of questionable halakhic relevance, as the procedures they addressed had in fact never occurred. We now have an unforeseen application of this literature. In our case, however, the extrapolation from the earlier discussion is not by analogy but is direct. Both cases are a testimony to the enduring value of halakhic analyses.

7. For a comprehensive contemporary halakhic discussion on uterine transplantation, see Tzvi Ryzman, *Ratz KaTzvi, Asufat Ma'amarim Pirkei Meḥkar Ve'Iyun: Poriyut, Yuḥsin Ishut* (Tzvi Ryzman, 2 Adar, 5776).

HaBe'er,[8] R. Posek opposed the entire procedure of reproductive organ transplant because it entails a violation of *havala* (sustaining unnecessary bodily harm) for both the donor and the recipient. R. Weinreb agreed that the donor would indeed violate the prohibition of *havala.*[9]

R. S. Weiss[10] raised a second issue of submitting to a procedure involving questionable risk.[11] The third issue raised was that of sterilization, or *sirus.* In the 1908 issue of the Hungarian journal *Vayelaket Yosef,*[12] R. Binyamin Arye Weiss states that reproductive organ donation is halakhically forbidden, for even if there were no danger to the patients involved, the donor would be undergoing sterilization (*sirus*), a prohibition which, at the very least, is of rabbinic origin.[13] In the journal *HaBe'er,*[14] R. Weinreb suggests that since the woman's role in the sterilization procedure is passive, and the prohibition of sterilization devolves only upon the one who actively performs the procedure, perhaps no prohibition would be violated by the passive donor.[15]

---

8. Year 6, vol. 3 (*Sivan*, 5691; May/June, 1931), 110–113. For the history of this journal, see I. Lewin, *Otzar Kitvei Et Torani'im* (New York, 5740), 46–48.
9. See below for his opinion regarding the recipient.
10. *Vayelaket Yosef,* Year 10, vol. 6 (Hanukka 5668/December, 1907), 21b. For the history of this journal, see I. Lewin, *Otzar Kitvei Et Torani'im* (New York, 5740), 88–95.
11. Regarding the permissibility of undergoing risky or unproved therapy, see J. D. Bleich, "Experimental Procedures: The Concept of *Refu'ah Bedukah,*" in his *Contemporary Halakhic Problems* 4 (Ktav, 1995), 203–217.
12. Year 10, vol. 9, no. 77 (*Shevat*, 5668; January, 1908), 29a. This response to R. Schwartz was subsequently published in R. Weiss' *Even Yekara,* n. 29.
13. For more on the prohibition of *sirus* see chapter, "The First Halakhic Discussion of Ovarian Transplantation," n. 70.
14. Year 7, vol. 2, nos. 70–71 (*Shevat*, 5692; January/February, 1932), 88–92.
15. As noted in the above chapter, "The First Halakhic Discussion of Ovarian Transplantation," the same *Minhat Hinukh* that R. Weinreb quotes (mitzva 291) also postulates (end of letter *aleph*) that even passive sterilization might be prohibited. The classic example of a passive recipient violating a prohibition is the prohibition of cutting the hair of the corners of the head (Vayikra 19:27 "*lo takifu pe'at roshkhem*"). The Gemara, in *Makkot* 20b, states that both the *makif* and the *nikaf* get lashes. Rashi s. v., "*de'amar lakh*" opines that one possible reason for this inclusion of the passive recipient in the prohibition is the plural language of the verse (*takifu*), which alludes to more than one person who is in violation of the prohibition (i.e., both the *makif* and the *nikaf*). Applying the same logic to the case of sterilization, since the verse is stated in plural

All three aforementioned issues of wounding, risk and sterilization are equally applicable to our modern case of uterine transplant,
but their respective relevance depends on the source of the donation.
There are also additional halakhic concerns not mentioned in the early
literature of reproductive organ transplant.

As with other transplants, the donated uterus can be harvested
from a living or cadaveric donor.

Live Uterine Donation

Living organ donation, for organs such as kidneys, is a common, halakhically sanctioned practice.[16] The donor has an obligation of *"lo ta'amod
al dam re'akha,"* and this obligation includes exposure to a limited
amount of risk. Furthermore, the concern for *ḥavala* (prohibition of
inflicting bodily harm) is superseded by the obligation of *"lo ta'amod."*[17]
The halakhic permissibility to subject oneself to the risk of organ donation, however, is predicated on the recipient's halakhic status of *pikuaḥ
nefesh*. The recipient of a uterus transplant would not appear to meet
the criteria of *pikuaḥ nefesh*, as neither her life span, nor her quality of
life are diminished (arguable) in the absence of the transplant. However,
while it is true that an infertile woman is technically not in a state of
pikuaḥ nefesh, it has been argued[18] that infertility may be akin to *pikuaḥ
nefesh*. Indeed, the comment of the Matriarch Rachel, "Give me a child,

---

(*"uve'artzekhem lo ta'asu"*), perhaps even the passive recipient is in violation. However,
since no other authorities seem to mention or concur with this analysis, the *Minḥat
Ḥinukh* does not consider this opinion binding.

16. Donations of partial livers and partial lungs are a matter of halakhic debate, as they
    involve a greater risk to the donor that is not well quantified.

17. On live organ donation, see, for example, M. Halperin, "Organ Transplants from
    Living Donors,"*Assia Jewish Medical Ethics* 2:1 (January, 1991), 29–37; R. Levi Yizchak
    Halperin, "Living Organ Donation," in his *Ma'aseh Ḥoshev* 4 (also titled *Inyanei Refua
    BeHalakha* volume 2) (Institute of Technology and Halakhah, 5757), 54–68 (Hebrew);
    J. David Bleich, "May Tissue Donations Be Compelled," in his *Contemporary Halakhic
    Problems* 4 (Ktav, 1995), 273–315.

18. R. Moshe Sternbuch, *"Akar Bli Banim BeHazra'a Melakhutit MiBaḥutz,"* *Ateret Shlomo*
    7 (5762), 146. It is not clear whether R. Sternbuch's logic is restricted to men. See also,
    J. Loike, M. D. Tendler, and I. Bedzow, "Does Halakhah Consider Female Infertility
    an Illness," *Hakirah* 25 (Fall 2018), 89–102.

for if not, it is as if I am dead," seems to support this. Furthermore, the nature of the donor's risk requires careful analysis in each case. There are at least three possible categories of live uterine transplant candidates, each requiring a separate halakhic analysis.

1) Medically Indicated Hysterectomy

In certain cases of live donation, there may be no halakhic obstacles for the donor. For example, if a woman undergoes a hysterectomy for treatment of a prolapsed uterus, the otherwise healthy uterus would usually be discarded. There is no issue of *havala* for the donor, as she is undergoing the procedure for medical reasons. While there is risk involved in the procedure, this is an acceptable risk for the medical benefit. Furthermore, the uterus does not require burial according to halakha, as limbs (*evarim*) removed from a living person are only customarily buried in order to prevent exposure of a *Kohen* to the impurity generated therefrom.[19] The uterus, which has no bones, does not constitute a legal limb (*ever*). Therefore, it does not generate impurity and does not, according to most authorities, require legal burial. Nor is there any prohibition of deriving benefit from the removed uterus, which is considered "*basar min hahai*" (mere flesh). It may, however, require placement in a proper, respectful place to prevent desecration.[20] Surely, transplantation of the uterus for restoring fertility would not constitute a desecration.

Regarding the issue of sterilization, this would be addressed in the original permission for undergoing the medical procedure, unrelated to the issue of donation. If a woman is allowed to have the hysterectomy for medical reasons, then sterilization is not an additional concern for donation.

2) Prophylactic Surgery for BRCA Gene Positivity

One category of possible candidates for uterine donation intersects with another new area of medical halakha: prophylactic surgery for carriers of

---

19. Abraham S. Abraham, *Nishmat Avraham*, v. 2 (*Y. D.*), p. 267. See also, J. D. Bleich, "Medical Experimentation Upon Severed Organs," in his *Contemporary Halakhic Problems* 1 (Ktav, 1977), 126.
20. *Iggerot Moshe, Y. D.*, 1:232; *Tzitz Eliezer* 10:25, chap. 8.

the breast and ovarian cancer genes, BRCA1 or BRCA2. It has been suggested[21] that women undergoing prophylactic removal of their ovaries to prevent ovarian cancer may wish to have a hysterectomy at the same time. This assumedly healthy uterus could then be donated for transplantation purposes. Leaving the halakhic issue of prophylactic ovarian resection aside,[22] if a woman is permitted to undergo the procedure to remove her ovaries, may she, in addition, have her uterus removed solely for donation purposes?

The surgery is being performed for a separate reason and is not being undertaken exclusively for the organ donation. The halakhically relevant risk in this case is the additional risk of removing just the uterus intra-operatively. This risk would seem negligible. Regarding *ḥavala*, R. Weinreb suggested that the prohibition of *ḥavala* might be mitigated since the procedure would be performed by expert surgeons. This would significantly minimize *ḥavala*.

Regarding sterilization, the donor is being rendered infertile by the primary surgery, the removal of the ovaries. Whether removal of the uterus in addition to the ovaries would, according to those who maintain that *sirus* applies to a woman, constitute an additional violation of *sirus* is a halakhic debate. According to R. Feinstein, legal culpability for sterilization after pre-existing sterilization (*sirus aḥar sirus*) does not apply to a woman.[23] Therefore, there would be no additional prohibition of *sirus* in performing the hysterectomy after the oophorectomy.

---

21. Albert Altchek, "Uterus Transplantation," *Mount Sinai Journal of Medicine* 70:3 (May 2003), 154–162.

22. See J. David Bleich, "Genetic Screening," *Tradition* 34:1 (Spring 2000). For an excellent review of the current state of prophylactic measures in cases BRCA positivity, see S. Galper Grossman, "BRCA Testing for All Ashkenazi Women: A Halakhic Inquiry," *Hakirah* 28 (2020), 257–283.

23. R. Moshe Feinstein, "Hysterectomy and Oophorectomy and Sirus," in R. Moshe Hershler, ed., *Halakha URefua* 4 (Regensberg Institute, 1985), 112–113 (Hebrew); also appears in *Iggerot Moshe*, C.M. 2:73, letter *zayin*. R. Feinstein addressed a case where a woman was undergoing a hysterectomy, and the physicians recommended that she have her ovaries and fallopian tubes removed at the same time to decrease the possibility of future ovarian cancer. The woman had no specific risk factors for cancer, and this occurred prior to the development of testing for BRCA 1 and BRCA 2. While the potential risk for cancer would be an additional reason to allow the

On balance, therefore, given the limited risk, absence of steriliza-tion, and possible *pikuaḥ nefesh* status of the recipient, it may be permit-ted for the woman to donate her uterus. This matter awaits a specific rabbinic ruling.

3) Uterine Donation from the Healthy Donor

A healthy woman in her childbearing years may choose to have a hysterectomy for no other reason than to serve as a uterus donor. It is for such a woman that all the issues of *ḥavala*, risk and steriliza-tion would coexist, apparently unmitigated. While there is a debate as to whether the prohibition of *sirus* applies to a woman, and if the prohibition is biblical or rabbinic in origin, unless there are compel-ling reasons to perform the procedure, most *poskim* would suggest against it.[24] The only factor, which would theoretically permit such a donation, would be the *pikuaḥ nefesh* status of the recipient. This would depend on how we would define the state of infertlity. Is it considered a halakhic illness, or not? Even if it were considered an illness, it is not life threatening. How literal are we to interpret the powerful statement of Rachel, "Give me a child, for, if not, it is as if I am dead."

If the donor were postmenopausal, the equation would change slightly, as the issue of *sirus* may not apply. The concerns regarding risk and *ḥavala*, however, would remain in place.[25]

---

oophorectomy, it does not appear to limit the statement of R. Feinstein that *sirus aḥar sirus* does not apply to a woman. See also R. Moshe Hershler, "Removing a Woman's Reproductive Organs (hysterectomy)," in R. Moshe Hershler, ed., *Halakha URefua*, 1 (Regensberg Institute, 1980), 332–335 (Hebrew). Regarding the prohibition of *sirus aḥar sirus* (sterilization after sterilization) for a man, see A. Steinberg, *Entzyclopedia Hilkhatit Refuit* 5 (Schlesinger Institute, 1996), 59–60.

24. R. Moshe Hershler, "Removing a Woman's Reproductive Organs (hysterectomy)," in R. Moshe Hershler, ed., *Halakha URefua*, 1 (Regensberg Institute, 1980) 332–335 (Hebrew).

25. While a postmenopausal woman is considered halakhically infertile, it is possible today, with ovum donation, for such a woman to carry and give birth to a child. Since this is not a natural process, it would not invalidate the halakhic status of post-menopausal women. See *Veshav Verafa* v. 2 *E. H.*, 69.

Cadaveric Uterine Donation

The issues of *ḥavala*, risk and sterilization are irrelevant to cadaveric donation,[26] as the deceased is no longer bound by halakha. There are, however, obligations and prohibitions relating to the disposition of the body, such as the prohibitions of desecration and deriving benefit from a corpse and the obligation for immediate burial.[27] R. Yeḥezkel Landau established the criteria that would allow these obligations to be suspended in a case of potential *pikuaḥ nefesh*, and required that there be direct and proximate benefit from the information or material gleaned.[28] Whether a woman suffering from infertility would meet these criteria is a matter for further discussion. As discussed, such a woman would clearly not fit the classical definition of *pikuaḥ nefesh*. This specific question awaits further rabbinic clarification.

With respect to the prohibition of desecration of the corpse (*nivul hamet*), if the hysterectomy is performed vaginally (as opposed to abdominally), there would be no external scarring on the body.[29] This, according to some, might not constitute a prohibition of *nivul*. For example, R. Unterman[30] ruled that cornea removal from a corpse for donation would not constitute *nivul* since the eyes are closed for burial and no external scar would be visible. Similarly, R. Feinstein did not consider a needle biopsy to constitute desecration because it leaves no major external scar.[31]

R. Dr. David Applebaum[32] suggests that cadaveric pituitary resection through an intranasal approach might not constitute a violation of

---

26. For this discussion, I assume the organs would be harvested from a non-heart beating cadaver. As opposed to other organs where the viability would be better if harvested from a brain-dead patient, this would likely not apply to the uterus. Thus, the brain death controversy would not factor into this discussion.

27. See A. Steinberg, *Entzyclopedia Hilkhatit Refuit* 4 (Schlesinger Institute, 1994), s. v., "*nituaḥ hamet*."

28. The term was coined as a "*ḥoleh lefaneinu*," a specific ill patient before us.

29. It very might be that in order to preserve the vessels for transplantation, the operation may not be able to be performed vaginally.

30. *Shevet MiYehuda*, 313–322.

31. *Iggerot Moshe Y. D.*, v. 2, n. 111.

32. R. Dr. David Applebaum, "Treatment with Growth Hormone According to Halakhah," in Moshe Hershler, ed., *Halakha URefua* 1 (Regensberg Institute, 1980) 262–271.

nivul for the same reason—no external scar is visible. R. Bleich, however, takes issue with Dr. Applebaum and considers the intranasal removal of the pituitary gland to indeed constitute *nivul*.[33] His logic bears particular relevance to our case. If Dr. Applebaum's approach is correct, R. Bleich argues, then a complete autopsy performed through a vaginal incision only, where all the internal organs are removed, would not constitute *nivul*, as no external scar remains. This cannot be, R. Bleich posits. It therefore must be that there are two components to the prohibition of *nivul*, the process and the result. Both corneal removal and organ biopsy involve no desecration either in process, as they are minor procedures, or in result. Pituitary removal, R. Bleich contends, while leaving no resulting external imprint, is nonetheless a repugnant process constituting a violation of *nivul*. It would therefore seem that R. Bleich would likewise consider a vaginal hysterectomy to constitute *nivul*, as the process of removing the uterus would be at least as halakhically repugnant as removing the pituitary gland.

R. Bleich discounts the position of R. Ettlinger[34] that if a procedure is performed as common medical practice on living human beings, such as a caesarean section, its performance postmortem does not constitute *nivul*. R. Ettlinger's position would seemingly allow for a postmortem vaginal hysterectomy, as the procedure is a commonly performed on living human beings.

III. UTERINE TRANPLANTATION—THE RECIPIENT

In the early halakhic literature on reproductive organ transplant, a number of issues were raised regarding the status of the recipient. These same issues merit consideration for our case of uterine transplantation.

Ḥavala—Wounding

In the journal *HaBe'er*, as mentioned above, R. Posek opposed the entire procedure of reproductive organ transplant because it entails a violation

---

33. "Pituitary Dwarfism," in his *Contemporary Halakhic Problems* 2 (Ktav, 1983), 64–68. R. Bleich further discusses the issue in a letter to *Tradition*, "Nivul Ha-Met," *Tradition* 37:3 (Fall 2003), 101.

34. Binyan Tzion cited in Applebaum, op. cit., 266.

of *ḥavala* for both the donor and the recipient. R. Weinreb, while concurring that *ḥavala* would apply to the donor, even if only minimal danger is involved, maintained that this prohibition does not apply to the recipient for two reasons. First, the procedure would be performed by expert surgeons, a fact that might minimize the *ḥavala*. Second, the prohibition might be waived for the sake of procreation and marital harmony.

In almost all cases of modern organ donation discussed in rabbinic literature, the halakhic issues for the recipient require little discussion. Since the recipients are in a category of *pikuaḥ nefesh*, they are permitted to undergo the procedure. The concern for *ḥavala* in the performance of surgery, as well as any other halakhic issues, is suspended. In the case of uterine transplant, since the organ recipient may not be in a state of *pikuaḥ nefesh*, we must consider the possibility of the surgical procedure constituting a prohibition of *ḥavala*.

The issue of undergoing surgery for bodily enhancement, in the absence of illness, has been addressed in the essays on plastic surgery in halakha.[35] These essays discuss the prohibition of *ḥavala* and its exclusions and limitations. Is uterine transplant for the treatment of infertility considered an elective, enhancing procedure analogous to plastic surgery, or is it a therapeutic intervention for the treatment of a disease? If the latter, then *ḥavala* would be permitted much the same as the *ḥavala* of surgery for the removal of an infected appendix is permitted. However, as opposed to appendicitis, where surgical appendectomy is the only

---

35. J. David Bleich, "Plastic Surgery," in his *Contemporary Halakhic Problems* 1 (Ktav, 1977), 119–123; R. Ḥayyim Eisenstein, "Plastic Surgery for Cosmetic Purposes in Halakhah," *Ateret Shlomo* 1 (5756), 57–72 (Hebrew); David B. Ettengoff, "Halachic Implications of Cosmetic Surgery," *Journal of Halacha and Contemporary Society* 15 (Spring 1988), 79; R. Moshe Feinstein, "Cosmetic Surgery for a Young Women to Improve her Appearance," in R. Moshe Hershler, ed., *Halakha URefua*, 1 (Regensberg Institute, 1980), 323–327 (Hebrew); R. Shlomo Yosef Zevin, "May One Person Grant Permission to Another to Injure Him?" in R. Moshe Hershler, ed., *Halakha URefua* 2 (Regensberg Institute, 1981) 93–100 (Hebrew); M. Westreich, "Orthodox Jewish Law (Halachah) and Plastic Surgery," *Plastic Reconstructive Surgery* 102:3 (September, 1998), 908–913. More recently, the principles of *ḥavala* have been employed to permit accepting money for organ donation. See, for example, "Rav Shaul Yisraeli—Organ Transplants: Responsa," in *Jewish Medical Ethics* 3:1, 14–17.

possible cure, infertility can be treated in less invasive and less halakhically problematic ways.

For example, if the woman has functional ovaries, she could use her eggs for in-vitro fertilization and contract the services of a surrogate to bear the child. However, while the subsequent progeny will be the genetic product of the husband and wife, the wife's (egg donor) claim to halakhic maternity may be in doubt.[36] Should we say that since the wife has no obligation of *peru urevu*, perhaps this is of little legal relevance? Or should we consider the wife's desire to have a legal child sufficient to outweigh the prohibition of *ḥavala* and allow her to undergo the procedure of uterine transplant?[37] If the child is not legally related to the wife, the child would have a different relationship with the woman, and, for example, would have no technical obligation of *kibud av va'em*.

Even if we consider uterine transplant a non-therapeutic intervention, similar to cosmetic surgery, some authorities have allowed *ḥavala* in the case of cosmetic surgery for psychological reasons.[38] Perhaps the psychological impact of restoring fertility may justify the *ḥavala* of uterine transplant surgery as well. In addition, as mentioned above, some ascribe to infertility a modified *pikuaḥ nefesh* status. In addition, as R. Weinreb mentioned in the earlier discussions, marital harmony is at stake. Perhaps the combination of all these factors would be sufficient to waive the prohibition of *ḥavala*.

Sakana—Risk

An additional issue is the inherent risk involved in the entire process of organ transplantation. In the early halakhic discussions, R. S. Weiss[39] briefly raised the concern of the recipient submitting herself to a procedure involving halakhically questionable risk.[40] For the case of uterine transplantation, as well as any other type of transplant, the risk includes

---

36. See discussion on the definition of maternity below.
37. See *Yevamot* 65b. A woman desires a child to assist her in her old age.
38. R. Feinstein, cited above.
39. *Vayelaket Yosef*, Year 10, vol. 6 (Ḥanukka 5668/December, 1907), 21b.
40. Regarding the permissibility of undergoing risky or unproved therapy, see J. D. Bleich, "Experimental Procedures: The Concept of *Refu'ah Bedukah*," in his *Contemporary Halakhic Problems* 4 (Ktav, 1995), 203–217.

the surgery itself, as well as the medications that are required to prevent the recipient from rejecting the donated organ. These so-called immunosuppressive medications, while preventing organ rejection, also suppress the patient's immune system. This makes the patient susceptible to serious, even fatal complications from even the most benign infectious diseases, such as the common cold. People receiving transplants such as kidney, liver or heart, are clearly halakhically allowed to subject themselves to the risks of surgery and immunosuppressive medications in order to prolong their lives. In the last few years, however, a number of transplants have been performed for non-life-threatening conditions, such as hand, larynx and uterine transplants.[41] These cases have been the subject of ethical debate in the medical literature for much the same reason that they present a halakhic problem.[42] Is it permissible to subject a patient to complicated surgery and prolonged immunosuppression for a medical condition that is not life threatening?

Furthermore, in uterine transplantation, the sole purpose of the transplant is to facilitate subsequent pregnancy. Pregnancy itself for patients on immunosuppressive medications may carry greater risks than a normal pregnancy.[43]

There is one mitigating factor unique to uterine transplant, however, which may minimize the halakhic concern about the risks of prolonged immunosuppressive therapy. While hand or larynx transplants necessitate lifelong immunosuppressive medicines, the uterus transplant is required only for bearing children. Once that objective has been accomplished, the uterus can be surgically removed and the medications stopped. Whether this fact would suffice to allow the transplant is a matter that requires further elucidation.

---

41. M. R. Hausman, et al., "Hand Transplantation: Current Status," *Mount Sinai Journal of Medicine* 70:3 (May, 2003), 148–153; E. M Genden and M. L. Urken, "Laryngeal and Tracheal Transplantation: Ethical Limitations," *Mount Sinai Journal of Medicine* 70:3 (May, 2003), 163–165; A. Altchek, "Uterine Transplantation," *Mount Sinai Journal of Medicine* 70:3 (May, 2003), 154–162.

42. G. J. Agich, "Extension of Organ Transplantation: Some Ethical Considerations," *Mount Sinai Journal of Medicine* 70:3 (May, 2003), 141–147.

43. Altchek, op. cit., 160–161.

Definition of Maternity

In the earlier discussion of reproductive organ transplant, the rabbis assumed that the ovaries, uterus and external genitalia were transplanted. As such, they grappled with the definition of maternity for the child born to the recipient. R. Weiss maintained that the halakhic mother of the offspring would be the organ recipient.[44] He brings proof for this position from the case in *Sota* 43b, where a branch of an *orla* tree, which is less than three years old and forbidden to eat, is grafted onto an older tree, whose fruit is permitted. The Gemara concludes that for halakhic purposes the branch becomes an integral part of the receiving tree and loses its original identity. Here, too, the transplanted organs would lose their identity and become an integral part of the recipient's body. The recipient would therefore be considered the sole halakhic mother.

R. Yeshaya Silverstein, head of the rabbinical court in Veitzen, likewise concluded that the transplanted organs, for halakhic purposes, become part of the recipient's body.[45] His proof is particularly relevant to our case as it specifically addresses uterine transplantation. He cites a passage in *Bekhorot* 28b regarding the *treifa* status of an animal whose uterus has been removed. In support of the position that such an animal is not a *treifa*, the Gemara mentions the practice in Alexandria, Egypt of removing the uteri of the cattle that were sold or exported.[46] Since these animals obviously lived for prolonged periods of time after the procedure (longer than twelve months), this is proof that the absence of a uterus does not constitute a *treifa*. R. Silverstein questions the Gemara's proof. If, by definition, the absence of a particular organ constitutes a *treifa*, then the animal's subsequent lifespan is irrelevant. Even should such an animal live longer than twelve months, it would still be considered a *treifa*.[47]

---

44. *Vayelaket Yosef*, Year 10, vol. 9, n. 77 (January, 1908), 29a.

45. *Tel Talpiyot*, Year 17, n. 19 (June, 1908), 169–171.

46. The cattle from this region were considered of superior quality. Removing the uterus would prevent the buyer from using the animal for breeding, thereby insuring the seller's control of the market.

47. This is the position of R. Yehezkel Landau in his commentary *Dagul MeR'vava*, Y. D., 29. Others maintain that the definition of *treifa* is restricted to animals that would invariably die within twelve months. See *Entzyclopedia Talmudit* 21, s. v., "*treifa*" (*ba'alei hayyim*) for extensive discussion on the laws of *treifa*.

R. Silverstein therefore understands the proof of the Gemara that the reason absence of the uterus is not a *treifa* is because the condition can be reversed with the transplantation of a uterus from another animal. *Treifa*, by definition, only applies to an irreversible ailment. If the removed organ can be effectively replaced, then its absence does not constitute a *treifa*. After transplantation the animal could return to complete health and fertility. Furthermore, the transplanted organs must be considered part of the recipient in order to sustain this proof; otherwise, the recipient would still be halakhically considered to have missing organs.

The definition of maternity in cases of surrogacy[48] remains one of the more complex areas of modern medical halakha.[49] The halakhic positions span the gamut and ascribe maternity to the genetic, gestational, and parturition (birth) mother, to no mother, and to many mothers. In the conventional case of the gestational host, where one woman donates the egg and the other carries the child, the two candidates vying for maternity are the genetic donor and the gestational or birth mother. The distinction between gestation and parturition (birth) is theoretical, since invariably, they are accomplished by the same person. In the case of uterine transplant, this distinction may become relevant,[50] depending on the status of the transplanted uterus. This may force us to reconsider the position that ascribes maternity to the gestational mother more carefully.

---

48. I refer here only to the case of the gestational host, where a woman carries in her womb the genetic child of another woman. The term surrogate motherhood, technically refers to a case where the surrogate is both the genetic and gestational mother, as was the case with Mary Beth Whitehead.

49. J. David Bleich, "Surrogate Motherhood," in his *Bioethical Dilemmas: A Jewish Perspective* (Ktav, 1998); E. Bick, "Ovum Donations: A Rabbinic Conceptual Model of Maternity," *Tradition* 28:1 (1993), 28–45; M. J. Broyde, "The Establishment of Maternity and Paternity in Jewish and American Law," *National Jewish Law Review* 3 (1988), 117–158; J. David Bleich, "In Vitro Fertilization, Maternal Identity and Conversion," in his *Contemporary Halakhic Problems* 4 (Ktav, 1995), 237–272; Y. Breitowitz, "Halakhic Alternatives in IVF Pregnancies: A Survey," *Jewish Law Annual* 14 (2003), 29–119, esp. 56–65; Avraham Kurtztag, "The Status of a Child Born from a Surrogate Mother," *Ateret Shlomo* 4 (5759), 173–183 (Hebrew); R. Aviad Trop, "Surrogate Motherhood," *Ateret Shlomo* 5 (5760), 100–122, esp. 113–116 (Hebrew).

50. The distinction is also relevant in a theoretical case where the embryo is transferred from one woman to another prior to birth. No such case has yet been reported in the medical literature.

If the transplanted uterus, wherein the gestation occurs, retains the identity of the donor, then the gestational mother, the donor, would be distinct from the birth mother, the recipient, who also happens to be the genetic mother. Both could then lay halakhic claim to maternity.[51] However, the preponderance of rabbinic opinion from the early halakhic literature maintained that any organ, once transplanted, assumes the identity of the recipient. If, indeed, the donor forgoes all rights to the organ once transplanted, and the organ acquires a new status in the recipient, then the uterus recipient is the genetic, parturition and birth mother, and is logically the only candidate for maternity.

Erva—Prohibited Physical Relationships

In the early halakhic discussions, where the rabbis assumed that all the internal and external reproductive organs were transplanted, the very first issue addressed in the first journal discussion is that of *erva*, as the husband of the transplant recipient would be having direct physical contact with the external reproductive organs of another woman.[52] R. Deutch considered this case to be halakhically comparable to having relations with a corpse; an act, although reprehensible and perhaps rabbinically prohibited, nonetheless does not constitute a biblical violation of *erva*.[53] The organs, once removed from the donor, are simply inanimate limbs of a corpse, rendering the prohibition of *erva* inapplicable

---

51. R. Z. N. Goldberg espouses the position that the gestational mother may be the halakhic mother in "*Yiḥus Amhut BiHashtalat Ubar BiReḥem Shel Aḥeret,*" *Teḥumin* 5 (5744), 248–259. See also J. David Bleich, "In Vitro Fertilization, Maternal Identity and Conversion," in his *Contemporary Halakhic Problems* 4 (Ktav, 1995), 248–251, and R. Aviad Trop, "Surrogate Motherhood," *Ateret Shlomo* 5 (5760), 113–116 (Hebrew). R. Bleich, in another essay, rejects the position ascribing maternity to a woman whose only contribution is gestation, and maintains that the definition of the gestational mother as the halakhic mother is predicated on that same mother's subsequent birthing of the child. See "*Be'Inyan Ḥalav Treifa UKeviat Amhut,*" in his *Benitivot HaHalakha,* v. 3 (*kuntres harefua*) (Ktav, 2000), 47–48.

52. *Vayelaket Yosef,* Year 10, vol. 3 (15 Ḥeshvan, 5668/October 23, 1907), 9a–9b.

53. *Yevamot* 55b and Maimonides, *Hil. Issurei Bi'ah* 1:12.

to them.[54] For more expansive discussion on the issue of *erva*, I refer you to the previous chapter.

In the current case of uterine transplant, the first issue to clarify is exactly which anatomical structures are being transplanted, and whether it is possible that a man having relations with a uterus recipient would have direct physical contact with the transplanted organ. Since the entire uterus, including the cervix, would be transplanted, it is indeed possible, as opposed to ovarian transplantation, that the husband of the recipient would have direct physical contact with the transplanted organ. Therefore, all the aforementioned discussions about the question of *erva* in reproductive organ transplantation could be directly assimilated to the current case of uterine transplant. As the majority of respondents considered the transplanted organs to acquire a new status in the recipient, the potential concern about the prohibition of *erva* is negated and should not be an impediment to uterine transplantation.

Bekhor—First Born

In the journal *Vayelaket Yosef*[55] R. Deutch addresses the issue of whether a child born from the organ transplant recipient would bear the status of a firstling, or *bekhor*. The Gemara, in *Ḥullin* 70a, brings a hypothetical case where the birth canal is so wide that the fetus can exit without direct physical contact with the uterine (or vaginal) walls. Is the air space of the uterus sufficient to generate the status of *bekhor*, the Gemara queries, or is direct physical contact with the uterine walls required? Maimonides maintains that the fetus in this case would be a questionable

---

54. The respondent acknowledges that in the case of a man having relations with a complete corpse, there is a rabbinic prohibition which was instituted to prevent one from extrapolating that, amongst other things, relations with a *treifa* would be permitted. However, once the body is no longer whole, as in this case, the decree would not apply. In addition, he argues that it must be the living body that generates *erva*, and not simply the reproductive organs. For if it were the latter, one could envision a scenario whereby one could circumvent the prohibition of *erva* with a woman by replacing her reproductive organs with those of a non-*erva*. Furthermore, he argues, that if the reproductive organs were the determinant for *erva*, doubt would be cast on all legal cases of *erva*. It would impossible for witnesses to ever verify whether the reproductive organs of the female were in fact her own, or those of a non-*erva*.

55. Year 10, vol. 4 (1 *Kislev* 5668/November 7, 1907), 12a–12b.

bekhor.[56] In our case, according to R. Deutch, the uterine walls belong to the donor, while the air space belongs to the recipient. Therefore, a child born to the organ recipient would be the first to pass through the air space of her birth canal, and, according to this logic, would be considered a questionable *bekhor*.

The discussion continued in the journal in two subsequent issues. Citing a passage from *Ḥullin*, R. Sheftel Weiss believed that he had found a remarkable talmudic analogy to our case of reproductive organ transplantation.[57] In the talmudic hypothetical, the uteri of two animals are adjacent to each other and the fetus moves from one uterus to the second before being born.[58] The Gemara ponders for which animal would this fetus would be considered a *bekhor*. R. S. Weiss does not elaborate, however, as to how this passage would be practically applied to our case.

In another journal, R. Katzburg discussed the issue of *bekhor*.[59] As mentioned above, he was of the opinion, even regarding the earlier case of reproductive organ transplant, that only the uterus was transplanted. His comments on the issue of *bekhor* are therefore directly relevant to our case. R. Katzburg claimed that even if this uterus, while part of the donor, had already borne fruit and previously produced a *bekhor*, since it takes on a new identity in the recipient, the first born for the recipient with the transplanted uterus would be considered a halakhic *bekhor*. Furthermore, he contends that the reason a caesarean birth precludes *bekhor* status is because the fetus must exit naturally through the birth canal.[60]

With respect to the current case of uterine transplant, R. Katzburg's position should apply directly to our case. According to this position, a first-born male child of the organ recipient should indeed be a full-fledged

---

56. *Hil. Bekhorot* 4:19.

57. Year 10, vol. 6 (Ḥanukka 5668/December, 1907), 21b.

58. It is unclear from the passage where the exact point of contact is. *Tosafot* s. v., "*ad*" in *Ketubot* 4b considers this case to be purely hypothetical ("*davar shelo ba le'olam*").

59. *Tel Talpiyot*, Year 17, no. 19 (*Sivan*, 5668/June, 1908), 169–171.

60. The Mishna in *Bekhorot* 47b excludes a child born by caesarean section from the laws of *bekhor*. The law is codified in *Y. D.*, 305:24. Regarding the history of caesarean section in Jewish sources see chapter, "A Matter of Life 'in' Death: Postmortem Caesarean Section in Jewish Law."

bekhor.[61] However, the current medical reality may render the entire discussion about *bekhor* in uterine transplantation moot, at least as it relates to the requirement of *pidyon haben.* The present protocol for all patients with a uterus transplant requires that they deliver through caesarean section. Normal spontaneous vaginal delivery would likely damage the anatomical connects and integrity of the transplanted uterus. A firstborn male child born through caesarean section is not required to undergo a *pidyon haben.*[62] Transplant surgeons, however, have recently begun to consider the possibility of vaginal delivery after uterus transplantation. If this comes to fruition, the aforementioned literature on *bekhor* would certainly be relevant.

Hana'at Hamet—Deriving Benefit from a Corpse

R. S. Weiss[63] briefly raised the concern about the prohibition of deriving benefit from a corpse.[64] If the uterine donation is cadaveric, then the recipient must indeed consider the prohibition of deriving benefit from a corpse.[65] There is debate as to whether this prohibition is rabbinic or biblical in nature, and this debate impacts on the case of uterine transplant. According to R. Yaacov Emden,[66] and R. Yehuda Rosanes,[67] the

---

61. See discussions on definition of maternity and *erva*. Regarding R. Deutch's source above and the air space of the womb, it would have to be clarified whether the air space in question refers exclusively to the air space of the uterus, or of the birth canal as well. If it includes the birth canal, then, according to R. Deutch, a child born from a uterine transplant recipient would likewise be a questionable *bekhor*.

62. See note 60 above.

63. *Vayelaket Yosef,* Year 10, vol. 6 (Ḥanukka 5668/December, 1907), 21b.

64. Most of the respondents in the earlier halakhic discussion, based on the initial question posed to them, assumed the organ donation to be from a live donor. R. Weiss entertained the possibility of cadaveric donation.

65. On the following, see J. D. Bleich, "Pituitary Dwarfism," in his *Contemporary Halakhic Problems* 2 (Ktav, 1983), 64–68.

66. *She'ilat Ya'avetz* 1:41. On a historical note, this *teshuva* was addressed to Benjamin Wolff Gintzburger, a medical student in Germany who wrote a treatise on biblical and talmudic medicine for his medical school dissertation. See F. Schiller, "Benjamin Wolff Gintzberger's Dissertation on Talmudic Medicine," *Koroth* 2:7–8 (1960), 307–318. On the field of biblical and talmudic medicine in general, see chapter, "Biblical and Talmudic Medicine: A Bibliographical Essay."

67. *Mishneh LeMelekh, Hil. Avel* 14:21. This passage deals with the ingestion of Egyptian mummy extract for medicinal purposes, which was common practice in the Middle

prohibition is rabbinic.[68] If so, perhaps the use of a cadaveric uterus would be permitted, as Rema rules that materials for which the prohibition of deriving benefit is only rabbinic in origin may be utilized for the treatment of any sick person, even those not in imminent danger.[69] However, the majority opinion rules that deriving benefit from a corpse is biblical in origin. Even amongst those who believe the prohibition to be biblical, some maintain that the material may be used for medical therapy if the particular use is unusual, or not characteristic for that object (*shelo kiderekh hana'a*),[70] or if the amount used is small (less than an olive size). While the size of the uterus is larger than this small amount, using the uterus for transplantation is not a halakhically usual or characteristic use for human tissue.[71]

If the donation comes from a non-Jewish cadaver, rabbinic authorities debate whether the specific prohibition of deriving benefit from a corpse applies to non-Jewish cadavers as well.[72]

Nidda – Ritual Impurity of Menstruation

In the early halakhic literature, R. Silverstein raised the issue of *nidda*, as one of the requirements for generating the *tum'ah* (impurity) of *nidda* is for the woman to actually sense the menstrual flow "*bivsara*" (i.e., in her flesh) as it exits her body.[73] If, as was the considered case

---

Ages and early Renaissance. For more on this chapter in medical halakhic history, see chapter, "The Impact of Medieval Medicine on Medical Halakha: The Case of Mumia."

68. On the derivation of the prohibition of deriving benefit from a corpse and the definition of *shelo kiderekh hana'a*, see *HaRefua L'Or HaHalakha*, vol. 2 (Makhon LeHeker HaRefua VeHalakhah: Jerusalem, 5743), 25–27 and 104–110.

69. *Y. D.*, 155:3.

70. Whether one allows use of a prohibited object *shelo kiderekh hana'a* may depend on the whether the derivation of the prohibition of deriving benefit from a corpse is from the laws of *egla arufa* or from *avoda zara*. See *HaRefua L'Or HaHalakha*, vol. 2 (Makhon LeHeker HaRefua VeHalakhah, 5743), 104–110.

71. The usual use of human flesh would be for human ingestion, similar to animal meats.

72. See *HaRefua L'Or HaHalakha*, vol. 2 (Makhon LeHeker HaRefua VeHalakhah, 5743), 33–40.

73. This halakha is derived from the term "*bivsara*" (in her flesh) in Vayikra 15:19. See *Nidda* 57b and *Y. D.*, 183:1.

then, the entire set of reproductive organs was transplanted, and the transplanted organs retained their legal association with the donor, the menstrual flow of the recipient might not technically meet the criterion of "*bivsara.*" Perhaps, then, the recipient would never become a *nidda.* This cannot be, contended R. Silverstein, as this would effectively circumvent all the laws of *nidda* for the recipient. Rather, the organs must become part of the recipient's body such that any flow would be considered "in her flesh."[74]

In the current case of uterine transplantation, even if the donated uterus retains the legal status of the donor, one might argue that the recipient would still become a *nidda,* since the menstrual flow would come into contact with the recipient's own reproductive organs when it exits the uterus.

Sirus—Sterilization

In the journal *HaBe'er,*[75] R. Weinreb responded to an earlier entry in the journal regarding the organ donor's violation of the prohibition of sterilization. Explaining why *sirus* does not apply to the recipient, whose ovaries are also removed before the transplant, R. Weinreb opines that the removal of nonfunctional reproductive organs may not constitute *sirus.*[76]

In the case of uterine transplant, if the recipient had undergone a medically indicated hysterectomy at an earlier stage, there would be no issue of *sirus* at the time of the transplant, as no further reproductive organs of the recipient are altered or removed at that time. If the recipient had congenital absence of the uterus, as in Rokitansky Syndrome, then there would surely be no issue of sirus.

---

74. Today, we understand sensation to be dependent on innervation. Even with uterine transplantation, the severed sensory nerves would likely not regain their function in the recipient. Even if the transplanted organs were halakhically considered an integral part of the recipient's body, the recipient would still be unable to actually sense the menstrual flow.

75. Year 7, vol. 2, nos. 70–71 (*Shevat,* 5692; January/February, 1932), 88–92.

76. See *Minḥat Ḥinukh,* mitzva 291.

IV. CONCLUSION

The mistaken question of R. Gordon in 1907 about reproductive organ transplantation has left us a fertile source of halakhic material that directly and indirectly addresses the contemporary case of uterine transplantation. While further analysis will be required to explore and resolve the halakhic dilemmas generated from this new procedure, the issues raised by our predecessors serve as an excellent starting point. This serves as a testimony to the enduring value of the halakhic discourse of every generation.

Shared Biological Paternity in Rabbinic Literature: From Goliath to Mitochondrial DNA and the Three-Parent Embryo

I. INTRODUCTION

Partible or shared paternity is a notion of paternity espoused by certain cultures, mainly in the Amazon region, whereby a child is believed to have more than one biological father.[1] Men who have had relations with a woman either before conception or during pregnancy are believed to contribute biological material to the child. In this chapter, we will discuss

---

1. S. Beckerman, et al., "The Bari Partible Paternity Project: Preliminary Results," *Current Anthropology* 39:1 (February, 1998), 164–168; S. Milius, "Who says only one sperm gets the prize?" *Science News* 155:5 (January 30, 1999), 71; S. Beckerman and P. Valentine, eds., *The Theory and Practice of Partible Paternity in South America* (University Press of Florida, 2002); W. Shapiro, *Partible Paternity and Anthropological Theory: The Construction of an Ethnographic Fantasy* (University Press of America, 2009); R. S. Walker, et al., "Evolutionary History of Partible Paternity in Lowland South America," *Proceedings of the National Academy of Sciences* 107:45 (2010), 19195–19200.

how this notion is reflected in rabbinic literature, and how its expression in rabbinic literature is distinct from that in other cultures. We will then address the rabbinic sources that explore the halakhic ramifications of this belief in different legal scenarios. Finally, we suggest how the rabbinic discussions on shared paternity might be applied to resolve a modern halakhic dilemma of genetically shared maternity, known as the three-parent embryo, where two women contribute biological material to one egg.

II. THE NOTION OF PARTIBLE OR SHARED PATERNITY

In a number of cultures, primarily in the Amazon, there is a pervasive societal belief that it is possible for one child to have more than one biological father. Shared paternity is considered a positive phenomenon with advantageous ramifications, including social and financial, and cohabitation of a pregnant woman with other men is encouraged based on this belief. All the "fathers" have a corresponding responsibility to provide care and support to this child.

The notion of shared biological paternity also finds its expression in rabbinic literature, though it is fundamentally different than that espoused by other cultures. In Jewish law, where it is absolutely forbidden for a married woman to cohabitate with another man, the notion of shared paternity is not a positive notion and is considered repulsive. In rabbinic sources, the notion of shared paternity is mentioned as a reflection of the moral depravity of other cultures, as contrasted and distinguished from the Jewish tradition.[2] It also finds its expression in relation to potential legal dilemmas that may result from the possibility of accidental shared paternity.

III. SHARED PATERNITY- RABBINIC SOURCES

The Talmud on the Birth of Goliath—The Locus Classicus

In its description of the birth of Goliath, the Bible says, "The man of *Beinayim* went out from the camp of the Philistines."[3] The talmudic

---

2. See, for example, Avraham ben Azarya Ḥakham, *Sefer Yizraeli* (Jerusalem, 5725), *Parashat Kedoshim*, 199; Yachya Albadiḥi, *Ḥen Tov* (Jerusalem, 5730), 55.

3. I Samuel 17:4.

discussion of this passage focuses on the interpretation and linguistic analysis of the word *"Beinayim."*[4]

> What means *"Beinayim?"* — Rav said: That he was built up [*mevuneh*] without any blemish. Shmuel said: He was the middle one [*beinoni*] of his brothers. In the School of R. Shila they explained: He was made like a building [*binyan*]. R. Yoḥanan said: He was the son of a hundred fathers and one mother [*ben nane*].

It is the interpretation of R. Yoḥanan that concerns us here.[5] According to R. Yoḥanan, the word *"beinayim"* reflects the fact that the mother of Goliath had relations with one hundred men, after which Goliath was conceived. Rashi explains that many men cohabited with the mother of Goliath in one night, but only one of them was considered his legal father.[6] All the others were adulterers. Rashi clearly assumes that shared paternity is not possible, as he explicitly states that despite the many men who had relations with Goliath's mother within a short period of time, legal paternity is assigned only to one. *Tosafot*, however, cites a position in the *Talmud Yerushalmi* that differs with Rashi.[7] Indeed, the *Talmud Yerushalmi* cites a position that clearly accepts the notion of shared paternity, and claims that all the men who cohabited with the mother of Goliath are biological fathers and share legal paternity.[8] It

---

4. *Sota* 42b.
5. According to some interpretations (see *Tosafot Sota* 42b s. v., *"me'ah"*), Goliath's mother also cohabited with a dog, which contributed materially to Goliath. See *Vayikra Rabba, Sefer Ha'Arukh*, s. v., *"ben bi-sof,"* and further analysis by Yosef Ḥayyim ben Eliyahu Ḥayyim MiBagdad, *Ben Yehoyada, Sota*, chapter 8, s. v., *"ben me'ah papi."* The author suggests literary allusions from the references to Goliath that he was derivative from a dog. The notion of an embryo composite of both human and animal DNA merits its own analysis and will not be considered here.
6. *Sota* 42b, s. v., *"bar me'ah."*
7. *Sota* 42b, s. v., *"me'ah papi."*
8. *Yerushalmi Yevamot* 4:2. While this passage in *Yerushalmi* is an explicit reference to the notion of shared paternity, R. Tamar brings a number of other passages in the *Yerushalmi* that he believes allude to the idea of shared paternity. See his *Alei Tamar: Yerushalmi Nashim* (Atir Publications, 1981), *Yevamot*, chapter 4, p. 16.

also records a dissenting opinion that maintains that, "a woman cannot conceive from two men at once."[9]

Three-Day Limitation on Shared Biological Paternity

R. Masya in the *Talmud Yerushalmi* clarifies that the debate about the possibility of shared paternity is limited to the time before the (male) seed putrefies. After one man cohabitates with a woman, if other men cohabitate with the same woman within three days, before the seed of the first man putrefies, then shared biological paternity is possible. After this period, all would agree that shared paternity is no longer possible. This idea of a time limitation of three days on the possibility of shared paternity appears to be unique to the rabbinic version of shared paternity and is not held by the other cultures that espouse the notion of shared paternity.[10]

Even within the rabbinic tradition this time limitation is debated. R. Yisakhar Tamar (twentieth century) questions this three-day limit from a Midrash that implies that shared paternity is possible even if coition occurs at a considerably later date.[11] The idea expressed in the Midrash is that God punishes an adulteress by making the child's appearance similar to the adulterer, even if the act of adultery occurs long after the woman is already pregnant from her husband.[12] R. Tamar considers

---

9. See A. Zilber, *Az Yashir* (Jerusalem, 5769), 229 who posits that according to the *Talmud Yerushalmi* it is possible for a woman to conceive from more than one male seed, while the *Bavli* may disagree with this fact. He also notes that Rashi himself holds that one cannot conceive from two men. See chapter, "Is There Life After Life: Superfetation in Medical, Historical and Rabbinic Literature" where I suggest a similar idea of disagreement between the two Talmuds in another area of reproductive physiology, the medical feasibility of superfetation (the possibility of a pregnant woman conceiving again from a subsequent ovulation).

10. See for example, S. Beckerman and P. Valentine, "The Concept of Partible Paternity Among Native South Americans," in S. Beckerman and P. Valentine, eds., *Cultures of Multiple Fathers: The Theory and Practice of Partible Paternity in Lowland South America* (University Press of Florida, 2002), 1–13. Confirmed by personal correspondence with S. Beckerman (December 29, 2014).

11. *Alei Tamar: Yerushalmi Nashim* (Atir Publications, 1981), *Yevamot*, chapter 4, p. 15ff.

12. R. Tamar cites another Midrash that implies that shared paternity may be limited to forty days after conception from her husband, as it is at forty days that the fetus begins to form. See *Bamidbar Rabba, Naso* 9:1, and *Eitz Yosef*, ad loc.

this a case of shared paternity and therefore questions the assumption of the *Talmud Yerushalmi* that shared paternity can only occur if the cohabitations are within three days of each other.

Shared Biological Paternity v. Maternal Impressions

I believe that R. Tamar[13] may be mistaken in his assumption that this passage of the Midrash refers to a case of shared paternity. It may possibly be referring to another phenomenon, known as maternal imprinting or impressions,[14] whereby the objects a woman sees during conception or pregnancy are believed to impact on the physical composition of her child.[15] In fact, one of the classic examples of the notion of maternal impressions in rabbinic literature is found in the very same chapter of the Midrash.[16] An Arabian king confided in R. Akiva that his wife, dark-skinned like himself, begat him a white-skinned child. As he considered this clear evidence of her infidelity, he intended to sentence her to death. R. Akiva asked the king if the sculptures in his palace were of white or dark color. When the king answered that they were white, R. Akiva explained that she likely set her eyes upon these white statues during the time of their relations, thus imprinting the white color on their child. This explanation appeased the king.

Furthermore, other rabbinic authorities explicitly link the Midrash mentioned by R. Tamar about the facial appearance of the child of an adulteress with the notion of maternal impressions.[17]

---

13. This would equally apply to the *Eitz Yosef*, cited by R. Tamar, who also clearly states that the midrashic case of adultery is a case of shared paternity.
14. Other synonymous terms include psychic maternal impressions, mental influence, and maternal imagination. For additional discussion, see chapter, "The First Halakhic Discussion of Ovarian Transplantation."
15. It is also possible that the Midrash addresses neither shared paternity nor maternal impression, but rather a unique divine punishment for adultery not based on either of these notions.
16. *Bamidbar Rabba, Naso* 9:32.
17. See "Rabbinic Court Decisions on the Determination of Paternity," (Hebrew) *Or Hamizraḥ* 4:3–4 (*Elul*, 5717), 35–40; Ḥayyim Pardes, "Facial Resemblance as a Proof of Paternity," (Hebrew) in his *Kevoda Shel Torah* 4 (5748), 81–84. See also, D. Barda, "Paternity Based on Facial Appearance," (Hebrew) *Zekhor LeAvraham* (5754–5755), 577–581.

The idea that maternal impressions serve as a public way of exposing adulterers or recalcitrant fathers was not unique to rabbinic tradition. There is a remarkable, if not highly imaginative, case recorded in the nineteenth century of a man who denied being the father of a woman's unborn child and reportedly gave his solemn oath that he would never acknowledge paternity for this child unless his name was literally written across the child's face. As is recorded, this fact made such an impression on the young woman that when the child was born, the name of the father appeared in legible letters in the child's eye. The account concludes with this cautionary message:

> This child has... been ...pronounced to be a most wonderful phenomenon of nature, and an astonishing dispensation of Providence in pointing out the truth against the wicked and perjured ways of men. An inspection of this child will, it is hoped, be a salutary warning to all young persons of both sexes, first to beware of all such doings and second, to beware of perjury in their attempts to conceal their shame.[18]

Maternal imprinting was believed to occur throughout pregnancy and was not limited to the first few days after conception. For example, if a pregnant woman would see a child with a cleft palate during pregnancy, it was believed that the child she bore would exhibit the same defect. In the case of the Midrash, the vision of the adulterer during pregnancy is imprinted on the fetus. This was a universally held belief since antiquity, and as opposed to shared paternity, which is held by a few select cultures, was virtually ubiquitous across the globe.[19] There is a rich lit-

---

18. T. E. C., Jr., "The Power of Maternal Impression Causes Alleged Father's Name to Appear in Legible Letters in His Infant Son's Right Eye (1817)," *Pediatrics* 58 (1976), 901.

19. See J. W. Ballantyne, "Teratogenesis: An Inquiry into the Causes of Monstrosities," *Transactions of the Edinburgh Obstetrical Society* 21 (1896), 220–232, 258– 296. There he writes, "As will be made abundantly evident when the history of the belief in maternal impressions comes under consideration, the notion is one of great antiquity; but it may here be pointed out that it is also one of practically world-wide distribution." See also J. Pearn and J. Sweet, "The Origins of Pregnancy Superstitions Relating to

erature on the history of this notion and scientists up to the pre-modern period have treated it seriously. Its ultimate origins may trace back to the biblical story of Jacob and the sheep, where the color of the sheep's progeny was apparently influenced by the colors and patterns the sheep observed during mating. Modern science has found no basis for the belief in maternal impressions, as least in this concrete iteration of the belief. Returning to the comment of R. Tamar that the Midrash is proof that shared paternity is possible even if subsequent cohabitations occur more than three days later, if the case of the adulterer in the Midrash is not in fact one of shared paternity, but rather of maternal impression, then the question on the three-day limit is rendered moot.

The Notion of Shared Paternity in Biblical Commentary

The notion of shared paternity is also reflected in a number of biblical commentaries. In the blessing of his first son, Yaakov says, "Reuven, you are my firstborn, my might, the first of my strength."[20] Rashi (*ad. loc.*) writes that Reuven was a product of the very first seed emitted by Yaakov. Maharal[21] notes a problem with this interpretation based on the talmudic pronouncement that a woman cannot conceive from her very first coition.[22] Maharal therefore suggests that in fact there were two coitions and Reuven was a product of the seed from both the first and second coition. Maharal accepts the possibility of a woman conceiving from two male seeds, though in this case they were from the same man.

Congenital Malformations," *Oceania* 48:2 (December, 1977), 146–153. For references to the notion of maternal impressions in rabbinic literature, see J. Preuss, *Biblical and Talmudic Medicine*, trans. F. Rosner (Hebrew Publishing Company, 1978), 391–392. S. Kottek, "*La Force de L'Imagination chez les femmes enceintes…*" *Revue D'Historie de la Medicine Hebraique* 27 (1974), 43–48. Preuss wrote a lengthy treatise on this topic, J. Preuss, "*Vom Versehen Der Schwangeren,*" *Berliner Klinik* (1892), 1–50.

20. Bereshit 49:3.

21. *Gur Aryeh*, ad loc.

22. *Yevamot* 34a. There is no known medical reason why a woman should not be able to conceive from a first coition. For discussion of this notion in rabbinic literature, see N. Gutal, *Sefer Hishtanut HaTeva'im* (Makhon Yaḥdav, 5758), 88–90.

Radak, in his commentary to *Sefer Shmuel*,[23] associates the birth of Goliath with the notion of shared paternity, though he does not reference the *Yerushalmi*. Additionally, he cites an opinion that Ahalivama, the wife of Esav, was also a product of shared paternity, explaining why she is cryptically referred to as the "daughter of Ana, the daughter of Tzivon." Why is Ahalivama described as the daughter of two men?[24] According to this interpretation, as the mother of Ahalivama had relations with both men, she was indeed the daughter of both of them. I was unable to find another source that clearly shared this version of Ahalivama's birth.[25]

Shared Paternity in Halakhic Literature

As mentioned above, shared paternity in rabbinic tradition is not a positive or encouraged circumstance. Irrespective of one's moral judgment, however, shared paternity, if indeed possible, would have legal ramifications. The halakhic discussions related to this notion refer to either accidental cases of possible shared paternity in a legally acceptable scenario, or to cases of adultery or rape. Furthermore, the halakhic discussions are entirely theoretical and are not responses to practical halakhic questions that were asked. The halakhic discussions relating to this notion are scarce, perhaps because the *Talmud Bavli* does not explicitly mention the notion of shared paternity.

R. Yitzhak Schmelkes (1828–1906) is one of the first to ponder the halakhic ramifications of shared paternity, based on the passage in *Yerushalmi*, in a purely hypothetical discussion.[26] He considers how the legal issues related to paternity would apply to all the possible multiple fathers, including, for example, the prohibition of striking one's father. In addition, if one of the fathers were a *Kohen*, how would laws of *tum'ah* apply to the child. Would he be required to refrain from exposure to *tum'ah*? He considers the question of whether partial paternity is equivalent to or treated similarly to complete paternity with respect to these

---

23. I Shmuel 17:23.
24. Tzivon was actually the father of Anah.
25. See *Midrash Tanhuma, Parashat Vayeshev* 1, which may possibly be alluding to a case of shared paternity, but the language is ambiguous.
26. *Beit Yitzhak, Y. D.*, 168.

laws. He finds precedent regarding the legal treatment of partial status from a talmudic discussion about hybrid animals,[27] and whether the progeny of a mixed breeding (e.g., a sheep and a deer) retains the identity of both parents—whether a partial sheep has the legal status of a full sheep.[28] He also references another case of partible legal status where a child is born to a Jewish man and a woman who is half slave-half free.

There is an important aspect of the halakhic analysis in these cases that R. Schmelkes raises—the element of doubt. As there was no DNA testing or even blood typing in the pre-modern era, there was no way to determine which man (or men) was with certainty a material contributor to the child, and which was not. As such, each man's legal status as a father is in question. R. Schmelkes debates the mechanics of *safek* (doubt) as it relates to this case.[29] He concludes that if an unmarried woman has relations with both a *Kohen* and *Yisrael*, the resultant child would be a doubtful *Kohen* and doubtful *Yisrael* with all the attendant halakhic ramifications. The same legal doubts would apply to an unmarried woman who had relations with both a legal bastard (*mamzer*) and a blemish-free man (*kasher*).[30]

---

27. *Ḥullin* 79b. The issue is whether we give consideration to the seed of the father (*hosheshin lezera ha'av*), and whether a partial *seh* (sheep or goat) has the status of a full *seh*. See *Entzyclopedia Talmudit*, s. v., "*hosheshin lezera ha-av*." R. J. David Bleich has written about how these notions reflect the rabbinic ideas of species identity. See his "Cloning: Homologous Reproduction and Jewish Law," *Tradition* 32:3 (1998), 47–86; "The Problem of Identity in Rashi, Rambam and the Tosafists," *Tradition* 41:2 (2008), 24–49.

28. The legal identity of an animal has significant halakhic ramifications for such laws as the prohibition of slaughtering an animal and its young on the same day (*oto ve'et b'no*), the prohibition of eating certain fats (*ḥelev*), and the obligation to cover the blood after slaughter (*kisuy dam*).

29. The issue of doubt and shared paternity is also discussed by a rough contemporary of R. Schmelkes, R. Eliyahu Kletzkin (1852–1932). See the latter's *Even HaRosha*, n. 48, regarding partible paternity and *safek bekhor*. He asserts that the Biblical phrase, "*bekhor banekha titen li*," implies a certain, not a doubtful firstborn, as would be true in the case of possible shared paternity.

30. R. Y. Tamar, in his *Alei Tamar*, op. cit., p. 16ff., also discusses potential halakhic ramifications of shared paternity and maintains, like R. Schmelkes, that if a woman has an adulterous relationship shortly after (within three days of) having relations with her husband, the child will be half *kasher* and half *mamzer*, rendering him unable to

Shared Paternity, Delaying Remarriage, and the Laws of Levirate

R. Schmelkes further applies the concept of shared paternity to analyze a talmudic passage on the laws of levirate marriage, otherwise known as *yibum*. If a man dies childless, his wife is required to marry the brother of the deceased (the levir). There is a requirement to wait a period of three months before remarrying (*havhana*). The reason for this delay is to determine with certainty whether the woman is pregnant from her first marriage before proceeding with the second marriage. By three months a pregnant woman begins to show physical signs of pregnancy. If she is pregnant from her husband, then the laws of levirate no longer apply and she is actually prohibited from marrying her husband's brother. This delay primarily serves to preclude a potentially prohibited union. If indeed the child is a product of her first marriage, then levirate would be biblically prohibited.

The Talmud entertains the possibility that a woman might disregard the required three-month delay for levirate and marry her husband's brother sooner. What would the status of her subsequent children then be? The Talmud states that the first child has no blemish and, if a *Kohen*, can become the High Priest; the second child, however, is a questionable bastard (*safek mamzer*). The reason the first child is blemish-free is because irrespective of who turns out to be the father, the child bears no legal stigma. If he is a product of the first marriage, he is a *kasher*, blemish-free, child; if he is a product of the second marriage, then it means that the woman had no issue from the first husband, thus *yibum* (levirate) was required, and the child is a product of a legal levirate marriage. Regarding the second child, however, the possibility exists that the first child was in fact the product of the first husband. If so, no levirate marriage would be required, thus rendering the woman's second marriage

---

marry either a daughter of Israel (as he is half *mamzer*) or another *mamzer* (as he is half Israelite). He also suggests that the child would have to honor both fathers, would receive inheritance from both (though he does not stipulate exact mathematical details of the distribution), and all other related matters regarding paternity would likewise apply. However, after his halakhic analysis, he adds that this is a novel idea which is found nowhere in the *Talmud Bavli* or codes. It must therefore be, he concludes, that the *Talmud Bavli* simply does not maintain that partible paternity is physiologically possible.

illicit, and the resultant child a *mamzer*. Since there is no way to confirm paternity of the first child, the second child is considered a *safek mamzer*.

R. Schmelkes focuses on the Talmud's unqualified pronouncement that the first child is *kasher*, blemish-free. If we accept the possibility of shared paternity, then if a woman has relations with the second man within a few days after the death of her husband, it is theoretically possible that the resultant child would be a product of both the first and second husbands, thus impacting on his legal status. Half of the child would be *kasher* (blemish-free) and half would possibly have the status of a *mamzer*. How could the Talmud then state unequivocally and without exception that the first child would always be blemish-free and permitted to become the High Priest?

A simple resolution could be that the *Talmud Bavli*, wherein we find this statement, simply does not accept the possibility of shared paternity.[31] R. Schmelkes, however, suggests another ingenious answer. In formulating this solution R. Schmelkes invokes the novel and remarkable position advanced by R. Yeḥezkel Landau on levirate marriage.[32] R. Landau questions the specifics of the laws of *havḥana*, the required three-month waiting period. It can take up to three days after intercourse for conception to occur. If so, then perhaps one should be required to wait a period of three months plus an additional three days, to ensure that three months after conception has elapsed. R. Landau therefore suggests a novel interpretation of the biblical phrase that establishes the requirement for levirate marriage. In order for levirate to apply, the husband must be childless. The Torah expresses this requirement with the phrase *"uvein ein lo"* (and he had no son).[33] According to R. Landau, this means that at the actual time of death, the deceased had no child or, relevant to our discussion, that conception had not yet occurred. According to this approach, if a man had relations with his wife and died before conception had occurred, he meets the criterion of *"uvein ein lo"* and

---

31. R. Yitzḥak Minkovsky (1784–1852) provides this answer in a brief mention of this same question. See his *Keren Orah, Yevamot* 37a, s. v., *"vetzarikh."* R. Schmelkes does not mention this reference.

32. *Noda BiYehuda, Even HaEzer* 1:69.

33. Devarim 25:5.

yibum is thus required, even if a child is born subsequently. The reason only an exact three months is required for the waiting period is because conception had to have already taken place before death.[34]

Based on the position of R. Landau, R. Shmelkes suggests an answer to his initial question as to how the Talmud could consider the first child born after the second marriage to be definitely *kasher*, ignoring concern for the possibility of shared paternity. In order for shared paternity to technically occur, based on the passage in the *Yerushalmi*, the coitions have to be in close proximity to each other, and according to R. Schmelkes' understanding, the fertilization of the female seed by the multiple male seeds must occur simultaneously. As the second husband only cohabitates with the woman after her first husband's death, for shared paternity to occur, conception/fertilization could not possibly have taken place before the death of the husband. According to R. Landau, the husband would then meet the criterion of *"uvein ein lo,"* *yibum* would be required, and the marriage to the second husband is legally valid. Therefore, remarkably, even if there were biologically shared paternity between the first and second husbands, the first child would be blemish-free and permitted to become the High Priest.[35]

Shared Paternity and Artificial Insemination

The talmudic discussions about the possibility of shared paternity address a case of more than one man having a physical relationship with one woman at different times. In the modern era, it has become possible to achieve conception through a process known as artificial insemination, whereby reproductive seed in injected directly into the reproductive tract of a woman. In the course of discussions on the halakhic ramifications

---

34. This novel interpretation applies only to the laws of levirate. With regard to others laws relating to paternity, such as inheritance, a child conceived after his father's death would be considered the man's legal child. (R. Landau himself is aware of the novelty of this interpretation and does not necessarily consider it halakhically binding.) This responsum is featured in contemporary halakhic discussions on postmortem insemination and the definition of paternity. See, for example, Y. B. Shafran, "*Avhut Aḥar Mita*," *Teḥumin* 20 (5760), 347–352.

35. R. Schmelkes ultimately rejects this answer, finding fault with the position of R. Landau for other reasons, and offers other possible answers to his question.

of these historically novel procedures, at least two modern rabbinic authorities invoked the notion of shared paternity.

In the early years of the performance of artificial insemination, for men whose reproductive seed was not sufficient either in number or motility, physicians would often mix their seed together with the seed of a donor. The intended purpose was to enhance the chances of success, and furthermore to provide for the theoretical, though usually remote, possibility that the husband would be the father of the child. As DNA testing was not possible at that time, there would have been no way to ascertain paternity with certainty. In this case the reproductive seed of two men would be simultaneously injected into the female reproductive tract of a woman. In addressing both the propriety and halakhic ramifications of such a procedure, R. Moshe Feinstein (1895–1986) considers the possibility of shared paternity.[36]

R. Feinstein assumes that this procedure was a mere ruse by physicians to facilitate the erroneous belief that the husband was possibly the father, when they in fact knew that this was not physiologically possible. Nevertheless, he considers the notion of shared paternity. While he quotes the position of Rashi in the *Talmud Bavli* that shared paternity is not possible, a position with which his son-in-law R. Moshe Tendler concurred, he avers as to how this case would be viewed according to the *Yerushalmi*, which accepts the notion of shared paternity. R. Feinstein suggests that even according to the *Yerushalmi*, shared paternity is only possible if the seed of the men are equal in quality. In this case, as the husband's seed is clearly inferior, even according to the *Yerushalmi*, shared paternity would not be possible. In this specific case, therefore, the notion of shared paternity has no legal consequence. R. Feinstein does leave the door open for the possibility of halakhic ramifications in other cases where the seed of the different donors is equal in quality, though to my knowledge he did not address this issue elsewhere.

R. Menashe Klein (1924–2011) addresses the topic of shared paternity in a responsum on whether the wife of a *Kohen* who undergoes artificial insemination with donor seed is subsequently

---

36. *Iggerot Moshe E. H.*, 1:71.

prohibited from returning to her husband, as perhaps the insemination with another man's seed is akin to adultery.[37] While R. Klein does not prohibit the woman from returning to her husband, he does maintain that the husband should refrain from marital relations with his wife both shortly before and during the entire pregnancy. In listing his reasons for this decision, he states, "I have other reasons that I cannot commit to writing, like the case of *me'ah papi* in *Sota* and others." I assume, that according to R. Klein, one reason, amongst a number of others, that he prohibits marital relations after artificial insemination is out of the concern of the theoretical possibility of shared paternity.[38]

Genetic Engineering

In the context of a discussion on the topic of genetic engineering of animals and plants, R. Ḥizkiyahu Yosef Kohen devotes a section to the notion of shared paternity as reflected in *Sota* and its impact on the identity of species that are genetically engineered from more than one plant or animal.[39]

Paternity Testing

The most expansive halakhic treatment of the notion of shared paternity of which I am aware is by R. Yitzḥak Zilberstein in an essay on the use of tissue/DNA testing to determine the paternity of a child born to a woman who had forced relations with two men.[40] He mentions the passage in *Yerushalmi* and that his father-in-law, R. Elyashiv *zt"l*, wondered what the halakhic status of the hundred fathers would be, had the involved parties been Jewish. He lists some possible halakhic ramifications:

---

37. *Mishneh Halakhot* 9:244, s. v., "*od.*"
38. In another responsum, R. Klein (*Mishneh Halakhot* 7:253 s. v., "*Ela dima*") briefly addresses the issue of shared paternity and its halakhic ramifications in the context of a case of a man who dies apparently childless but is subsequently found to have a daughter from an unmarried woman, whether this absolves his wife from *yibum*.
39. "*Handasa Genetit,*" *Ateret Shlomo* 5 (5760), 123–155, section 3.
40. *Shiurei Torah LeRofim* 4 (5772), 351–355.

1) Regarding *yibum* (levirate marriage), if one died without children from his marriage, but was one of the hundred men who shared paternity for one child, is it considered as if he had a child such that his wife is absolved from the obligation of *yibum* (or *halitzah*)?
2) Does the resulting son inherit a portion of the estate of all the fathers?
3) Does a son who hits one of the fathers violate the prohibition of striking one's father?
4) Would Goliath perform the levirate marriage for the wife of one of his (partial) paternal brothers if the brother died childless?
5) If one of the fathers were a *Kohen* and the other a *Yisrael*, would the child be permitted to marry a divorcee? Would the child be considered a *Kohen* with respect to receiving the first *aliya* to the Torah and performing the priestly blessing?
6) If one of the fathers was a *Kohen*, would the child be absolved from the mitzva of *pidyon haben* (redemption of the first born)?
7) The Torah provides a license for a person to kill an intruder based on the notion of self-defense. This license does not apply to a son when his father is the intruder, as the father would never kill his own son. Does this exception apply to any of the hundred fathers?
8) The Talmud (*Bava Batra* 42a) gives unique status to a son with regard to his consumption of food or materials from his father's estate. Does this apply in this case?
9) The Talmud assumes a special affinity of a father for his son, such that if he transfers his estate to another party, but later finds out that he has a son, the transaction is nullified. (*Bava Batra* 146b). Would this special relationship be recognized in this case as well?

To resolve the halakhic issues related to shared paternity, R. Zilberstein, like his predecessor R. Schmelkes, cites the talmudic passage on the legal implications of the birth of a hybrid animal.[41] For certain purposes an animal that is only part sheep is halakhically considered a full sheep. Perhaps this should apply in this case of shared paternity, he argues, and that the son, though only a partial son, is considered a full son for each father?

---

41. *Ḥullin* 79b.

R. Zilberstein further probes the passage in *Yerushalmi* accepting shared paternity and questions whether the paternity is shared equally, or perhaps one man is the primary father, while the others are but minor contributors.[42] This issue has ramifications with respect to tissue testing in the case at hand, as well as for the proof for shared paternity from the talmudic passage mentioned above, which might only be applicable if there is equal sharing of paternity, as with the case of the sheep.

Though the medical expert consulted by R. Zilberstein concludes that based on contemporary medical knowledge shared biological paternity is not possible, he nonetheless offers a physiological explanation as to how shared paternity would be possible and leaves the door open that the position of *Yerushalmi* could be relevant today.[43]

One feature in common with all the above halakhic discussions is that, irrespective of whether one accepts the possibility of shared paternity or not, they are all hypothetical. It has never been possible to prove with certainty that any one individual was indeed the product of multiple fathers. From our modern vantage point this is true because shared biological paternity is not physiologically possible, in consonance with the position of Rashi in the *Talmud Bavli*. As such, there has never been a true "practical" halakhic question about shared paternity—until now.

IV. APPLICATION TO THE THREE-PARENT EMBRYO

The rabbinic sources above all discuss the notion of shared paternity, a notion held by other cultures throughout history as well. The talmudic sources are split as to whether it is physiologically possible. Medically, there is no feasible explanation for shared paternity, though some rabbinic authorities may differ. Today, however, there is a genuine case of biologically shared maternity that is intentionally created to prevent the propagation of disease. This new form of shared parenthood, in

---

42. R. Zilberstein marshals support for this position from *Sefer Kerem Neta, Sota* 42b. The author ponders in essence the same questions about shared paternity in a case of *yibum* or adultery. I was unable to locate the section that specifically addresses the proportionality of the division of paternity.
43. Perhaps R. Menashe Klein was of the same opinion.

this case maternity, merits its own analysis and may also benefit from an evaluation of the rabbinic literature discussed above on shared paternity.

The Three-Parent Embryo and Mitochondrial Disease

While the majority of the DNA of the human egg resides in the nucleus of the cell, a small percentage is found within a structure called the mitochondria, which floats in the fluid (cytoplasm) of the egg cell. Mitochondrial DNA can only be transmitted by the female, as it is found in the egg. A male child can receive mitochondrial DNA from his mother, but he cannot pass it on. Rarely, the mitochondrial DNA can be defective and can cause neurological or cardiological disease in the offspring. Scientists have devised a method to prevent the transmission and propagation of these diseases through the following procedure. The nucleus of the egg of woman "A", with mitochondrial disease, is extracted and inserted into the egg of woman "B", with normal mitochondrial DNA (from which the nucleus was previously removed). The resulting composite egg has the nuclear DNA of woman "A" and "normal" mitochondrial DNA of woman "B". The egg is then fertilized and implanted, producing a child with two genetic mothers—true shared biological maternity.

Halakhic Issues of the Three-Parent Embryo

The notion of more than one mother vying for the status of maternity in Jewish law is not new. Earlier chapters in this book address the definition of maternity from various perspectives, and halakhic discussions of the definition of maternity in cases of surrogate motherhood (technically gestational hosthood) are commonplace today. This issue still remains one of the most complex areas of contemporary medical halakha. There is no consensus, and positions span from assigning legal maternity to the egg donor alone, to the birth mother alone, to both or to neither.[44] Perhaps we could take the existing debates and simply substitute "mitochondrial donor" for "surrogate mother." This of course would not do justice to the intricacies and nuances of this complex issue,

---

44. For a summary of positions, see, A. Steinberg, *Encyclopedia of Jewish Medical Ethics* 2, trans. F. Rosner (Feldheim Publishers, 2003), s. v., "in-vitro fertilization."

and it appears a new body of halakhic analysis will need to be written for this technology.

The location for this new body of analysis will be within the section on the authorities who consider genetics as the halakhic determinant of maternity. For the other positions, which do not acknowledge, or minimize, the halakhic significance of the genetic contributor, the substitution of a small percentage of DNA will have no legal consequence.

For those who identify the genetic contributor (egg donor) as the halakhic mother, who is considered the halakhic mother in our case? Here there are two genetic contributors. Do we consider the contribution of mitochondrial DNA to be halakhically significant such that the donor would share legal maternity? If so, would it be an equal or asymmetric share of the maternal status, as the mitochondrial DNA comprises only a small percentage of the human genome? What if the mitochondrial DNA or nuclear DNA comes from a non-Jewish woman? Would the child need conversion? What if the mitochondrial DNA comes from the daughter of a *Kohen* or *Levi*, whose children are usually excluded from the requirement of redemption of the firstborn (*pidyon haben*), would a resulting firstborn male child require a *pidyon haben*?[45]

The rabbinic literature on shared paternity could inform our discussions and possibly serve as legal precedent for the case of shared maternity in mitochondrial DNA donation. This literature discusses whether the laws regarding a parent (striking a parent, honoring a parent, etc.) would apply to all the contributors. Questions of asymmetric parental status are entertained. In the case of Goliath, there were one hundred contributors. Each provides only a fraction of the material, similar in concept to a mitochondrial donor, yet they are given consideration as possible legal parents. Is each participant granted full, or only partial paternal status? R. Y. Tamar discusses this very issue and maintains that the laws of paternity only apply to a full father, not to a partial father. If so,

---

45. For a discussion of how advances in modern medicine, including the three-parent embryo, the *Kohen* gene, ectogenesis, ovarian or uterine transplantation, and artificial reproductive seed impact on the mitzva of *pidyon haben*, see E. Reichman, "*Pidyon Ha-Ben* (Redemption of the Firstborn) in the 21st Century: An Appendix to *Shulhan Arukh*," *Verapo Yerapei: Journal of Torah and Medicine of the Albert Einstein College of Medicine Synagogue* 5 (2014), 261–287.

perhaps the mitochondrial donor has no maternal status. R. Zilberstein specifically addresses the issue of asymmetric contributions, though he does not develop definitive conclusions for such a scenario.

In the halakhic discussions of R. Schmelkes, the analysis revolves mainly around the issue of doubt, as there was no way to ascertain whether paternity was actually shared or not. In the case of the three-parent embryo, however, the fact of biologically shared maternity is unquestioned, so his analyses of the laws of *safek* might not apply in this case. There are, however, two ways the laws of *safek* could be applied: doubt as to whether shared paternity/maternity has occurred; or assuming shared paternity/maternity has definitely occurred, doubt as to whether the legal status of parenthood is conferred upon all the contributors. This latter form of doubt might be applied in the modern case and would in essence lead to the same legal conclusions as R. Schmelkes.

To be sure, there are a number of differences between the case of the three-parent embryo and the cases discussed in the earlier halakhic literature. First, this is a case of shared maternity, as opposed to paternity. While the issues of honoring or striking a parent could be assimilated here, the issue of *yibum* would not, as levirate is a paternal issue. Furthermore, as the tribal status of a child is transmitted paternally, the issues of *Kohen* status would generally not be applicable here, with one exception. With respect to *pidyon haben*, if the mother is a *bat-Kohen* or *bat-Levi*, the child is absolved from the requirement for *pidyon haben*. If one of the female genetic contributors is a *bat-Kohen* and the other a *Yisrael*, would a first-born male issue require redemption or not?

If the mitochondrial donor is married, would the fact that her DNA is combined with that of another man constitute adultery and render the child a *mamzer* or part *mamzer*, part *kasher*? In this case, the shared maternity is achieved through microscopic manipulation and in the absence of any physical relationship between the mitochondrial donor and the husband. The issue of adultery and bastardy has been addressed with respect to artificial insemination with donor sperm.[46]

---

46. A. Steinberg, *Encyclopedia of Jewish Medical Ethics 1*, trans. F. Rosner (Jerusalem: Feldheim Publishers, 2003), s. v., "artificial insemination."

In this case as well, it is only biological adultery, not physical. R. Yoel Teitelbaum, the Satmar Rebbe, argued that indeed this constitutes biblically prohibited adultery and the resulting progeny would be a *mamzer*. R. Moshe Feinstein countered that adultery does not apply in the absence of a physical relationship, and, as such, any progeny would not carry any stigma of bastardy and would be entirely blemish-free. These same arguments could potentially be applied here as well.[47]

A major and fundamental difference between shared paternity and shared maternity is the fact that Jewishness is determined through matrilineal descent. In the current cases of surrogate motherhood, if either the egg donor (genetic mother) or the gestational host (birth mother) is not Jewish, there is genuine halakhic concern as to the legal status and Jewishness of the child. In the case of the three-parent embryo, if one of the genetic donors is not Jewish how does this impact the legal status of the child? Is it possible for the child to be part Jewish and part non-Jewish?

A full treatment of the halakhic issues relating to the three-parent embryo is beyond the scope of this article. Rabbinic authorities are just now beginning to address this new technology. R. Moshe Tendler and Dr. John Loike briefly address the issue of the three-parent embryo in a recent article and maintain that it is a *safek* whether the mitochondrial donor has maternal status.[48] R. Asher Weiss addresses this issue as

---

47. Some rabbinic authorities invoke a specific scriptural source for the prohibition of performing artificial insemination with donor seed—"*lo titen shekhavtekha lezara.*" While this verse is generally understood to mean that one should not have an intimate relationship with one's neighbor's wife, R. Y. L. Zirelsohn, *MiArkhei Lev* 73, in discussing donor insemination, comments on the fact that the phraseology of this verse differs from the previous prohibitions regarding illicit relations. He therefore interprets the phrase literally, to mean that in any way one deposits seed into the woman, including through artificial insemination (even in the absence of any physical relationship), one has violated this prohibition. This unique analysis is limited to the deposition of male, not female, seed, and as such, would not apply to our case of mitochondrial DNA donation.

48. "Creating Human Embryos Using Reproductive Cloning Technologies," *Journal of Halacha and Contemporary Society* (Spring 2014), 37–60, esp. 56–58. They mention the case of Goliath in a footnote and comment, "It is unclear from Rashi and *Tosafot*

well,[49] and absent any other clear halakhic precedent, bases his analysis of this case on the principle of *"rov*," or majority. As the nuclear DNA is clearly in the overwhelming majority, he therefore considers the nuclear DNA donor to be the primary and exclusive halakhic mother.[50] Nonetheless, he requires a conversion if the mitochondrial donor is a non-Jew, though the nature of the conversion is solely to imbue the child with *"kedushat Yisrael*," (sanctity and holiness). As this is not a standard conversion, but is done for concern of the *"kedushat Yisrael"* status of the child, he would not preclude a girl born from this arrangement from subsequently marrying a *Kohen*.[51] R. J. David Bleich takes issue with R. Weiss' analysis and rejects the analogy to the principle of *rov* (majority) as irrelevant to the determination of legal status.[52] He offers his own thorough analysis, though concludes that it remains a matter of significant dispute.

Advances in the technology of the three-parent embryo, as well as the possibility of gene splicing, will necessitate a more thorough analysis of the issue of shared genetic parenthood. Perhaps the existing rabbinic literature on shared paternity can assist the rabbinic authorities in navigating these complex halakhic dilemmas.

V. CONCLUSION

Rabbinic discussions on shared paternity represent a curious, obscure and arcane chapter in rabbinic literature. Beginning with the possible

---

whether they are arguing biologically or halakhically or if these discussions only impart a moral message." From our discussion it is clear that many construed these discussions about shared paternity literally.

49. https://drive.google.com/file/d/oB8pV_AB_KYvpU3Y3aHRsaEY3YkU/view.

50. Applying the principles gleaned from the halakhic discussions of shared paternity might give more weight to the contribution of the mitochondrial donor, though the percentage contribution of the mitochondrial donor is significantly less than that of one of the hundred fathers.

51. While he does not explicitly address the converse case, I assume that, according to R. Weiss, if the nuclear DNA donor is non-Jewish, the minority contribution of a Jewish mitochondrial donor would not be sufficient to alter the non-Jewish status of the child.

52. R. J. David Bleich, "Mitochondrial DNA Replacement: How Many Mothers?" *Tradition* 48:4 (2015), 60–84.

biological origins of the birth of a biblical villain, rabbinic authorities, in classic talmudic tradition, explored an array of hypothetical legal dilemmas generated by the notion of shared paternity. It is only now, in the twenty-first century that these purely hypothetical discussions have been transformed into a source of potential practical halakhic relevance in addressing advances in reproductive medicine. This chapter represents yet another example of how pre-modern hypothetical rabbinic discussions can be resuscitated and applied to modern halakhic dilemmas.[53]

---

53. See chapters, "Midrash, Miracles and Motherhood: The Birth of Dinah and the Definition of Maternity," and "The Resuscitation of Halakha: An Animated Discussion."

Anatomy and Physiology

The Anatomy of the Human Body in Rabbinic Literature: The 248 *"Evarim"*

The most basic aspect of medicine is human anatomy. The practice of medicine is based on its understanding. In the next chaper, "The Anatomy of Halakha," we discuss the history of anatomical dissection from talmudic times onwards. In this chapter, we focus on one aspect of the history of anatomy in rabbinic literature, the number of limbs in the body.

A number of physicians over the centuries, including Hippocrates, Galen and Avicenna, have enumerated the bones of the human body. The attempts at enumeration were neither precise nor exhaustive, perhaps because there was no clinical relevance to the absolute number of bones or limbs. This is not the case in rabbinic literature. In the Mishna in *Ohalot*[1] we find such an enumeration, where it lists 248 *evarim*. The meaning of this term, *evarim*, has been the subject of debate in rabbinic literature. The Talmud is not a medical or anatomical text. Why, then,

---

1. 1:8.

does it discuss anatomical matters? The answer lies in the halakhic relevance of this information. The Mishna mentions these facts inasmuch as they relate to the specific laws of impurity. According to Jewish law, exposure to a corpse, or parts thereof, either by direct contact, or by presence under the same enclosure, generates impurity. The laws of impurity were of daily concern for the Jews of the Temple period, as entrance to the Temple in Jerusalem was restricted for those who were ritually impure. According to Jewish law, even if a majority of the number of *evarim* of one corpse were located in one enclosure, anyone under the same enclosure would be rendered impure. To determine the majority of *evarim*, one must know the total number. Hence the Mishna enumerates the 248 *evarim*, the majority of which, 125, would convey impurity.

This number was verified experimentally in a remarkable passage in the Talmud[2] where we find an account of the students of R. Yishmael who performed some form of dissection on a woman who was sentenced to death by the secular authorities. The verb used for the treatment of the body is "*shalak*," which has been variously translated as boiled or dissected. This passage is one of the earliest recorded human dissections. After completion of their careful anatomical observations, they arrived at the grand total of 252 *evarim*. The discrepancy between this number and that of the Mishna, 248, is addressed in this passage, and the difference is attributed to the fact that it was a female body that was dissected. One thing is clear from this passage: *evarim* does not refer to bones, as the number of bones in the female skeleton is identical to that of the male. The angles of the skeleton may differ, especially in the spinal and pelvic areas, but the total number of bones is identical.

It is unclear whether the Mishna in *Ohalot*, which counts 248 limbs, is in consonance or disagreement with the aforementioned talmudic passage, which arrives at a different sum total of limbs. Some resolve the discrepancy between the two counts by asserting that only 248 limbs, as enumerated in the Mishna, convey impurity, while the additional limbs of the woman mentioned in the Talmud do not convey impurity. The Jerusalem Talmud[3] states the when the woman suspected

---

2. *Bekhorot* 45a.
3. *Sota*, chapter 5, 20a.

of adultery drinks the waters that are bitter, "*hame'arerim*," the very word alludes to the fact that both the woman, as well as her male partner, are being tested. This is reflected in the fact that the numerical value of the word "*hame'arerim*" equals 496, or two times 248—one set of 248 limbs representing the woman, and one set of 248 limbs representing the man. This tradition obviously does not assume that the woman has 252 *evarim*.

The distinction between the number of *evarim* of the man and woman has been the source of a number of rabbinic discussions relating to Jewish liturgy.[4] The prayer that is recited for the sick, known as the "*Mi SheBeirakh*," specifically states that an ill person should have a complete recovery for their 248 *evarim*. If, as the talmudic passage states, a woman does not have 248 *evarim*, how could this text be recited for her? It would not be accurate. Indeed, there are divergent traditions as to whether the phrase "248 *evarim*" should be recited for both men and women. To this day, some communities use this phrase, while other substitute, "she should have a complete recovery to *all her evarim*," instead of the specific number.[5]

R. Yeḥezkel Shraga Lipschutz Halberstam contends that the "*Mi SheBeirakh*" text should be amended to say "all *evarim*" for both men and woman. He argues that since the *evarim* mentioned in the Mishna refer exclusively to limbs that have bones, and many of the organs without bones could also be afflicted with disease, a prayer restricted to the 248 *evarim* would be insufficient to cover all the organs that may be in need of a cure. This logic applies to both men and women.[6]

Another area of the liturgy where the number 248 is granted significance is the *Shema* prayer.[7] The prayer, an expression of faith, contains 245 words. When the *Shema* is recited as part of communal prayer, the cantor, or *ḥazan*, adds an additional three words, *Hashem Elokeikhem emet*, so that the total number of words of the prayer adds up to 248 words. When recited in private, the individual adds three words at the beginning of the

---

4. For further discussion, see chapter, "The Anatomy of Prayer."
5. See *HaElef Lekha Shlomo, Oraḥ Ḥayyim* 120; *Rivevot Ephraim, Oraḥ Ḥayyim*, vol. 3, 200; *Ravaz, Yoreh De'ah*, 111.
6. *Otzrot Yerushalayim* 105 (5732), 69.
7. On the origins of the association of the *Shema* with the number 248, see, for example, S. K. Mirsky, *Talpiyot*, Year 1, Volume 2, Issue 1 (*Tevet-Adar*, 5704) 239–244.

prayer (*Kel melekh ne'eman*) to achieve the same objective of reaching a total of 248 words. The intentional association of the words of *Shema* with the number of limbs of the human body has its origin in the *Midrash Tanḥuma*,[8] where it states that if man observes (or watches over) the precepts of the Torah, God will in turn watch over man, i.e., his 248 limbs. The question has been raised as to the necessity of women adding the additional three words if they do not, in fact, have 248 *evarim*.[9]

One source finds a hint to the nature of the obligation to procreate in the numerical value of the biblical words *peru urevu* (be fruitful and multiply). The obligation is to beget both a male and a female child. The numerical value of this phrase equals 500–248 for a male child and 252 for a female child.[10]

How do the 248 limbs mentioned in the Mishna correlate with our modern understanding of anatomy? This question has occupied many over the centuries. R. David Nieto (1654–1728), philosopher and Ḥakham of the Spanish and Portuguese Synagogue in London (1701–28), graduate of the medical school of the University of Padua, authored the *Kuzari Hasheni* (or *Mateh Dan*), a defense of the Jewish oral tradition against attacks by Karaites and skeptics, wherein he has the following passage:[11]

> Regarding the number of limbs in the body, there is a small difference between the rabbis and the anatomists. But do not be concerned with this discrepancy, as each one is involved with their respective disciplines, without contradiction... The purpose of the anatomists is to identify the human limbs as they relate to the

---

8. *Parashat Kedoshim.*
9. See *Minḥat Elazar* 28; R. R. Avers, *VeShav VeRafa*, v. 2, *Oraḥ Ḥayyim*, n. 7. On the origins of the recitation of "*kel melekh ne'eman*" see Y. Ta-Shma, "*Kel Melekh Ne'eman: Gilgulo Shel Minhag*," *Tarbitz* 39:2 (*Tevet*, 5730), 184–194, and follow up comment on Ta-Shma by S. Z. Havlin in *Tarbitz* 40:1 (*Tishrei*, 5731), 107–109.
10. See Ḥayyim Yosef Dov Azulai, known as Ḥida, *Sefer Devash Lefi*, letter *aleph*, section 9. For additional rabbinic sources on the differences in the number of *evarim* between men and women, see *Pardes Yosef, Mishpatim* 23:7, s. v., "*ma she'omrim*"; Abraham S. Abraham, *Nishmat Avraham* 5 (Rimonim), 9–11.
11. See M. Levin's annotated translation of this work, *The Rabbis' Advocate: Chacham David Nieto and The Second Kuzari* (Yashar Press, 2007).

practice of medicine, and the purpose of the rabbis is (to identify the limbs) as they relate to the conferring of ritual impurity.[12]

In the mid-nineteenth century, R. Samuel David Luzzatto briefly
addressed the Mishna in *Ohalot*, trying to identify the limbs of the fore-
arm mentioned in the Mishna.[13] His analysis, which entertained the
possibility that the Rabbis enumerated the bones at different developmental stages, foreshadowed the better-known work of Dr. Katznelson
discussed below.[14] R. Luzzatto further contended that while the number 248 was an ancient received tradition, the exact composition of this
number was not. Therefore, one could speculate as to which *evarim* were
included, and which were not.

In 1886, Dr. Binyamin Sharshevsky published a medical book
in Hebrew on anatomy and medicine entitled *Mishnat Olam Katan:
Masekhet Nituaḥ*. Amongst other discussions on anatomy, the author
listed the number of limbs in the human body. The fact that the number
of limbs detailed by Dr. Sharshevsky did not coincide with the number
mentioned by the rabbis of the Talmud was not lost on R. Michal Pines,
whose introduction to the book devotes much attention to this issue.
The book was reviewed the year of its publication in *HaMelitz*, a Hebrew
language journal in Russia known for its anti-religious sentiment, where
R. Pines' comments were highlighted:

> It has not eluded me that with respect to the number of bones
> in the human being, your work contradicts that of Ḥazal in *Oha-
> lot*... as Ḥazal enumerate 248 limbs in the human body, while

---

12. Argument number 4. I consulted the Mosad HaRav Kook edition (5718), 106.
13. This letter was published in *Kerem Ḥemed*, section 7 (Prague, 1843), 42–44. (reference
    cited in R. Kippervasser, "*Ramaḥ Evarim*," BDD 8 (Winter 5759), 29–64.)
14. For additional discussion on the 248 limbs, see J. Preuss, *Biblical and Talmudic Medi-
    cine*, trans. F. Rosner (Hebrew Publishing Co., 1978), 60–67; R. Yair Weinstock, *Sefer
    Mareh Ha'Adam* (Jerusalem, 5755) (I thank Menachem Butler for this reference); R.
    Kippervasser, "*Ramaḥ Evarim*," BDD 8 (Winter 5759), 29–64; M. Bar Ilan, "Medicine
    in Israel in the Early Years of the Common Era," *Katedra* 91 (*Nisan*, 5759), 31–78. The
    excellent articles of Kippervasser and Bar Ilan expand upon a number of the issues
    discussed in this chapter, including the definition of the term *ever*, and the different
    approaches to the explanation of the 248 *evarim*.

your book states, "there are 211 limbs in the human body." I have expended great effort to resolve this discrepancy so there should be no contradiction between the rabbis and the anatomists on a factual matter. But I have not been successful. Nonetheless, I see no diminution (in the words of the rabbis). I am not an expert in this field and have not seen a human skeleton. My heart tells me that if a skeleton should come into my possession, I would understand that what the rabbis counted as one, we count as two, and vice versa.[15]

The book review elicited two comments published in a subsequent issue of *HaMelitz*,[16] where one writer brings to our attention that another physician, a certain Dr. A. Porjes, in his *Torat Haberiut*, struggled to reconcile the number of limbs with those listed by the rabbis. The author he is referring to is Aaran ben Meir Asher Zelig Hacohen Porjes (1848–1919), born in Lvov. The work, *Torat HaBeriut*, was published as a monograph in the journal *HeAsif* in 1884[17] and comprises a brief overview of anatomy and physiology.[18] As the author states in the prosaic introduction, the work was intended to educate the masses in order to effectively facilitate the practice of preventative medicine. One of the main reasons people do not take proper care of their health, he claims, is due to their lack of knowledge about the basic functions of the human body. This monograph is an attempt to remedy this deficiency. In the context of his overview of anatomy in chapter 3, at page 10, he enumerates the bones of the human body, and arrives at the final tally of 242. In a footnote, he comments that Ḥazal counted 248 *evarim*. To account for the discrepancy, he posits that if one considers the pelvis as being comprised of more than one bone, as it is fused from multiple components,

---

15. *HaMelitz* 24 (24 March, 1886), 382–383.

16. *HaMelitz.* 30 (1886), 470.

17. Warsaw, year 5645 (1884), section 8.

18. Porjes states that the monograph would contain three sections: the composition of the human body, guidelines for the practice of preventative medicine, and a description of common ailments and diseases. This journal issue deals primarily with the first section.

and if one adds the two wisdom teeth, this would bring the final tally to 248, in line with the count of the rabbis.[19]

The author of the letter is quick to point out, that while Dr. Porjes was well intentioned, his efforts were in vain, as the Mishna clearly excludes teeth from its list of limbs. Thus, the discrepancy between the rabbis and the physicians remains. Despite this fact, he continues to attest to the veracity of the number 248 based on the fact that the rabbis of the Talmud clarified the number with an experimental dissection (see above). Furthermore, the fact that Maimonides, who often deviates from the Talmud in areas where he believed the science did not correlate, mentions the number 248. If there were not 248 identifiable limbs, Maimonides would surely have at least omitted this number from his writings, if not corrected it.

Another letter in the same issue mentions the work of the famous nineteenth century anatomist, Joseph Hyrtl, and aligns his calculation, with some minor adjustments, with that of the rabbis.

Dr. Yehuda Leib Katznelson penned an entire volume devoted to this issue entitled *Ramaḥ Evarim*, published in 1887.[20] He indicates in the introduction to this work that the aforementioned work by Dr. Sharshevsky, as well as the ensuing exchange in *HaMelitz*, at least in part, induced him to write this book. This work was subsequently incorporated into his more expansive *HaTalmud VeHokhmat HaRefua*.[21] Dr. Katznelson contends that the number 248 was primarily based on the dissection of the body of a teenager, roughly sixteen or seventeen years old, as recorded in *Masekhet Bekhorot* (see above). The larger bones

---

19. In this essay, Porjes footnotes his previous work, *Torat HaHayyim* (Vienna, 1880), an expansive work on human physiology, including discussions on heat, electricity, chemistry, physics and magnetism. Of note, this work mentions the wonders of the recently invented telegraph and compares its function to that of the nervous system.

20. The year of publication in the Jewish calendar is 5648. When written in Hebrew in the conventional fashion, the last three letters are *resh, mem, ḥet,* of *ramaḥ*, corresponding to the 248 limbs. I wonder how long the author waited, or perhaps rushed, to achieve this publication date.

21. This work was published posthumously in Berlin, 1928. The only addition to the chapter on *ramaḥ evarim* in the book is an essay responding to the criticism of the original monograph that appeared in an article in *HaTzefira* in 1887 by a man identified as Axelrod. See pp. 297–303.

of the body grow from the center outwards, with three distinct bone centers—the diaphysis and two epiphyses. The rate of complete fusion of the different bones of the body varies. In the adult, these centers ultimately all fuse into one indistinguishable bone. If the body of an adolescent were subjected to boiling, as the talmudic passage recounts, the three bone growth centers would be separated and considered as three separate *evarim*. It is this novel approach that Dr. Katznelson applies in a very detailed fashion to reconcile the Mishnaic number of 248 with our current knowledge of anatomy.

Dr. Katznelson summarizes his conclusions:

1) The number of bones in the body is not fixed from the beginning of human embryological development, rather it changes with time and varies with chronological age.

2) The fewest number of bones appear in the neonate, as ossification has not yet been completed. From roughly fifteen years of age, the number of bones decreases, as the growth plates begin to fuse between bones.

3) *Ḥazal* determined the number of bones by scientific experimentation, not by estimation or philosophical considerations.

4) *Ḥazal*'s inspection of the body followed a boiling process, which separated the growth plates and increased the number of bones.

5) From the number of bones enumerated by *Ḥazal*, it is clear that their anatomical inspection was of a body of the age of sixteen or seventeen years.

6) He reaffirms that his objective was not to falsely assume that *Ḥazal* were aware of all future developments that would occur in the understanding and development of human anatomy, rather, it was to demonstrate that in areas relating to halakha, *Ḥazal* relied not on prophesy, but on observation and experimentation to the fullest extent of their capability.

Many have taken issue with the creative theory of Dr. Katznelson, including Dr. Julius Preuss, author of the classic work, *Biblisch-Talmudische Medizin*, first published in 1911, and later translated into English by

Dr. Fred Rosner.[22] Preuss was skeptical of the validity of the theory for two main reasons. First, he argues that the age limits of ossification are not as constant as Katznelson states. Second, Preuss is dissatisfied that Katznelson attributes any inconsistencies in his theory to the inexperience of the rabbinic investigators and their methodologies. In sum, he writes:

> Katznelson first arranged his hypothesis; whenever the facts did not coincide with his hypothesis, he did not abandon or even modify his assumptions; rather he ascribed the error to his source, whereas the real guilty one, naturally, was he. As a result, his entire work, so painstakingly prepared, loses its validity and reliability.[23]

Preuss offers no substitute theory to account for the exact number of limbs but does offer comments on many of the difficult aspects of the Mishnaic text.

In his 1927 publication, *Binat Nevonim*, R. Nisan Markel devotes an entire chapter to clarifying and identifying the 248 limbs. He analyzes the commentary on the Mishna in *Ohalot* of R. Israel Lipschutz's (1782–1860), from which he radically deviates. R. Markel assumes that R. Lipschutz could not have actually seen a skeleton when he penned his commentary on the Mishna, as some of his comments are clearly not in consonance with reality.

In order to arrive at 248, R. Markel invokes two ideas. The first involves the understanding of osteology and the embryological development of the bones of the human body. He asserts that some bones, like the sternum, are comprised of multiple smaller bones and fuse later in life. This approach is reminiscent of that of Dr. Katznelson, although he does not cite his work. As this idea alone is insufficient to account for all the discrepancies, R. Markel advances an additional theory involving the sesamoid bones. While the number and location of sesamoid bones currently vary greatly, he posits that it is possible that in previous

---

22. *Biblical and Talmudic Medicine* (Hebrew Publishing Company, 1978). For Preuss' discussion of the 248 *evarim*, see pp. 60–67.
23. Ibid., 62.

generations sesamoid bones were uniformly found in certain parts of the body, such as in each digit of the foot. With these theories, R. Markel is satisfied that he has discharged his obligation to reconcile the words of the rabbis to the best of his ability.

More recently, Dr. David Margalit rejected the theories of Dr. Katznelson,[24] finding it hard to believe that the number 248, which is so integral to rabbinic literature, and which served as the foundation for the enumeration of the 248 positive commandments, could have been based on one anecdotal dissection of a seventeen-year-old girl.[25] Dr. Margalit offers his own theory, which challenges the assumption, or axiom, in his words, that an *ever* must, by definition, include bone. He marshals ample evidence that the word *ever* is used frequently throughout rabbinic literature to refer to non-osseous organs, as well as those containing bones, such as the heart and the tongue. His essay is followed by a lengthy footnote listing the 248 *evarim* according to his calculation, and including visceral, non-osseous organs.

In fact, the idea that the 248 *evarim* included non-osseous organs did not originate with Dr. Margalit. Dr. I. M. Rabbinowicz, in his *La Medecine du Talmud*, published in Paris in 1880, suggested the very same notion.[26] Dr. Katznelson, devotes an entire appendix in his *Ramaḥ Evarim* to addressing the theory of R. Rabbinowicz[27] and vehemently rejects the notion that the number 248 includes non-osseous structures. This refutation would have applied equally to the theory of Dr. Margalit.

While R. Markel was satisfied that he had discharged his obligation to the best of his ability, I believe there is yet unexplored territory in this fascinating area of the history of the rabbinic understanding of human anatomy. I do hope that this brief survey, with its attendant references, will spark further research and clarification of what remains an unsolved mystery.

---

24. D. Margalit, "*Pirkei Anatomia Lifnim BeYisrael VeHayom*," *Koroth* 1:11–12 (June-July, 1957), 378–391.
25. Dr. Katznelson, perhaps anticipating this criticism, offers an explanation for this aspect of his theory. See his *Ramaḥ Evarim*, pages 50–51.
26. See pp. 101–105.
27. *Ramaḥ Evarim*, pp. 115–125.

The Anatomy of Halakha

INTRODUCTION

This chapter explores the impact and relationship of the history of autopsy and anatomical dissection on Jewish history and rabbinic literature. Familiar sources will be viewed in a new, rarified light, and new sources—both historical and halakhic—will be presented.

I. THE HISTORICAL PERIOD OF THE HALAKHIC DISCUSSIONS ON ANATOMY

The earliest responsa to address autopsy and anatomical dissection appeared in the eighteenth century by R. Yaakov Emden and R. Yeḥezkel Landau. The oft-ignored question about these anatomical *teshuvot* concerns their historical period: Why does Maimonides (twelfth century), the ultimate rabbi/physician, make no mention of the halakhic issues of dissection or autopsy in any of his medical or halakhic works? Likewise, in his *Shulḥan Arukh*, R. Yosef Karo (sixteenth century) covers all aspects of human existence, including burial practices and bodily exhumation, but makes no reference to autopsy or dissection. The reason for these omissions lies not in their neglect, but in the historical reality. Systematic human cadaver dissection, while practiced briefly in antiquity[1] and

---

1. Mundinus (1270–1326) is recognized to have introduced human anatomical dissection into the medical curriculum. See, for example, C. D. O'Malley, *Andreas Vesalius of*

sporadically throughout the centuries, did not become an integral part of medical student training until the Renaissance.

The figure most often credited with establishing anatomical dissection as part of medical training is Andreas Vesalius (1514–1564).[2] Vesalius's relationship to the Jews, albeit limited, deserves mention. The anatomical terms detailed in his works—the *Tabulae Anatomicae* and later the classic *De Humani Corporis Fabrica*—are presented in multiple languages, including Hebrew.[3]

Exactly who is responsible for the Hebrew translations in the *Tabulae Anatomicae* is unknown. Vesalius may have attended lectures on the Hebrew language by Joannes van Campen at the Pedagogium Trilingue in Louvain.[4] With the Hebrew terminology for the *Fabrica*, however, Vesalius duly acknowledges some assistance:

Brussels (University of California Press, 1964), 1–20; Ludwig Edelstein, "The History of Anatomy in Antiquity," in O. Temkin and C. L. Temkin, eds., *Ancient Medicine* (Johns Hopkins University Press, 1967), 247–302; Charles Singer, *A Short History of Anatomy and Physiology from the Greeks to Harvey* (New York, 1957); Mary Niven Alston, "The Attitude of the Church towards Dissection before 1500," *Bulletin of the History of Medicine* 16:3 (October 1944), 221–238; T. V. N. Persaud, *Early History of Human Anatomy: From Antiquity to the Beginning of the Modern Era* (Charles C. Thomas Pub. Ltd.,1984).

2. On Vesalius, see O'Malley, *Andreas Vesalius of Brussels*. The classic bibliography of works about Vesalius by Harvey Cushing was recently updated by Dr. Maurits Biesbrouck, *Vesaliana: An Updated Bibliography* (Roeselare, 2019).

3. On the use of Hebrew in medical literature throughout history, see the excellent survey of H. Friedenwald, "The Use of the Hebrew Language in Medical Literature," *Bulletin of the History of Medicine* 2 (1934), 77–111. See also J. J. Barcia Goyanes, "Medieval Hebrew Anatomical Names: A Contribution to Their History," *Koroth* 8:11–12 (1985), 192–201; A. Goldstein, "Historical Development of Hebrew Medical Terminology," *Koroth* 3:11–12 (May 1966); Goldstein, 4:1–2 (December 1966), 122; 4:5–7 (December 1967), 452; 4:11–12 (December 1968), 773. On the use of Hebrew in universities during this period, see, for example, Z. Y. Flashkas, "The Hebrew Language in the Universities of the Middle Ages," *Koroth* 2:9–10 (May 1961), 494–495.

4. O'Malley, *Vesalius of Brussels*, op. cit., 33. For a list of professors of the Hebrew language at the Collegium Trilingue (University of Leuven) during Vesalius's stay there, see Valerius Andreas, *Fasti Academici Studii Generalis Lovaniensis* (List of the Academics of the University of Louvain) (Lovanii, apud Hieronymum Nempaeum, 1650), p. 284. I thank Dr. Maurits Biesbrouck for graciously providing me with a copy of the relevant passage in this reference.

I have decided to give in the index principally a simple list of the names of the bones, first presenting those I use in the text; then the Greek; then, any others in Latin taken from authoritative writers, and all that in such way that it may have value. After these will follow the Hebrew, but also some Arabic, almost all taken from the Hebrew translation of Avicenna[5] through the efforts of Lazarus de Frigeis, a distinguished Jewish physician and close friend with whom I have been accustomed to translate Avicenna.[6]

This Hebrew contribution has been studied by both historians and linguists.[7] Some have been less than complimentary. As one scholar notes:

> If, however, we are to suppose that both the Hebrew equivalents and their transliterations were written for Vesalius by his Hebrew friend Lazarus de Frigeis… then we must credit the latter with little knowledge of Hebrew, since some of the grammatical mistakes are inexcusable for a connoisseur of the language.[8]

Vesalius credits Lazarus de Frigeis, "a distinguished Jewish physician and close friend," with assisting him with the Hebrew translation in the

---

5. On *Avicenna* (aka Ibn Sina) in Hebrew, see J. O. Leibowitz, "The Preface of Nathan Ha-Meati to his Hebrew Translation (1279) of Ibn-Sina's Canon," *Koroth* 7:1–2 (April 1976), 1–7; Leibowitz, "Ibn Sina in Hebrew," *Koroth* 8:1–2 (June 1981), 3; B. Richler, "Manuscripts of Avicenna's Canon in Hebrew Translation: A Revised and Up-to-Date List," *Koroth* 8:3–4 (August 1982), 145–168; S. Kottek, "The Hebrew Manuscript of Avicenna's Canon" (French), *Medicina Nei Secoli* 8:1 (1996), 13–29.

6. *De Humani Corporis Fabrica* (1543), 166, translated in O'Malley, *Vesalius of Brussels,* op. cit., 120.

7. M. Etziony, "The Hebrew-Aramaic Element in Vesalius's *Tabulae Anatomicae Sex,*" *Bulletin of the History of Medicine* 18 (1945), 413–424; Etziony, "The Hebrew-Aramaic Element in Vesalius: A Critical Analysis," *Bulletin of the History of Medicine* 20 (1946), 36–57; Jacques Pines, "La Nomenclature Hebraique dans le Oeuvres Anatomiques d'Andre Vesale," *Le Scalpel* 118 (1965), 85–92; Juan Jose Barcia Goyanes, "Los Terminos Osteologicos de la 'Fabrica' y la Evolucion del Lenguaje Anatomico Hebreo en la Edad Media," *Sefarad* 42 (1982), 299–326.

8. Etziony, "Hebrew-Aramaic Element in Vesalius," op. cit., 36.

Fabrica.[9] While some evidence has come to light about this friend, his exact identity still eludes scholars.[10] De Frigeis is believed to be depicted in the classic illustration on the frontispiece of the *Fabrica*, wearing characteristically Jewish garb.[11] While Vesalius mentions De Frigeis in the second edition of the *Fabrica*, the latter's Jewish identity is conspicuously omitted. It is possible that external social pressures led to this emendation. Alternatively, De Frigies may have converted to Christianity by the time of the publication of this edition and was thus not identified as a Jew.[12]

Another relationship between Vesalius and the Jews[13] is inferred from his tenure as a lecturer at the University of Padua.[14] This famous university[15] was one of the only institutions of higher learning in the medieval and Renaissance periods that admitted Jews.[16] Most universities

---

9. For unclear reasons, the phrase "distinguished Jewish physician" was omitted from the second edition of the *Fabrica*. See O'Malley, *Vesalius of Brussels*, op. cit., 120.

10. S. Franco, "Ricerche su Lazzaro Ebreo de Frigeis, Medico Insigne ed Amico di Andre Vesal," *La Rassegna Mensile di Israel* 15 (1949), 495–515; J. Pines, "Lazarus Hebraeus of Frigeis, Collaborator and Close Friend of Andreas Vesalius" (French), *Le Scalpel* 117 (January, 1964), 5–12; Balazs Bugyi, "Rilievi Critici sul Medico Traduttore di Vesalio, Lazarus de Frigeis," *Acta Medicae Historiae Patavinae* 11 (1964–1965), 203–205; B. Bugyi, "Critical Notes about Lazarus de Frigeis: Vesalius's Advisor in Hebrew Terminology," *Koroth* 3:11–12 (May 1966), 613–615; Francesco Piovan, "Nuovo Documenti sul Medico Ebreo Lazzaro 'De Frigeis' Collaboratore di Andrea Vesalio," *Quaderni per la Storia Dell'Universita di Padova* 21 (1988), 67–74; D. Carpi, "Alcune Nuove Considerazione su Lazzaro di Raphael 'de Frigiis,'" *Quaderni per la Storia Dell'Universita di Padova* 30 (1997), 218–226.

11. See O'Malley, *Vesalius of Brussels*, 142.

12. For more of the identity and history of De Frigies, see M. Nevins, "A Face in the Crowd: Vesalius' Jewish Friend," *Koroth* 23 (2015–2016), 237–256.

13. Vesalius also addresses a midrashic tradition that an indestructible *luz* bone will be the nidus, or origin, of the resurrection of the body in Messianic times. He attributes this notion to an Arabic or magical tradition. He rejects this belief as neither verifiable nor consistent with anatomical observation. See chapter, "The Illusive and Elusive Luz Bone."

14. See O'Malley, *Vesalius of Brussels*, op. cit., 73–110.

15. On the University of Padua in general, see, for example, H. Rashdall, *The Universities of Europe in the Middle Ages*, 3 vols. (Oxford University Press, reissued 1987); L. Rosetti, *The University of Padua: An Outline of Its History*, trans. Alice W. Maladorno Hargraves (Edizioni Lint, 1987).

16. On the Jews and the University of Padua, see A Ciscato, *Gli Ebrei in Padova* (1300–1800) (Arnaldo Forni Editore, 1901); Cecil Roth, "The Medieval University and the Jew," *Menora* 9:2 (1930), 128–141; S. Dubnov, "Jewish Students at the University of Padua," *Sefer*

required graduates to avow their belief in Christianity as a prerequisite to obtaining their degree and subsequent licensure, thereby effectively precluding Jews from university-based medical training. Despite its proximity to the Vatican, the University of Padua was part of the free Venetian state and relaxed this requirement. As a result, many European Jews attended.[17] This university, one of the greatest in European history, was home to the likes of William Harvey (1578–1657), Galileo (1564–1642), and Giovanni Battista Morgagni (1682–1771),[18] in addition to Vesalius. It is more than likely that Jews attended his classic dissections. As we shall see, the Jewish medical students at the University of Padua had to go to great lengths to prevent Jewish bodies from reaching the dissection table.[19]

Hashanah: American Hebrew Yearbook (1931), 216–219; Jacob Shatzky, "On Jewish Medical Students of Padua," *Journal of the History of Medicine* 5 (1950), 444–447; Cecil Roth, "The Qualification of Jewish Physicians in the Middle Ages," *Speculum* 28 (1953), 834–843; David B. Ruderman, "The Impact of Science on Jewish Culture and Society in Venice (with Special Reference to Jewish Graduates of Padua's Medical School)," in *Gli Ebrei e Venezia*, Secoli xiv–xviii (Atti del Convegno Internazionale Organizzato D'all'Instituto di Storia della Sociata e della Stato Veneziano dell a Fondazione Giorgio Cini, Venezia, 1983), 417–448, reprinted in Ruderman, *Jewish Thought and Scientific Discovery in Early Modern Europe* (New Haven, 1995); S. Massry et al., "Jewish Medicine and the University of Padua: Contribution of the Padua Graduate Toviah Cohen to Nephrology," *American Journal of Nephrology* 19:2 (1999), 213–221; S. M. Shasha and S. G. Massry, "The Medical School of Padua and Its Jewish Graduates" (Hebrew), *HaRefua* 141:4 (April 2002), 388–394; E. Reichman, "The Valmadonna Trust Broadsides: A Virtual Reunion of the Jewish Medical Students of the University of Padua," *Verapo Yerapei: The Journal of Torah and Medicine of the Albert Einstein College of Medicine Synagogue* 7 (2017), 55–76.

17. For a list of Jewish graduates from the University of Padua Medical School in past centuries, see Abdelkader Modena and Edgardo Morpugo, *Medici E Chirurghi Ebrei Dottorati E Licenziati Dell'Universita Di Padova dal 1617 al 1816* (Bologna, 1967); E. V. Ceseracciu, "Ebrei laureate a Padova nel cinquecento," *Quaderni per la storia Dell'Universita di Padova* 13 (1980), 151–168.

18. Morgagni's *The Seats and Causes of Diseases* (Venice, 1771) established him as the father of modern anatomical pathology. The diploma of Cervo Conigliano, a Jewish medical student at the University of Padua, bears Morgagni's signature. See Bruno Kisch, "Cervo Conigliano: A Jewish Graduate of Padua in 1743," *Journal of the History of Medicine* 4 (1949), 450–459.

19. A ducal document from 1549, during Vesalius's tenure in Padua, condemns grave robbing but does not single out the Jews. See Ciscato, *Gli Ebrei in Padova*, p. 297. Later documents, as discussed below, address body snatching in the Jewish community specifically.

In addition, some of these Jewish students may have left the anatomical theater of Vesalius to attend a lecture in the yeshiva of Meir ben
Isaac Katzenellenbogen, Maharam MiPadua (1473–1565).[20] Avtalyon
Modena, a brilliant Talmudist and student at the University of Padua medical school, learned with Maharam MiPadua.[21] R. Yehuda Arye DeModena
(Modena's nephew), another prominent Italian rabbinic figure, also had
significant contact with the Jewish medical students of Padua.[22]

More direct evidence that Jewish medical students and physicians
studied the works of Vesalius lies in the existence of a rare manuscript of
the *Fabrica* in Yiddish, dating from the late 1500s.[23] Its survival is clear
proof of Jewish interest in Vesalius, and this very manuscript may have
been used by anatomy students in Padua.

Thus, in response to our initial question about the historical
period of the first responsa on anatomy, based on the foregoing discussion, it is clear why neither Maimonides nor R. Yosef Karo addressed the
issue of dissection. It simply was not routinely practiced during these
historical periods. Since the study of anatomy became popular only in

---

20. R. Katzenellenbogen's own grandson, Shaul Wahl, attended the University of Padua.
    See Byron L. Sherwin, *Sparks amidst the Ashes: The Spiritual Legacy of Polish Jewry*
    (Oxford University Press, 1997), 68.
21. See Judah Saltaro Fano, *Mikveh Yisrael* (Venice, 1607), 35a, 36b.
22. M. R. Cohen, ed. and trans., *The Autobiography of a Seventeenth-Century Venetian
    Rabbi: Leon Modena's Life of Judah* (Princeton University Press, 1988), 30, 190. R.
    Modena also edited a volume of poems and letters marking the graduation of Joseph
    Hamitz from the medical school in Padua. See Cohen, *Leon Modena's Life*, 126 and
    233. Composition of poems and songs for such occasions was not uncommon in
    Renaissance Italy. See, for example, M. Benayahu, "Songs on the Occasion of the
    Graduation of the Physician Yehuda Matzliach Padova," *Koroth* 7:1–2 (April 1976),
    39–49. In the introduction to his *Ziknei Yehudah*, R. Modena mentions a number of
    physicians with whom he had contact. Perhaps his most famous student was Yosef
    Shlomo Delmedigo, author of *Sefer Elim*. On Delmedigo, see D. A. Friedman, "Joseph
    Shelomoh Delmedigo," *Medical Leaves* 4 (1942), 83–95; G. Alter, *Two Renaissance
    Astronomers* (Czechoslovakia Academy, 1958); I. Barzilay, *Yosef Shlomo Delmedigo
    (Yashar of Candia): His Life, Works and Times* (Brill, 1997).
23. This extremely rare manuscript of a unique and unpublished Yiddish translation of Vesa-
    lius's work on anatomy is one of only fifty surviving Yiddish manuscripts predating 1600,
    of which only five address medical subjects, the other four containing medical recipes
    and folkloric cures. The manuscript was gifted to the University of Pennsylvania (Rare
    Book & Manuscript Library LJS 485) in 2015 and is available in digital format online.

the Renaissance, it is understandable that the first recorded responsa on dissection did not appear before this time.

II. NOTES ON THE EARLIEST RESPONSA ON ANATOMICAL DISSECTION

The first of the earliest two responsa on anatomical dissection was written by R. Yaakov Emden in reply to a medical student at the University of Gottingen, in Germany.[24] The masterfully poetic prose of the question, as well as the attempt at halakhic analysis, is testimony to the quality of the student's education. The student queried whether he could participate in anatomy lab on the Sabbath and details how, when human cadavers were not available, animals were often substituted.[25] (This shortage of human cadavers for the training of medical students is a matter to which we return later.) Oft ignored in the medical halakhic literature is the identity of this student: Benjamin Wolff Gintzburger, who is known to us from another source as well. Gintzburger wrote his dissertation, a requirement for the completion of his medical degree,[26] on talmudic medicine, one of the earliest contributions of its kind in the history of medical halakhic literature.[27] The work is extant and has been translated into English.[28]

---

24. R. Yaakov Emden, *She'elat Yavetz*, 41.

25. For the history of the supply of bodies for medical school training, with specific mention of the University of Gottingen, see T. Buklijas "Cultures of Death and Politics of Corpse Supply: Anatomy in Vienna, 1848–1914," *Bulletin of the History of Medicine* 82 (2008), 570–607.

26. On the history of Jewish medical student dissertations, see E. Reichman, "The History of the Jewish Medical Student Dissertation: An Evolving Jewish Tradition," in J. Karp and M. Schaikewitz, eds., *Sacred Training: A Halakhic Guidebook for Medical Students and Residents* (Ammud Press, 2018), xvii- xxxvii.

27. Benjamin Mussafia, a graduate of the Padua medical school, wrote *Dicti Sacro-Medicae Sententiae* (Hamburg, 1640), the earliest known work by a Jewish physician on the Bible, collecting and explaining medically related passages from *Tanakh*. See H. Friedenwald, *The Jews and Medicine*, vol. 1 (Ktav, 1967), 112. Benedetto Frizzi, a physician in Mantua in the late eighteenth century, wrote a number of works on biblical and talmudic medicine published from 1787 to 1799. See S. Simonsohn, *History of the Jews in the Duchy of Mantua* (Kiryat Sefer, 1977), 649, n. 226; Friedenwald, *Jews and Medicine*, 115.

28. F. Schiller, "Benjamin Wolff Gintzburger's Dissertation on Talmudic Medicine," *Koroth* 9:7–8 (Fall 1988), 579–600. For biographical notes on Gintzburger, see N. M. Gelber,

The other, better-known responsum to address autopsy is by R. Yeḥezkel Landau in his *Noda BiYehuda*.[29] The case presented to R. Landau involved a patient who died after an operation for "cutting of the stone." Many erroneously consider this to be a case of gallstones, but in fact, it was clearly a case of urinary bladder stones.[30] (There is potential halakhic relevance to this disease identification.) Perhaps not coincidentally, surgeons in England—from whence the responsum originated—were experimenting with new stone-cutting techniques during this period.[31] R. Landau famously concluded that the prohibitions and obligations that devolve upon the human body after death can be waived if there is a "*ḥoleh lefaneinu*," a patient who can directly and immediately benefit from the information gleaned.

The application of this principle in the modern context remains a matter of rabbinic debate and interpretation. Some argue that a prevalent disease would constitute a "*ḥoleh lefaneinu*" situation and justify violation or suspension of Torah prohibitions according to R. Landau. Indeed, this was the extrapolation of the Ḥazon Ish in applying R. Landau's principle in a time of plague.[32] Prof. Abraham

"History of Jewish Physicians in Poland in the Eighteenth Century" (Hebrew), in Y. Tirosh, ed., *Shai Li-Yeshayahu: Sefer Yovel le-Rav Yehoshua Wolfsberg*" (*HaMerkaz LeTarbut shel HaPoel HaMizraḥi*, 5716), 347–371, esp. 356; *Koroth* 9, *Proceedings of the Third Symposium on Medicine in the Bible and Talmud* (special issue, 1988), 255–261.

29. *Mahadura Tinyana, Yoreh De'ah* 210.

30. For more expansive discussion of this topic, see chapter, "A Tale of Two Stones." For a review of the rabbinic literature dealing with stones in the urogenital system, see Abraham Ofir Shemesh, "*Ḥoleh HaEven: Avanim BeDarkei HaSheten*," *Assia* 79–80 (January 2007), 57–76.

31. See, for example, William Cheselden, "A Remarkable Case of a Person Cut for the Stone in the New Way," *Philosophical Transactions* 44 (1746). In 1727, Cheselden performed the first lateral lithotomy to remove bladder stones. This procedure lasted minutes instead of hours and had a significantly lower mortality rate (less than 10%).

32. Ḥazon Ish, *Ohalot* 22:32. In the 1951 jubilee volume of *HaPardes* (138–141), R. Shlomo Yitzchok Levin of Minneapolis argues for an autopsy where the patient died of a contagious disease, possibly affecting his living relatives. R. Levin neglects to cite the Ḥazon Ish in support. He also considers generally expanding R. Landau's permissive ruling in the case of "*ḥoleh lefaneinu*," as the results of an autopsy could be broadcast on the radio, potentially saving other lives. This argument is obviously stronger today with the development of communications systems far superior to radio.

S. Abraham cites in the name of R. Shlomo Zalman Auerbach that "the Ḥazon Ish meant that even if the seriously ill patient was not present, if the disease was so prevalent that a similar patient was certain to be present elsewhere and could immediately be helped by the autopsy, it would be permitted."[33] It should therefore be noted that bladder stones were indeed extremely common in the eighteenth century, as was surgical stone removal.[34] Yet R. Landau still prohibited an autopsy in the responsum mentioned above. This ruling might lead one to limit rather than expand the applicability of his responsum. How one defines "prevalent" is the issue. This information may be helpful for the *posek* in extrapolating from R. Landau's opinion to today's medical reality. To be sure, one could clearly distinguish between a plague—which is highly contagious, likely to affect people in the same geographical area, and arguably constitutes a case of "*holeh lefaneinu*"—and bladder stones, which, although highly prevalent then, are not contagious. The history of the understanding of contagion in rabbinic sources requires further study.[35]

III. ANATOMICAL DISSECTION AND BODY SNATCHING

With the incorporation of systematic anatomical dissection into medical training in the Renaissance, a need for the supply of human cadavers rapidly developed. As there was initially no legal means of obtaining such specimens, the universities employed novel procurement methods. In certain cases, medical students were obliged to provide cadavers from their respective communities. This demand impacted on the Jewish medical students and the broader Jewish community, who obviously opposed the desecration of the body for this purpose.

---

33. Abraham S. Abraham, *Nishmat Avraham*, 2nd expanded ed. (Schlesinger Institute, 2007), 2:349.
34. On the general history of bladder stones, including surgical interventions and prevalence of the disease, see H. Ellis, *A History of Bladder Stone* (Blackwell Scientific Publications, 1969).
35. See, for example, Ramban on Bereshit 19:17, Rabbenu Baḥya on Bamidbar 16:21; *Yoreh De'ah* 116:5; *Shu"t Beit David*, 22; *Nishmat Kol Ḥai, Ḥoshen Mishpat* 49; *Shevut Yaakov* 2:97.

In Padua, the Jewish medical students suffered harassment at the hands of their peers, who requested Jewish cadavers for dissection.[36] To prevent this request from being met, the Jewish students received special dispensation from the Senate to exempt and protect the bodies in the Jewish cemeteries. For this privilege, they paid handsomely. Nonetheless attempts were made to kidnap Jewish corpses and violate Jewish cemeteries.

In 1624, students interrupted a Jewish funeral and began removing the body from the coffin. Only the protestations of citizen onlookers stopped the crime. In February 1680, following the murder of young Graziadio Levi, armed students stormed the Jewish ghetto in great numbers, kidnapped the corpse and placed the body on the dissection table. Again, much effort was marshaled to rescue the body and provide a proper Jewish burial. A ducal letter dated February 27 of that year rued the incident and reaffirmed the commitment to protect Jewish corpses.[37]

It reached a point where gravely ill patients would be transported out of Padua for fear of being dissected upon their death.[38] In other cities, the dead were buried under the cover of night.[39] In the ghetto, the

---

36. For the following, see Ciscato, *Gli Ebrei in Padova*, op. cit., 209–212; Cecil Roth, *Venice* (Jewish Publication Society of America, 1930), 286–287.

37. See Ciscato, *Gli Ebrei in Padova*, op. cit., 299–300; *Hebraische Bibliographie* 16(1876), p. 37, which identifies the murdered Jew as Chananel ben Israel ha-Levi. The latter reference discusses an unpublished manuscript by Ḥayyim (Vital) Moshe ben Elisha Cantarini that details this incident. I have been unsuccessful in locating this manuscript. Cantarini, member of an illustrious Italian family comprising many rabbis/ physicians, graduated from the medical school in Padua and apparently taught in a yeshiva there as well. However, this incident is described in great detail by Isaac Ḥayyim Cantarini in his *Paḥad Yitzḥak* (Amsterdam, 1694).

38. This practice might have violated the prohibition of moving a *gosses*, the halakhic equivalent to a "dying person." A similar question was posed to R. Moshe Stern: Could one move a critically ill patient out of the hospital for fear that, upon his death, his body would be taken for autopsy and dissection without family consent? R. Stern ruled in the negative. See his *Be'er Moshe* 8, nos. 239, 240, 241, 243. Likewise, R. Moshe Lemberger was asked whether a *Kohen* physician could expose himself to *tum'ah* in order to establish cause of death and prevent a likely autopsy. R. Lemberger argues that the *Kohen must* do so, as this case is akin to a *met mitzva* (one who dies without family or friends to bury him). See Lemberger, *Ateret Moshe, Yoreh De'ah* 2:244.

39. *Hebraische Bibliographie* 16(1876), 37.

Jews hid bodies until their funerals. As late as 1721, confirmation of the prior Jewish immunity was required.[40]

When students could not provide sufficient cadavers, schools often relied on grave robbers or body snatchers.[41] The impact of this practice on the Jewish community has not been well documented.

The demand for Jewish cadavers in medical education continued into the twentieth century throughout Europe. In Warsaw in the 1920s, a medical school requested Jewish bodies for dissection. Some community members were willing to provide cadavers, lest refusal lead to exclusion of Jewish students from medical training or, worse, to larger anti-Jewish backlash.[42] R. Ḥayyim Elazar Shapira (1871–1937), the Munkatch Rebbe, vehemently opposed this acquiescence.[43] Likewise, at Denver's Tuberculosis Hospital in 1916, rabbis refused to furnish Jewish bodies for dissection.[44]

---

40. Roth, *Venice*, op. cit.

41. See Norman Adams, *Dead and Buried: The Horrible History of Body Snatching* (Aberdeen University Press, 1972); J. M. Ball, *The Body Snatchers: Doctors, Grave Robbers and the Law* (Dorset: New York, 1989); Martin Fido, *Bodysnatchers: A History of the Resurrectionists, 1742–1832* (Weidenfeld & Nicolson, 1988); Ruth Richardson, *Death, Dissection and the Destitute* (Weidenfeld & Nicolson, 2001); Suzanne Shultz, *Body Snatching: The Robbing of Graves for the Education of Physicians in Early-Nineteenth-Century America* (McFarland and Co., 1992); M. Sappol, *A Traffic of Dead Bodies: Anatomy and Embodied Social Identity in Nineteenth-Century America* (Princeton University Press, 2002).

42. Regarding the acquisition and dissection of Jewish bodies for medical training in Poland and Germany in the early twentieth century, see M. Graber, *Nituach ha-Metim le-Tzarchei Limud ve-Chakira* (Palestine, 1948). This work contains a wealth of information about the halakhic discussions of this period, including the famous cases in Warsaw and Denver. See also the archival research of Natalia Aleksiun, "Christian Corpses for Christians! Dissecting the Anti-Semitism Behind the Cadaver Affair of the Second Polish Republic," *Eastern European Politics and Societies* 25:3 (2011), 393–409; idem, "Jewish Students and Christian Corpses in Interwar Poland: Playing with the Language of Blood Libel," *Jewish History* 26 (2012), 327–342.

43. *Minḥat Elazar*, addendum to 4:28. See also *Dovev Mesharim* 1:58.

44. On the Denver episode, see Graber, *Nituaḥ HaMetim*, p. 41ff. For a scathing critique of the American rabbinate's handling of this case, see Ḥayyim Hirschensohn, *Malki BaKodesh* 3:4. See also Yosef Goldman, *Hebrew Printing in America 1735–1926: A History and Annotated Bibliography* (YG Books, 2006). I thank Menachem Butler for this reference.

IV. GRAVE ROBBING BY JEWS

At least two sources—one literary, one historical—implicate the Jews themselves in the heinous practice of providing bodies to medical schools. The first source is Thomas Nashe's 1594 novel, *The Unfortunate Traveler, or the Life of Jack Wilton*, where we read the following (spelling modernized):

> It was then the law in Rome that if a felon fell into any man's hands, either by breaking into his house or by robbing him on the highway, he might choose whether he would make him his bondman or hang him. Zadoch (like all Jews, covetous), thinking to himself that he should have no benefit by casting me off the ladder [hanging], had another idea in his head. He went to one doctor, Zacharie the Pope's physician,[45] who was a Jew and his countryman likewise, and told him he had the finest bargain for him that might be. "It is not concealed from [me]," said he, "that the time of your accustomed yearly anatomy is at hand, which behooves you… to make provisions. The infection is great and will hardly get you a sound body to deal upon. You are my countryman; therefore, I come to you first. … I have a young man at home fallen to me for my bondman… you are an honorable man, and one of the scattered children of Abraham; you shall have him for five hundred crowns…."

The narrator recounts how Zadoch the Jew almost sold him to the Pope's physician, also a Jew, for the purpose of anatomical dissection. The narrator was guilty of a criminal offense, theft, and delivery into the hands of the anatomists was one possible punishment. Before the establishment of laws allowing the legal procurement of bodies, many subjects for dissection were obtained through the criminal justice system.

---

45. Despite repeated papal decrees that Christians should not be treated by Jewish physicians, many popes throughout history maintained a Jewish physician on staff. See J. Pines, "Des Medecins Juifs au Service de la Papaute du XII au XVII Siecle," *Le Scalpel* 114 (May, 1961), 462–470.

The second source appears in the late nineteenth century in the *Diary of a Resurrectionist*,[46] depicting a year in the life of a leading body snatcher. He and his cronies attempted to sabotage others who sold cadavers to the local medical school. In August 1812, we find the following entries regarding Jewish involvement in the body trade:

Monday, August 24

me and Ben went in the cart to different places to look out. coming back from Charing Cross met the Jews Drag. touted till dark and lost scent. came home.

Tuesday, August 25

understood the Jew had brought a male to Bartholomew. met by appointment at the above place.

J. B. Bailey, who published the diary in 1896, identified this unnamed Jew as Israel Chapman, a known grave robber.[47] Historians[48] don't know whether Chapman dealt only in Jewish corpses, but these were certainly highly sought-after by schools, since the ideal bodies for dissection are those buried soon after death, and the Jewish practice is to bury as soon as possible after death, based on the biblical commandment of "you shall

---

46. James Blake Bailey, *Diary of a Resurrectionist, 1811–1812* (Swan Sonnenschein, 1896). The grave robbers or body snatchers were also called resurrectionists, as they raised the bodies from their graves.

47. On Chapman's activities as a resurrectionist, see Fido, *Bodysnatchers*, index. At the time of the writing of this diary, Chapman was 18 years old. Six years later, on January 14, 1818, he was sentenced to death for highway robbery, but the sentence was commuted to deportation to Australia. See *The Proceedings of the Old Bailey*, Ref: t18180114-25. In Australia, Chapman became a famous figure in Jewish history and the continent's first detective. See G. F. J. Bergman, "Israel Chapman (1794–1868): Australia's First Police Detective, and Noel Chapman, Chief Constable," *Journal of the Australian Jewish Historical Society*, 6, part 7 (December 1969), 392–410; J. S. Levi and G. F. J. Bergman, "Izzy the 'Noted Trap Man,'" in their *Australian Genesis: Jewish Convicts and Settlers 1788–1860* (Melbourne University Press, 2002), 69–77 and notes on 335–336; Grace Karskens, "Resurrecting Chapman," *Journal of the Australian Jewish Historical Society*, 18, part 1 (June 2006, 8–21). I thank Prof. Karskens for furnishing me with a copy of her article.

48. Richardson, *Death, Dissection and the Destitute*, op. cit., 62.

surely bury him on that day" (Deuteronomy 21:23). An anonymous address to the public in 1829 states, "as the Jews bury early, their cemetery [yields] the best and freshest subjects, equal in freshness to the body sent to the venal undertaker, who having interred sand, inwardly chuckles at the solemn words 'dust to dust.'"[49]

V. METHODS OF PREVENTING BODY SNATCHING

In response to the epidemic of body snatching, the Jewish community was forced to take measures to prevent violation of the sacred graves. One approach was to expand the role of the keeper of the burial ground, requiring his presence there after sunset.[50] This tactic proved insufficient, so others were adopted. In his *History of the Great Synagogue*, Cecil Roth writes:

> A mere ground-keeper was found later on to be an insufficient safeguard. It was the age of the "resurrection men," who removed recently interred corpses and sold them to the medical schools for dissection. Accordingly, as with other cemeteries, Christian as well as Jewish, a system of watch and ward was devised. A sort of wheeled sentry box was provided, which was moved about the ground and placed near newly-made graves, which were watched from it so long as was necessary. At the Great Synagogue, a law was passed to the effect that all members of the congregation between the ages of eighteen and seventy were to be obliged to lend their services in rotation. Each night, therefore, three of them, armed with blunderbusses, performed this cold and rather gruesome duty, from as early as four o'clock on winter evenings to seven in the morning. At intervals, they had to ring the bell of the watchtower to show they were alert: In some grounds, they

---

49. Ibid. Jeffrey Levine has suggested that one of the illustrations in Vesalius' Fabrica indicates that he obtained bodies specifically from a Jewish cemetery. See his, "Jewish History in Vesalius' Fabrica (September 17, 2014), http://jmlevinemd.com/jewish-history-vesalius-fabrica/ (accessed May 21, 2021).

50. Jessica Wyman, *West London Synagogue of British Jews* (issued by West London Synagogue in commemoration of its 150th anniversary). Accessed May 21, 2021, at http://www.jewishgen.org/jcr-uk/London/wls/history.htm.

were supposed to walk about every hour and to call, "All's well," if they found nothing amiss. Among the Synagogal records there are preserved rosters of the roll of service, "for the guarding of the House of Life." It was possible to obtain exemption only on the payment of a substantial fine, of which too the records are preserved. This system continued to obtain until well on in the nineteenth century.[51]

Wealthy Jews provided from their estates for a watchman over their grave. According to the *Times* of February 10, 1800, the Jew A. de Matto Mocatta left 200 guineas to have his grave in the burial ground of the Spanish and Portuguese Jews watched for twelve months.[52]

Grave robbing was by no means restricted to Europe. American Jewish communities faced similar issues. Following the Civil War, for instance, an unprecedented enrollment in Ohio medical schools[53] led to great demand for cadavers. With no other recourse, schools turned to professional body snatchers, or "resurrectionists." Roughly five thousand bodies were exhumed in Ohio in the nineteenth century for dissection purposes. Unique patents for devices designed to prevent grave robbing were submitted from this state. These included a terra cotta burial case and the "torpedo" coffin, the latter rigged with explosives set to detonate upon disturbance of the casket.[54]

R. Schachne Isaacs, a congregational rabbi in Cincinnati in the late nineteenth century,[55] wrote the following question to R. Ben Tzion b. Arye Leib Sternfeld of Calveria, the European community adjacent to Isaacs' native Liubava, Lithuania:

---

51. Cecil Roth, *History of the Great Synagogue London 1690–1940* (Edward Goldston and Son, 1950).

52. Roth, *Great Synagogue*.

53. For what follows, see L. F. Edwards, "Body Snatching in Ohio in the Nineteenth Century," *Ohio History* 59:4 (October 1950), 330–351.

54. Another classic device of this kind was the so-called mortsafe tomb, a covering made of wrought-iron bars. Nineteenth-century graves of this kind can be seen today in the Greyfriars graveyard in Edinburgh.

55. On Isaacs, see Jonathan D. Sarna and Nancy Klein, *The Jews of Cincinnati* (Center for the Study of the American Jewish Experience, 1989); Leo Jung, *Men of the Spirit* (Kymson Publishing Co., 1964), 575–576. I thank Prof. Sarna for these references.

In our city (Cincinnati) there is a plague, the mere mention of which will cause one to guard his ears. In our city there are many medical schools with students studying anatomy, for which they require human cadavers. It has come to light that they have removed hundreds, perhaps thousands of bodies from their graves. This is also a source of commerce, as they preserve the bodies and send them to different states. The gentiles have made caves adjacent to the cemetery, wherein they carve out cavities to place the bodies temporarily until reinterment in the summer. The wealthy people in our community arrange for watchmen over their grave for some time… but this is at great expense. Even this is for naught, as we have spoken with physicians who state that, even two to three weeks after burial, the bodies are still useful for the dissection table. We therefore ask if we can do as [the gentiles]. Since this is a novel matter, we do not wish to do this on our own authority, though we believe it to be permitted. … We would like to build a special, cavernous structure in which to deposit the body temporarily, until permanent burial can take place in the summer.[56]

With Jewish cemeteries at risk, R. Isaacs considered allowing temporary interment above ground, in a mausoleum, with subsequent burial in the earth. The adoption of this gentile practice would accomplish at least two objectives. First, full burial could be postponed until after the university semester, when the need for cadavers would diminish. Second, the appeal of the Jewish cemeteries was the "freshness" of the cadavers; delaying formal burial would make the bodies less desirable. While R. Isaacs opined that a deviation from normal traditional Jewish burial practices was halakhically justified, due to the gravity of the matter, he forwarded the query to R. Sternfeld.

R. Sternfeld addressed the prohibition of delaying burial, *"lo talin,"* since interment in a mausoleum might not constitute halakhic burial.[57]

---

56. *Sha'arei Tzion* 31 (Hebrew).
57. R. Sternfeld considers grave robbing a form of *"ḥatutei shikhvi,"* an expression found in *Yevamot* 63b and in subsequent halakhic literature. This phrase could be loosely translated as "body snatchers" and misapplied to grave robbing for anatomical

However, he recalled the ancient Jewish tradition of burial in caves (*kukhin*). Thus, interment in a mausoleum, similar to a *kukh*, might be considered an appropriate primary halakhic burial. As for reinterment, Sternfeld noted that *Shulḥan Arukh* expressly permits it[58] as long as such was the original intent. In conclusion, he approved R. Isaacs' request, provided that some earth be placed directly on the body and that the casket rest on earth as opposed to stone.

R. Sternfeld also apparently sent his conclusions to another great rabbinic figure, R. Yitzchak Elchanan Spektor, for review and approval.[59] While R. Sternfeld's published responsum nowhere indicates that he consulted R. Spektor, nor is there any mention of R. Sternfeld in R. Spektor's response to this question in his *Ein Yitzḥak*, it appears evident to this author that R. Spektor was indeed replying to R. Sternfeld.[60] In any case, R. Spektor likewise concurred with the temporary burial suggested by R. Isaacs, adding that the casket need not rest on earth,

---

dissection. However, the term refers primarily to anti-Semitic desecration of Jewish cemeteries. It is found in responsa literature throughout the centuries and has been used to describe the relocation of Israeli cemeteries or graves during the course of construction. Nonetheless, nineteenth-century responsa employing this term may in fact refer to grave robbing. For example, in *LeYitzḥak Reyaḥ* (Yitzḥak ben Shmuel ibn Donan, Livorno, 1902), letter *shin*, s. v., "*kevurah*" (the fourth entry), we find a question concerning a man's wife who was buried but subsequently exhumed by "*ḥatutei shikhvi*." Since the shrouds had been removed, was reburial obligatory? Ibn Donan refers to the oft-quoted *Tashbetz* 2:111 on this exact question. The law protected the property of the deceased but not the body itself. Grave robbers therefore commonly removed all clothing and took only the corpse. Thus, the case in question might have involved grave robbing.

58. *Yoreh De'ah* 363:1.

59. *Ein Yitzḥak*, vol. 1, *Yoreh De'ah* 33.

60. To my knowledge, the connection between these two responsa has not been made. For example, in Ephraim Shimoff's *Rabbi Isaac Elchanan Spektor: His Life and Works* (1959), he writes, "An American rabbi also sought Rabbi Isaac Elchanan's counsel in an unusual problem which concerned the pilfering of cemeteries. Neither the name of the community nor the name of the rabbi is mentioned in the responsum. It seems, however, that the rabbi came from a large city, since the inquirer states that there are many medical schools in his community." However, Y. D. Eisenstein, in his *Otzar Zichronotai* (New York, 5690), 356, states that the manuscript of R. Specktor's responsum (dated 5 *Kislev* 5640) addresses R. Binyamin Bainish Zelkind Rabbiner. I thank Menachem Butler for these references.

as stone is also halakhically considered connected to the ground. R. Spektor also preferred that the earth placed upon the deceased should derive from Eretz Yisrael.

VI. THE PRESERVATION OF THE HUMAN BODY

The resurgence of anatomical dissection led to responsa about the preservation of human bodies. Two such treatises deal with buildings that housed preserved human remains. Were *Kohanim* permitted to traverse these enclosures, possibly exposing themselves to *tum'ah* (ritual impurity)? In the responsa of Dayan Aryeh Leib Grossnass, we read:

> I was asked by some *Kohanim*, who are students at a certain university in England, if they are permitted to traverse the halls of the university out of concern for the presence of *tum'ah* therein. The body of a certain non-Jewish professor, one of the founders of the university, rests in a large, wooden cabinet adjacent to the wall in the hallway.[61]

The professor in question is the Utilitarian philosopher Jeremy Bentham (1748–1832), and the "certain university" refers to University College, London. How Bentham's body ended up in the hall of University College in London, where it remains to this day, is related to the history of anatomy.[62] Bentham was directly responsible for the development of the Anatomy Act of 1831 in England, which laid the foundation for the legal provision of bodies to medical schools.[63] American legislation followed suit. A staunch advocate of dissection, Bentham stipulated in

---

61. *Lev Aryeh* 15. While Bentham died in 1832, his body remained for several years in the office of Dr. Thomas Southwood Smith, who performed the public autopsy on him. Then it was stored at University College, London. It became a halakhic concern only some years later, when the body went on display.
62. C. F. A. Marmoy, "The 'Auto-Icon' of Jeremy Bentham at University College London," *Medical History* 2 (1958), 77–86; Ruth Richardson and Brian Hurwitz, "Jeremy Bentham's Self-Image: An Exemplary Request for Dissection," *British Medical Journal* 295 (18 July 1987), 195–198.
63. Ruth Richardson, "Bentham and Bodies for Dissection," *The Bentham Newsletter* 10 (June 1986), 22–33.

his will that his body be dissected in a public forum and that the elite of British society be invited to the event.[64] His bones were then to be rearticulated, dressed in the clothes, hat, and cane he designated for this purpose, and displayed. Bentham's request was honored. The "auto-icon," as it is called, ultimately found its resting place at the end of the South Cloisters of the main building of University College, which precipitated the question to Dayan Grossnass.

Bentham's body sits in a double enclosure of glass and wood. In addition, the display head was formed of wax, while the original was placed in another case at the foot of the body. Among other issues, R. Grossnass considered whether non-Jewish bodies generate *tum'at ohel* (impurity under the same enclosure); whether the enclosure prevents escape of *tum'ah* (*ḥotzetz bifnei hatum'ah*); whether the display case itself has the halakhic status of a grave; the halakhic status of glass with respect to *tum'ah*; and the status of the case-enclosed head. After lengthy analysis of these matters—taking into account their rabbinic or biblical status—Grossnass ruled that, in cases of great need, *Kohanim* may enter the university hall.[65] He cited the responsum of R. Spektor (mentioned above) as support that burial above ground, as was the case with the

---

64. The text of the invitation reads as follows:

> Sir,
>
> It was the earnest desire of the late Jeremy Bentham that his Body should be appropriated to an illustration of the Structure and Functions of the Human Frame. In compliance with this wish, Dr. Southwood Smith will deliver a Lecture, over the Body, on the Usefulness of Knowledge of this kind to the Community. The Lecture will be delivered at the Webb-street School of Anatomy and Medicine, Webb-street, Borough, Tomorrow, at three o'clock; at which the honour of your presence, and that of any two friends who may wish to accompany you, is requested.
>
> Friday, 8th June, 1832.

65. R. Grossnass discussed his conclusions with R. Dov Ber Weidenfeld, author of *Dovev Mesharim*, Chief Rabbi of Tchebein and, later, resident of Jerusalem. R. Weidenfeld informed him of a similar responsum by Maharsham (R. Shalom Mordechai Schwadron [1835–1911]), 1:215. The question, submitted by R. Ḥanokh Ehrentreu of Munich (1854–1927) concerned an exhibit of Egyptian mummies under a glass enclosure. Based on analyses similar to those employed by R. Grossnass, Maharsham permitted *Kohanim* to enter adjoining rooms though not the exhibit itself.

Bentham auto-icon, may under certain circumstances be considered halakhically valid.[66]

The Bentham case is not the only recorded question about preserved human remains and *tum'ah*. With the renaissance in anatomical training, and the proliferation of medical schools in the eighteenth and nineteenth centuries, came the frequent public display of human remains and the development of the anatomical museum.[67] Most such museums were an integral part of medical schools, but many were independent. In addition, the lay public had an insatiable curiosity about anatomy, including the most grotesque human deformities. As a result, many universities, institutions, and public buildings housed human remains, presenting halakhic concerns for visiting *Kohanim*.

R. Moshe Tzvi Fuchs (1843–1911) received an inquiry from R. Shimon Krauss of Hungary about whether a *Kohen* student was allowed to enter a school/university building housing a human skeleton.[68] R. Fuchs ruled in accordance with the opinion that non-Jewish bodies convey *tum'at ohel*, so he prohibited the entry of a *Kohen* into the building. R. Tzvi Pesach Frank was asked whether a *Kohen* is permitted to occupy a room next to a place where a human skull is housed, if the door between them is closed.[69]

Other responsa address the permissibility of preserving human remains for display. Two halakhic discussions relate to the preservation of fetal specimens. R. Yaakov Ettlinger (1798–1871) was asked whether a Jewish physician was allowed to preserve the formed fetus of a Jewish patient who had miscarried. The fetus was intended to be "preserved for a long period for teaching purposes, as is the practice of physicians."[70] R. Ettlinger delineates three halakhic concerns. The first two, the obligation of burial (with its attendant prohibition of *lo talin*) and the

---

66. *Lev Aryeh* 15, sec. 6.
67. See F. J. Cole, *History of the Anatomical Museum* (Constable, 1914). English popular anatomical museums are discussed in Richard D. Altick's *The Shows of London* (Cambridge, Mass., 1978). For the development of anatomy museums in the United States during this period, see Sappol, *Traffic of Dead Bodies*, 274–312.
68. *Yad Rama, Yoreh De'ah*, 129.
69. *Har Tzvi, Yoreh De'ah*, 283
70. *Binyan Tzion* 119, 120.

prohibition of deriving benefit from a cadaver, are both deemed inapplicable to a fetus. The third concern, however, that the fetus generates *tum'at ohel* and would constitute an impediment for a *Kohen* who enters the same enclosure, was sufficient for R. Ettlinger to forbid the practice.

While these examples reflect the development of anatomical museums associated with the medical profession, "cabinets of curiosity" also fascinated the lay public during this period. These small exhibitions were often displayed in the homes of wealthy collectors and included strange, beautiful, and outlandish objects. Preserved bodies, often fetuses, were frequently accompanied by the stuff of fairy tales—mermaids, dragons, or the clothes or footsteps of giants. Collections also featured examples of rare and misunderstood deformities. Frederik Ruysch (1638–1731), a Dutch botanist and anatomist, is remembered for his developments in anatomical preservation and the creation of dioramas incorporating human parts, many derived from fetuses.[71]

R. Yonatan Eybeschuetz (1690–1764) discusses the case of a man whose wife miscarried a grossly deformed fetus. The man, being destitute, wished to exhibit the fetus for money. R. Eybeschuetz forbade the practice as constituting a violation of deriving benefit from a cadaver, which in his opinion includes a fetus as well.[72]

While few permanent anatomical museums exist today,[73] the tradition continues with the proliferation of exhibits on the human body

---

71. On Ruysch, see A. M. Luyendijk-Elshout, "Death Enlightened: A Study of Frederik Ruysch," *Journal of the American Medical Association* 212:1 (April 1970), 121–126.

72. *Bina Leіttim* (Lvov, 5617), 12a (*Hil. Yom Tov* 1:23).

73. These include the Mutter Museum (Philadelphia); the Hunterian Museum (London); the Warren Anatomical Museum (part of the Countway Library of Medicine's Center for the History of Medicine in Boston); the Army Medical Museum (Washington, D.C.); the Wellcome Museum of Anatomy and Pathology (London, England); the Harry Brooks Allen Museum of Anatomy and Pathology, associated with the University of Melbourne; and the Pathological-Anatomical Museum (Vienna). Another result of the dearth of bodies for dissection from the Renaissance onward was the use of wax anatomical models in lieu of human cadavers. A number of museums house these historical specimens: La Specola—The Museum of Wax Anatomical Specimens (Florence); and the University Citadel of Cagliari Museum. See T. N. Haviland and L. C. Parish, "A Brief Account of the Use of Wax Models in the Study of Medicine," *Journal of the History of Medicine and Allied Sciences* 25:1 (1970), 52–75; M. Lemire,

comprised of genuine human specimens. Gunther Von Hagen's *Body Worlds*, as well as the similar *Bodies* exhibit, have been displayed in the world's most prominent museums. While these showcases, designed to simulate motion or normal, human activity, are perceived by the modern observer to be novel, they are indeed direct descendants of their eighteenth-century predecessors.[74]

R. Bleich has addressed the halakhic ramifications of these displays,[75] focusing on the derivation of benefit from a corpse.

VII. CONCLUSION

The understanding of the human body is an integral part of the practice of medicine. Since the introduction of formal anatomical training into the medical curriculum in the sixteenth century, a wide variety of halakhic issues have arisen in rabbinic literature. There is little doubt that related issues will arise in the future, for as long as there are humans, there will be those interested in their composition. It is therefore important to place these issues in their appropriate historical and halakhic context.

"Representation of the Human Body: The Colored Wax Anatomical Models of the Eighteenth and Nineteenth Centuries in the Revival of Medical Instruction," *Surgical and Radiologic Anatomy* 14:4 (1992), 283–291.

74. For a comparison of the *Body Worlds* exhibit to strikingly similar eighteenth-century anatomical displays, see J. Simon, "The Theater of Anatomy: The Anatomical Preparations of Honore Fragonard," *Eighteenth Century Studies* 36:1 (2002), 63–79.

75. J. D. Bleich, "Cadavers on Display," *Tradition* 40:1 (Spring 2007), 87–97. In his discussion of "unusual" benefit as it relates to a corpse, R. Bleich cites Radbaz and *Mishneh LeMelekh*. As in most halakhic discussions, the conclusions are analyzed, but reference to the original question is absent. Both the aforementioned sources address the use of a medicinal substance called mumia, which, during a limited period in history, derived from ancient Egyptian embalmed mummies. The very word "mummy" owes its origin to this bituminous substance. See chapter, "The Impact of Medieval Medicine on Medical Halakha: The Case of Mumia."

The Anatomy of Prayer[1]

The organs that You set within us, and the spirit and soul that You breathed into our nostrils, and the tongue that You placed in our mouth—all of them shall thank and bless, praise and glorify, exalt and revere, sanctify and declare the sovereignty of Your name, our King. For every mouth shall offer thanks to You; every tongue shall vow allegiance to You; every knee shall bend to You; every erect spine shall prostrate itself before You; all hearts shall fear You, and every stomach and kidney[2] shall sing praises to Your Name, as it is written: "All my bones shall say, *Hashem*, who is like You."

(*Nishmat* prayer from *Shabbat Shaḥarit*)[3]

The inspiration for this chapter is drawn from two articles that appeared neither in the midrashic literature, nor in any rabbinic or halakhic source for that matter, but in the academic medical literature. In fact,

---

1. This chapter is dedicated to the memory of my dear father, Barukh ben Yitzḥak Isaac, z"l, who was *oleh le'olam ha'emet* during its writing. *Yehay zikhro barukh.*
2. I deviate here from the Artscroll rendition, "all innermost feelings," and offer the literal translation to preserve our anatomical focus.
3. Translation adapted from the N. Scherman, trans. and ed., *The Complete Artscroll Siddur* (Mesorah Publications, 1984), 403.

both articles appeared in the same premier publication, the *Journal of the American Medical Association*, though separated by some eighty years. The first, by Dr. Charles Spivak, entitled, "An Anatomic Prayer," was published in 1916; the second, by Dr. Kenneth Prager, entitled, "For Everything a Blessing," in 1997. Though disparate in time, they share the same core Jewish tradition about a key element of prayer. Both of these illustrious Jewish physicians reflected on the relationship between prayer and the human body. It is this dimension of prayer, and its relationship to the human body, that we will superficially dissect in this brief essay.

The association of prayer with the anatomy of the human body is found both explicitly and implicitly in a number of prayers.[4] Some have even suggested the very architectural design of the *Mishkan*, the conduit for our earthly prayers, is patterned after the human body.[5] The idea is most succinctly encapsulated in the phrase from *Tehillim*,[6] uttered as part of the *Nishmat* prayer on *Shabbat*, "*kol atzmotai tomarna Hashem mi khamokha*," "All of my bones shall say, '*Hashem*, who is like You?'" This phrase, at once poetic and halakhic, has served as the title of a beautiful poem on prayer by Avraham ibn Ezra,[7] as well as the source for the required movement of the spine during the recitation of the silent *Shemoneh Esreh* prayer.[8] Below we discuss a number of prayers where either the recitation, or content of the prayer is specifically related to human anatomy.

I. THE 248 EVARIM (LIMBS)

Charles David Spivak, originally Ḥayyim Dovid Spivakofsky, fled Russia in 1882 and became a prominent physician and leader in the treatment of tuberculosis. He helped found the Jewish Consumptive Relief Society

---

4. For a discussion of general medical references in prayer, see M. Etziony, "Medicine in the Hebrew Daily Prayer," *Canadian Medical Association Journal* 71 (October, 1954), 396–398.
5. For discussion of this idea, see audio lecture, Hanan Balk, "The Mishkan as an Expression of the Human Body," http://www.yutorah.org/lectures/lecture.cfm/733493#.
6. 35:10.
7. Published online by the Ben Yehuda Project, http://benyehuda.org/ibnezra_a/78.html.
8. *Yerushalmi Berakhot* 4:3.

(JCRS) in 1904. His contribution to the field of Judaism and medicine is reflected in his work, *The History of Medicine in the Bible and Talmud*.

On September 30, 1916, in anticipation of the upcoming holiday of Rosh Hashana,[9] the *Journal of the American Medical Association* published an article by Dr. Spivak titled, "An Anatomic Prayer: A Hymn Based On an Ancient Fragment of Osteology." Dr. Spivak's contribution is a translation and explanation of a *piyyut* (hymn) that is part of the Rosh Hashana *Mussaf* service. Despite the appearance of this unique *piyyut* in the ubiquitous Artscroll High Holiday prayer book,[10] albeit in the supplementary section, I suspect its existence, and content, has escaped most of us.

The *piyyut* is introduced as follows:

> O deign to hear the voice of those who glorify Thee with all their limbs (*evareihem*), according to the number of the 248 positive commandments.

The poet then proceeds to list ceremonial tasks that are performed for the new year whose numerical value correspond to the groups of limbs in the human body. Thus, for example:

> In this month they blow thirty sounds [of the *shofar*] according to the thirty limbs in the sole of their foot; there are ten additional sacrifices of the day [Rosh Hashana] corresponding to the ten [limbs] in the ankles.

This *piyyut* indicates that every limb of the body has its corresponding mitzva, an idea that is reflected in the fact that the number of positive commandments is identical to the number of limbs listed in the Mishna.[11]

---

9. While the date of publication is September 30, and the first day Rosh Hashana was September 28 in 1916, medical journals are typically released prior to their publication date. In this case, it would have been in advance of the upcoming Rosh Hashana holiday.

10. N. Scherman, trans. and ed., *The Complete Artscroll Machzor Rosh Hashanah* (Mesorah Publications, 1985), 683.

11. *Ohalot* 1:8.

In fact, while many assume that the establishment of the number of positive commandments as 248 predates the enumeration of the 248 limbs, some have argued the opposite—that the tradition of the number of *evarim* is ancient, and later authorities endeavored to correlate the number of positive commandments to the pre-existing known number of limbs, each in his own way.[12]

The structure of this *piyyut* is clearly based on the Mishna in *Ohalot*[13] which enumerates the 248 *evarim* in the body. The very definition of the halakhic term "*ever*," the identification of each of the enumerated *evarim*,[14] and the correlation with our modern understanding of anatomy have challenged Rabbinic authorities and scholars for centuries with no definitive resolution.[15] For our purposes, we will use the term "limbs" and "*evarim*" interchangeably. The focus of this section, however, is to highlight the areas in *tefilla* where this number is reflected or incorporated, the aforementioned *piyyut* being one clear example. While this *piyyut* is the most famous, there are a number of other *piyyutim* that use the Mishnaic list of limbs as the backbone, or spine, of their literary structure.[16]

Parenthetically, Dr. Spivak's preoccupation with the 248 limbs extended even after his death, as he bequeathed his body to science for the purpose of medical dissection.[17] Most Rabbinic authorities would

---

12. David Margalit, "*Pirkei Anotomia Lifnim BiYisrael VeHayom,*" *Koroth* 1:11–12 (June-July, 1957), 378–391. With respect to this specific *piyyutim*, Margalit points out that the author includes non-osseous organs that are not included in the Mishnaic list. He uses this as a support for his thesis to redefine the understanding of the term "*ever*," and to correlate the Mishnaic list with our modern anatomical understanding.

13. 1:8.

14. For a discussion on the halakhic definition of "*ever*," see *Entzyclopedia Talmudit*, s. v., "*evarim.*"

15. On the 248 limbs, see chapter, "The Anatomy of the Human Body in Rabbinic Literature: The 248 '*Evarim.*'"

16. See Malakhi Beit Aryeh, "*Birkhot Evarim,*" *Tarbitz* 56 (5747), 265–272, esp. note 8 on page 267. I thank my dear friend Jay Zachter for this reference. The relationship of the limbs and prayer in the works of the Rokeach, and in particular in the prayer *Anim Zemirot*, will be addressed by Zachter in his forthcoming work.

17. The paragraph of his will dealing with the disposition of his body reads as follows:
    I request my wife and heirs to permit of the disposal of my remains after my death in this way:

only allow dissection of the body after death for an immediate life saving purpose,[18] thus precluding its use in routine student dissection, though some authorities have permitted donation of one's body to science.[19]

Below we discuss other prayers wherein the 248 limbs find their expression.

Shema

The recitation of one of the most central and fundamental prayers in our entire liturgy is governed by the need for its word tally to arrive at the anatomical number of 248.[20] The custom to say 248 words when reciting the *Shema* is found in the Midrash.[21]

The body should be embalmed and shipped to the nearest medical college for an equal number of non-Jewish and Jewish students to carefully dissect. After my body has been dissected the bones should be articulated by an expert and the skeleton shipped to the University of Jerusalem with a request that the same be used for demonstration purposes in the department of anatomy.

The will was reportedly executed as written and Dr. Spivak's body was delivered to the University of Colorado for student dissection. (*Jewish Daily Bulletin*, November 2, 1927)

18. For a general discussion on the laws of autopsy and dissection, see A. Steinberg, *Encyclopedia of Jewish Medical Ethics*, trans. F. Rosner (Feldheim Publishers, 2003), s. v., "autopsy."

19. R. Dr. Immanuel Jakobovits, in his classic *Jewish Medical Ethics* (Bloch Publishing Co.: New York, 1959), 150, quotes R. Herzog, "The Plenary Council of the Chief Rabbinate of Israel ... do not object to the use of bodies of persons who gave their consent in writing of their own free will during their lifetime for anatomical dissections as required for medical studies, provided the dissected parts are carefully preserved so as to be eventually buried with due respect according to Jewish law." See also R. Asher Grones, *Peri Asher*, n. 3.

20. For discussion on this topic, see, Macy Nulman, *Encyclopedia of Jewish Prayer* (Jason Aronson, 1993), s. v., "*Shema*," and Refael Avers, *VeShav VeRafa* 2:7.

21. *Midrash Tanḥuma, Parashat Kedoshim.* On the origins of the association of the *Shema* with the number 248, see, for example, Shmuel Mirsky, *Talpiyot*, Year 1, Volume 2, Issue 1 (*Tevet-Adar*, 5704), 239–244; Yisrael Ta-Shma, *Minhag Ashkenaz HaKadmon* (Jerusalem, 5749), 285–298. On numerology in general and its impact on *tefilla*, see Daniel Sperber, *Minhagei Yisrael*, 2 (Mosad HaRav Kook, 5751), 157–188 and idem, *Minhagei Yisrael*, 4 (Mosad HaRav Kook, 5755), 291–299.

The recitation of *Shema* should not be considered light in your eyes, as it contains 248 words, and there are 248 *evarim* in the body. *Hashem* said, "watch over that which is mine, and I will watch over that which is yours."

In reciting the *Shema*, the *ḥazan* repeats the words "*Hashem Elokeikhem emet*" at the end. The sole purpose of this repetition is to complete a total of 248 words. Indeed, when the prayer is recited without a *minyan*, an additional three words, "*Kel melekh ne'eman*," are added at the beginning of the prayer to accomplish the same numerical objective.[22]

This simple three-word phrase inserted to achieve a numerical objective has generated some halakhic discussion regarding the appropriateness of its position in the order of prayers.[23] For example, Naḥmanides[24] considers the prayer immediately preceding the *Shema*, *ahavat olam*, a *birkat mitzva*, a necessary prefatory blessing prior to the *Shema*. As such, utterance of "*Kel melekh ne'eman*," the equivalent of saying *amen* (the acronym for these three words) would constitute a clear *hefsek* (legal interruption) and would be prohibited.[25]

The Meiri records that the custom of inserting "*Kel melekh ne'eman*" was widespread amongst the sages prior to Naḥmanides, and he defends the practice as a fulfillment of *hoda'a* (praise), being consonant with the theme, and an integral part of, *Shema*, consequently not constituting a legal interruption.

---

22. On the origins of the recitation of "*Kel melekh ne'eman*" see Yisrael Ta-Shma, "*Kel Melekh Ne'eman: Gilgulo Shel Minhag*," *Tarbitz* 39:2 (*Tevet*, 5730), 184–194, and follow up comment on Ta-Shma by Shlomo Zalman Havlin in *Tarbitz* 40:1 (*Tishrei*, 5731), 107–109.

23. For the following I rely primarily on Avers, op. cit.

24. Commentary on *Berakhot* 11b.

25. At an earlier period in history, the *ḥazan* would recite all the blessings and the congregation would only recite the obligatory *Shema*. As listeners to the blessings, they could technically answer *amen*. In order to complete the 248 words as mentioned in the *Midrash*, they would say the full words which the acronym *amen* represented, *Kel melekh ne'eman*. However, it is clear according to Naḥmanides that one who says all the blessings together with the *Shema*, whether *beyaḥid* (as an individual), or with the *tzibur* (congregation), should not add any additional words before the *Shema*.

The Kaf HaHayyim states in the name of Rama that the recitation of "*Kel melekh ne'eman*" presents three problems: 1) It is an interruption between the *berakha* and recitation of *Shema*. 2) It constitutes saying God's name in vain, as the phrase bears no particular relevance to that which comes before or after it. 3) It is an unsanctioned addition to the prayer.

Based on the above concerns, some suggested another option to complete the 248 words—repeating the phrase "*Hashem Elokeikhem emet*" at the end of *Shema*.[26] However, the Ashkenazi custom is to complete the 248 words by inserting "*Kel melekh ne'eman*" at the beginning of *Shema* when reciting it independently (*beyahid*). R. Yaakov Emden, in his *Siddur Beit Yaakov*, recommends reciting the phrase "*Kel melekh ne'eman*" even when reciting the *Shema* with the congregation (*betzibur*).[27]

The "*To'elet Evarim*" (function of the limbs) Prayer

There is a practice described by medieval authorities to daily recite a list of every limb of the body, along with its purpose or function, the so-called "*to'elet evarim*," as a means achieving or enhancing the obligation of "and you shall love the Lord your God."[28]

Moshe MiCoucy, author of the *Sefer Mitzvot Gadol* (*SeMaG*), in his discussion of positive commandment number three, "and you shall love...," suggests this very approach as a means of fulfilling this obligation. Maimonides, in his *Moreh Nevukhim*, and Bahya ibn Pakuda in his *Hovot HaLevavot*, present the same approach.[29] Embedding the number of limbs into the very prayer containing "*ve'ahavta*," "and you shall love," is an effective means of insuring the proper fulfillment of the mitzva, and perhaps it is possible that the application of this specific anatomical correlation with the *Shema*, the central prayer of belief, is a correlate to the "*To'elet Evarim*" paradigm.

---

26. See *Minhat Elazar* 2:28 who quotes the *Birkei Yosef* that this was the custom followed by the *Ari z"l*.
27. For further discussion see Avers, op. cit., 40.
28. Mordechai Meir, op. cit., p. 37, note 62.
29. See articles by Shraga Abramson in *Sinai* 80 (5737), 207–216 (in the context of his analysis of the *Sefer Mitzvot Gadol*) and "*To'elet Evarim*," *Sinai* 82 (5738), 7–11.

In a similar vein, *Sefer Ḥasidim* recounts the story of a *"ḥasid"* who recited a blessing on each *ever* of the body that it should properly worship its Creator and not be the vehicle of sin.[30] While no similar list of blessings has been incorporated into our standard prayer book, a fourteenth-century manuscript of such a rubric has been published. The so-called *"Birkhot Evarim,"* blessings of the limbs, are stylistically similar to the *Birkhot HaShaḥar*.[31]

The Healing Power of Shema

The *Beit Yosef* on the *Tur* elaborates on the association of the *Shema* with the anatomy of the human body and cites in the name of the *Midrash Ne'elam* the practical relevance of the 248 words of *Shema*.[32] Each limb is associated with, and has a corresponding word of, the *Shema*. For one who recites *Shema* with proper intent, each word will affect a cure to its corresponding limb.

The healing powers and the anatomical correlation of *Shema* are reflected in a story recounted in *Nitei Eitan*[33] about two rabbinic sages of a previous generation. R. Ḥayyim Aryeh Leib Rottenberg-Mishkovsky, rabbi of Stavisk (1836–1898), once observed R. Avraham Shmuel of Aishishok, author of the *Amudei Esh*, enter the *beit midrash* with one side of his jaw severely swollen. He inquired of R. Avraham Shmuel as to what had led to this condition. R. Avraham Shmuel attributed his ailment to his lack of proper *kavana* (concentration) in his recitation of *Shema* in the *Ma'ariv* service the previous night. He hastened to add that he would rectify the situation by reciting the *Shema* in *Shaḥarit* with additional *kavana*. And so it was, as the story is recounted, that after the recitation of the morning *Shema* the swelling of the jaw receded and returned to normal.

Women and Ramaḥ[34]

As we discussed above in our chapter on the 248 *evarim*, while the Mishna lists the *evarim* without differentiating between genders, the

---

30. *Sefer Ḥasidim* (Mosad HaRav Kook, 5717), n. 155.
31. See Malakhi Beit Aryeh, *"Birkhot Evarim,"* *Tarbitz* 56 (5748), 265–272.
32. *O. Ḥ.,* 61:3.
33. Avraham Zakheim, *Nitei Eitan* (Horev Press, 5694), n. 30.
34. For an excellent article on the impact of the different tally of the limbs of the female body on prayer, see Mordechai Meir, *"Minyan Evareha Shel Isha VeHashlaḥotav Al Nusaḥ HaTefilla,"* *HaMa'ayan* 45:3 (Nisan, 5765), 27–37.

Talmud in *Bekhorot*[35] indicates otherwise. In order to verify the 248 *evarim* listed in *Ohalot*, the students of R. Yishmael performed a modified anatomical dissection of a woman who had been sentenced to death by the secular authorities. The inspection of the body revealed 252[36] *evarim*, an obvious discrepancy from the comprehensive list in *Ohalot*.[37] The difference is attributed by the Talmud to gender. The dissection was performed on a woman, and a woman has a number of additional limbs not found in a man. This purported difference means that the female body deviates from the number 248, which is the structural foundation for the aforementioned prayers. If so, is a woman obligated to recite these "248" prayers and to conform to this literary structure? Perhaps the number tally needs adjustment if a woman is reciting the prayer?

Women and the Recitation of Shema

As discussed above, according to the Talmud in *Bekhorot*, the female body is not comprised of exactly 248 limbs, but rather of a higher number. The author of *Sefer Leket HaKemaḥ HaḤadash*[38] therefore suggests that perhaps women should not add the phrase "*Kel melekh ne'eman*," at the beginning of *Shema*, as they do not have exactly 248 limbs (especially since there are authorities that consider this phrase to constitute a legal interruption). However, the *Ari z"l* asserts that the number 248 in the *Midrash* does not correspond to the earthly human body, but rather to the limbs of the spiritual body, "*ze'eir anpin.*" As such, a woman can recite the phrase "*Kel melekh ne'eman*," as it is just as relevant for her as it is for a man.[39]

R. Ovadia Yosef *zt"l* was unique in suggesting women make specific additions to the *Shema* so they can say a total of 252 words,

---

35. 45b. See chapter, "The Anatomy of the Human Body in Rabbinic Literature: The 248 'Evarim.'"
36. Commentators mention varying numbers for the limbs of a woman, including 251 and 253. See Maimonides, *Tum'at Met* 2:7 who mentions that a woman has 251 limbs, and *Kesef Mishna*, ad. loc. See also, Yisachar Tamar, *Alei Tamar: Seder Nashim* (1981), 211 for a novel explanation of Maimonides.
37. For halakhic ramifications and approaches to the discrepancy between the number of limbs enumerated in the Mishna in *Ohalot* and *Bekhorot*, see Mordechai Meir, op. cit., 30.
38. 61:12.
39. This idea is expressed in *Minḥat Elazar* 2:28.

corresponding to their specific bodily composition. He suggests this while acknowledging that women are not obligated to recite the *Shema*, though if they choose to, this is the preferred method.[40]

Women and the *Mi SheBeirakh* Prayer for the Sick

A similar question is raised with respect to the *Mi SheBeirakh* prayer for the sick. The standard text reads, "and they should have a complete recovery to their 248 *evarim*." As women do not have exactly 248 limbs, perhaps this text should be amended when recited for an ill woman.[41] Indeed, there are two varying customs today regarding the recitation of the *Mi SheBeirakh* prayer for women. Some congregations recite one text for both men and woman, perhaps based on the position of the *Ari z"l* above. Alternatively, R. Shlomo Kluger asserts[42] that when we say the *Mi SheBeirakh*, we invoke the merit of our forefathers, and since they had 248 limbs, it is irrelevant if the person uttering the prayer does not, as in the case of a woman.

Other congregations recite a separate text for women, which contains essentially one emendation. Instead of requesting a complete recovery for the "248 *evarim* ..." it reads "for all her *evarim*," as, based on the Gemara in *Bekhorot*, a woman has more than 248 limbs.[43]

R. Yeḥezkel Shraga Lipschutz Halberstam[44] contends that the *Mi SheBeirakh* text should be amended to say "all *evarim*" for

---

40. R. Ovadya Yosef, *Otzar Dinim Le'Isha ULeBat* (Eish Pituḥim Publications, 5765), 100. Another specific reference to the 252 limbs of a woman is mentioned by the *Ari z"l* in his *siddur* at the beginning section of the paragraph in *Shemoneh Esreh*, "*Re'eh na ve'anyeinu*." He points out that as the beginning letters of these three words are "*resh*," "*nun*," and "*bet*," equaling the 252 limbs of a woman, one should pray at this point specifically for concerns regarding women. See manuscript edition of *Siddur HaAri* from the Ḥayyim Elozor Reich Renaissance Hebraica Collection at http://hebrewbooks.org/pdfpager. aspx?req=45008&st=&pgnum=119. R. Shay Schacter cited this reference in his *shiur*, "The Proper Way to Daven for a Sick Woman," delivered August 4, 2013, http://www.yutorah.org/lectures/lecture.cfm/796656/Rabbi_Shay_Schachter/ Proper_Way_to_Daven_For_a_Sick_Woman#.
41. For further discussion, see *HaElef Lekha Shlomo*, *O. Ḥ.* 120; *Rivevot Ephraim*, *O. Ḥ.*, vol. 3, 200; *Ravaz*, *Y.D.*, 111.
42. *HaElef Lekha Shlomo*, *O. Ḥ.*, 120.
43. This is the suggested text of R. Moshe Feinstein *zt"l* in his *Iggerot Moshe*, *O. Ḥ.*, 4:67.
44. *Otzrot Yerushalayim* 105 (5732), 69.

both men and women. He argues that since the limbs mentioned in the Mishna refer exclusively to limbs that have bones, and many of the organs without bones could also be afflicted with disease, a prayer restricted to the 248 *evarim* would be insufficient to cover all the organs that may be in need of a cure. This logic applies to both men and women.

One authority suggests amending the woman's *Mi SheBeirakh* to say, "for her 252 limbs."[45] In sum, in light of the anatomical differences between men and women, virtually every possible permutation of the *Mi SheBeirakh* prayer has been proposed.

Anatomical Defects and the *Mi SheBeirakh* Prayer for the Sick

It is not only the anatomical composition of a woman that generated discussion about the text of the prayer for the sick. The *Pardes Yosef*,[46] in his discussion of the prohibition of distancing oneself from falsehood, responds to a query as to whether one who has undergone a limb amputation can recite a prayer for his recovery that explicitly refers to his 248 limbs. As he in fact does not have 248 limbs, perhaps this constitutes a violation of the aforementioned prohibition. He offers two reasons why such a person can maintain the traditional rubric of the text with no fear of uttering a falsehood. His first suggestion, of a metaphysical nature, argues that the 248 limbs refers also to the "limbs" of the *neshama* (soul), which remain intact irrespective of any physical amputation.[47] He also offers a creative embryological approach. While the limb may have been physically amputated, its potential is unimpaired, as evidenced by the fact that the progeny of an amputee will possess the missing limb.

II. *SHEMONEH ESREH*, THE SPINAL VERTEBRAE, AND THE *LUZ* BONE

In *Berakhot* 28b, it states that the eighteen blessings of *Shemoneh Esreh* correspond to the spinal vertebrae, of which, according to the

---

45. Mordechai Meir, op. cit., p. 37, note 62.

46. Shemot, *Mishpatim* 23:7.

47. Similar to the position of the *Ari z"l* and the *Minhat Elazar* cited above.

list in *Ohalot*, there are eighteen. There has been debate about the correlation of this number with modern anatomical understanding, the references to which I refer the reader.[48] The contemporary anatomical correlate notwithstanding, the Talmud queries about the later-added nineteenth blessing of *VeLamalshinim*. If each blessing has its spinal companion, what then is the anatomical companion to this later-added blessing? The Talmud answers that there is an additional small nineteenth vertebra that corresponds to the small bone at the base of the spine. While the Talmud does not identify this bone and simply calls it "the small bone in the spine," it has been identified by many authorities with the bone called "*luz.*"[49] In the next chapter, we will elaborate on both the anatomical and halakhic aspects of the *luz* bone.

III. *ASHER YATZAR* PRAYER[50]

We conclude our survey with a discussion of the *Asher Yatzar* prayer, recited after one performs the normal bodily excretion functions. This prayer explicitly refers to anatomy and physiology and provides a means of appreciating, thanking and praising God through our understanding of these processes. In Abudraham's classic work on prayer, he uses this prayer as a springboard for an extensive discussion on the physiology and anatomy of the human body.[51]

---

48. See Preuss and Katznelson cited above. On orthopedics in rabbinic literature, see Irwin M. Siegel, "Orthopedics in the Torah," *Surgery, Gynecology and Obstetrics* 136 (January, 1973), 107–110; Samuel W. Boorstein, "Orthopedic Passages in the Bible and Talmud," *Medical Leaves* 5 (1943), 49–55. On the number of spinal vertebrae mentioned in the Talmud, see Robert Shapiro, "Talmudic and Other Ancient Concepts of the Number of Vertebrae in the Human Spine," *Spine*, 15:3 1990), 24–25. For a lengthy analysis of the halakhic sources on the vertebrae and ribs, see Nisan Markel, *Binat Nevonim* (Pietrikov, 1927), chapters 27–28.

49. See, for example, Barukh Shimon Schneerson, ed., *HaRokeaḥ HaGadol* (Jerusalem, 5727), 218.

50. For a thorough hashkafic and halakhic treatment of this prayer, see Beni Gesundheit, "*Birkat Asher Yatzar*," *Assia* 16:3–4 (5759), 124–137.

51. *Abudraham*, s. v., "*asher yatzar.*" Abudraham's entry must be understood in its historical context, as he incorporates a number of scientific theories of the Middle Ages. One such theory is the notion of the seven-chamber uterus. On this notion,

There is a linguistic oddity in this prayer, which has drawn the attention of the rabbinic commentaries. It repeats the words *ḥalulim* (cavities). In explaining the necessity for this repetition, the *Midrash Tanḥuma*[52] points out that the numerical value of the two words *ḥalulim, ḥalulim* equals 248, equivalent to the limbs in the body. While this desire to associate the number 248 with prayer is reflected above, it is all the more relevant in a prayer focusing specifically on human anatomy.

I wish to leave the reader with a thought not on the technicalities of prayer, but on their emotional and psychological impact, specifically related to the *Asher Yatzar* prayer, as so beautifully reflected in an essay penned by Dr. Kenneth Prager, a prominent contemporary physician and ethicist.[53] Dr. Prager discusses the beginnings of his true appreciation of the *Asher Yatzar* prayer during his medical school training, when learning about pathophysiology, and how this prayer became an opportunity for him to offer thanks not just for the proper functioning of the excretory organs, but for overall good health. He concludes with a personal story:

> There was one unforgettable patient whose story reinforced the truth and beauty of the *Asher Yatzar* for me forever. Josh was a twenty-year-old student who sustained an unstable fracture of his third and fourth cervical vertebrae in a motor vehicle crash. He nearly died from his injury and required emergency intubation and ventilatory support. He was initially totally quadriplegic but for weak flexion of his right biceps.
>
> A long and difficult period of stabilization and rehabilitation followed. There were promising signs of neurological recovery over the first few months that came suddenly and unexpectedly: movement of a finger here, flexion of a toe there, return of

---

see chapter, "The Doctrine of the Seven-Chamber Uterus." He also discusses the famous rabbinic notion of reproductive physiology that when a woman is *"mazra'at"* first, she will give birth to a male child. We discuss this notion in detail in chapter, *"Parashat Tazria* and Childbirth: An Open and Shut Case."

52. *Parashat Shemini*, n. 8 (Warsaw edition). See also *Tur, O. Ḥ.,* 6, who cites the association of the word repetition with the 248 limbs. R. Yosef Karo did not copy this statement of the *Tur* in his *Shulḥan Arukh.*

53. *Journal of the American Medical Association* 277:20 (May 28, 1997), 1589.

sensation here, adduction of a muscle group there. With incredible courage, hard work, and an excellent physical therapist, Josh improved day by day. In time, and after what seemed like a miracle, he was able to walk slowly with a leg brace and a cane.

But Josh continued to require intermittent catheterization. I know only too well the problems and perils this young man would face for the rest of his life because of a neurogenic bladder. The urologists were very pessimistic about his chances for not requiring catheterization. They had not seen this occur after a spinal cord injury of this severity.

Then the impossible happened. I was there the day Josh no longer required a urinary catheter. I thought of Abayei's *Asher Yatzar* prayer. Pointing out that I could not imagine a more meaningful scenario for its recitation, I suggested to Josh, who was also a yeshiva graduate, that he say the prayer. He agreed. As he recited the ancient *berakha*, tears welled in my eyes.

Josh is my son.

This sentiment is indeed the ideal fulfillment and modern iteration of the *"To'elet Evarim"* prayers—how the appreciation of the function of the human body through prayer is the vehicle through which we can achieve spiritual heights and fulfill the obligation of "and you shall love the Lord your God." So concludes our superficial dissection of the relationship of human anatomy to prayer.

The Illusive and Elusive *Luz* Bone

DEDICATION

This chapter is dedicated to my dear wife Sara, as the *luz* bone is partially responsible for our engagement. A number of the references I encountered in my research of this topic are in Latin. I consulted Professor Louis Feldman, *z"l*, a professor of Latin and Greek at Yeshiva University and prominent Classics scholar, to assist me in translation. When I dropped off the materials at his house, his lovely daughter Sara answered the door. We were soon engaged, and the rest is (medical) history.

I. INTRODUCTION

In this book there are a number of essays on anatomy in rabbinic literature. One essay deals with the 248 limbs and their identification. There is one curious bone mentioned frequently in rabbinic literature that is nowhere to be found in the comprehensive list of the 248 limbs in the Mishna in *Ohalot*—the bone called *luz*. Both its name and location have been a matter of discussion for thousands of years. In this essay we explore the many aspects of this diminutive ossicle and how it has both enamored and mystified rabbis, physicians and theologians for millennia.

The Hebrew or Aramaic word *luz* has several meanings. It refers to a city in ancient Israel and another city in the land of the Hittites. It also means nut, almond, hazel, hazelnut, or nut tree. *Luz* also means to turn, twist or bend. It also connotes libel or disrespectful talk.[1] Finally, *luz* refers to a bone, which is the subject of this essay.

II. THE CITY OF LUZ

Luz is the Canaanite name of the city known to the Israelites as Beit-El (literally: House of God) because of Jacob's dream there.[2] Beit-El is also called Luz when Jacob returned there.[3] In his blessing of Joseph's sons, Jacob again refers to Luz where God appeared to him.[4]

In the description of the borders of Ephraim, Beit-El and Luz seem to be separate entities as it is written: "And it went out from Beit-El to Luz and passed along unto the border of the Archites to Ataroth."[5] The biblical commentary by R. David Kimchi (1160–1235) suggests that this was a different Beit-El. Another interpretation is that Beit-El was outside the city of Luz and represented the outskirts of the city. This thesis is supported by a later biblical verse: "And the border passed along from thence to Luz, to the side of Luz—the same is Beit-El—southward."[6] Thus, when Jacob had his dream, he spent the night on the outskirts of Luz to avoid the danger of entering a strange town at night.[7]

Another city called Luz was built by one of its inhabitants in the land of the Hittites, one of the seven nations of Canaan. This man delivered the city as described in the Bible:

> And the house of Joseph, they also went up against Beit-El; and the Lord was with them. And the house of Joseph sent to spy out Beit-El—now the name of the city beforetime was Luz. And the

---

1. M. Jastrow, *Dictionary of the Targumim, the Talmud Bavli and Yerushalmi, and the Midrashic Literature* (Pardes Publishing House, 1950), vol. 2, 695–96, R. Alcalay, *The Complete Hebrew English Dictionary* (Prayer Book Press, 1965), 1106.
2. Bereshit 28:19.
3. Bereshit 35:6.
4. Bereshit 48:3.
5. Yehoshua 16:2.
6. Yehoshua 18:13.
7. J. H. Hertz, *The Pentateuch and Haftorahs* (Oxford University Press, 1929), vol. 1, Genesis, 244.

watchers saw a man come forth out of the city, and they said unto him: "Show us, we pray you, the entrance into the city, and we will deal kindly with you." And he showed them the entrance into the city, and they smote the city with the edge of the sword; but they let the man go and all his family. And the man went into the land of the Hittites, and built a city, and called the name thereof Luz, which is the name thereof unto this day.[8]

This explains how a city by the name of Luz could have existed in the days of the Judges so far away from Canaan. It was built in memory of the original Luz. According to later sources such as Eusebius, Luz and Beit-El are the same city. Some scholars conclude from the above biblical references that Luz remained the name of the city until the time of Jeroboam and that Beit-El was originally the name of the Sanctuary to the east of it. More probable is the view that Luz was the ancient name of the neighboring town of Ai and that Beit-El inherited the role and area of Ai.[9]

Later legend invested the city of Luz with marvelous powers. Sennacherib and Nebuchadnezzar were unable to conquer it, and no one who stayed within its walls died because the angel of death had no power there.[10] It is also the place where the blue dye (*tekhelet*) was made for the fringes of *tzitzit*.[11] The pertinent talmudic passage is as follows:

And the man went into the land of the Hittites, and built a city, and called the name thereof Luz: which is the name thereof unto this day. It has been taught: That is the Luz in which they dye the blue; that is the Luz against which Sennacherib marched without destroying it, and even the Angel of Death has no permission to

---

8. Shoftim 1:22–26.
9. C. Roth, ed., *Encyclopedia Judaica* 11 (Keter Publishing House, 1971), 593.
10. I. Landman, ed., *The Universal Jewish Encyclopedia* 7 (New York, 1942), 244. See Y. Y. Fish, "Luz: The City and Bone," (Hebrew) *Mikabtziel Journal* 24 (Adar 1, 5757), 307–311 for a discussion about the kabbalistic relationship between the indestructible city and the indestructible bone.
11. *Sota* 46b.

pass through it, but when the old men there become tired of life they go outside the wall and then die.[12]

The Talmud proves from the words, "which is the name thereof unto this day," that the city survived destruction and still exists. This indestructibility of the city of Luz is probably the source for the legend that the bone called *luz* is also indestructible as described below.

III. THE BONE CALLED *LUZ* IN THE MIDRASH AND TALMUD

The Midrash describes the *luz* as an indestructible bone of the spinal column, probably shaped like an almond. It is from this bone that the resurrection of the dead will take place. Even if the rest of the body decays and disintegrates, the *luz* bone remains intact and will provide the starting point for the reintegration of the body at the time of the resurrection. Commenting on the biblical verse, "And the almond tree shall blossom,"[13] the Midrash states the following:

> R. Levi says it refers to the nut (*luz*) of the spinal column. Hadrian, may his bones be crushed, asked R. Yehoshua ben Ḥananiah: whence will man sprout in the Hereafter? He replied: from the nut (*luz*) of the spinal column. He said to him: prove it to me. He had one brought; he placed it in water, but it did not dissolve; he put it in fire, but it was not burnt; he put it in a mill, but it was not ground. He placed it on an anvil and struck it with a hammer; the anvil split and the hammer was broken, but all this had no effect on the *luz*.[14]

A nearly identical Midrash is found elsewhere including the conversation between Hadrian and R. Yehoshua.[15] Only once in recorded history was the *luz* bone destroyed and that was during the Flood when the

---

12. Ibid.
13. Eikha 12:5.
14. *Kohelet Rabba* 12:5.
15. *Vayikra Rabba* 18:1.

Lord destroyed the entire world except for Noah and his family and the animals in the ark. The Bible records that the Lord said, "I will blot out man whom I created."[16] The Midrash comments on this verse as follows:

R. Levi said in R. Yohanan's name:

> Even the nether stone of the millstone was dissolved…R. Yohanan said in the name of R. Shimon B. Yehotzadak: even the nut (*luz*) of the spinal column from which the Holy One Blessed be He will cause man to blossom forth in the future [that is, at the resurrection] was dissolved.[17]

IV. LOCATION OF THE *LUZ* BONE

The location of the *luz* bone has been long debated. From the above sources it appears that the *luz* bone is located in the spinal column and is shaped like an almond. Whether the *luz* is identified with the coccyx or lowest bone in the spinal column, as many writers suggest, cannot be established with certainty.

The 248 bones of the human body are enumerated in the Mishna.[18] It is unclear from whence the Rabbis derived this number. In the only talmudic case which resembles a postmortem examination, 252 limbs or bones were found.[19] Although the bone called *luz* is not mentioned in the two aforementioned passages, there is mention in the Talmud[20] of a small bone at the end of the spine. Some have identified this bone as the *luz* bone.[21] According to Preuss, this unusual little bone, which can only refer to the coccyx, was sought in various sites of the body by the anatomists of the Middle Ages without their being able to find it.[22]

Other non-spinal locations have been suggested for the elusive *luz* bone, including in the occipital area of the skull (wormian bones),

---

16. Bereshit 6:7.
17. *Bereshit Rabba* 28:3.
18. *Ohalot* 1:8.
19. *Bekhorot* 45a.
20. *Berakhot* 28b.
21. E. Rokeah, *Sefer Rokeah Hagadol*, laws of prayer.
22. J. Preuss, *Biblical and Talmudic Medicine*, trans. F. Rosner (Hebrew Publishing Co., 1978), 65.

where the *tefillin* for the head is placed; and inside the skull, not con-nected to other bones.[23] Modern authors have reaffirmed the lack of consensus on the exact location of the *luz* bone.[24]

Non-Jewish scholars in the Middle Ages also accepted the leg-end of the indestructibility of the bone called *luz* and spoke of the Jews' bone, or *Juden-knoechlein*. They likewise debated the exact location of the bone.[25] These sources are discussed in detail below.

Between the rabbinic and secular sources, the locations vying for the honor of the *luz* bone include the coccyx, the sacrum, the twelfth dorsal vertebra, the seventh cervical vertebra, the wormian bones of the skull, and the sesamoid bone of the great toe.

V. ORIGIN AND NUTRITIONAL SOURCE FOR THE *LUZ* BONE

The *luz* bone does not acquire its nutrition through normal methods; rather, its requirements are said to be minimal and are provided exclu-sively from the food ingested at the *melaveh malka* meal after Shabbat. This nutritional fact, as well as the longevity of the bone, is linked to the bone's supposed origins.[26]

The body of Adam was comprised not of earthly dust but of a celestial substance from *Gan Eden* which was immune from mortality. After the sin, the only remaining material from this original body was the

---

23. See D. Y. Weiss, *Megadim Ḥadashim* (Jerusalem, 5772), Bamidbar, 483–486, esp. 485. The Rokeaḥ specifically identifies the Luz bone as the coccyx. See M. Tal, "Luz," (Hebrew) *Assia* 57–58 (November, 1996), 213, who identifies the *luz* as the dens of the axis (the second cervical vertebra).

24. R. Harel, S. Kottek and A. Steinberg, "The Luz Bone," (Hebrew) *Assia* 56 (September, 1995), 125–126.

25. F. H. Garrison, "The Bone called 'Luz'," *New York Medical Journal* 92 (July 23, 1910), 149–151. See "The Bone Called 'Luz'," *Lancet* (October 1, 1910), 1029. This anonymous, brief entry, published a few months after Garrison, mentions many of the latter's sources though does not cite him. J. C. Miller, "Ossiculum Lus," *Anatomical Record* 8:8 (August, 1914), 415–419, also has an excellent discussion on the different possible locations of the *luz* bone.

26. A. Meisels, "The Resurrection Bone Called Luz," (Hebrew) *Or Yisrael* 7:2 (*Kislev*, 5762), 216 cited from *Sefer Gilgulim* of R. Ḥayyim Vital. This is the most compre-hensive study of the *luz* bone I have seen.

luz bone. This bone is transmitted from generation to generation, retains its immortality and is the ultimate source of the body's resurrection.

Death was given as a punishment to man after Adam partook of the Tree of Knowledge. Since this bone is designed to benefit only from the food of the *melaveh malka*, it did not benefit when Adam ingested the fruit of the tree. The curse of death only devolved upon the parts of the body that benefited from the sin. As the *luz* bone did not partake or benefit from the sin, it likewise did not receive the punishment of death. This bone therefore remains immortal.[27]

VI. DIFFERENT NAMES FOR THE *LUZ* BONE

The indestructible *luz* bone has been called by other names in rabbinic literature.

Betuel HaRamai (Betuel the Cheater/Deceiver)

The Zohar identifies the *luz* bone by the name of *"Betual Rema'a"* and explains that the bone is deceptive (just like Betuel) in not requiring as much nutrition as other bones and being able to survive even after death as the ultimate source of the resurrection of the body.[28] The Zohar also states that the bone is shaped like the head of a snake, which would fit with its anatomical identification as the sacrum, as opposed to the other suggestions of the identity of the bone.

Niskoy

Another name for the bone is *"niskoy."*[29] R. Yaakov Emden was baffled by the names Betuel and *niskoy* being associated with the *luz* bone. He offered his own explanation, based partially on *gematria* (numerical value of Hebrew letters), as to how these three terms are actually synonyms for the same indestructible bone and are thematically related to each other. It is necessary for a piece of the body to remain after death so that at the time of the resurrection the resurrected body is connected

---

27. See, for example, A. Polshnitzky, *Atkinu Seudata* (Jerusalem, 5762), 36, in the name of Ḥanukkat HaBayit.
28. *Parashat Toldot.*
29. See, for example, *Arukh HaShulḥan*, O. Ḥ., 300:2.

to the person who lived before. Of course, God is capable of creating the body *de novo*, but such a creation would be viewed as a new person with no relationship to the one who lived previously. The *luz*/Betuel/*niskoy* bone serves this purpose and the different names and their corresponding numerical values correspond to the fact that this deceptive bone though "close to death" is actually very much alive.[30]

The confusion of the names for this special bone was appreciated by Eliezer Ben-Yehuda, the author of the modern Hebrew dictionary, when he queried R. Kook, the then-chief rabbi, as to whether he should list the terms *luz* and *niskoy* separately or as one unified entry in his work.[31]

VII. DOES THE *LUZ* BONE CONVEY *TUM'AH*?

As discussed above, the *luz* bone is not mentioned in the list of 248 limbs in the Mishna in *Ohalot*. This is a list of limbs that convey *tum'at ohel* (impurity under an enclosure). As the *luz* bone is omitted from the list, perhaps it does not convey *tum'at ohel*? This is indeed the conclusion of a number of rabbinic authorities.[32] It may not qualify as a "limb" as perhaps it is not associated with flesh and sinew (*gidim*). Others suggest that the reason for the exemption from *tum'ah* relates to the fact that the *luz* bone is fundamentally different than other bones, due to its indestructability and its relation to resurrection. As such, it does not convey *tum'ah*.[33]

The issue of *tum'ah* for the *luz* bone was also raised in practical halakhic discussions. Ḥatam Sofer was asked about potential *tum'ah* for a building that occupied land where a cemetery may have existed over five hundred years previously. It was assumed that while most of the flesh and bones would have decomposed by that time, the indestructible *luz* bone would have remained intact. Ḥatam Sofer (*Y. D.*, 337) considers whether the *luz* conveys *tum'at ohel*, and if so, would this be a sufficient amount to render the entire house impure. This concern is

---

30. See *siddur* of R. Yaakov Emden, *motza'ei Shabbat*.
31. See. N. Gutal, "Between Luz and Niskoy: A Letter from Rabbi Avraham Yitzḥak HaKohen Kook to Ben Yehuda," (Hebrew) *Assia* 59–60 (June, 1997), 84–89.
32. See, for example, *Minḥat Ḥinuch* 263:10; *Sidrei Taharot Ohalot*, 25b.
33. For further discussion, see, for example, D. Y. Weiss, *Megadim Ḥadashim* (Jerusalem, 5772), Bamidbar, 483–486.

raised by Ḥatam Sofer not only for the one house in question, but to geographical locations of historical national tragedies as well, such as the flood and the destruction wrought by Nebuchadnezzar, where the remnants of thousands of bodies could create *tum'ah* problems today. Here also, the existence intact of the *luz* bones from all these bodies could potentially convey *tum'ah*.

R. D. Y. Weiss invokes the *luz* to explain an enigmatic practice of Rav Yoḥanan, who tragically lost ten children in his lifetime.[34] According to the Talmud, Rav Yoḥanan carried with him a bone from his tenth child, and when he would visit mourners he would show them the bone as a means of comforting them. This practice appears problematic both on halakhic and psychological grounds. How could he carry a continuous source of *tum'ah* on his person, and furthermore, how could this possibly be of comfort to a mourner. R. Weiss suggests that R. Yoḥanan carried the *luz* bone of his tenth son with him. Not only is no *tum'ah* conveyed through the *luz* bone (according to many), but the *luz* bone represents the resurrection. Showing a mourner who just lost a loved one that ultimately, they will return in the time of the resurrection is indeed a source of *niḥum* (comfort).

Some suggest a creative reason as to why the *luz* bone should not convey any form of *tum'ah* (touching—*maga*, supporting—*masa*, or under the same enclosure—*ohel*). *Tum'ah* is associated with the death of a person. The indestructible *luz* bone never "dies" and is forever living. It is the ultimate source of the resurrection. Since the notion of death does not adhere to the *luz* bone in any way, it is per force precluded from any laws of *tum'ah*.[35]

VIII. *LUZ* BONE AND CREMATION

In the midrashic description of the resilience of the *luz* bone, it specifically states that it can withstand fire without burning. This particular trait led to discussions about the *luz* bone in cases of cremation, both in secular and halakhic literature.

---

34. A. Meisels, op. cit., "The 'Resurrection Bone' Called Luz," independently suggests the same explanation.
35. D. Y. Weiss, *Megudim Ḥadashim* (Jerusalem, 5772), Bamidbar, 488.

The anatomist Jean Riolan (1580–1657) was so curious about the tradition of an indestructible bone that he was "driven to pay a formal visit to the public executioner for the purpose of asking this very important functionary whether he had observed, in his extensive experience of the combustion of human bodies, that the ultimate osseous item of the spinal column was really fireproof."[36]

In a homily given by R. Shaul Brach, rabbi of Kasho, Hungary (1865–1940) after a Shabbat in 1933, he discussed the *luz* bone.[37] In the course of his discussion, he cites an article he had recently read in the Czechoslovakian newspaper, *Morganzeitung*. The article was by the director of a local crematorium who happened to notice a small bone amongst the ashes of the human remains. After further inquiry he concluded that this bone was not consumed by fire. In the course of time, he discovered many other similar bones and kept a box filled with these bones in his office. R. Brach brought this as corroboration of the veracity of rabbinic tradition of the *luz* bone.

The nature of the halakhic discussions on cremation and the *luz* bone requires introduction to a unique legal concept regarding *tum'ah* and the cremated body. While the body after death is clearly a source of *tum'ah*, when the body is converted to ash through fire/cremation, it can lose its *tum'ah* status. Both the *Talmud Bavli* and *Yerushalmi* debate this halakha and there is a difference if the cremated body retains its form or shape (*sheldo kayam*).[38] In many of the discussions about cre-

---

36. J. Knott, "Some Remarks on the Epiphyses of the Long Bones, and their Bearings on the Operation of Resection" *New Zealand Medical Journal* 3:12 (1904), 408–417. Another example of non-Jews seizing an opportunity to verify the Jewish notion of the *luz* bone is recorded in "Cemeteries and Catacombs of Paris," *Quarterly Review* 21:42 (1819), 365, "During the Pontificate of Urban VIII a large burial ground of the Jews at Rome was broken up to make room for some new fortifications; and the Jews were particularly anxious to collect all the bones, paying the laborer a dear price for them. But not a single specimen of the *luz* could they produce to their enemy Bartolocci when he called for it upon so favourable an opportunity."

37. Yisrael Erlich, *Shaul Beḥir Hashem: Biography of Rabbi Shaul Brach* (Netanya, 5736), 198.

38. See, for example, B. Z. Shevchik, *Teshuva al Da'at Eifer HaNisrafim* (5649), footnote spanning pages 13–16.

mation the question is raised as to whether the *luz* bone, which should survive cremation, impacts on the *tum'ah* status of the remaining body.[39]

The discussions on cremation were applied to the biblical case of Nadav and Avihu, whose bodies, according to the Midrash, were burned in the Holy Temple. The issue debated is whether the *Kohanim* Mishael and Eltzafan were exposed to *tum'ah* in the course of their removal of the bodies.[40]

The cremation debate became a matter of practical halakha when cremation became an acceptable method of disposing of the body after death in the secular world. Of note, the overwhelming majority of rabbinic authorities prohibited cremation.[41]

In the post-WWII era, the discussions about the *luz* bone and cremation took on a different tone, as rabbinic authorities considered the halakhic ramifications of the remains of those who perished in the crematoria of the Holocaust. Did the *luz* bones of the *kedoshim* (victims of the Holocaust) survive, and if so, what are the halakhic ramifications?[42]

R. Yaakov Yisrael Zuber addresses the question of when the period of mourning begins in a case of cremation—from the time of cremation; from the time of placement of the ashes in an earthenware (stone) vessel; or when the ashes are buried in the ground.[43] He cites *Lehem HaPanim* in the name of *Paneah Raza* who questions why a cremated body should generate *tum'ah* or require burial. He concludes that after cremation a body requires a conventional burial because of the remaining *luz* bone. Based on this idea one would argue that mourning

---

39. See Shevchik, op. cit., who argues that while *tum'at ohel* does not apply to the *luz* bone, both *tum'at maga* and *tum'at masa* do. He uses this fact to answer potential contradictions in other rabbinic sources.

40. See, for example, B. Z. Shevchik, *Eifer HaNisrafin* (London, 5649), 13; D. Y. Weiss, *Megadim Hadashim, Bamidbar* (Jerusalem, 5772), 487–488.

41. On cremation in rabbinic literature, see, for example, E. Ben Amozeg, *Ya'aneh B'Aish* (Livorno, 1906); D. Malkiel, "Technology and Culture Regarding Cremation: A Historical and Phenomenological Analysis," (Hebrew) *Italia* 10 (5753), 37–70; A. Ferziger, "Ashes to Outcasts: Cremation, Jewish Law, and Identity in Early 20th Century Germany," *AJS Review* 36:1 (April, 2012), 71–102.

42. See, for example, *Hesed Yehoshua* 1:4.

43. *She'elot UTeshuvot Zikhron Yaakov* n. 15.

should begin only after burial. R. Zuber dismisses this position primarily because it is a minority opinion not cited by major rabbinic authorities.[44]

R. Yaakov Breisch addresses the case of cremated remains discovered to be buried under a house, and whether this would preclude the entry of a *Kohen* into the house. He concludes that there is no concern for *tum'at ohel* for ashes that remain after cremation. However, one should be concerned for *tum'ah* generated by direct contact, in part due to the possibility of contact with the *luz* bone, which would not be converted to ash in the process.[45]

The Time of Cremation

In the context of a question whether a *Kohen* from a town in Europe can transfer his family's ashes for burial in Israel, R. S. Efrati mentions a novel concept regarding the susceptibility of ashes to *tum'ah*.[46] According to *Shevet Shimon*, the debate about ashes being free of *tum'ah* applies only to a case when the person was burned while alive. If the person died before cremation, then the status of *tum'ah* already devolves upon the body and will not be removed through cremation. R. Efrati refutes this idea.

One author considers whether different types of fire affect the *luz* bone differently.[47] While the *luz* bone may remain unscathed after exposure to natural fire, it may indeed be destroyed by fire of a miraculous origin, such as that which consumed Nadav and Avihu. He also suggests that the industrial strength fire of the crematoria may have also caused disintegration of the *luz* bones.[48]

---

44. See also, *Har Tzvi*, Y. D., 275, who discusses whether the ashes require a legal burial and considers the *luz* bone in the analysis.
45. Ḥelkat Yaakov Y. D., 217.
46. *MeEmek HaBakha* 2.
47. *Emek Halakha* 2:49–50. He also debates the same idea as the *Shevet Shimon* regarding whether cremation occurs before or after death.
48. Regardless, he posits that the size of the *luz* may be less than a wheat kernel (*se'ora*), thus being too small to convey even *tum'at maga*. In the case at hand, he discounts the relevance of the *luz* bone as perhaps it was not included in the sample of ash gathered, and even if present, might not meet the requisite volume to convey *tum'ah*. It is therefore permitted for a *Kohen* to touch and be under the same enclosure as these ashes.

Soap from Human Remains

A number of authorities discuss halakhic issues related to the soap that was purportedly fashioned from human remains by the Nazis *yimaḥ shemam*. The *luz* bone surfaces in these responsa as well.[49]

IX. THE *LUZ* BONE IN NON-JEWISH SOURCES

A number of non-Jewish sources discuss the notion of an indestructible bone. The sources vary from theological to literary to anatomical. Some of these sources attribute the notion to rabbinic tradition, while others do not. As each source merits its own discussion, they are addressed individually and in chronological order.[50]

Sebastian Muenster (1489–1552)[51]

Sebastian Muenster was an outstanding Christian Hebraist of the sixteenth century. His proficiency in the Hebrew language earned him the position of professor of Hebrew at Basel University in 1528. He authored a number of grammatical treatises as well as Latin translations of Hebrew works, including the Bible. Amongst his many works is a small book of Christian-Jewish polemics entitled *Sefer HaVikuaḥ*, or *The Messiah of the Christians and the Jews*.[52] This work is a continuation of the tradition of Jewish-Christian debate in the Middle Ages and is derivative from earlier

---

49. See *Tzitz Eliezer* 8:35; *Shu"t Shem HaKohen* 15.
50. See the brief discussion by Anders Retzius (1796–1860), Professor of Anatomy at the Karolinska Institute, in *Dublin Quarterly Journal of Medical Science* 22 (1856), 253–255; F. H. Garrison, "The Bone called 'Luz'," *New York Medical Journal* 92 (1910), 149–151; J. P. McMurrich, "The Legend of the 'Resurrection Bone'," *Transactions of the Canadian Institute* 9 (1913), 45–51; J. C. Miller, "*Ossiculum Lus*," *Anatomical Record* 8:8 (August, 1914), 415–419. The famous anatomist of the University of Vienna, Joseph Hyrtl (1810–1894), has a lengthy discussion of the Luz in his *Das Arabische und Hebraische in der Anatomie* (Wilhelm Braumuller: Vienna, 1879), chapter 73, 165–168.
51. See Roth, op. cit., *Encyclopedia Judaica*, vol. 12, 505–06.
52. Sebastian Muenster, *Sefer HaVikuaḥ* (Basel, 1539). This book was originally published as one volume in both Hebrew and Latin. However, a number of libraries, including the British Library and the New York Public Library, possess only the Hebrew section of this work. For further bibliographical details, see J. Prijs, *Die Basler Hebraischer Drucke* (1492–1866) (Urs Graf-Verlag, Olten und Freiburg: Basel 1964), 91–93.

similar works.[53] It is in the context of this work that there appears a passage on the indestructible bone.[54] The work is structured as a dialogue between a Christian and a Jew and this section is excerpted from the statement of the Christian:

> But in the world to come and resurrection of the dead, it is farre otherwaies [sic] with us; for then man shall be by the resurrection, a new creature, and renewed upon their former bones, like that vision in Ezekiel, when the Lord God did raise up His people, saying I will lay sinews upon you, and will bring up flesh upon you, and will cover you with skin, and put breath in you, and ye shall live. Wherefore, your Rabbis have said in the secrets of the Law, that there is in the neibe,[55] a very stiffe bone, which being put in the fire, is not hurt by it, and being put into the ground, doth not putrifie, and they affirm the resurrection of the body doth increase by that. So also it is in Genesis, and the Lord made; I say upon the bone, sinewes, flesh and skin, and breathed into her the breath of life, and brought her to Adam, that by this mystery he might foreshew, although man should dye, yet he should rise in the same body and should be made a building of nerves, bones, and flesh joined together, which should not be dissolved, wherefore Adam called her bone of my bone, because the resurrection of man should be in his first bones of eternal life.[56]

---

53. Prijs, op. cit., *Hebraischer Drucke*, 92. See also, D. Berger, *The Jewish-Christian Debate in the High Middle Ages* (a critical edition of the *Nizzahon Vetus* with an introduction, translation, and commentary by David Berger) (Jewish Publication Society of America, 1979), 377.

54. This passage does not appear in the British Library copy of *Sefer HaVikuah*, which lacks a title page, consists of only the Hebrew section of this work, and appears to be an abridged version of Muenster's original. I was unable to make a direct comparison between the British Library copy and other copies.

55. The Hebrew term is *tzavar*, which means neck. It is unclear as to the etymology of the word "neibe," and I have been unable to locate it in either English or Latin language dictionaries.

56. This passage is excerpted from the translation of Muenster's work by Paul Isaiah (London, 1655).

Muenster refers to the indestructible bone but does not ascribe to it the name *luz*. In addition, he quotes the source of this notion as being from the "secrets of the law" which likely refers to mystical or kabbalistic literature.[57] Muenster was familiar with the works of Menahem Recanati, an early fourteenth-century Italian kabbalist and halakhic authority, but his notion of the indestructible bone could not have derived from Recanati, as the latter places the bone at the bottom of the spine, not in the neck.[58] Other kabbalistic sources, however, do describe the bone as being in the neck.[59]

Andreas Vesalius (1514–1564)[60]

Vesalius, the master of Renaissance anatomy, makes mention of an indestructible bone in his monumental work *De Humani Corporis Fabrica*.[61] The relevant passage is found in a discussion on the sesamoid bones of the foot:

> Another one of these bones is that which the magicians and followers of occult philosophy so often call to mind as being fashioned like a chickpea, liable to no decay, and which, buried in the earth after death, will (they affirm) reproduce man like a seed on the day of the Last Judgment. This may perhaps be the bone on either side, but is more likely to be the exterior, which is somewhat like a pea; for on bringing both bones in apposition we should obtain a whole pea. Then the internal ossicle is so large in men of great stature that a die might easily be made out of it. These bones differ, however, from those noted by the Arabs in that they may be burned or broken like

---

57. E. I. J. Rosenthal, "Sebastian Muenster's Knowledge and Use of Jewish Exegesis," in I. Epstein, et al., eds., *Essays in Honor of the Very Rev. Dr. J. H. Hertz* (Edward Goldston and Son, 1942), 351–69, especially 355.

58. See Commentary of Menahem Recanati to Exodus 25:30. I thank Jay Zachter for this reference.

59. Aaron ben Moses Modena, *Ma'avar Yabok* (Yashpe, 1966), 201– 202.

60. For a comprehensive biography, see C. D. O'Malley, *Andreas Vesalius of Brussels, 1514–1564* (University of California Press, 1965).

61. Andreas Vesalius, *De Humani Corporis Fabrica* (Joannis Oporini, 1543), 126.

other bones, as well as in being surely liable to decay to some extent, although of durable structure. But the dogma which asserts that man will be regenerated from this bone, of which we have just narrated the immense fiction, may be left for elucidation to those philosophers who reserve to themselves alone the right to free discussion and pronouncement upon the resurrection and the immortality of the soul. And even on their account we should attach no importance whatever to the miraculous and occult powers ascribed to the internal ossicle of the right great toe, however much one may be concerned about it. At our public dissections and even as an amateur, we have often obtained a better supply of these bones than those truculent male strumpets of the Venetian horde, who to obtain the bone for purposes of comparison, as also the heart of an unpolluted male infant [pueruli virginis masculi], lately killed a child, put the heart from its living body, and was punished, as they richly deserved, for the foulest of crimes. Moreover, this ossicle, called Albadaran by the Arabs and the truly occult and obscure philosophers alluded to, is less known to actual students of anatomy than to certain superstitious men who are capable of likening the fourth carpal bone [quartum brachialis os] to a chickpea.[62]

Vesalius mentions the notion of the indestructible bone and the belief that it serves as the nidus for resurrection on the day of the Last Judgment. However, he cites it as a tradition of the magicians and occult philosophers, and later mentions it in the name of Arabic tradition. It is quite possible that by this time the *luz* bone of rabbinic teachings had been filtered through Arabic sources.[63]

---

62. Translation by Garrison, op. cit., 151.
63. Ibid. Garrison also quotes an introduction to the Koran published in 1821 which mentions the incorruptible bone, the seed for the future edifice, as being part of Islamic teachings. They call the bone *al ajb*, which is synonymous with the coccyx.

What is particularly interesting is that Vesalius himself employs Hebrew terminology in this very work, *De Humani Corporis Fabrica*, as well as in the early anatomical work, *Tabulae Anatomica Sex.*[64] One might, therefore, expect Vesalius to have been familiar with Jewish anatomical tradition, in which case he should have quoted the tradition as one of Jewish origin, referred to the bone as the *luz*[65] instead of Albadaran, and located it in the neck or spine rather than in the big toe of the foot.

What was, in fact, the nature of Vesalius' training, if any, in the Hebrew language? It is speculated that he may have attended the lectures on Hebrew by Joannes van Campen[66] at the Pedagogium Triingue in Louvain.[67] What is known with certainty is that Vesalius was tutored in Hebrew by Lazarus de Frigeis, who assisted him with the Hebrew terminology used for the Fabrica.[68] Vesalius explicitly acknowledges his assistance in the introduction to this work.[69]

Returning to the notion of the indestructible bone, Vesalius categorically rejects it because "these bones… may be burned or broken like other bones." He leaves the discussion of resurrection to the domain of the philosophers. Vesalius' attention to dissection and experimentation enabled him to rectify a number of errors perpetuated by the teachings of Galen.[70]

---

64. For a detailed study of the Hebrew terminology used by Vesalius, see the articles by Mordecai Etziony, "The Hebrew-Aramaic element in Vesalius' Tabulae Anatomicae Sex," *Bulletin of the History of Medicine* 18 (1945), 413–24; idem, "The Hebrew Aramaic element in Vesalius," *Bulletin of the History of Medicine* 20 (1946), 36–57.

65. Although Vesalius himself does not mention the term "*luz*," some historians refer to the above quoted passage as the passage of the bone of Luz. See L. Clendening, *Source Book of Medical History* (Dover Publications, 1942), 150.

66. See Roth, op. cit., *Encyclopedia Judaica*, vol. 5, 76.

67. O'Malley, op. cit., *Andreas Vesalius*, 33.

68. Ibid., 119–120. De Frigeis apparently appears as one of the observers of Vesalius' dissection on the famous frontispiece of the *Fabrica*. See ibid., 142.

69. For further discussion on Vesalius, Hebrew and the Jews, see chapter, "The Anatomy of Halakha."

70. F. H. Garrison, *An Introduction to the History of Medicine*, 4th ed. (W. B. Saunders, 1929), 219.

Girolamo Maggi (d. 1572)[71]

Biographical information on Maggi is scant,[72] but it is known that he was an Italian engineer who wrote a number of books on theology, including *De Mundi Exustione et Die Judicii* (Concerning the Burning of the World and the Day of Judgment). This book was published in Basel by the same printer who, some twenty-three years earlier, printed *Sefer HaVikuah*.[73] The passage relevant to our discussion is found in Book Five, Chapter One, on the topic of resurrection:

> Some occult philosophies, or rather followers of Philomoria [lit., "Love of Foolishness"], indeed admit resurrection, but they say that a man must be restored from a certain bone of the foot, as if from a seed. Andreas Vesalius, chapter 1, summary of his books concerning the structure of the human body, speaks thus on this topic... The heretical Talmudists and other Hebrew authors blab out not dissimilar things. For they think that on the last day a man must be restored and regenerate from a certain uncorruptible bone (this, they have written, is indeed, next to the base of the calvaria, or in the base itself or the so-called nut [nuca]; others say that it is the first of the twelve vertebrae from which the thorax has its beginning, which when we bend our head and neck, sticks out and swells out a very great deal) which they themselves call Luz. But it will be worthy of effort to refer to what is written in chapter 28 of the book which is called *Bereshit Rabba*, in explanation of these words of Genesis, chapter 6 which we cite: I shall destroy from the face of the earth the man whom I have created, etc. R. Yoḥanan in the name of R. Shimon

---

71. Maggi is also known synonymously as Hieronymus Magnus.
72. See Benjamin Vincent, ed., *Dictionary of Biography Past and Present* (London: Moxon, 1877), 371; Mario Emilio Cosenza, *Biographical and Bibliographical Dictionary of the Italian Humanists and the World of Classical Scholarship in Italy, 1300–1800* (G. K. Hall, 1962), 2070–2071; De M. Le D'Hoefer, ed., *Nouvelle Biographie Generale* (Paris: Firmin Didot Frères, 1863), 698–699.
73. Girolamo Maggi, *De Mundi Exustione et Judicii* (Henric Petrie, 1562). I thank Professor Louis Feldman, z"l, for translating both the title and the subsequent passage from the original Latin.

the son of Yehotzadak mentioned also that the bone of the back and that vertebra whose name is Luz has been destroyed, from which the Lord God, at the future time of resurrection, will cause a man to shoot up. Hadrian asked R. Yehoshua, son of Hanina, from which thing the Lord God in the future time is going to produce a man. He replied: from a certain bone of the human back, which is called *luz*. When Hadrian asked him, whence he knew this, Yehoshua asked him to order the aforementioned bone to be brought and that he would reveal the matter through an experiment. That bone which is below the jawbone was not able to be rubbed away and rubbed out; when placed in fire it was not burned; when cast into water it was not dissolved; and finally, when it was placed on a forge and struck with a hammer it was so far from being able to be worn out and diminished in any part that the anvil was split and dashed to pieces and the hammer was broken before anything was lacking to the bone. The author of that book says these things: that they are true no one is going to persuade me, for although bones according to the witness of Plato, are especially long lasting, nevertheless we see every day that they are crushed and rubbed out by stones and hammer by a slight effort into the shape of dust, that they are dissolved by the force of water and old age into dirt, and turned into ashes by flames, unless teeth (as Pliny in Book 7, chapter 16, testifies and antiquity noticed and observed) survive, which at last a longer-lasting fire, like all remaining things, subdues and abolishes. But let the Hebrews depart with their lies; let us return to our subject.[74]

Maggi cites Vesalius but then mentions the independent rabbinic tradition of the indestructible bone. Maggi is the first of our secular sources to explicitly use the term *luz*.[75] In addition, he quotes the exact rabbinic source for this tradition. As little is known of his education, we can

---

74. Ibid., 170–171.

75. In Maggi 's work, which was printed in Latin, the word luz is printed in Hebrew characters, as are the words *Bereshit Rabba*. In the entire book, there are perhaps less than ten words printed in Hebrew characters. As mentioned above, Maggi's *De*

only speculate as to how he obtained such detailed knowledge of rabbinic sources.[76] Apparently, Maggi, at some point, worked in the printing shops of Venice.[77] Venice was a major center of Jewish culture and Hebrew printing in the Renaissance. Ironically, Christians owned and operated many of the Hebrew printing shops where Jewish scholars were employed as editors.[78] It is possible that Maggi came into contact with some of these scholars, or perhaps simply befriended Italian Jews, who comprised a significant portion of the Italian population at that time. We need not even postulate that Maggi had contact with the Jews, for this was a thriving period for Christian Hebraists, many of whom also worked at Italian printing shops.[79]

Regarding the location of the *luz* bone, Maggi cites two differing opinions, both in the name of the Hebrew or talmudic tradition. Some say it is located at the base of the skull or the so-called nut (nuca), while others identify it as the first of the twelve thoracic vertebrae. The term nucha or nuchal is used by anatomists to refer to the nape of the neck. The word nucha means nut, as does the word *luz* (hazelnut). In addition, it is true, as Maggi and Muenster state, that some rabbinic sources locate the *luz* in the area of the nape of the neck. It is, therefore, possible that the anatomical term "nucha" may ultimately derive from the rabbinic bone of *luz*.

Similar to Vesalius, Maggi rejects the notion of an indestructible bone because it does not stand the test of experimentation. In addition, he has less than kind words to say about the Jewish tradition. He concludes, "but let the Hebrews depart with their lies."

Mundi was printed by Henric Petrie, who also printed Hebrew language works at his press. Hebrew letters were therefore likely available for discriminate usage in the printing of *De Mundi*.

76. Maggi quotes rabbinic sources multiple times throughout his work and, in his index of sources, which appears after the table of contents, a number of rabbinic sources can be found.

77. Cosenza, op. cit., *Dictionary*, 2071.

78. See, e.g., David Amram, *The Makers of Hebrew Books in Italy* (Holland Press, 1963).

79. Roth, op. cit., *Encyclopedia Judaica*, vol. 8, 9–71.

Caspar Bauhinus (1560–1624)

Bauhinus was a native of Basel, where he ultimately became professor of anatomy and botany in 1589. His work on anatomy, *Theatrum Anatomicum*, was a popular text in its day because it was systematic and provided adequate coverage of the ancient authorities.[80] According to Fielding Garrison, the first reference to the name *luz* in any work on anatomy is to be found in the 1621 edition of the aforementioned work by Bauhinus.[81]

However, in his book, *History of Medicine*, Garrison erroneously states that Bauhinus' work is the first in which the term *luz* appears outside rabbinic literature.[82] The publication of Maggi's *De Mundi*, discussed above, predates the *Theatricum Anatomicum* by fifty-nine years. Bauhinus writes as follows:

> Hebrew writers affirm that there is a bone in the human body just below the eighteenth vertebra which cannot be destroyed by fire, water, or any other element, nor be broken or bruised by any force; this bone God shall, in His exceeding wisdom, water with the celestial dew, whence the other members shall be joined to it, coalescing to form the body, which breathed upon by the Divine Spirit, shall be raised up alive. Such a bone they call *lus* [not *luz*]; and its site, they say, is in the spine, from the eighteenth vertebra to the femur. The author of this fable is the R. Uschaia, who lived 210 A.D., about which time he wrote the book called *Bereshit Rabba*, i.e., *Glossa magna in Pentateuchum*, from which many later Rabbis have taken this fiction. This bone, they say, can never be burned or corrupted in all eternity, for its ground substance is of celestial

---

80. Leslie W. Dunlap, ed., *Heirs of Hippocrates: The Development of Medicine in a Catalogue of Historic Books in the Health Sciences Library, the University of Iowa* (Friends of the University of Iowa Libraries, 1980), 123–24.

81. Garrison, op. cit., 149. Garrison points out that the passage about *luz* does not appear in the earlier editions of Bauhinus' Theatrum Anatomicum. I was able to consult the 1605 edition, where in fact, this passage does not appear. I was unable, however, to obtain a copy of the 1592 edition, which coincidentally was printed in Basel by none other than Henric Petri, the printer of Meunster's *Sefer HaVikuaḥ* and Maggi's *De Mundi*.

82. Garrison, op. cit., *History of Medicine*, 230.

origin and watered with the heavenly dew wherewith God shall make the dead to rise, as with yeast in a mass of dough. They insist, moreover, that this bone will outlast all the others because it does not assimilate food as they do and because it is harder than the rest, being the fundamental part of the body, from which it is built up. We read further that the Emperor Hadrian once asked R. Yehoshua, the son of Chanin, how God would resurrect man in the world to come. He made answer: From the bone *luz* in the spinal column. Whence Hadrian asked him how he came by this knowledge and how he could prove it. Whereupon R. Yehoshua produced the bone so that he could see it. When placed in water it could not be softened; it was not destroyed by fire, nor could it be ground by any weight; when placed on an anvil and struck with a hammer, the anvil was broken in sunder but the bone remained intact. Munsterus says the Rabbins believe it to be located in the neck. But Vesalius writes that this ossicle is called Albadaran by the Arabs, resembling a chickpea in size and shape, and he questions whether, being notably hard, it may not be the ossicle between the two bones of the great toe. Heironymus Magius represents that, according to the talmudists and other Hebrew commentators, the real bone is near the base of the skull, whether it be in the base itself or in the spine. To others it stands apart as the twelfth of the dorsal vertebrae with which we incline the head and bend the neck. But what R. Yehoshua said to Hadrian the Emperor, no one can be persuaded to believe. For if bones as Plato bears witness, are highly durable, nevertheless we see daily that they can be pulverized by hammer or stones or reduced to ashes by fire; as Plato [Plinius][83] testifies and the ancients point out, only the teeth can survive, being more enduring than the fire which subdues and effaces all other remains.[84]

---

83. Garrison inadvertently wrote Plato instead of Pliny, which appears in the original text. This is obviously borrowed from Maggi.

84. Up to this point, the translation is by Garrison, op. cit., 149. The passage beginning with "thus" was not translated by Garrison in his article and was translated by Dr. Louis Feldman, *z"l*.

Thus, these circumcised fathers are accustomed, when they are unable to explain the true reason of a more difficult thing, to take refuge in fables which they gulp down on behalf of the articles of their holy faith, lest they seem to have been ignorant of anything. But let the Hebrews depart with their lies; also let the magicians and the followers of occult philosophy depart; let the Cabbalist depart who both jest and impose so impudently in manifest matters.[85]

Bauhinus quotes all three of the aforementioned sources, two of which are theological and not anatomical. He cites the same reference from *Bereshit Rabba* as does Maggi, but differs in his information about the rabbinic tradition regarding the bone's location. Bauhinus says, "Hebrew writers affirm that there is a bone in the human body just below the eighteenth vertebra which cannot be destroyed ..." It is clear that Bauhinus' information about the rabbinic teachings did not derive exclusively from the works of Maggi and Muenster as neither of these sources identify the *luz* bone in this location. As with Maggi, we can only speculate about his education in Jewish literature. In his youth Bauhinus trained in Padua. For various reasons the University of Padua was the major center of medical training for European Jews during the Renaissance.[86] Could the young Bauhinus have interacted with Jewish students at the university and thereby gained his knowledge of rabbinic sources? It is possible. Alternatively, his knowledge might well have been obtained in Basel, which, although not a center for medical training, was a center for Hebrew printing in the sixteenth and seventeenth centuries.[87] As, by law, no Jews were allowed to reside in Basel at this time, special permits had to be secured for Jewish scholars who came to Basel to proofread

---

85. Caspar Bauhinus, *Theatrum Anatomicum*, 3rd ed. (Henric Petri, 1621). Dunlap, op. cit., *Heirs*, 123.

86. For further discussion on the University of Padua and the Jews see chapter, "The Anatomy of Halakha," and E. Reichman, "The Valmadonna Trust Broadside Collection and a Virtual Reunion of the Jewish Medical Students of Padua," *Verapo Yerapei: Journal of Torah and Medicine of the Albert Einstein College of Medicine Synagogue* 7 (2017).

87. See Roth, op. cit., *Encyclopedia Judaica*, vol. 4, 304. See also Prijs, op. cit., *Hebraischer Drucke*.

the Hebrew works printed at the Christian printing presses.[88] In addition, the tenure of Bauhinus at the University of Basel coincided with that of Johannes Buxtorf I (1564–1629), a renowned Christian Hebraist who, in 1591, became professor of Hebrew at the university, a position held earlier in the century by Sebastian Muenster.[89] Buxtorf was well versed in the full spectrum of rabbinic literature and could easily have been the provider of information for Bauhinus.

Like Maggi, Bauhinus concludes his discussion of the *luz* bone with less than kind words for the Jewish tradition. He even quotes a phrase verbatim from *De Mundi*, "but let the Hebrews depart with their lies."

Samuel Butler (1612–1680)

Another reference to the *luz* bone outside rabbinic literature appears in the literary work of Samuel Butler entitled *Hudibras*. In the context of this satirical poem lampooning Puritan rule, Butler has occasion to employ the rabbinic *luz* bone for the purpose of metaphor:

> The learned Rabbins of the Jews
> Write there's a bone which they call *luz*
> In the rump of man, of such a virtue, no force of nature can do
> hurt to; And therefore at the last great day,
> All the other members shall, they say,
> Spring out of this, as from a seed
> All sorts of vegetals proceed;
> From whence the learned sons of art
> Os sacrum justly style that part. Then what can better represent
> Than this Rump Bone, the Parliament, that after several rude
> ejections,
> And as prodigious resurrections,
> With new reversions of nine lives,
> Starts up and like a cat survives?[90]

---

88. Roth, op. cit., *Encyclopedia Judaica*, vol. 4, 304.

89. Ibid., vol. 4, 1543.

90. Garrison, op. cit., also quotes this passage from Butler, which appears in Part 3, Canto 2 of *Hudibras*. Samuel Butler, *Hudibras* (London, 1663–78). Garrison misquotes the

Butler clearly identifies the os sacrum as the *luz* bone. As this bone (*luz*) is associated with resurrection, the use of the religious term, "the sacred bone," makes this identification palatable (see below).

X. THE *LUZ* BONE IN OTHER RELIGIONS AND CULTURES

The notion of a "resurrection bone" is not restricted to the Jewish religion.[91] Other religions and cultures have similar notions. Heinrich Cornelius Agrippa (1486–1535) is one of the most influential writers of Renaissance esoterica. He devotes a chapter in his book *de Occulta Philosophia* on magic and esoteric traditions to the resurrection bone. Islamic tradition has a very similar idea of an indestructible bone from which resurrection will take place. Muhammad identified the coccyx as the equivalent of the Jewish *luz* bone. A modern Islamic scientist wrote a lengthy, learned treatise on this bone[92] and finds interesting parallels between the coccyx and a plant seed, both of which ultimately sprout to produce life. Some Mayan cultures espouse the idea of a resurrection bone and identify it as the sacrum. The etymology of this bone derives from the word "sacred" which can possibly be identified with the religious significance of the resurrection bone.[93]

---

date of this work as being 1615–1630. In fact, Butler was only born in 1612 and the 3rd part of *Hudibras* appeared in 1678. See M. H. Abrams, ed., *Norton Anthology of English Literature*, 3rd ed. 1 (New York, 1974), 1965.

91. There is a debate as to whether the *luz* is found universally, or whether it is present exclusively in the Jewish body, See, for example, *siddur* of *Ari z"l* (*mizmor liDavid bishanoto*). If the latter, one would need to address the issue of whether the *luz* bone would be found in a convert. If yes, how would this be accomplished? See also D. Y. Weiss, *Megadim Ḥadashim* (Jerusalem, 5772), Bamidbar, 485–486, who questions how the *Ari's* position applies to the *Midrash Rabba* story of Andrianus and R. Yehoshua. See also A. Meisels, "The Resurrection Bone Called Luz," (Hebrew) *Or Yisrael* 7:2 (*Kislev*, 5762), 224–225.

92. See Zaid Ghazzawi, *Scientific Miracles in the Noble Quran: Resurrection of Humans on the Day of Judgment as Viewed from a Scientific Point of View*, self-publication.

93. See B. Stross, "The Mesoamerican Sacrum Bone: Doorway to the Otherworld," *Famsi Journal of the Ancient Americas* (August 23, 2007). See J. C. Miller, "Ossiculum Lus," *Anatomical Record* 8:8 (August, 1914), 415–419, who discusses many explanations of the term os sacrum, and why it is not necessarily related to the *luz*.

XI. A MODERN UNDERSTANDING OF THE LUZ BONE

A modern understanding of the *luz* bone is beautifully articulated by R. Aryeh Kaplan.[94] In his discussion of a passage from the Zohar about resurrection, R. Kaplan writes:

> The Zohar combines both of these traditions. The *luz* bone, one for each person, will be placed in the dew of resurrection, and it will grow into the body of that particular person... These allusions to the mechanics of the resurrection can be understood scientifically. God will reveal the genetic code required for duplication to a divinely inspired group of peoples, who will place the *luz* containing the RNA into the "dew of resurrection," a nutrient fluid. Under the right conditions, an exact duplicate of any human body could be grown. The final stage of the process will be completed by God, when He restores the soul to the body. This will be the true miracle of resurrection.

This passage was published in 1990, some years before cloning was performed for the first time. The twenty-first-century reader will surely appreciate that the entire body can be reconstructed from just one molecule of DNA.

XII. CONCLUSION

The notion of the bone called *luz*, or the analogous concept of the indestructible bone, is clearly of rabbinic origin. Although it has been ascribed to other traditions, including those of mystics, philosophers, and other religions, the earliest recorded source is that of the Midrash (400–600 C. E.), and all subsequent sources either quote the Midrash explicitly or allude to it, whether knowingly or unwittingly.

The theological import of this bone, by virtue of its association with resurrection, has fueled continued discussion about it throughout the ages. Despite its religious significance, however, it is quite evident from the above sources that the location of this elusive bone remains

---

94. "When Bones Rise Again," in his *Encounters* (Moznaim Publishing, 1990), 125–128.

obscure, even to this day. Clarification of this latter issue may have to wait until the very time of the resurrection.

I conclude our study with two beautiful metaphors for the *luz* bone advanced by modern authors.

Some liken Eliyahu to the *luz* bone, as Eliyahu, like the bone, never died. This is also why Eliyahu is associated with the resurrection. In addition, we invoke Eliyahu HaNavi on *motza'ei Shabbat*, as the food of the *melaveh malka* nourishes the *luz* bone, from which the resurrection, heralded by Eliyahu, will begin.[95]

R. Eliezer Waldenberg applies the concept of the *luz* bone to the Western Wall. The Western Wall is the "*luz*" which is indestructible and survives from the body of the *Beit HaMikdash*. From this remnant the future *Beit HaMikdash* will rise and we will witness the ultimate redemption.[96]

May we merit both the return of Eliyahu HaNavi accompanied by the rebuilding of the *Beit HaMikdash* in our lifetimes, and may we also witness the activation of the *luz* bone, wherever in the body it may lie.

---

95. See, for example, P. Shapiro, *Imrei Pinḥas HaShalem* 1 (Yeḥezkel Frankel, 5763), 477.
96. *Tzitz Eliezer* 11:15, s. v., "*v'amnam ken.*"

Are Two Heads Really Better Than One? Halakhic Issues Relating to Conjoined Twins and a Two-Headed Person

I. INTRODUCTION

Conjoined twins are identical twins whose bodies are joined, or do not fully separate in utero. They can be joined along virtually any part of the body and are categorized by the specific point of connection, such as the chest, abdomen, back or head, and have been known to exist since antiquity.[1] In the modern era, it has become possible to successfully

---

1. On the history of conjoined twins, see G. M. Gould and W. L. Pyle, *Anomalies and Curiosities of Medicine* (Bell Publishing, 1896), 167–189; H. H. Wilder, "Duplicate Twins and Double Monsters," *American Journal of Anatomy* 3:4 (1904), 388–472 (includes a discussion on the physiological theories of development of conjoined twins); J. Bondeson, *The Two-Headed Boy and Other Medical Marvels* (Cornell University Press, 2000). See also the National Library of Medicine online exhibit, "From Monsters to Modern Medical Miracles: Selected Moments in the History of Conjoined Twins from Medieval to Modern Times," http://www.nlm.nih.gov/hmd/conjoined (accessed May 23, 2021). The Mutter Museum in Philadelphia has a permanent exhibit with artifacts and images explaining how conjoined twins develop, including examples of famous conjoined twins of the past and present. The autopsy of the famous Siamese twins, Eng and Chang Bunker was performed at this museum, and a cast of their bodies is on display. For a current review of incidence

separate conjoined twins, depending on the nature of the shared vital organs. Such procedures, which invariably attract media attention, are among the most complex in the surgical arsenal and require a concert of interdisciplinary services. These cases often create correspondingly complex ethical dilemmas.[2]

While there has been occasional discussion of the phenomenon of conjoined twins in halakhic literature,[3] contemporary discussions focus primarily on the issue of surgical separation, with reference to

---

of conjoined twins, see O. M. Mutchinick, et al., "Conjoined Twins: A Worldwide Collaborative Epidemiological Study of the International Clearinghouse for Birth Defects Surveillance and Research," *American Journal of Medical Genetics, Part C, Seminars in Medical Genetics* 157C:4 (November 15, 2011), 274–287.

2. For recent examples, see M. Lee, et al., "The Bioethics of Separating Conjoined Twins in Plastic Surgery," *Plastic and Reconstructive Surgery* 128:4 (October, 2011), 328e–334e; B. M. Cummings, et al., "Case 33-2107: 22-Month-Old Conjoined Twins," *New England Journal of Medicine* 377:17 (October 26, 2017), 1667–1677.

3. For discussions of conjoined twins in rabbinic literature, see Tuvia Cohen, *Ma'aseh Tuvia* (Venice, 1708), section *Olam Katan*, chapter 6; Y. Reischer, *Shevut Yaakov* 1:4; C. Y. D. Azulai, *Mahzik Berakha Y. D.* 13, letter *heh*; Y. Y. Shmelkes, *Beit Yitzhak, Y. D.*, 2:99, letters *gimmel* and *dalet*; Y. M. Glassberg, *Zekhor Brit LeRishonim* (*Helek Miluim*), chapter 5 (Yosef Fisher: Cracow, 5652); H. J. Zimmels, *Magicians, Theologians and Doctors* (Edward Goldston and Son, 1952), 71–73; W. M. Feldman, *The Jewish Child* (Bailliere, Tindall and Cox: London, 1917), 129–130 and 137–139; Y. Ba-Gad, "On the Two-Headed Baby," in his *Nahalei haEshkolot* 1 (self-publication), 74–89 (Hebrew); D. Sperber, "Two-Headed Monsters," in his *Magic and Folklore in Rabbinic Literature* (Bar-Ilan University Press, 1994), 13–14; Yosef Potzanovsky, *Pardes Yosef, Bereshit*, letter 38; D. A. Mandelbaum, *Pardes Yosef HaHadash, Bamidbar* p. 13, letter 14; N. Slifkin, "Two-Headed Men and Other Mutants," in his *Sacred Monsters* (Zoo Torah, 2007), 209–216. Dr. Abraham Abraham has a number of substantive halakhic discussions on issues relating to conjoined twins in the second edition of his *Nishmat Avraham* (Jerusalem, 2007). See index, "*t'umei sayam.*" The most comprehensive essay on conjoined twins in rabbinic literature is J. D. Bleich, "Conjoined Twins," in his *Bioethical Dilemmas* (Ktav, 1998), 283–328. The present chapter contains much new material not discussed in the aforementioned sources and should be considered a supplement to these excellent contributions.

There is a midrashic approach that Adam and Havva were created as conjoined beings, as mentioned in *Eruvin* 18a. This definitionally is not a case of conjoined twins, as the latter are believed to be derivative from one embryo and are thus always identical twins, though scientists have debated this. For a discussion of a sixteenth century illustration of a pair of male-female conjoined twins, see I. Blickstein, "The

a specific case, which will be addressed below. This body of halakhic material has been thoroughly addressed and will only be referenced here. There are however other halakhic issues that relate to conjoined twins, and whether they have the status of one or two people. This chapter will focus on these issues.[4]

II. *PIDYON HABEN*

A variant of conjoined twins is the two-headed person, or dicephalic type, where there are two heads, but no duplication of other major organs.[5] If such a child were a firstborn to an Israelite family, what would the halakha be regarding *pidyon haben*, redemption of the firstborn? This issue is discussed in what is perhaps the most famous passage in early rabbinic literature dealing with conjoined twins:[6]

> Palimo inquired of Rebbe: In the case of one who has two heads, on which of them does he don *tefillin*? Rebbe indignantly said to him: either rise and go into exile or accept excommunication upon yourself! Meanwhile, a certain man came and said to Rebbe: A child who has two heads was recently born to me. How much money must I give to the *Kohen* for this firstborn's redemption? A certain elder then came and taught Rebbe as follows: The father is obligated to give the *Kohen* ten *selaim*.

The Gemara then discusses the basis for the ruling. A child who is *nitraf* (see below for definition) within thirty days does not require redemption.

Conjoined Twins of Lowen," *Twin Research* 3 (2000), 185–188. The formation of the human being at the very time of creation is to be viewed with a different lens. We therefore do not explore this Midrashic thesis in this chapter.

4. The halakhic discussions on conjoined twins have also been applied to other halakhic matters. For example, R. Eliyahu Posek, in his work on the laws of lulav and etrog, *Etz HaSadeh* (published by his son in 5697), uses the case in *Menaḥot* 37a, as well as the responsum of *Shevut Yaakov* on conjoined twins as proofs in his discussion on the halakhic status of a "twin" lulav and a "twin" etrog.

5. For a history of dicephalic twins specifically, see J. Bondeson, "The Tocci Brothers, and Other Dicephali," in his *The Two-Headed Boy and Other Medical Marvels* (Cornell University Press, 2000), 160–188.

6. *Menaḥot* 37a–37b (based on Artscroll translation).

A child with two heads should be similar to this excluded category of *nitraf* within thirty days and should not require any redemption, let alone a double redemption. Why then is a payment of ten *selaim* required? The Gemara answers that the Torah makes the mitzva specifically contingent on the head count [*gulgolet*]. As there are two heads in this case, each head requires redemption.

There are number of interpretations of this passage, some based on the different definitions of the word "*nitraf.*" Rashi defines the word as "killed," while *Tosafot*[7] consider it etymologically related to *treifa,*[8] the term for a person diagnosed with a terminal illness with a limited prognosis.

R. Neumark posits a novel, though in my opinion, historically anachronistic approach to the passage in *Menaḥot.*[9] He contends that the passage refers not to a child with one body and two heads, but to a set of full, conjoined twins, with two full bodies and two heads. Furthermore, it is a form of conjoined twins that is surgically separable, though will not survive connected. Since they are two full separable bodies, any discussion about or application of the specific law of *treifa* would likely not apply in this case. This principle only applies to one body with duplicate organs, not to two separable bodies. The question of the Gemara then is based on a doubt if this set of twins is considered a *treifa,* since, without intervention, they would die soon. If separated, however, they could live full lives. R. Neumark posited his novel thesis in 1960, when surgery for separation of conjoined twins had recently

---

7. For lengthy discussion on the point of argument between Rashi and Rabbenu Tam, see Yaakov Schick, *Yashresh Yaakov* (Budapest, 5684), 14–16; S. Goldman, "Explanation of the Positions of Rashi and Rabbenu Tam for a Firstborn Who Becomes a *Treifah* Within Thirty Days and Redemption of a Firstborn With Two Heads," *HaDarom* 72–73 (*Elul*, 5762), 139–149 (Hebrew); A. Y. Neumark, "Born With Two Heads," *Kol Torah* Year 14 (31), Volume 11 (*Av*, 5720), 5–6 (Hebrew).

8. *Treifa* is a category/status of animals that are diagnosed with terminal conditions with a prognosis of less than twelve months. For discussion of how the term *treifa* applies to humans, and whether it is exactly analogous to animals or not, see A. Steinberg, *Entzyclopedia Hilkhatit Refuit,* s. v., "*treifa*"; Y. Robinson, "*Treifah* for Human Beings," *Assia* 56 (September, 1995), 30–34 (Hebrew).

9. A. Y. Neumark, "Born With Two Heads," *Kol Torah* Year 14 (31), Volume 11 (*Av*, 5720), 5–6 (Hebrew).

become a reality. Such a complex surgery would simply not have been possible in talmudic times.

Irrespective of the interpretation of the passage, the conclusion appears to be that for a two-headed child one is required to give the *Kohen* ten *selaim* (coins). Rashi explains that in a case of twins only five *selaim* are given, since one head opens the womb first. In the case of dicephalic twins, it is possible for both heads to exit the womb simultaneously, thus ten *selaim* are required. Regarding practical halakha, the *Tur*[10] accepts the passage in *Menaḥot* above as dispositive and maintains that for a two-headed child ten *selaim* are indeed given to the *Kohen*.[11] However, this conclusion is not mentioned either by Maimonides or in the *Shulḥan Arukh*. R. Yaakov Reischer, in his responsum on a case of twins conjoined at the head (known as craniopagus twins), states, that despite the connection of the skulls, they are clearly two distinct individuals with two distinct bodies and faces. Thus, if they are delivered feet first (breech), only *five* selaim would be required, as one head would clearly exit the birth canal first. However, if both heads exit the birth canal simultaneously ten *selaim* would be required for redemption. Parenthetically, given the anatomical configuration of the craniopagus twins described by R. Reischer, they would certainly have been born breech and would have required only five *selaim* for redemption.

Dr. Abraham points out that today, the question of *pidyon haben* for a two-headed baby has no practical relevance, as these babies are invariably delivered by caesarean section, thus exempted from the requirement of redemption.[12]

III. *TEFILLIN* FOR CONJOINED TWINS

The initial question which begins the famous talmudic passage about the two-headed child is about *tefillin*, but after the appearance of the father of a newborn two-headed child, the discussion quickly shifts to the topic of *pidyon haben*, never again to return to the orginal question. Alas, the Gemara's question about which head should don the *tefillin*

---

10. *Y. D.*, 305.

11. See also *Rosh* on *Bekhorot* 8:5; *Ḥatam Sofer Y. D.*, 294.

12. A. S. Abraham, *Nishmat Avraham*, 2nd ed. (Jerusalem, 5767), *Y. D.*, 305, letter *heh*, n. 4.

shel rosh remains unanswered. A number of rabbinic authorities have ventured to resolve this halakhic dilemma.

R. Moshe Rosen in his *Nezer HaKodesh*[13] points out the inconsistency in the way the Gemara addresses *pidyon haben* and *tefillin* for the two-headed child. While the Gemara queries whether one should pay for the redemption of one or two children in the case of the two-headed child, with respect to *tefillin*, the Gemara assumes only one of the heads should don the *tefillin shel rosh* and simply asks, "on which [head] should he place the *tefillin*?" Why is it obvious that only one head should bear the *tefillin*? Perhaps both heads are required to wear the *tefillin*. He posits that perhaps since it is but one body, the placement of a second *tefillin shel rosh* would constitute a violation of *bal tosif* (inappropriately adding to the mitzva).

If only one *tefillin shel rosh* is to be worn, the question then turns to preference. Just as there is a primary and secondary hand, perhaps there is a primary and secondary head. In addition, perhaps the *tefillin shel rosh* should be placed on the head in closer proximity to the hand that bears the *tefillin shel yad*. Alternatively, as the right always has greater importance in many areas of halakha, perhaps the right head should bear the *tefillin*. It is for this reason, the absence of clear guidelines, according to R. Rosen, that the Gemara asks, "on which [head] should he place the *tefillin*?"

R. Binyamin Fleischer likewise mentions the notion that *bal tosif* would preclude the wearing of *tefillin* on both heads.[14] However, if each head is to be viewed as an independent person, he counters, then *bal tosif* would not apply. He rejects this counterargument by citing the *Shita Mekubetzet* to *Menaḥot*, which recounts the story of Shlomo HaMelekh (see below) pouring water on one head of a two-headed person, and the other head experienced the pain as well. This seemingly proves that the two heads are in fact one unified body. As such, the concern for *bal tosif* would still apply.[15]

---

13. (New York, 5719), n. 59.

14. *Shavei Binyamin* (New York, 5694), n. 14.

15. See also Y. Y. Schmelkes, *Beit Yitzḥak Y. D.* 2:99, who compares the case of a child born with two male reproductive organs, and the requirement to undergo two circumcisions, to the case of *tefillin* for the two-headed boy. Similar to Rabbis Rosen and Fleischer, he adopts the approach of *bal tosif.*

R. Ephraim Greenblatt was troubled by the same question as R. Rosen (though he does not quote him), and uses the case of the two-headed child in *Menaḥot* to offer a whimsical proof that it is not possible to read the *haftara* twice on the same Shabbat.[16] (One can only speculate if Rebbe's response to this proof of R. Greenblatt would have been similar to his response to Palimo, though I suspect Rebbe would have thoroughly appreciated the intellectual exercise.) Why is it, he asks, that while the Gemara allows for the possibility of requiring redemption for both heads, when it comes to *tefillin*, the assumption is that only one head should bear the *tefillin*? After all, it states that they (*tefillin shel rosh*) should be a sign between your eyes, and both heads possess a pair of eyes? Both heads should therefore be obligated in *tefillin*. (Note that this same logic might dictate the necessity for two pairs of *tzitzit* for a two-headed person, as it says *"velo taturu... aḥarei eineikhem,"* Do not stray after your eyes. Since each head possesses a separate pair of eyes, each would require a separate pair of *tzitzit*. However, since the torso is shared, there would only be one garment worn. I have not seen anyone address this issue, arguably for obvious reasons.) It therefore must be that the sole reason the mitzva of *tefillin* is restricted to one head is to prevent the future potential conflict at the bar mitzva of the two-headed child. If each head were allowed to wear *tefillin*, then each would claim the right to recite the bar mitzva *haftara* with its attendant blessings. This is clearly not permissible. For if it were, then both heads would be able to don *tefillin*, and both would be able to recite the *haftara* and its blessing one after the other.

R. Greenblatt does suggest a serious reason why only one head should wear the *tefillin*, based on the principle prevalent in the laws of *treifot* that all duplicate organs are considered as removed or absent. Thus, one would not fulfill the mitzva if the *tefillin* are placed on a head which is considered halakhically absent.

A Possible *Nafka Mina* (Practical Difference)

As described above, there are two main positions explaining why only one head can don *tefillin*—the position of Rabbis Rosen and Fleischer,

---

16. *Rivevot Ephraim O. Ḥ.*, 5:211.

who claim that the reason is because of *bal tosif,* inappropriately adding to the mitzva; and the position of R. Greenblatt, that the reason is due to the principle that duplicated organs are considered absent. I would suggest a possible practical difference between these two positions—if a two-headed person wished to wear Rashi *tefillin* on one head, and simultaneously, Rabbenu Tam *tefillin* on the other head. According to Rabbis Rosen and Fleischer, this might not constitute a violation of *bal tosif,* as you would only fulfill your obligation with one of the two pairs. One could therefore simultaneously wear the *tefillin* of Rashi on one head and those of Rabbenu Tam on the other and fulfill the obligation for both. However, according to R. Greenblatt, donning two pairs of *tefillin* simultaneously has no halakhic value, as one of the heads is considered legally absent. Thus, there would be no halakhic utility in placing both the *tefillin* of Rashi and Rabbenu Tam on the two heads.

The above discussions are examples of legal analyses of the talmudic passage about a two-headed child. However, a number of rabbinic authorities have discussed the issue of *tefillin* with respect to specific cases of conjoined twins that they themselves observed. While the twins mentioned in these cases are not Jewish, the question is addressed as if they were. R. Yaakov Reischer discussed the question of *tefillin* in his responsum on a case of craniopagus twins. He concludes that without doubt, as there are two complete bodies, each should don *tefillin* on their respective head.

R. Hayyim Elazar Shapira observed a case of twins on display in Vienna with two upper bodies, but one shared body from the waist down (a form of dicephalous twins).[17] Based on the anatomic description, location and historical period, I suspect he observed the famous Tocci brothers, who were exhibited widely at that time. In his work on the laws of *tefillin,* R. Shapira finds it difficult to consider this anomaly as one legal person, since there are two separate hearts and heads. He therefore concludes that each twin should don his own *tefillin shel rosh,* with the *tefillin shel yad* worn on the corresponding left hand, adjoining their respective hearts.[18]

---

17. *Ot Hayyim VeShalom,* section *Ot Hayyim* (on *tefillin*) *siman* 27, *se'if* 9, letter 13.
18. R. Shapira offers other explanations as to why both heads should don *tefillin.*

IV. THE REASON FOR REBBE'S RESPONSE

When Palimo inquires of Rebbe about the applicability of the laws of *tefillin* to a two-headed child, Rebbe responds in a way reminiscent of a teacher frustrated with a difficult student whose absurd question distracts the class from the day's intended lesson. "Either go into exile or accept upon yourself a curse!" The simple explanation is that Rebbe assumed Palimo was mocking or making folly of the halakha[19] by mentioning a ludicrous example, one that could not possibly occur. In fact, *Tosafot* comments that "in this world there is no such thing."[20] Similarly, R. Yitzhak Or Zarua (thirteenth century) includes this case of the two-headed baby in a list of talmudic cases that he considers purely hypothetical with no basis in factual reality.[21] These comments are somewhat difficult in light of the fact that the passage continues with a story of a man who had a two-headed child.[22] As to the historical veracity of this statement, while there were sporadic, rare cases of conjoined twins noted from antiquity onwards, it is quite possible that many areas of the world were indeed unfamiliar with this congenital anomaly until accounts were published and disseminated in the medical literature. For example, there is an illustration of conjoined twins in one of the first printed treatises on obstetrics, the Rosengarten, by Eucharius Rosslin, printed in 1513.

While a student's distraction may merit a response, Rebbe's particular response seems more severe than such a common circumstance would dictate. What, then, compelled Rebbe's extreme rebuke? Commentaries have suggested anatomical, homiletic and magical explanations.

To understand the explanation of R. Menashe Klein, a brief preface on a specific aspect of the laws of *treifa* is in order. A *treifa* is a person or animal that has a terminal condition with a prognosis of less than twelve months. Most rabbinic authorities maintain that by definition a *treifa* cannot survive more that twelve months, and if it does, it is

---

19. See Rashi, *Menahot* 37a, s. v., "*oh.*"

20. *Menahot* 37a, s. v., "*oh.*"

21. *Or Zarua*, v. 2, *Hil. Aveilut*, end of n. 424 (p. 173–174 in the Zhitomer, 5622 edition)

22. See D. Sperber, "Two-Headed Monsters," in his *Magic and Folklore in Rabbinic Literature* (Bar-Ilan University Press, 1994), 13–14, where this question is discussed.

a reflection that the original *treifa* designation was invalid. One of the anatomical categories of *treifa* is called *yeter*, when there is an additional or duplicate organ in the body. The accepted legal principle is that "*kol yeter kenatul dami*," additional or duplicate organs are considered as if removed or absent. A legally absent vital organ would render the animal a *treifa*. Palimo's case of the two-headed child would be included in the category of *yeter*.

Additionally, there is a debate as to whether this specific category of *yeter* has a unique status and is treated differently than all other *treifa* categories. According to Rashba, those in the *yeter* category alone, are able to survive longer than the twelve-month period, yet, despite this fact, are still considered to have a full legal status of a *treifa*. Others disagree, and claim that the *yeter* category is no different than other *treifa* categories, and such a *treifa* could not survive beyond twelve months.

R. Klein uses this debate about the category of *treifa* to explain the exchange between Rebbe and Palimo. Palimo asked about the halakha of *tefillin* for a two-headed person. According to all, a two-headed person would fit into the *treifa* category of *yeter*, as there are two heads. Palimo, in accordance with Rashba, maintained that it is possible for one in the *yeter* category of *treifa* to live longer than twelve months while still being considered a *treifa*. It was therefore appropriate for him to ask about a law that would apply to the child only when he reached thirteen years of age. Rebbe, however, per the approach of R. Klein, did not agree with the position of Rashba, and held that as a *treifa*, even in the category of *yeter*, this child could not possibly survive to bar mitzva, when the question of *tefillin* would become relevant. Rebbe therefore considered Palimo's question heretical. Palimo was assuming that the child would live beyond twelve months, thereby overtly rejecting the words of Ḥazal, as Rebbe understood them. Such a heretical statement merited the extreme response of Rebbe.[23]

R. Klein further suggests that *Hashem* orchestrated the presentation of the man with the two-headed child, and the subsequent statement of "*hahu saba*," who has been identified with Eliyahu HaNavi, to affirm that Palimo's position is in fact not heretical and is in accordance

---

23. A similar approach is suggested by S. Goldman, op. cit.

with halakhic tradition that this type of *treifa* can indeed survive to the age of bar mitzva.

R. Yaakov Epstein bypasses the anatomical discussion, preferring a homiletic interpretation of Rebbe's response instead.[24] He interprets the question of Palimo as follows: If one is of two heads, or two minds, with his thoughts both on the heavenly matters of prayer, but also on worldly matters as well, is he allowed to put on *tefillin*? This explains the severity of the response by Rebbe to Palimo, immediately ostracizing him. Since one clearly should refrain from wearing *tefillin* if his thoughts are impure, Rebbe answered angrily that one should subjugate his thoughts and his heart, expel any impure thoughts, and be receptive to the holy thoughts of prayer.

While R. Greenblatt discussed a potential problem that may arise at a bar mitzva of a two-headed child, R. Meyer Blumenfeld invoked the case in *Menaḥot* of the two-headed boy to teach a lesson to a one-headed bar mitzva boy.[25] In a bar mitzva sermon on the *haftara* of Bamidbar, R. Blumenfeld employs a homiletic idea similar in concept to R. Epstein and likens the different lands of the Diaspora to the two heads of one body. If, as in the case of Shlomo HaMelekh, when hot water or suffering is endured by one head (or Jews in one land), and the other head (Jews in the other lands) cries out in pain, this is a sure sign that we are ready for the redemption. This is reflected, he suggests, in the phrase "and they will become one head."

He further applies the idea of two heads to certain Jews whose behavior reflects a dichotomy between their presence in both the Jewish and non-Jewish world at the same time—a split personality, as if living with two heads. The question goes beyond whether they can put on *tefillin*, he argues, and is a fundamental question as to the nature of their Judaism. Is it possible to remain a Jew with two heads? Turning his attention to the bar mitzva boy, R. Blumenfeld concludes that the people who received the Torah on Mount Sinai were of one head, and he enjoins the young boy to continue in that vein.

---

24. *Beit Yaakov*, 1933.
25. M. Blumenfeld, *Netivot Nevi'im* 2 (Balshan Press, 1965), 97–99.

R. Ḥayyim Elazar Shapira, known pseudonymously as the Minḥat Elazar, suggests another explanation of the unexpected nature of Rebbe's response.[26] *Tosafot* mention the case of the two-headed child presented to Shlomo HaMelekh as originating from Ashmadai, the king of the demons. Such a creature was therefore considered a product of demons, witchcraft and sorcery, matters clearly prohibited by the Torah. Rebbe's response reflected his complete and utter rejection of these prohibited endeavors, the ultimate source of such a creature. R. Shapira brings proof that Palimo was concerned about the existence of such sorcery amongst the Jewish people, thus prompting him to ask such a question.

An alternate explanation reinterprets the phrase "rise and go into exile" as a suggestion rather than a punishment. This is based on the *Seder Hadorot*, quoting the Zohar, that in the place when Kayin was banished to exile, the children had two heads. When Rebbe said "rise and go into exile," he meant go to the same place of exile that Kayin went to. There, where people have two heads, you will be better able to find an answer to your question.[27]

V. INHERITANCE

The issue of inheritance, while not mentioned in the talmudic discussion, is raised by *Tosafot* in a brief recounting of a midrashic story.[28] According to the expanded version of the Midrash,[29] Ashmedai, the king of the demons, raised up from the netherworld a man with two heads to present to Shlomo HaMelekh. Shlomo requested that he return the person to his place of origin, but this was apparently no longer possible. The two-headed person remained in this world, married a woman, and begat children of both the two-headed and one-headed variety. Upon the death of the father, the two-headed son requested two portions of inheritance. When brought before Shlomo, he covered one of the heads and poured scalding water on the other. When both heads simultaneously cried out

---

26. *Nimukei Oraḥ Ḥayyim, siman 27, se'if "tet".*

27. J. D. Bleich, "Conjoined Twins," in his *Bioethical Dilemmas* (Ktav, 1998), 283–328, esp. 311 at n. 25.

28. *Tosafot Menaḥot 37a, s. v., "kume gali."*

29. *Otzar HaMidrashim* (Eisenstein), p. 533.

in pain, Shlomo declared them one person, with one share of inheritance. The logic behind this proof is not explicitly stated. Perhaps Shlomo's sole purpose was to experimentally determine if they had two separate nervous systems, as he believed this to be the criterion for their individuality. It is equally possible that this was a dramatic method of publicly verifying a decision that Shlomo had arrived at for other reasons.

The German government in the early twentieth century concurred with the decision of Shlomo HaMelekh, though for different reasons. The parents of a set of dicephalous twins petitioned the German government for public assistance for two mouths to feed. Despite support from the medical community, the government rejected their claim stating that twins that could not be surgically separated were legally considered as one person.[30]

R. Yitzḥak Yehuda Schmelkes heard of a case on display in Vienna of twins with one shared lower body, likely the Tocci brothers who were personally seen by R. Shapira.[31] Unlike the talmudic case of one body with two heads, these twins were possessed of separate upper bodies. He seems inclined to consider them as two halakhically separate people for matters such as counting for a minyan and entitlement to inheritance, as they have separate hearts and upper bodies.

R. Reischer addresses a case of twins conjoined at the head, with two complete bodies, and states that as two complete individuals, they are obviously each entitled to separate shares of inheritance.[32]

R. Yaakov Chagiz (seventeenth century) comments on the halakhic status of a unique form of conjoined twins he observed in Italy.[33] One twin appeared as a normal adult, while the second, smaller twin was connected at the waste with its legs reaching only to the knees of the other. He reports that this smaller, so-called parasitic twin had no apparent sensation. R. Chagiz considered this twin a *gosses* (a person on the verge of death) with its attendant halakhic ramifications, including

---

30. J. Bondeson, "The Tocci Brothers and Other Dicephali," in his *The Two-Headed Boy and Other Medical Marvels* (Cornell University Press, 2000), 160–188, esp. 182.
31. See above.
32. *Shevut Yaakov* 1:4.
33. *Halakhot Ketanot* 1:245.

rights to inheritance. It is remarkable that R. Chagiz labeled the parasitic twin a *gosses*, a term given to one whose death is imminent, given the fact this twin survived for many years. He also considers whether the parasitic twin would require a *mila* and whether, upon seeing this unusual being, one should recite the blessing of *meshaneh habriyot*, which is recited upon unique or unusual creatures.

We thus have discussions in rabbinic literature about inheritance for four unique types of conjoined twins—two forms of dicephalous, craniopagus, and parasitic.

VI. MARRIAGE OF CONJOINED TWINS

The famous Siamese conjoined twins, Chang and Eng Bunker, who were joined at the chest wall but had completely separate bodies, married different wives, sisters in fact, and maintained separate families. The Godina twins, born in 1908, were joined at the sacrum (pyopagus) and married identical, though not conjoined, twins. The success with which these sets of twins navigated this unique marital arrangement was apparently not shared by another earlier set of conjoined twins. Rabbenu Gershon ben Shlomo of Arles (thirteenth century), father of Ralbag, in his encyclopedic *Sha'ar HaShamayim*[34] records a story in the name of Avicenna (the Persian physician) about a pair of female conjoined twins anatomically similar to the Bunker twins.[35] One of the twins wished to marry, but the other refused out of concern for her modesty during the course of marital relations. When the twins presented the case before a judge, the judge devised a Solomonic solution to determine if one twin had the right to marry against the will of the other. After the twins were seated, he asked one to rise and walk across the room. With great effort, she was able to partially stand, but her sister remained seated. He then asked the other sister, who had requested to marry, to perform the same action. She stood with ease forcibly carrying her sister with her across the room. Having satisfactorily determined that the sister requesting marriage was the dominant twin, the judge acceded to her request and

---

34. *Ma'amar shemini.*
35. This story is repeated by others. See, for example, Tuvia Cohen, *Ma'aseh Tuvia* (Venice, 1708), section *Olam Katan*, chapter 6.

allowed the marriage. Shortly thereafter, however, the non-dominant twin died, purportedly due to anger and shame. With her passing and decomposition of the body, the remaining dominant twin died as well.

R. Yaakov Reischer, in his responsum on a case of craniopagus twins, addresses the halakhic issues that arise regarding marriage. For a case of male conjoined twins, he maintains that it is prohibited for [one of] them to marry, as the woman's lying in bed, by necessity, with the other twin might potentially lead to adultery. Furthermore, there is a general prohibition against cohabitation in the presence or view of others. For this latter reason, it would likewise be prohibited for a set of female-female conjoined twins to marry,[36] even though the concern for adultery may not technically apply. He adds that even in a place where it is accepted custom for one to have two wives, it would still be prohibited to marry conjoined twins since cohabitation in the presence of another is prohibited.

According to Yosef Potzenovsky,[37] the *beit midrash* in the European city of Liske housed an old copy of R. Reischer's *Shvut Yaakov* that contained the handwritten marginalia of R. Akiva Eiger. In R. Eiger's notes, he queries that if the twins were female, there would be a prohibition of marrying two sisters, and one needn't resort to the secondary prohibition of public marital relations.

In his approbation to the published responsa of R. Reischer, R. Yosef Shaul Nathanson asks the identical question as R. Eiger. R. Nathanson wonders why R. Reischer didn't invoke the prohibition of marrying two sisters as an obvious reason why marrying conjoined twin sisters would be prohibited. He suggests that perhaps conjoined twins are considered a legal *treifa* and, based on *Nidda* 23, the prohibition of marrying two sisters does not apply to a *treifa*.

R. Yosef Dzialofsky,[38] however, claims that R. Nathanson extrapolated incorrectly from the passage in *Nidda*, and the reason the marriage

---

36. R. Reischer also applies this logic to a set of male-female conjoined twins, though this combination is not physiologically possible. Conjoined twins are the product of the splitting of a single embryo and, by definition, are always identical, and of the same gender.
37. *Pardes Yosef, Bereshit*, n. 38.
38. *Yad Yosef* (Lublin, 1911), *hashmatot* n. 86.

is not valid for the sister in that case is because the fetus was nonviable. In the case of conjoined twins, where the sisters are healthy, even if they may be considered a *treifa*, there is no reason why the prohibition of marrying two sisters should not apply. The question of Rabbis Eiger and Nathanson thus still remains.[39]

I would suggest a different answer to the question of Rabbis Eiger and Nathanson as to why R. Reischer did not mention the prohibition of marrying two sisters. R. Reischer introduces the concept of engaging in marital relations in front of others as the main reason to prohibit a set of male conjoined twins from marrying one woman. He extends this logic to a set of female conjoined twins as well. The biblical prohibition is to marry two sisters. As the conjoined twins (of the configuration discussed by R. Reischer) are separate individuals, it is technically halakhically permissible for a man to marry one of them. The only issue that would preclude this arrangement is, as R. Reischer mentions, the prohibition of public marital relations violated by the conjoined sister. Even in locations where it is customary to marry two women, he adds, one is still prohibited from engaging in relations in front of the second wife.[40] The prohibition of marrying two sisters would not in any way preclude a man from marrying *one* of the twins, thus R. Reischer did not deem it necessary to mention this prohibition.

There is one reported case in the early twentieth century of a set of pyopagus twins (fully formed twins, joined at the sacrum and positioned back to back), Rosa and Josepha Blazek, who were rumored to have married the same man.[41] In this case, had the characters been Jewish, the man would have been in violation of the prohibition of marrying two sisters, as well as the prohibition of engaging in relations in public.

---

39. For another approach to the question of R. Nathanson, suggesting that this was a case of conjoined twins who converted, see R. E. Waldenberg, *Tzitz Eliezer* 17:49, and his discussion of *Beit Yitzhak* there.
40. This is my interpretation of the phrase "even in locations where one can marry two women." I recently saw that R. Schmelkes provides a similar answer in *Beit Yitzhak* Y. D., 2:99, letter *dalet*.
41. J. Bondeson, "The Biddenden Maids," in his *The Two-Headed Boy and Other Medical Marvels* (Cornell University Press, 2000), 141–159, esp. 154.

All of the aforementioned discussions about the marriage of con-joined twins refer to twins with complete, though connected, bodies. The marriage of dicephalous twins, with two heads and one body, would require a different analysis. While the case that was brought before Shlomo HaMelekh was of a two-headed child that was the product of the marriage of a woman with a two-headed man, there is no specific discussion about the halakhic aspects of such a marriage, perhaps since this was a creature of the netherworld. There is a historical account of dicephalous twins who married a single wife, "with whom they were said to live in harmony."[42]

A two-headed person has only one set of reproductive organs and, according to the decision of Shlomo HaMelekh, is legally considered one person with two heads. There is therefore no concern about adultery or the marriage of two sisters as discussed above. However, it remains a question as to whether R. Reischer's concern for cohabitation in public would apply in this case. Technically, the spouse of a two-headed person is engaging in relations with one individual, yet each head has a differ-ent brain, personality, and set of eyes.

The famous Tocci brothers married two separate women. They had two separate bodies above the waist and one shared common lower body, with one set of reproductive organs. Bondeson mentions discus-sion in the contemporary newspapers and medical journals about the legal ramifications of this marriage, including questions of inheritance and paternity, such as which twin would be the father of which child.[43] This configuration would require yet another unique analysis with respect to marriage. R. Yitzḥak Yehuda Schmelkes engages in just such an analysis, precipitated by his hearing of an exhibit in Vienna of what was quite likely of the Tocci brothers themselves.[44] He argues that if this configuration were present for female sisters the *kiddushin* of either one of the sisters would be invalid as it would be a marriage for which consummation is legally impossible. As the sisters would share one set

---

42. J. Bondeson, "The Tocci Brothers and Other Dicephali," in his *The Two-Headed Boy and Other Medical Marvels* (Cornell University Press, 2000), 160–188, esp. 167.

43. Ibid., 181.

44. *Beit Yitzḥak Y. D.*, 2:99, letter *dalet*.

of reproductive organs, the man would violate the prohibition of cohabitation with his wife's sister. This is a form of adultery and a more severe violation than cohabitation in public.

VII. CRIMINALITY AND CONJOINED TWINS

R. Chagiz, in his discussion of the case of a parasitic twin, ponders what the punishment would be for one who murders the parasitic twin. He concludes that the parasitic twin would be considered a *gosses*, with all its ramifications. One is guilty of homicide for the murder of a *gosses*, despite the poor prognosis.

Based on the historical period, location, and description of R. Chagiz, it is clear that he is referring to the Colloredo brothers, Lazarus and his parasitic twin, Baptista, who were born in Italy in 1617.[45] While R. Chagiz had pontificated on the punishment for murdering the parasitic twin, this actually had practical relevance for the Colloredo brothers. There are accounts of Lazarus, the normal size twin, striking a man and killing him after the man had teased him in public. Lazarus was sentenced to death but was reprieved after he claimed that if he were killed, his brother, who was innocent of this crime, would be unjustly murdered as a result.[46] A similar case of obfuscation of criminal culpability relating to conjoined twins is found in the fictional work of Mark Twain, *Those Extraordinary Twins*. The dicephalus twins, Count Angelo and Count Luigi Capello, were accused of kicking another person and were put on trial for assault. The defense lawyer, Pudd'nhead Wilson, in seeking acquittal, claimed that it is impossible to say which of the twins did the kicking and that the guilty twin could not be punished without incarcerating the innocent brother.[47]

---

45. On the Colloredo brothers, including illustrations and poems about their life, see, J. Bondeson, "The Two Inseparable Brothers and a Preface," in his *The Two-Headed Boy and Other Medical Marvels* (Cornell University Press, 2000), vii-xxii.

46. Ibid., ix-x. For further discussion of this legal quandary, see D. Engber, "If a Siamese Twin Commits Murder, Does His Brother Get Punished, Too?" *Slate Magazine* (January 5, 2010).

47. See M. Twain, *Those Extraordinary Twins*, chapter 5. Twain based his story on a famous contemporary set of dicephalous twins, the Tocci brothers. See J. Bondeson, "The Tocci Brothers and Other Dicephali," in his *The Two-Headed Boy and Other Medical Marvels* (Cornell University Press, 2000), 180.

R. Schmelkes[48] ruled as the judge in the Colloredo case, that if one of the conjoined twins committed a sin punishable by lashes or death, one could not administer the punishment, as an innocent person (the non-guilty conjoined twin) would be punished as a result. He compares this to the case of a pregnant woman who is sentenced to death for a capital crime, where the fetus is killed prior to the execution of the death sentence. However, once the woman is in labor and the fetus is a separate entity, one no longer has license to take its life and must wait until after birth to execute the mother. Since the twins are halakhically separate people, one cannot punish the innocent twin on account of the guilty one.

VIII. SEPARATION OF CONJOINED TWINS

There are rare accounts of attempts at separating conjoined twins in pre-modern times, one dating back as early as 945 C. E.[49] With advances in imaging and surgical techniques over the last few decades, the separation of conjoined twins has become less rare, though not common. The halakhic aspects of the separation of conjoined twins have been amply explored in the medical halakha literature, and will not be revisited here.

The index case which sparked interest in the halakhic world was the birth of a set of twins joined at a six-chamber heart who were born to a religious Jewish couple in Lakewood, New Jersey in 1977. It was determined that without surgical intervention, the twins would die. Furthermore, surgery could possibly save one of the twins, though this required the sacrifice of the other. The medical and halakhic issues were varied and complex, but the main ethical/halakhic issue was whether it was permitted to sacrifice one twin to save the other. R. Moshe Feinstein *zt"l* was approached by the couple to render a decision in this case. Rav Moshe's lengthy discussions with the chief surgeon, Dr. C. Everett Koop, over the days before the operation are now part of the medical halakha

---

48. *Beit Yitzḥak Y. D.*, 2:99, letter *dalet*.
49. See G. M. Gould and W. L. Pyle, *Anomalies and Curiosities of Medicine* (Bell Publishing: New York, 1896), 172–173; R. M. Van der Weiden, "The First Successful Separation of Conjoined Twins (1689)," *Twin Research* 7:2 (April 2004), 125–127.

lore.[50] The decision was made to allow separation. For reasons unknown to me, Rav Moshe did not commit this decision to writing in his published responsa, *Iggerot Moshe*, though his son-in-law, R. Moshe Tendler, later published an account of the decision process.[51] Despite the lack of a printed responsum, rabbinic authorities subsequently commented on what was known to be the decision of Rav Moshe.[52] Dr. Koop reminisced about this landmark case in a discussion with students at the Chabad Center of Dartmouth College.[53]

IX. ABORTION OF CONJOINED TWINS

The halakhic literature on conjoined twins dates back to talmudic times, and topics of discussion have included inheritance, marriage, *tefillin*, and *pidyon haben*; yet there is one issue relating to conjoined twins which appears nowhere in pre-modern rabbinic literature—abortion. While

---

50. The article from the Philadelphia inquirer describing this episode, D. Drake, "The Surgery: An Agonizing Choice—Parents, Doctors, Rabbis In Dilemma," *Philadelphia Inquirer* (October 16, 1977) has been reprinted in *Jewish Medical Ethics* 4:1 (February, 2001), 14–21.

51. R. Moshe Tendler, "*KisheDochin Nefesh Mipnei Nefesh*," *LeTorah VeHora'a: Sefer Zikaron* (New York, 5749), 114–122; idem, "Unpublished Responsum: 'So One May Live,'" in his *Responsa of Rav Moshe Feinstein: Care for the Critically Ill* (Ktav, 1996), 125–133 and 209–213.

52. R. Dovid Povarsky, *Bad Kodesh* 4: 51; R. J. D. Bleich, "The Separation of Conjoined Twins Joined at the Heart," *Benitivot haHalakha*, v. 3 (*Kuntres HaRefua*) (Hebrew); idem, "Conjoined Twins," in his *Bioethical Dilemmas* (Ktav, 1998), 283–328; M. Halperin, "Siamese Twins: Rav Feinstein's Ruling and the Subsequent Controversy," *Jewish Medical Ethics* 4:1 (February, 2001), 26–27. For other halakhic discussions on the separation of conjoined twins, see, R. M. Sternbuch, *Teshuvot VeHanhagot, C. M.*, 893; A. Steinberg, "Siamese Twins," in *Sefer Assia* 2 (Jerusalem, 5741), 246–251 (Hebrew); R. M. M. Klausner, "Killing One Fetus to Save the Remaining Ones," *Ateret Shlomo* 1 (5756), 255–266; (Hebrew); D. Stein, "On the Topic of Conjoined Twins," *Beit Yizḥak* 32 (2000) (Hebrew); A. N. Tzuker, "On the Topic of Conjoined Twins," *Hakirah* 5 (Fall 2007), Hebrew section 33–39; A. Enker, "Necessity: Do Numbers Ever Count," in his *Ikarin BeMishpato HaPelili HaIvri* (*Fundamentals of Jewish Criminal Law*) (Jerusalem, 2007), 389–448. (Hebrew)

53. See A. Levy, "'Former Surgeon General Looks Back at Hallmark Case Influenced by Rabbinic Law," (April 24, 2009) at http://www.chabad.org/news/article_cdo/aid/880801/jewish/Surgeon-General-Addresses-Dartmouth-Students.htm (accessed May 23, 2021).

rabbinic discussions on abortion date back to antiquity, the issue of abortion for conjoined twins is a product of the modern era and the advent of ultrasound imaging.[54] An ultrasound allows visualization of the anatomic features of the fetus or fetuses in utero. In the premodern era, a woman could not have known prior to birth if she was carrying a set of conjoined twins. A number of contemporary rabbinic authorities address the halakhic permissibility of aborting fetal conjoined twins.

R. Levi Yitzḥak Halperin was asked whether a woman carrying conjoined twins is allowed to perform an abortion, or whether she should carry the twins to term and attempt surgical separation.[55] Initially, he queries as to whether they are considered two separate beings, or one being with duplicate organs. He brings proof from the story of Adam and Ḥavva, who according to some, were created as conjoined beings. Citing the case of the two-headed child presented to Shlomo HaMelekh, he wonders if Shlomo's test reflected a specific attempt to determine whether each twin had a unique and separate sensori-nervous system, which is what defines an individual being, or whether this was simply an effective, dramatic demonstration of his decision, which was based on other criteria.

R. Halperin distinguishes between the nature of the anatomical connection. If the twins are not connected by any vital organs, and would be relatively easily separated surgically, then they would be considered two separate, potentially viable fetuses. As such, abortion would be prohibited. If, however, they shared vital organs, like a heart, as well as a common nervous system, there could be a number of possibilities. R. Halperin enumerates three possible scenarios and approaches, hastening to add that this is a very general overview, and that any actual case would require much greater analysis given the complexity of the issue.

---

54. See, for example, T. C., Mackenzie, et al., "The Natural History of Prenatally Diagnosed Conjoined Twins," *Journal of Pediatric Surgery* 37:3 (March, 2002), 303–309; R. M. Nomura, et al., "Conjoined Twins and Legal Authorization for Abortion," *Revista da Associacao Medica Braileira* 57:2 (March-April, 2011), 205–210.

55. See L. Y. Halperin, "Pregnancy Termination for Siamese Twins," in his *Ma'aseh Ḥoshev* 3 (Jerusalem, 5757), chapter 8, pp. 147–150 (Hebrew).

1) Considered as Two Fetuses, with One Healthy and One a *Treifa*

This approach would apply to a case similar to that of the Lakewood twins, where the shared heart rested primarily in the chest of one twin (of course this is a simplification, and anatomical position does not necessarily reflect physiological dominance), with one twin considered dominant or primary, and the other one weaker and secondary. The dominant twin is viewed as a "*shalem*," healthy fetus, while the secondary twin carries the legal status of a *treifa*. In this approach, according to R. Halperin, abortion would be prohibited without exception as there is no *heter* to sacrifice the healthy fetus along with the *treifa*. However, it would be permitted to selectively abort the secondary twin if it were possible to preserve the dominant fetus in the process. To my knowledge, such a procedure has not yet been attempted.

2) Considered as Two Fetuses, Both with the Status of *Treifa*

According to this position, even if one twin were dominant and the other secondary, we would consider both twins to have the status of *treifa*. In this case, there would be room to consider the possibility of abortion. However, it is possible that surgical separation of the twins after birth would change the status of one twin from a *treifa* to a "*shalem*." Would we consider this potential upgrade in legal status, which would only possibly occur through a risky surgical operation after birth, enough to preclude an abortion in utero? R. Halperin leaves this difficult question unanswered.

3) Considered as One Fetus with the Status of *Treifa*

If we consider the conjoined bodies as one fetus with some duplicate organs, then it would have the status of a *treifa*. (based on the principle that "*yeter kenatul dami*," a duplicate organ is considered as if that organ is removed or absent. The legal absence of these organs would render the fetus a *treifa*.) Given the poor prognosis both in utero, as well as if the fetus survives to birth, R. Halperin would in principle allow an abortion in this case. However, each case would require its own unique legal analysis before any decision is rendered.

While R. Halperin's discussion above is hypothetical, when he was asked in a specific case of conjoined twins who shared a heart whether it was permitted to perform an abortion, his answer was affirmative. He added an important proviso that another rabbinic judicial authority must concur with the decision.[56]

R. Menashe Klein was also asked a practical question about the permissibility of abortion for a woman who was found on ultrasound to be carrying a child with two heads (and one body). As a preface to his consideration of terminating the pregnancy of a deformed or defective child, he cites three references reflecting the attitude and actions of rabbinic figures when faced with the birth of a child with congenital anomalies or with halakhic stigmata. Rav Ada bar Ahava had a child with an anatomical defect of his genitalia rendering him a *petzua daka* and infertile. He fasted for him, and the child died.[57] Similarly, according to some, when a legal bastard (*mamzer*) is born there is a custom to not recite the usual prayer, "sustain this child ..." as we do not genuinely wish to sustain such a child. Some suggest that one should even specifically pray that this child should die. Along the same vein, R. Yitzhak ben Yehuda Halevi mentions that with the birth of a severely deformed child people often pray for the child's death.[58] R. Klein makes it clear that while there may be cases where one is permitted to pray for death, under no circumstances is it permitted to physically hasten the death of a child with any deformity or stigma.

With this preface, he launches into a discussion about the status of a two-headed fetus, defining such a fetus as a *treifa*, and therefore entertaining the possibility of abortion. He concludes, in accordance with the position of Rashba, that even though a two-headed fetus is designated as a *treifa*, it can still potentially live well beyond the twelve-month period. Given the projected longevity, R. Klein concludes that abortion is clearly prohibited.

---

56. See Y. Stein and L. Y. Halperin, "Siamese Twins Seen on Ultrasound During Pregnancy," *HaBerakha* 6 (*Tammuz*, 5771), 15–18 (Hebrew).
57. *Yerushalmi Shabbat*, chapter 19, 17a, halakha 2, cited in *Rabbenu Hananel* on *Shabbat* 135a. It is not clear if R. Ada bar Ahava fasted or if R. Abin fasted.
58. *Paneah Raza*, end of *Beha'alotekha* on the verse "*al na tehi kamet.*"

X. CONCLUSION

There is more to the rabbinic literature on conjoined twins than separation alone. Rabbinic authorities over the centuries have observed, and commented on, a variety of types of conjoined twins, including craniopagus, dicephalus and parasitic. Issues such as redemption of the firstborn, *tefillin*, inheritance and criminal liability were addressed in pre-modern times, while modern authorities have newly addressed the issues of separation and abortion. The two-headed twins in Mark Twain's *Those Amazing Twins* would ask to get paid for two when they worked but traveled the railway with just one ticket. Depending on the anatomical configuration and the issue under consideration, conjoined twins have been considered at times either one or two people.

I would suggest that we might learn about the separate identity of conjoined twins from a Midrash about the events at Mount Sinai. The Midrash states that the Jews at Mount Sinai were united, *"k'ish ehad b'lev ehad"* (as one person with one heart). One could perhaps learn from here that in order to be considered *ish ehad*, one person, one would have to have *lev ehad*, one heart, and it is the heart that creates the separate identity. This conclusion is in agreement with the position of Shlomo HaMelech, who considered the two-headed person one being, perhaps since there was only one heart. This would also be consistent with the *pesak* of Rav Moshe Feinstein allowing the sacrifice of one twin to save the other, though for a different reason. Since, in that case, they were joined at and shared one heart, albeit a 6–chambered heart, they would be considered *ish echad*, one person. It is permitted to amputate part of the body to save the rest of the body. I think I have a good idea how Rebbe would have responded to me had I mentioned this idea in his class.

But eschewing the legal application of this idea and invoking the conceptual and homiletic analysis, in the vein of Rabbis Blumenthal and Epstein above, we look forward to the time when the disparate heads of the Diaspora and the divergent halakhic approaches reflected in the two heads will one day unite under a single-minded Sanhedrin, when we will genuinely be *"k'ish ehad b'lev ehad."* with the rebuilding of the Beit HaMikdash speedily in our time.

The Incorporation of Pre-Modern Scientific Theories into Rabbinic Literature: The Case of Innate Heat

I. INTRODUCTION

Rabbinic commentators throughout the ages utilized many disciplines of human knowledge for their exegetical enterprise in the hope of achieving optimal textual and legal clarification. For passages that explicitly refer or allude to anatomical or physiological notions, commentators often drew upon contemporaneous medical and scientific theories to enhance or supplement their understanding of a passage. While the methodology of employing scientific theories for rabbinic exegesis is ubiquitous throughout the centuries, the particular theories used are a product of the exegete's generation. Clearly, the medieval doctrines of human physiology are not those of today, and consequently, medieval commentators may invoke scientific principles which are unfamiliar or enigmatic to the modern reader. Only knowledge of medical history can assist the reader in understanding an author's application of scientific teachings in his commentary. The reader must understand the medicine and science as understood by the author himself in order to appreciate the author's true exegetical intent.

The very notion that the rabbis based, or supplemented, their interpretations on scientific information that we now consider invalid raises profound theological and halakhic implications, and this issue has been addressed elsewhere.[1] However, the fact that the rabbis incorporated these theories should in no way be surprising. Modern rabbinic authorities engage in the same process, seeking out the most up-to-date information about the latest medical advances in order to interpret a text or rule in a case of law. The question, therefore, is not *if* the rabbis incorporated early scientific theories, but *when* and with *what* exegetical and halakhic intent. If the scientific information is merely supplementary or homiletic, its obsolescence is of little theological import. However, if it constitutes the core of a halakhic decision, its antiquation may alter the contemporary applicability of the source. It must be noted, however, that according to some opinions, even if the medical information were to constitute the essence of the halakhic decision, it would in no way alter the relevance or applicability of the normative halakha.[2] This weighty matter is for rabbinic authorities to decide and is beyond the scope of this discussion. But, in any case, it is incumbent upon us to understand how these early theories are applied in rabbinic literature, and the context within which they were understood. Only then can a decision be made as to the relevance and applicability of an earlier source to contemporary discourse.

---

1. See D. Cohen, "*Shinuy Hateva*: An Analysis of the Halachic Process," *Journal of Halacha and Contemporary Society* 31 (Spring 1996); S. Sprecher, "*Divrei Ḥazal VeYedi'ot Mada'iyot*," B.D.D. 2 (Winter 1996), 2–39; S. Z. Leiman, "R. Israel Lipshutz and the Mouse that is Half Flesh and Half Earth: A Note on Torah U-Madda in the Nineteenth Century," in *Ḥazon Nachum* (Yeshiva University Press, 1997), 449–458; N. Gutal, *Sefer Hishtanut HaTeva'im BeHalakha* (Makhon Yahdav, 5758); A. Steinberg, *Encyclopedia of Jewish Medical Ethics*, trans. F. Rosner (Feldheim, 2003), s. v., "change in nature"; N. Slifkin, *Mysterious Creatures* (Targum Press, 2003), 17–41; Yehuda Levi, *The Science in Torah: The Scientific Knowledge of the Sages* (Feldheim, 2004); M. Meiselman, *Torah, Chazal and Science* (Israel Bookshop, 2013).

2. See Slifkin, op. cit.

This chapter deals with one unique pre-modern physiological notion, the doctrine of innate heat, which finds its expression throughout rabbinic literature. After providing a brief medical historical overview of this physiological principle, I will provide examples of rabbinic passages in which it has been employed, beginning with selections from biblical exegesis, followed by references from aggadic and halakhic literature. This exercise illustrates how an understanding of medical history can be a valuable supplement for the study of rabbinic literature.

II. THE DOCTRINE OF INNATE HEAT

Since the beginnings of scientific inquiry, research efforts have focused on defining the unique physiological properties of warm-blooded animals and, in particular, the human being. One such fundamental property is the ability of the human being to maintain its core body temperature despite fluctuations in the outside environment. This principle, in conjunction with the movement of the blood and the passage of air during respiration, has always served as a cornerstone of physiology. While a corpse soon accommodates its temperature to that of its surrounding environment, a living being succeeds in maintaining its body temperature with only very slight variability. What accounts for this remarkable phenomenon? We now understand the origin of the body's heat on a molecular level, being generated by the interplay of multiple complex biochemical reactions. But how did the pre-modern scientist, unequipped with a microscope and ignorant of biochemistry, microbiology and cellular physiology, explain this phenomenon?

In order to account for the body's ability to maintain a temperature above its environment, scientists of antiquity postulated the presence of a heat source within the body. As the exact nature of this heat was elusive, intense debates regarding its identity, quantity, and regulation raged on for centuries. Here I mention only some of the issues and principles of this so-called "innate heat," as it relates to our analysis of the rabbinic sources.[3] It must be understood, however, that the innate

---

3. For discussions on innate heat, see C. R. S. Harris, *The Heart and the Vascular System in Ancient Greek Medicine* (Oxford, 1973), esp. 374–378; Margaret Tallmadge May, *Galen*

heat is but one piece of the complex puzzle of human cardiac and respiratory physiology as understood in antiquity.

Issues regarding innate heat addressed in the history of medicine include the location of the heat, whether it was equally disseminated throughout the body or centralized in one location; the relationship between the innate heat and the soul; the mechanism of transmission of the innate heat to one's progeny; the regulation of the heat; and the relationship between fever and innate heat, whether fever represents an increase in the pre-existing innate heat or the influence of an extrinsic heat superimposed on the innate heat. While many theories evolved in early antiquity to explain the different aspects of innate heat,[4] the formulation of Galen, who incorporated aspects from, among others, Hippocrates[5] and Aristotle, superseded those of his predecessors. Galen's theories of human physiology, including innate heat, remained prevalent, with only minor variations, into the eighteenth century.

According to Galen, heat is the most important element in the body, facilitating the existence of life. Innate heat is housed within the heart[6] where the heat is the greatest,[7] and from where the heat is

---

on the Usefullness of the Parts of the Body 1 (Ithaca, 1968), 50–54; G. J. Goodfield, *The Growth of Scientific Physiology: Physiological Method and the Mechanist-Vitalist Controversy, Illustrated by the Problems of Respiration and Animal Heat* (London, 1960); David J. Furley and J. S. Wilkie, *Galen on Respiration and the Arteries* (Princeton, 1984), 3–46.

4. D. J. Furley and J. S. Wilkey, op. cit., 3–40.

5. It is now accepted as fact that the Hippocratic corpus does not represent the work of one man, but is rather the collection of a group of disparate, and occasionally contradictory, works penned by multiple authors, but related in theme. As a result, since the works of Hippocrates are not unified, it is not always possible to say that there is one Hippocratic theory on a particular topic. D. J. Furley and J. S. Wilkey, op. cit., 11–14, grapple with this problem in their discussion of the Hippocratic theories of respiration and innate heat.

6. M. T. May, op. cit., 52–53. More specifically, the heat was thought to reside in the left ventricle. Galen accepted this notion from Hippocrates. See G. E. R. Lloyd, ed., *Hippocratic Writings* (Middlesex, 1978), 349.

7. The heart, in fact, does not have a higher temperature than the rest of the body, but this notion persisted until it was disproved by Alfonso Borelli in the seventeenth century with the use of a thermometer. See M. T. May, op. cit., 53.

disseminated to the rest of the body.[8] By means of this innate heat all the major physiological functions of the body are accomplished, including growth, digestion and production and regulation of the humors.

In attempting to elucidate the nature of innate heat, Galen draws a tentative analogy to the flame of an ordinary fire,[9] noting that while an ordinary flame consumes the material which sustains it, innate heat preserves and protects it.[10] However, despite Galen's hesitant use of the fire analogy, others employed it to explain the aging process. Innate heat, they maintained, was like a fire nourished by wet logs. "For newly born animals are all damp, and they grow slowly, just as a fire almost choked by the dampness of the logs with which it is fed grows slowly, while it is overcoming the dampness. When it has succeeded in doing this, it burns brightly until it has consumed all its fuel. It then dies down through lack of fuel, and quenches itself, this latter process corresponding to old age and death."[11]

Heat is not only required for the preservation of life, according to Galen, but for its generation as well. Heat is therefore found in the semen. Regarding the regulation of innate heat, Galen maintained that the heat must be cooled and contained by respiration if the source of life is to persist, for in the absence of this cooling mechanism, the heat will consume itself, and the person will die.[12]

One aspect of innate heat which plagued physiologists for centuries is its relationship to the condition of excess temperature, or fever. Despite Galen's extensive writings on human physiology, he left no clear

---

8. The mechanism of dissemination throughout the body is itself a matter of debate, as it depends upon how one understands the constitution of the blood vessels and arteries, and the interrelationship between respiration and circulation. As circulation was not clearly understood until the time of Harvey (seventeenth century), the function and identity of the veins, arteries and nerves was not agreed upon. Furthermore, many believed that air passed through the vessels, either in conjunction with or to the exclusion of blood. For extensive discussion of these issues see C. R. S. Harris, D. J. Furley and J. S. Wilkey.

9. See J. Halevi, *Kuzari* 2:26 for a similar analogy.

10. Aristotle also struggled with the exact relationship between the innate heat and ordinary fire. See D. J. Furley and J. S. Wilkey, op. cit., 15–17.

11. C. R. S. Harris, op. cit., 375.

12. M. T. May, op. cit., 51.

definition of fever, except that, in contradistinction to innate heat, it was considered a "heat contrary to nature."[13] This ambiguity led to centuries of debate as to the essence, origin and regulation of febrile heat. Observations of fevers varying in intensity, duration and periodicity led to the evolution of a fever taxonomy prevalent in the Middle Ages, which included the three major genera of ephemeral, putrid and hectic fevers. Theories on fever pathology and taxonomy occupy a prominent role in pre-modern medical literature.[14]

III. RABBINIC REFERENCES TO INNATE HEAT

The doctrine of innate heat, a physiological notion universally accepted until recent times, is mentioned in a number of areas of rabbinic literature, and is variously referred to as *hom hativ'i, hom hatoladi,* and *hom halev.* Being that a number of different aspects of innate heat are discussed in these sources, such as its diminution with age, its association with fever and disease, and its presence in the semen, it is essential to have a familiarity with these particular aspects in order to appreciate each source independently.

A) BIBLICAL COMMENTARIES

The doctrine of innate heat appears in biblical commentaries throughout *Tanakh,* and the following section is arranged by topic, according to biblical chronology. The understanding of the use of the doctrine of innate heat enhances our general understanding of rabbinic biblical interpretation in a number of ways. On the microcosmic level, it helps explain passages that heretofore may not have been fully understood. On the macrocosmic level, it reveals the breadth of the biblical commentators in their integration of scientific theory into their works. The following section reveals that the application of the doctrine of innate heat was not restricted to one or two cases, or to peripheral commentators. Rather, it was consistently applied, in numerous cases, by the most prominent

13. See Iain M. Lonie, "Fever Pathology in the Sixteenth Century: Tradition and Innovation," in W. F. Bynum and V. Nutton, eds., *Theories of Fever from Antiquity to the Enlightenment* (London, 1981), 19–44.

14. See W. F. Bynum and V. Nutton, op. cit.

of exegetes. In addition, the thematic, literary and etymological ways in which the doctrine was applied is a testimony to rabbinic creativity.

Furthermore, as the passages cited below are largely examples of homiletic exegesis, the incorporation of the doctrine of innate heat, a doctrine supplanted by modern theories, may appear to be of little theological consequence. However, in some cases, the interpretations are adapted to halakhic contexts. Accurate interpretation of these passages is therefore crucial in order to facilitate proper extrapolation to the realm of halakha.

The Creation of Man

The second account of the creation of man reads, "And the Lord God formed man of the dust of the ground and breathed into his nostrils the breath of life; and man became a living soul" (Bereshit 2:7)." While most commentaries on this verse focus on the process by which man received his soul, R. Abraham ibn Ezra (1089–1164) addresses the relationship between the nostrils and the creation of life: "The reason it says, 'into his nostrils,' for it is by their virtue that man lives. They remove the warm air from the [innate] heat of the heart and replace it with other air." As described above, respiration of air through the nostrils was thought to be essential for the cooling and regulation of the innate heat of the heart. If this cooling mechanism failed, it was believed that the innate heat would consume the body.

This comment of Ibn Ezra was cited by R. Tzvi Ashkenazi (1656–1718), known as Ḥakham Tzvi, in his famous responsum on the halakhic status of a chicken that was found to be lacking a heart,[15] and is an example of the application of homiletic exegesis to the realm of halakha. In this responsum of R. Ashkenazi, which emphasizes the physiological and halakhic importance of the heart, the understanding that the heart is the center of the innate heat figures prominently in the discussion, and many of Ḥakham Tzvi's prooftexts regarding the centrality of the heart, including that of Ibn Ezra, rely on this physiological notion. This particular responsum has been applied to the contemporary halakhic

---

15. *She'elot UTeshuvot Ḥakham Zvi* #77.

debate regarding the definition of death,[16] an area where a medical historical analysis of the rabbinic sources can be particularly helpful.[17] The aforementioned interpretation of Ibn Ezra, as quoted by R. Ashkenazi, also appears in other modern responsa.[18]

Returning to the homiletic realm, the aforementioned verse regarding the creation of man was adapted by the prophet Isaiah in the following statement: "Cease from man, though his breath be in his nostrils (*neshama be'apo*) for in what is he to be accounted of?" (2:22). In his commentary on this verse, R. David Kimhi (also known as Radak, 1160–1235) explains the verse in the same vein as did Ibn Ezra: "and it says 'in his nostrils' because the spirit (*ruah*) of life depends on the nose. It is through the nostrils that innate heat of the heart exits, and likewise it is through the nostrils that the cooling air enters."[19]

The Fainting of Jacob

Upon hearing that his son Joseph was still alive, Jacob's response was dramatic: "And they told him, saying, Joseph is still alive, and he is governor over all the land of Egypt. V*ayafag libo*, for he believed them not. And they told him all the words of Joseph which he had said to them. And when he saw the wagons which Joseph had sent to carry him, the *ruah* of Jacob their father revived" (Bereshit 45:26–27).

Rashi (1040–1105) explains the phrase *vayafag libo* to mean that Jacob turned his heart away in disbelief, but after seeing the wagons and realizing the truth, the power of prophecy, or the presence of the *Shekhina* (i.e., *ruah*) was rekindled within him. According to *Siftei Hakhamim*, Rashi was compelled to interpret the phrase to mean that Jacob regained his powers of prophecy because the word *ruah* is used, and this word, in other contexts, refers to prophecy. Nahmanides (1194–1270), as we

---

16. See, for example, M. D. Tendler, *Responsa of Rav Moshe Feinstein: Care of the Critically Ill* (Hoboken, 1996), 75. R. Tendler is sensitive to the medical historical context of the responsum of R. Ashkenazi.

17. See chapter below, "The Halakhic Definition of Death in Light of Medical History."

18. Y. Y. Weiss, *She'elot UTeshuvot Minhat Yitzhak* 9:120.

19. See also Radak to Jeremiah 2:24, where R. Kimhi applies the same physiological explanation to another verse similar to Bereshit 2:7.

will see, does not feel bound by the same definitional constraints and interprets the term *ruaḥ* differently.

This exegetical debate is an example of a larger problem regarding the ambiguous definition of the term "spirit," and its Hebrew analogue, " *ruaḥ*." G. J. Goodfield notes that in the history of medicine the word "spirits" "could at one and the same time mean a gas, a volatile fluid, a soul, an animating principle, something which was the cause of nervous energy in the animal, something which was the cause of its being alive, and something which when mixed with various other substances was the cause of heat in the animal."[20] The term had material and immaterial, descriptive and explanatory implications. Goodfield further quotes Aristotle who clearly acknowledges the ambiguous usage and nature of the word. A similar ambiguity exists with the usage of the analogous word "*ruaḥ*" in Hebrew. For example, Maimonides details the multiple meanings of the word.[21]

Returning to the interpretation of the biblical passage, Naḥmanides argues for a different etymology for the word "*vayafag*," meaning cessation or arrest, as well as for the word "*ruaḥ*." With these different meanings, Naḥmanides advances the following novel interpretation:

> ... here *vayafag libo* means that his heart arrested and his breathing ceased, for the heartbeat stopped and he appeared as dead.... And it is mentioned in the medical books that the elderly and infirm often faint when confronted with a sudden surprise. The heart expands and suddenly opens, the natural heat (*ḥom hatoladi*) escapes and dissipates, and the heart, thereby cooled, ceases activity. The aged man then collapses as if dead. And it says "for he believed them not" to indicate that he remained unconscious for a long time because he did not believe them. For it is known that the treatment for this type of fainting is to shout at him and

---

20. See above.
21. *Guide for the Perplexed* 1:40. For the usage in rabbinic literature of the words *ruaḥ*, *neshama* and *nefesh*, which are plagued with ambiguity and often used interchangeably, see Samuel S. Kottek, "The Seat of the Soul: Contribution to the History of Jewish Medieval Psycho-Physiology," *Clio Medica* 13:3–4 (1978), 219–246.

accustom him to the surprise until he is calmed. This is why it says "and they told him all the words of Joseph, which he had said to them. And when he saw the wagons which Joseph had sent to carry him…," for they were shouting into his ears the words of Joseph and bringing before him the wagons. Only then was his respiration (*ruah*) restored and he awoke and regained consciousness, as it says, "the *ruah* of Jacob their father revived."[22]

Here Nahmanides applies the physiological principle of innate, or natural, heat (i.e., *hom hatoladi*) in order to provide what, in his opinion, is the most logical and literal interpretation of the passage.[23] Parenthetically, Maimonides (1138–1204), in his commentary on Galen entitled *Pirkei Moshe*, devotes a section to the causes of fainting wherein he also notes that the surprise mention of good news can lead to the dissipation of innate heat.[24]

The Aging and Illness of King David

The book of Melakhim opens with an account of the aging of King David, and states that, despite his layered clothing, "he could not become warm" (I Melakhim 1:1). In his commentary, R. David Kimhi attempts to explain the nature of King David's deficiency of heat and makes the following comment: "In his old age he became infirm and bedridden… and as long as the aging process progresses, the innate heat (*hom hativ'i*) continues to diminish, therefore, 'and they covered him with clothes, but he could not become warm.'" As mentioned above, this notion of the diminution of innate heat with age was a commonly held belief.

---

22. *Nahmanides Commentary on the Torah, Bereshit* 45:26. Rabbenu Bahya, ad loc., repeats the same interpretation as his teacher, Nahmanides, and uses this physiological explanation of the fainting associated with surprise to explain a passage in *Ketubot* 62b (see below).

23. While our current understanding of the mechanism of fainting, or syncope, may differ from that of Ramban, this does not preclude acceptance of his basic interpretation that Jacob fainted and was revived.

24. See Suessmann Muntner, ed., *Rambam: Kitvei Refua* 2 (Jerusalem, 1961). The section devoted to the causes of fainting begins on p. 92, and the relevant passage appears on p. 114, at n. 32. Maimonides makes no reference there to this story of Jacob, but, then again, there are few, if any, biblical or halakhic references in his medical works.

Metzudat David (eighteenth century) understands King David's illness in the same vein and uses this to explain why Avishag HaShunamit was present in the King's quarters when Bat Sheva paid him a visit. "Lest we think that she [Bat Sheva] came to lie with the King, it says, 'and the king was very old.' His innate heat had diminished, and Avishag was serving the King by providing warmth."[25]

Resuscitation Episodes of Eliyahu and Elisha

There are two accounts of resuscitation in *Tanakh*, both performed by prophets, with the actual resuscitation procedures being similar. The first was performed by Eliyahu on the son of the widow from Tzarfat: "And he stretched himself upon the child three times, and cried to the Lord and said, 'O Lord my God, I pray thee, let this child's soul return to him again', and he revived" (I Melakhim 17:21–22).[26] The second was performed by Elisha on the son on the Shunamite woman: "And he went up, and lay upon the child, and put his mouth upon his mouth, and his eyes upon his eyes, and his hands upon his hands and he stretched himself upon the child; and the flesh of the child was warmed. Then he returned and walked in the house to and fro; and went up and stretched himself upon him, and the child sneezed seven times, and the child opened his eyes" (II Melakhim 4:34–35).

---

25. *Metzudat David* on I Melakhim 1:14–15.
26. There is debate amongst the commentaries whether the child had actually died, or whether his condition was so grave that he appeared to be dead but was, in fact, barely alive. See, for example, *Radak*, ad loc.; Maimonides, *Guide for the Perplexed* 1:42; *She'elot UTeshuvot Ḥatam Sofer, Yoreh De'ah* #338. *Targum Yonatan* implies that the child may not have died, and Josephus (*Antiquities* 8, 13:3.325) is explicit in saying that the child's illness was so severe that he "ceased to breathe and seemed to be dead." This debate has a number of halakhic ramifications. According to rabbinic tradition, Eliyahu was thought to be the embodiment of Pinḥas. As Pinḥas was a *Kohen*, it is logical to assume that this distinction would have likewise been conferred upon Eliyahu. If he was, in fact, a *Kohen*, it would have been forbidden for him to come into contact with a corpse. How, then, could he have performed the resuscitation? This issue is addressed in *She'elot UTeshuvot HaRadbaz* #2203. Furthermore, this discussion impacts on the halakhic definition of death. See *She'elot UTeshuvot Ḥatam Sofer*, cited above. For a discussion on how an understanding of medical history impacts on the halakhic definition of death, see chapter, "The Halakhic Definition of Death in Light of Medical History." For more on these resuscitation episodes, see chapter, "The Resuscitation of Halakha: An Animated Discussion."

While many have drawn upon our modern understanding of physiology and resuscitation in order to shed light on these episodes,[27] I would like to focus on how the pre-modern commentator understood the strange maneuvers of Eliyahu and Elisha. While the miraculous element of both resuscitations seems clear, R. David Kimḥi (Radak) suggests that the method of resuscitation was chosen so that these miracles, like others in *Tanakh*, would have some basis in the natural world order.[28] He therefore posits, based on his contemporary understanding of nature, that the prophets positioned their mouths against those of the victims in order to transmit their innate heat, via respiration and exhalation, into the victims' lifeless bodies. The inspired air was thought to travel directly to the heart, where it came in contact with the innate heat. When the air was released during exhalation, it was now a higher temperature, having been warmed by the heat of the heart. As innate heat is required for the generation and preservation of life, the method employed by both Eliyahu and Elisha represents, according to Radak, a natural physiological basis for resuscitation upon which the miracle was based.

The Healing of Na'aman from *Tzara'at*

Na'aman, the military commander for the king of Aram, is one of a few specific people mentioned in *Tanakh* to have been stricken with the disease of *tzara'at*.[29] While *tzara'at* is mentioned many times throughout

---

27. F. Rosner, "Artificial Respiration in Biblical Times," *New York State Journal of Medicine* 69:8 (April 15, 1969), 1104–1105; Z. Rosen, "Rhinological Aspects of Biblical Resuscitation," *Archives of Otolaryngology* 95:5 (May, 1972), 488–489; Z. Rosen and J. Davidson, "Respiratory Resuscitation in Ancient Hebrew Sources," *Anesthesia and Analgesia* 51:4 (July-August, 1972), 502–505; L. Wislicki, "A Biblical Case of Hypothermia-Resuscitation by Rewarming (Elisha's Method)," *Clio Medica* 9:3 (September, 1974), 213–214; R. B. Howard, "...And There is Nothing New Under the Sun," *Postgraduate Medicine* 65:3 (March, 1979), 25; J. H. Comroe, Jr., "...In Comes the Good Air," *American Review of Respiratory Diseases* 119:6 (June, 1979), 1025–1031; A. S. Abraham, "*Hanshama Melakhutit BeTanakh*," *Ha-Ma'ayan* 28:3 (Nisan, 5748), 72–76; J. A. Paraskos, "Biblical Accounts of Resuscitation," *Journal of the History of Medicine and Allied Sciences* 47:3 (July, 1992), 310–321.
28. See Radak on I Melakhim 17:21 and II Melakhim 4:34.
29. I intentionally do not identify *tzara'at* with the disease known today as leprosy, or Hanson's Disease, because the biblical *tzara'at* is clearly a disease of a different

Tanakh, there is one literary aspect of the story of Na'aman which attracted the attention of biblical commentaries. The discussions of *tzara'at* in Leviticus focus largely on the diagnosis of the disease, while the story of Na'aman focuses on its treatment. Throughout the passage in II Melakhim, the enigmatic word *asaf* is consistently employed to refer to the cure for *tzara'at*, (*va'asafto mitzara'ato* [5:6], *le'esof ish mi'tzara'ato* [5:7], *ve'asaf hametzora* [5:11]). The usual term for healing is *le'rapot*, not *le'esof*. Both Rashi and Radak explain the usage of the verb *asaf* based on the unique social and halakhic dimension of the disease of *tzara'at*. The word *asaf* means to gather, or be gathered. When stricken with *tzara'at*, a person is ostracized, both socially and physically, from the camp of Israel. Once cured, the person can now return to the camp, and again gather with his people.[30]

R. Levi ben Gershon (Ralbag; 1288–1344) also contends that the cure for *tzara'at* is unique, and therefore merits the use of a verb other than *lerapot*. However, his justification for the use of the verb *asaf* is based on the physiological, rather than halakhic or social, uniqueness of the disease:

> "The cure for *tzara'at* is called *asifa* because *tzara'at* makes from one, many. The domination of the putrid fever or heat (*hom ha'ipushi*) weakens the innate heat, which is normally responsible for binding and unifying the limbs of the body. Consequently, in the *metzora* [who lacks this unifying force] we often find that their limbs fall off. Therefore [Elisha] says, regarding the healing, that 'thy flesh shall be restored to thee, and thou shalt be clean,' for the *metzora* lacks the substance or power which normally allows the flesh to adhere to the body."[31]

Ralbag operates with the premise that was widely accepted throughout history, that biblical *tzara'at* was identified as leprosy. He therefore

---

nature. The bibliography on the exact medical definition of *tzara'at* is extensive and continually growing. See A. D. Rabinowitz and Bezalel Naor, "The Medical Aspects of Tzara'at: Selected Bibliography," *Orot* 1 (1991), 30–32, for a sampling.

30. See their commentaries to II Melakhim 5:6 and II Melakhim 5:3 respectively.

31. See his commentary to II Melakhim 5:6. Translation by the author.

applies the principles of the pathology of leprosy, as understood in his time, to the explanation of this abnormal verb usage. The notion that leprosy was in part due to the decline of the unifying and adhesive force of the innate heat was already advanced by Galen.[32]

Cheese Analogy of Job

Nestled among the conversations of Job we find a number of metaphors for the creation of man: "Remember, I beseech Thee, that Thou hast made me like clay; and wilt Thou bring me back to dust? Hast Thou not poured me out like milk, and curdled me like cheese?" (*Iyov* 10:10). In his commentary on this verse, Ralbag applies the physiological principle of innate heat in order to explain the cheese analogy, stating that the innate heat found in the seed of the male congeals or solidifies the seed of the female with which it comes in contact.

This analogy of the formation of the human embryo to the process of making cheese was already advanced by Aristotle: "The action of the semen of the male in setting the female's secretion in the uterus is similar to that of rennet upon milk. Rennet is milk which contains vital heat, as semen does... As the nature of milk and the menstrual fluid is one and the same, the action of the semen upon the substance of the menstrual fluid is the same as that of rennet upon milk."[33]

R. Isaac ben Sheshet (1326–1408) is aware of the Greek origins of the cheese analogy, and, in fact, comments that this physiological understanding is in contradiction to rabbinic teachings which state that both the male and female contribute material to the fetus.[34]

---

32. See A. J. Brock, trans., *Galen: On the Natural Faculties* (London, 1916), 41. Another rabbinic passage addressing the pathology of *tzara'at* will be discussed below in the halakhic references.

33. A. L. Peck, trans., *Aristotle: Generation of Animals* (Cambridge, 1942), 739b, 21–29. For more on the cheese analogy see J. Needham, *A History of Embryology* (New York, 1959), 26, 50, 64, 66, 76, 82–85; C. R. S. Harris, op. cit., 139.

34. *She'elot UTeshuvot HaRivash* #447. See also S. Sternberg, op. cit., 90–102, who discusses a number of notions from the history of anatomy and physiology as they relate to the laws of *treifot*.

B) AGGADIC LITERATURE

Much like the previous section on biblical commentaries, the use of the doctrine of innate heat in the aggadic literature is homiletic in nature. We gain further appreciation of both the widespread use of the doctrine as it is applied to different areas of rabbinic literature as well as the interpretive ingenuity of the rabbis.

The Fainting of R. Ḥanina's Wife

There is a story told of R. Ḥanina b. Ḥakhinai which appears in the Talmud and, with slight variations, in the *Midrash*.[35] According to the story, R. Ḥanina left his family to study in a yeshiva for twelve years. When he returned from his journey and entered his house, his wife was occupied with sifting flour. When she lifted up her eyes and noticed the presence of her husband, she was overcome with joy and fainted. R. Ḥanina prayed for mercy on his wife's behalf and she revived. The phrase used to describe the wife's fainting differs between the Talmud, where it states that *"para ruḥa"* and the Midrash, which states *"yatza nishmata."* The terms *ruaḥ* and *neshama* could be interpreted metaphysically, to mean spirit and soul respectively, or physiologically, to refer to cessation of respiration.[36]

This episode is reminiscent of the fainting of Jacob as explained above according to Naḥmanides, which was also associated with a surprise, and, in fact, a number of commentators interpret this passage in the same vein. According to R. Ḥanokh Zundel, in his commentary to the Midrash, the wife's faint was caused by the sudden surprise, which expanded her heart, causing the innate heat to dissipate and thereby cool it.[37] While R. Zundel makes no reference to the fainting of Jacob, Rabbenu Baḥya (thirteenth century) links the two events in his biblical commentary,[38] claiming that both episodes of fainting were caused by the same physiological mechanism of the dissipation of innate heat.

---

35. See *Ketubot* 62b; *Vayikra Rabba* 21:7.
36. See discussion above on the ambiguity of the term *ruaḥ* in the context of the fainting of Jacob.
37. *Etz Yosef* on *Vayikra Rabba* 21:7, s. v., *"ad sheyazta."*
38. *Rabbenu Baḥya, Commentary on the Torah, Bereshit* 45:26.

The Miracle of Healing

R. Zundel uses the doctrine of innate heat to interpret another aggadic passage in the Talmud: "Said R. Alexandri in the name of R. Ḥiya bar Abba, 'Greater is the miracle performed for the sick than the miracle performed for Ḥananya, Misha'el and Azarya, for in the case of Ḥananya, Misha'el and Azarya, the fire was ordinary [*hedyot*] and anything could extinguish it, but in the case of the sick person, it [the fire] is heavenly, and who can extinguish it?'" (*Nedarim* 41a). R. Zundel makes the following comment on this passage: "If man considers the frequent miracles that exist in nature... innate heat is a perfect example. It is truly a heat of heavenly [*shamaymi*] origin, for the power of this man-centered fire is far greater than that of an ordinary fire. However, even though water is unable to extinguish its flames, still, other contrary forces can overcome it." The latter statement regarding contrary forces overcoming the innate heat is likely a reference to the pathology of fever, which was thought to be caused by a force or heat contrary to nature, as opposed to innate heat, which was thought to be a natural force.

C) HALAKHIC LITERATURE

As opposed to the aforementioned references to the doctrine of innate heat which were largely devoted to textual interpretation and explication and are homiletic in nature, the sources in the next section employ the doctrine for the purposes of legal and conceptual clarification. It is in the realm of halakha that the incorporation of early scientific theories has its greatest potential theological import. The following references are taken from three areas of halakha, all of which rely, to varying extents, on medical and scientific knowledge: the laws of *treifot*, the laws of *nidda*, and the definition of the disease *tzara'at*. In fact, the laws of *treifot* serve as the basis for many halakhic discussions about the conflict between contemporary and rabbinic scientific knowledge.[39]

The Laws of *Treifot*

There are at least three areas within the laws of *treifot* where the doctrine of innate heat has been invoked. The first relates to the interpretation of

---

39. See N. Gutal, op. cit., 32–39.

the law regarding the finding of perforations in the lung of an animal in conjunction with worms on its surface. R. Yosef Karo states that such an animal is kosher, on the assumption that it was after the slaughtering that the worms burrowed in and made the perforations. Perforations of the lung made during the animal's lifetime, however, would render the animal a *treifa*.[40] R. Shabtai Meir HaCohen (Shakh; 1621–1662) comments that while R. Karo states, without qualification, that the finding of both perforations and worms on the lung does not render the animal a *treifa*, other authorities require the performance of a special test with the worm-ridden lung in order to determine its halakhic status.[41] While the nuances of the debate are not of concern here, the nature of the test, and the logic behind its performance are relevant to our discussion.

The Shakh cites *Hilkhot Treifot* of Rabbenu Gershon Me'or HaGola (960–1040), where it states, "if a lung is found infested with worms, one should place the lung out in the sun. If [the worms] exit to the surface of the lung as it is heated, the animal is kosher; if not, [the animal is a] *treifa*." The Shakh proceeds to explain the logic of the test as follows: "If one finds the lung perforated, and suspects that the perforations were made by worms, as worms are also found on the lung's surface, he should place the lung in the sun. If the worms come to the lung's surface as it is warmed by the sun, then we assume the perforations were made by the worms. For just as the worms crawl to the surface to seek the sun's heat, so too, after the animal was slaughtered, the worms, sensing the loss of innate heat with the death of the animal, burrowed into the lung seeking another source of innate heat." Innate heat was perceived as a life-sustaining force even for animals and insects, and the doctrine was adapted in explaining this unique test of the laws of *treifa*.[42] It is important to ascertain whether the interpretation of this test is predicated exclusively on the doctrine of innate heat, or whether the doctrine is mentioned only in a supplementary role. Although the sun test is not required by R. Karo, this represents an incorporation of

---

40. *Yoreh De'ah* 36:5.
41. *Shakh, Yoreh De'ah* 36:18.
42. The author of the *Kol Bo* also applies the doctrine of innate heat to the sun test. See *Kol Bo, Hil. Treifot*, chap. 101.

an early scientific doctrine into the realm of halakhic *pesak*. More recent authorities perpetuate this explanation of the sun test.[43]

Another aspect of the doctrine of innate heat has been invoked regarding the debate as to the procreative status of a *treifa* animal. According to some, inability to procreate is a required characteristic for the definition of *treifa* while, according to others, ability to procreate in no way affects this status.[44] R. Judah b. Israel Assad (1794–1866) employs the doctrine of innate heat as a possible explanation of this debate: "It appears to me that the ones who maintain that a [female] *treifa* cannot procreate contend that once the animal becomes a *treifa*, her innate heat becomes weakened and she loses the power necessary for gestation. Those who maintain that a [female] *treifa* can give birth contend that since the male suffers no weakening of his innate heat, the female can receive his seed and conceive."[45] As mentioned above, the semen was thought to possess innate heat. Since the innate heat which is responsible for the generation of life remains intact within the semen of the male who is not a *treifa*, the female *treifa* should logically be able to conceive.

The third reference to the doctrine of innate heat is made by Maimonides. According to rabbinic tradition, there are only eighteen pathological conditions that constitute a *treifa*.[46] Maimonides, however, adds one to the list that is not found in the Talmud, i.e., absence of the upper jaw or maxilla.[47] This enigmatic inclusion provoked a query from the sages of Lunel, who asked Maimonides to explain his unique position. Invoking the doctrine of innate heat to explain his contention that absence of the upper jaw constitutes a *treifa*, Maimonides makes the following comment: "The upper jaw serves as a roof over the trachea to prevent the cold air from entering... If the upper jaw is removed, and the trachea is exposed, excess air will enter with every breath... it will

---

43. See, for example, R. Moses Sofer, *She'elot UTeshuvot Ḥatam Sofer, Yoreh De'ah* #44, and R. Ovadia Yosef, *Yabia Omer* 1, *Yoreh De'ah* #2.

44. For a summary of the opinions on this issue see *Entzyclopedia Talmudit* 21 (Jerusalem, 1993), cols. 77–79.

45. R. Judah b. Israel Assad, *Yehuda Ya'aleh* 1, *Yoreh De'ah* #377.

46. *Ḥullin* 42a–43a.

47. *Mishneh Torah, Hil. Sheḥita* 8:23.

cool the lungs and the heart, and the animal will die."[48] R. Yosef Karo states that one should be concerned for the position of Maimonides,[49] implying that absence of the upper jaw should be considered a *treifa*.

Maimonides relies on the doctrine of innate heat to explain why absence of the upper jaw would constitute a *treifa*. Therefore, since we now understand the physiology of respiration differently, theoretically, excess air should in no way be harmful to an animal. However, to be sure, there may be other reasons why absence of the upper jaw could be detrimental. How does this impact on the laws of *treifa*? Should the absence of the upper jaw still be included in the list? Is Maimonides' physiological explanation crucial to his decision, or did he have other reasons to prohibit such a pathological condition, aside from those relating to the doctrine of innate heat? Even if Maimonides relied exclusively on the doctrine of innate heat in deciding to add an additional category of *treifa* to the traditionally accepted list, does this affect the validity of his decision? These questions, as stated above, are the province of the rabbinic decisor.

The Laws of *Nidda*

In order for menstrual blood to generate *tum'ah* it must derive from the uterus and be the product of a natural physiological occurrence. Blood which derives from a uterine laceration or lesion does not generate *tum'ah*.[50] The problem, however, is that it is not always possible to ascertain the source of the bleeding.

A problem relating to this distinction was presented to R. Yeḥezkel Landau, who, *inter alia*, discussed the physiology of menses and its cessation during menopause. The case involved a postmenopausal woman who suffered from a prolapsed, or fallen, uterus, and who subsequently resumed uterine bleeding. The question was whether this renewed bleeding is to be considered a natural flow, in which case she

---

48. See Y. Blau, ed., *Teshuvot HaRambam* 2 (Jerusalem, 1989), #315. The responsum is also cited by R. Y. Karo in his commentary to Maimonides' *Mishneh Torah, Kesef Mishna, ad loc.*

49. *Hil. Treifot, Yoreh De'ah* 23:2.

50. See *Yoreh De'ah* 187:5.

would be a *nidda*, or whether, since it is the product of a wound, she would not. R. Landau wrote:

> In truth, the physicians do not understand the origins of menstrual bleeding, neither its onset at puberty, nor its cessation with old age. Their belief, however, is that the origin and onset of menses is related to the innate heat in the uterus. Therefore, in old age, when the innate heat diminishes and the uterus becomes cool, menses ceases. It is possible to say that this logic is applicable only when the uterus sits in its proper, spacious anatomical location. However, if a woman suffers prolapse of her uterus in old age, and the uterus, now detached from its usual location, occupies the narrow space between her thighs, perhaps the narrowness of the location, along with the friction created by walking, will regenerate sufficient innate heat to cause her to resume her natural menses. If such is the case, then the resulting flow is true *nidda* blood [which is *tamei*] and not blood deriving from a wound [which is not *tamei*].[51]

While the final decision in this case does not rely on the doctrine of innate heat, R. Landau nonetheless incorporates the doctrine into his analysis in a way that could theoretically have practical halakhic ramifications.

The Definition of *Tzara'at* and the Obligation to Divorce

As mentioned above in the section on biblical commentaries, Ralbag employs the doctrine of innate heat to explain a difficult verb usage in conjunction with the treatment of *tzara'at*. Another rabbinic authority, R. Yosef Trani (1568–1639), discussed the pathology of leprosy in a more detailed fashion, also drawing upon the doctrine of innate heat, regarding the halakhic obligation of a leper to divorce his wife. A prerequisite for the invoking of this law is the accurate diagnosis of the husband with leprosy. In the course of his detailed diagnostic discussion, R. Trani asserted that leprosy affects the liver's ability to properly control

---

51. *She'elot UTeshuvot Noda BiYehuda, Mahadura Tinyana, Yoreh De'ah* #114.

digestion. The body, therefore, develops an excess of waste, which is expelled through the skin as boils or other skin lesions. However, if the innate heat is diminished, the waste becomes too great and pieces of skin and flesh begin to fall off the body.[52] This notion that the diminution of innate heat ultimately leads to the loss of flesh and limbs in leprosy is consistent with the comment of Ralbag and the teachings of Galen, and the reference to the liver's role in leprosy is consistent with contemporary teachings.[53]

The specific cause for the decrease in innate heat mentioned by R. Trani is intercourse. As the semen itself was thought to contain innate heat, intercourse was logically thought to decrease the total body innate heat. The reason intercourse specifically is mentioned is because the halakhic issue at hand is whether a marital relationship should be maintained or dissolved. One of the marital obligations of the husband is *ona* (i.e., engaging in marital relations). The fact that the fulfillment of the obligation of *ona* will cause physical harm to the husband, by virtue of its diminution of his innate heat, factors into R. Trani's decision regarding whether or not a divorce is obligatory. The potential detriment of intercourse for those stricken with leprosy was debated by medical authorities throughout the ages, with some actually considering intercourse to be therapeutic rather than harmful. In any case, one must ask here, as with the other halakhic sources which incorporate early scientific theories, whether the scientific information incorporated by R. Trani is peripheral or integral to his decision. This is especially important in this case since the responsum of R. Trani, with its detailed medical and diagnostic discussion of leprosy, is cited by a number of later rabbinic authorities in their discussions on the grounds for obligatory divorce.[54]

---

52. *She'elot UTeshuvot Maharit, Even HaEzer* #14.

53. See Luke Demaitre, "The Relevance of Futility: Jordanus de Turre (fl. 1313–1335) on the Treatment of Leprosy," *Bulletin of the History of Medicine* 71:1 (1996): 25–61, esp. p. 45. A more detailed analysis of the rabbinic diagnosis of leprosy, as compared to the contemporaneous medical theories, would make for a valuable study. R. Trani, himself, in the aforementioned responsum, addresses the inherent problems regarding the halakhic diagnosis of biblical *tzara'at*, as compared to the disease known by physicians as leprosy.

54. See, for example, R. Judah b. Israel Assad, *Yehuda Ya'aleh* 2:79; R. Eliezer J. Waldenberg, *Tzitz Eliezer* 6:22, *Orḥot HaMishpatim*, chap. 5; *Piskei Din Rabani'im*, 3, p. 126.

IV. CONCLUSION

The above references are examples of how the fundamental, pre-modern physiological belief in the doctrine of innate heat finds its expression in different areas of rabbinic literature.[55] This chapter illustrates the importance of medical history for the study of rabbinic literature in general, and should specifically enable the reader to better understand other passages which incorporate this doctrine.

---

55. For other examples in biblical exegesis, see *Ralbag* on 2 *Shmuel* 2:23 and 20:10, *Mishlei* 17:22 and 25:25, and *Iyov* 31:40; *Metzudat David* on *Iyov* 41:10–11. For other examples in halakhic literature, see J. Chagiz, *Teshuvot Halakhot Ketanot*, 1:267; R. Judah b. Israel Assad, *Yehuda Ya'aleh* 1, *Yoreh De'ah* #66 and 1, *Orah Hayyim* #127; R. Yitzhak Y. Weiss, *Minhat Yitzhak*, 4:13.

Diseases and Therapeutics

The Impact of Medieval Medicine on Medical Halakha: The Case of Mumia

I. INTRODUCTION

The medical halakhic literature from the post-talmudic to the pre-modern period serves as a foundation of modern medical halakha inasmuch as halakha is a precedent-oriented system. A *posek* or rabbinic decisor, in whatever generation he may live, invariably looks to the writings of his predecessors in order to see how they grappled with comparable problems.

Today, a number of books are devoted exclusively to medical halakha. Had such books been written in previous centuries, their tables of contents would read quite differently than those of today. Had such a book been authored in the tenth century, it would have included, for the first time, a chapter on the prohibition of using the medical remedies of the Talmud.[1] In the fourteenth century, such a text would have included

---

1. During the period of the *Gaonim* a ban was enacted on the use of talmudic remedies. This ban is found in a number of collections of Gaonic literature. See, for example, *Otzar HaGaonim* on *Masekhet Gittin* edited by M. B. Levin (Jerusalem, 1941), 78. Other

a chapter on the use of astrology in medicine;[2] in the sixteenth century, a chapter on the use of mummies for medicinal purposes (the topic of this chapter); and in the eighteenth century, a chapter on smallpox innoculation and vaccination.[3]

To be sure, a number of topics in today's medical halakhic works, such as contraception, abortion, and euthanasia, might have appeared in works of previous generations. Yet, the treatment of these topics would have differed relative to the medical understanding of each era.

This evolution of medicine and science poses difficulty for the modern reader of the pre-modern medical halakhic literature. Each passage or responsum, depending on its period, as well as its author, deals with a different medical reality, a reality sometimes hidden from the modern reader and impeding proper contextual understanding. The modern reader often unintentionally interpolates modern medical theories into the texts of his predecessors thereby yielding anachronistic and possibly erroneous interpretations.

Thus, when discussing the halakhic determination of death, it is important to realize that the conceptions of cardiac and respiratory

---

sources are quoted in J. Shatzmiller, *Jews, Medicine and Medieval Society* (University of California Press, 1994), 148, n. 48. This ban was mentioned subsequently by R. Jacob Molin in *Likutei Maharil* and R. Akiva Eiger in his glosses on *Shulḥan Arukh*. On this topic see also *Havot Yair* by R. Yair Bacharach (n. 20) and the commentary of R. Solomon Luria to the eighth chapter of *Masekhet Ḥullin*, no. 12.

2. See H. J. Zimmels, *Magicians, Theologians, and Doctors* (Edward Goldston and Son, 1952), 137–139 and 163–164. Naḥmanides apparently used a medallion with the likeness of an astrological lion for the treatment of a kidney ailment. This is attested to by his student, R. Shlomo ibn Adret (*Rashba*) in his responsa, n. 413.

On this topic see J. Shatzmiller, "In Search of the 'Book of Figures': Medicine and Astrology in Montpellier at the Turn of the Fourteenth Century," *AJS Review* 7–8 (1982–3), 383–407; idem, "*Tzurat Aryeh LeKlayot VeHaMakhloket al Limudei HaHokhmot Bereshit HaMe'ah Ha-14*," *Mekhkerei Yerushalayim* 9 (1990), 397–408; David Horwitz, *The Role of Philosophy and Kabbalah in the Works of the Rashba*, unpublished Master's thesis, Bernard Revel Graduate School (Yeshiva University, 1986), 43–72 and 153–174.

Maimonides is one of the only rabbinic authorities in the medieval period to have opposed the use of astrology. See Alexander Marx, "The Correspondence Between the Rabbis of Southern France and Maimonides About Astrology," *Hebrew Union College Annual* 3 (1926), 311–358.

3. See chapter, "Lessons from the First Halakhic Analysis of Vaccination."

physiology have changed radically over the centuries. The circulation of the blood was only first accurately described in the sixteenth century. It was also believed that the inspired air traveled directly to the heart, until the advances in respiratory physiology in the seventeenth and eighteenth centuries disproved this notion.[4]

Additionally, regarding the medical halakhic issues of infertility, such as artificial insemination and in-vitro fertilization, it should be noted that the understanding of reproductive anatomy and physiology has evolved over centuries. The existence of the human female egg was only affirmed in the sixteenth century, and the egg itself was not visualized until 1867.[5]

To illustrate the importance of understanding medical history in order to better appreciate the post-talmudic medical halakhic literature, I offer a chapter that would have appeared in a book on medical halakha between the sixteenth and nineteenth centuries.

II. MUMIA: AN HISTORIC OVERVIEW

Introduction

In the sixteenth and seventeenth centuries, mumia was a commonly prescribed drug for ailments ranging from liver disorders to bone fractures. While in antiquity, mumia consisted of natural bitumen, at this period in history, the drug called mumia was primarily a derivative of parts of ancient Egyptian mummies, or other more recently embalmed or dessicated bodies. How this came to be is a tale of mistranslations and transference, as we shall see, and led to some confusion as to the true identity of mumia, as well as to questions regarding its therapeutic value.

Understanding the history of mumia facilitates a greater appreciation of the Jewish, and especially halakhic, literature in a number of ways. It explains why the halakhic literature on this topic is restricted to a certain historical period. It provides an historical context for a selection of sources that reflect not isolated incidents but, rather, a major historical chapter in both Egyptology and medical history. As a result,

---

4. See chapter, "The Halakhic Definition of Death in Light of Medical History."
5. See chapter, "The Rabbinic Conception of Conception."

secular and Jewish sources work in a complementary fashion to provide a more comprehensive picture of the history of mumia. Most importantly, an appreciation of the medical history of mumia illuminates the medical details of the rabbinic discussions which may seem enigmatic, at best, to the contemporary reader. By revealing practical or factual background information, one gains insight into the reasons for certain halakhic decisions.

Mumia (Bitumen) in Antiquity

In antiquity, bituminous or asphalt-like substances were used for multiple purposes.[6] Both Strabo (d.24 CE) and Diodorus Siculus (50 CE) give full accounts of a major source of this bitumen—the Dead Sea area—and each mentions how this substance was exported to Egypt for use in the embalming of human bodies.[7] Josephus attests to the varied uses of the bitumen of the Dead Sea, asserting that it was not only useful for the caulking of ships, but for the cure of men's ailments. Accordingly, it was "mixed in a great many medicines."[8]

Asphalt was used for building in antiquity. The Bible records that Noah's ark[9] and Moses' basket[10] were constructed with the use of asphalt-like substances. The Talmud is also replete with references to the use of asphalt-like materials,[11] reflecting its common usage.

---

6. See Charles Singer, E. J. Holmyard and A. R. Hall, eds., *A History of Technology*, vol. 1 (Oxford University Press, 1954), 250–256.
7. See Menahem Stern, *Greek and Latin Authors on Jews and Judaism* (Academic Press: Jerusalem, 1974), vol. 1, 178 and 304. See also p. 181 where Stern comments that since Diodorus and Strabo say the same thing, "It is, therefore, useless to deny that, at least in the Graeco-Roman period, the asphalt of the Dead Sea was used in embalming." See D. Kaplan, "*Al HaTechnologia shel Ḥomrei Bitumen BiYisrael BiY'mei Kedem*," *Koroth* 3:1–2 (Oct 1962), 80–83; ibid., "*HaḤomer BiYam HaMelaḥ VeHaShimush Bo BiY'mei Kedem*," *Koroth* 3:5–6 (Feb-March 1964), 230–237; Carl Ritter, *The Comparative Geography of Palestine and the Sinaitic Peninsula*, trans. William Cage, (Haskell House Publishers, 1969), 150–158. See also Karl H. Dannenfeldt, "Egyptian Mumia: The Sixteenth Century Experience and Debate," *The Sixteenth Century Journal*, 16:2 (1985), 163–180, esp. 166.
8. *Wars of the Jews*, Book 4, Chap. 8, No. 4.
9. Bereshit 5:14. See also D. Kaplan, op. cit.
10. Shemot 2:3.
11. See articles by D. Kaplan, op. cit.

As for the medicinal value of bitumen, Pliny (d.79 CE) hailed its use for cataracts, leprosy, gout, toothaches, coughs, dysentery, and wounds.[12] Galen (c. 130 CE–c. 200 CE) considered the asphalt of the Dead Sea to be the most beautiful of bitumens and thought it useful for the closing of bleeding wounds.[13] Dioscorides established the use of bituminous substances in Europe. In his classic work, *Materia Medica*, he refers to the bitumen of the Dead Sea, bitumen Judaicum, as the best bitumen for medicines.[14]

The Persians called this substance "mumia," derived from the Persian word *mum*, wax.[15] According to some historians, the term "mummy" comes from mumia, since mumia was apparently used in the embalming process in ancient Egypt, as we shall see.

Mumia in the Middle Ages

In the Middle Ages, the Dead Sea bitumen was no longer considered the most valuable. Rather, the black asphalt from a certain mountain in Persia was considered by the Arabs to be ideal for therapeutic use.[16]

---

12. *Natural History*, 35, 180–182, quoted in Karl Dannenfeldt, "Egyptian Mumia: The Sixteenth Century Experience and Debate," *The Sixteenth Century Journal* 16:2 (1985), 163–180. For the subsequent discussion of the mistranslations and transference of the term mumia, I am largely indebted to this work.

    A general history on the use of mumia as a drug is provided by Thomas Pettigrew, *A History of Egyptian Mummies* (Longman, Rees, Orme, Brown, Green and Longman: London, 1834), 1–12. See also Warren R. Dawson, *The Bridle of Pegasus* (London,1930), 162–173.

    For other references to the use of mumia, or mummy, as a drug, see, for example, Warren R. Dawson, "Mummy as a Drug," *Proceedings of the Royal Society of Medicine* (November, 1927), 34–39; Howard W. Haggard, *Devils, Drugs, and Doctors* (Blue Ribbon Books, 1929), 324; Arno Karlen, *Napoleon's Glands and Other Ventures in Biohistory* (Little Brown and Company, 1984), 96–119; E. A. Wallis Budge, *The Mummy: A Handbook of Egyptian Funerary Archeology* (Dover Publications, 1989), 202–203.

13. See M. Stern, op. cit., vol. 2, 324.

14. Ibid., 164.

15. See Dawson, op. cit.; Carrubba, op. cit., 464; Dannenfeldt, op. cit., 463.

16. Although medieval Arabic writers like Rhazes and Avicenna make reference to this Persian source of mumia, it was not until the early eighteenth century that we find an accurate historical account of the ceremonial collection of mumia by the Persian royalty from a remote mountain in the province of Darab. See Robert W. Carrubba, "The First Detailed Report of Persian Mummy," *Physis* 23 (1981), 459–471.

Dannenfeldt states that Rhazes (d.923) was the first to use the word mumia for bituminous substances.[17] A century later, the famous Persian physician Avicenna likewise used the term mumia to describe the medicinal bitumen.[18] He refers to the bituminous waters as Judaic waters,[19] likely borrowing the term from Dioscorides.

Thereafter began a transference of the term mumia from natural bitumen to an exudate, similar in appearance, derived from the embalmed bodies in the tombs of Egypt. As mentioned above, both Strabo and Diodorus claimed that the bitumen of the Dead Sea, which was later called mumia by Arab writers, was used in the embalming process in Egypt. This transference, therefore, seems logical.[20]

Dannenfeldt points out that in the sixteenth century, physicians and scholars began to protest the use of mumia as a drug. They noted the change in the identity of the drug and attributed the transference to a series of mistranslations of works by Rhazes and Serapion the Younger (c. 1070), among others. While these authors were logically referring to the natural bitumen, textual ambiguities led tranlators to expand on the original texts and identify mumia with the exudates of embalmed bodies, an identification common in their day. Furthermore, Dannenfeldt views the transference as occurring in a stepwise fashion. Initially, mumia was associated only with the fluids or exudates that flowed from the embalmed body. Ultimately, however, mumia became associated with the very flesh of the corpse, for this too was impregnated with the valuable bitumen.[21]

---

17. Dannenfeldt, op. cit., 164.
18. Ibid. See also Pettigrew, op. cit., 9.
19. O. Cameron Gruner, trans., *A Treatise on the Canon of Medicine of Avicenna Incorporating a Translation of the First Book* (Luzac and Co., 1930), 237.
20. Of note, Dawson maintains that bitumen was never used in the embalming process: "The resin, which was used in large quantities in mummies of late periods, was applied in a molten condition, and in this state often closely simulates both pitch and bitumen but must not be confounded with these substances as is usually done; there is no evidence as yet that bitumen was ever used." See Warren R. Dawson, "Making A Mummy," *Journal of Egyptian Archeology* 13 (1927), 40–49, quoted in Carrubba, op. cit., 460, n. 4.
21. Dannenfeldt, op. cit., 164–170.

Trade of Mumia

The first to prescribe Egyptian mummy, or mumia, for medicinal use was the expert Jewish physician named Elmagar.[22] It is recorded in *Les Diverses Lecons de L. Guyon* (1625) that Elmagar lived around 1100, (or possibly 1300 according to some authors), and prescribed mumia to the Christians and Muslims then fighting for Palestine. Other physicians followed suit and so began the widespread use of mumia. The Jewish merchants of Egypt soon entered the trade. Some of these merchants, in order to fill the growing demand, took the bodies of executed criminals, or other bodies they could obtain, filled them with inexpensive simple asphalt, bound them up tightly, and exposed them to the heat of the sun for rapid drying. They then sold these counterfeit mummies in place of the genuine, properly embalmed ones. These freshly prepared mummies were apparently sold to the Christians.[23]

Although purportedly first prescribed in the Middle Ages, Egyptian mumia only became popular in the sixteenth century, when it was widely prescribed by physicians.[24] In 1564, Guy De la Fontaine, physician

---

22. I have found no reference to this physician outside of this statement of Guyon. Regarding medieval Jewish physicians in Arabic countries, see, for example, Max Meyerhof, "Mediaeval Jewish Physicians in the Near East, from Arabic Sources," *ISIS* 27–28 (1937–38), 432–460; idem, "Jewish Physicians Under the Reign of the Fatimid Caliphs in Egypt (969–1171)," *Medical Leaves* (1939), 131–139; S. D. Goitein, "The Medical Profession in Light of the Cairo Geniza Documents," *Hebrew Union College Annual* 34 (1963), 177–194; R. Y. Ebied, *Bibliography of Mediaeval Arabic and Jewish Medicine and Allied Sciences* (Wellcome Institute for the History of Medicine: London, 1971); Moshe Perlman, "Notes on the Position of Jewish Physicians in Medieval Muslim Countries," *Journal of Israel Oriental Studies* 2 (1972), 315–319; H. D. Isaacs, "Medieval Judaeo-Arabic Medicine as Described in the Cairo Geniza," *Journal of the Royal Society of Medicine* 83 (November, 1990), 734–737; idem, "A Medieval Arab Medical Certificate," *Medical History* 35 (1991), 250–257; idem, *Medical and Para-Medical Manuscripts in the Cambridge Geniza Collections* (Cambridge University Press, 1994).
23. Cited by Pettigrew, op. cit., 7–8. The anatomist William Williams Keen also mentioned this practice of the Jews in his historical work, *A Sketch of the Early History of Practical Anatomy* (Philadelphia, 1874), 37, stating that when the demand for mumia exceeded the supply of the real article, a substitute was sold "at enormous profits by avaricious Jews of Alexandria." This passage is quoted in James Moores Ball, *The Body Snatchers* (Dorset Press, 1989), xxiv-xxv.
24. Dannenfeldt, op. cit.

to the king of Navarre, journeyed to Egypt. While in Alexandria, he sought out the principal Jew in charge of the mummy trade and inquired from him as to the origin of his supply and the nature of the ancient burial and embalming practices. The merchant showed him some thirty or forty bodies, and explained with amusement that all those bodies had been prepared over the last four years. When De la Fontaine asked as to what nation they belonged, or whether the bodies were diseased, the merchant said that he cared not, for once the bodies were embalmed, they all appeared the same. The merchant further marveled that the Christians, "so daintily mouthed," could eat of the bodies of the dead.[25]

De la Fontaine related this encounter to his friend Ambrose Pare, the celebrated French military surgeon, who subsequently incorporated the information into his medical works. Pare quotes Louis de Paradis, a French surgeon who visited Cairo, that the Egyptians refused to permit any of their embalmed bodies to be exported, saying that the Christians are unworthy of eating their dead bodies. If the bodies did end up outside the country, he said, it was likely by means of some Jews, who smuggled them out by stripping the bodies and packing them with their merchandise.[26] Pare also wrote an entire treatise, *On Mumia*, published in 1582, in which he refers to a Jewish physician prescribing mumia.[27]

Regarding the duration of the mumia trade, Louis Guyon relates an anecdote which may account for the diminution of the trade of counterfeit mumia, or perhaps even the cessation of the Jewish mumia trade altogether. A Jew of Damietta, Egypt, who manufactured counterfeit mummies, had a Christian slave whom he wished to convert to Judaism. When the slave refused to undergo the required circumcision, their relationship turned adversarial, and the merchant began to mistreat the slave. As a result, the slave informed the authorities of his master's illicit practices. The merchant was imprisoned but was able to secure his release with the payment of three hundred sultanins of gold. When

---

25. Cited by Pettigrew, op. cit., 8, without quoting a source, and by Dannenfeldt, op. cit., 170 and n. 28.
26. Dannenfeldt, op. cit., 7–8.
27. Geoffrey Keynes, ed., *The Apologie and Treatise of Ambrose Pare* (Dover Publications, 1968), 143–146.

the governors of the neighboring cities, including Alexandria, Rosetta, Aleppo, and other cities in Egypt, heard of these events, they delighted in the prospect of easily obtaining money for their respective treasuries. Forthwith, they began collecting ransom from all Jews involved in the mummy trade. Historians recount that from this time onwards the trade of mumia ceased, since the Jews were fearful of being subjected to further oppression.[28]

Although this account was published in 1625, it is unclear exactly when the trade stopped. In 1718, John Quincy wrote that although mumia could still be found in medicinal catalogues, it was rarely prescribed.[29] Despite this attestation, the use of mumia seems to have continued, albeit on a limited basis, into the eighteenth[30] and nineteenth centuries.[31]

In summary, the history of the drug mumia is somewhat convoluted, having undergone a transference from the natural bitumen of the Dead Sea and Persia to the embalmed or dessicated bodies of Egypt. This transference resulted in confusion as to the true identity of mumia and led to the questioning of its therapeutic efficacy.

III. MUMIA IN JEWISH SOURCES[32]

With this brief overview, we can now address the Jewish sources on the use of mumia. The sources can be divided into two categories, those that simply provide an account of the use of mumia, and those that address the halakhic implications of its use.

---

28. Pettigrew, op. cit., 11, and Dannenfeldt, op. cit., 171.

29. Dannenfeldt, op. cit., 179.

30. Pettigrew, whose work was published in 1834, states that during his day Arabs still used mummy powder.

31. Dannenfeldt, op. cit., 179–180.

32. The use of mumia in Jewish sources has been dealt with in the following works: H. J. Zimmels, *Magicians, Theologians and Doctors* (London, 1952), 126–128 and 244–245; Raphael Patai, "Indulco and Mumia," *Journal of American Folklore*, 77 (January-March, 1964), 3–11; Daniel Sperber, *Minhagei Yisrael* 2 (Mosad HaRav Kook, 1991), 61, n. 28. Abraham Ofir Shemesh has a lengthy discussion on mumia in his *Medical Materials in Medieval and Modern Jewish Literature* (Bar-Ilan University Press, 2013) (Hebrew), 54ff.

Accounts of Mumia in Extralegal Sources

Historians refer to the Jewish physician Elmagar, who is dated between 1100 and 1300, as being the first to prescribe Egyptian mumia. What went unnoticed is the fact that Maimonides, who lived during this very time period (1138–1204), mentions mumia amongst a list of medications in his medical treatise, *Pirkei Moshe*.[33] In this work, Maimonides simply states the term "mumia" without qualification, making it difficult to ascertain whether he refers to mumia the bitumen or mumia the embalmed body. However, in his dictionary of medical terms, Maimonides translates mumia as *"el-k'buria,"*[34] reflecting mumia's association with graves, and perhaps with embalmed bodies. Even this term, however, is ambiguous. Is Maimonides referring to the bitumen, which could commonly be found in the graves, as it was used in embalming, or is he referring to the corpse itself, which could likewise be found in the grave? Maimonides does not translate the term mumia explicitly as either bitumen or as parts of embalmed corpses.

In any case, this is an important source, as it reflects a step in the transference of the term mumia, here being associated, in the twelfth century, with the burial process. In addition, if Maimonides refers to bitumen,[35] this source reflects one of two possibilities. Perhaps Elmagar

---

33. In personal communication Dr. Gerrit Bos confirms that the term mumia appears in the original Arabic edition (ms. Gotha) of *Pirkei Moshe*, aphorisms, 21:80. See S. Muntner, trans. and ed., *Rambam: Kitvei Refuah* 2 (Mosad HaRav Kook, 1961), 262.

34. S. Muntner, ed. and trans., *Biur Shemot HaRefuot* in *Rambam: Kitvei Refua* 4 (Mosad HaRav Kook, 1969), 71. In Muntner's notes on *Pirkei Moshe*, ibid., n. 385, he translates *"el-k'buria"* as body parts from ancient corpses. In addition, he states that mumia also refers to pissasphalt (bitumen), thereby alluding to the confusion and transference of the term.

     The term *"el-k'buria"* was used in conjunction with the term mumia in folk remedy prescriptions well beyond the time of Maimonides. See Avraham Ben-Yaakov, *HaRefua HaAmamit Etzel Yehudei Bavel* 1 (Yerid HaSefarim, 1991), 533–534.

35. The term mumia used by Maimonides more likely refers to bitumen for a number of reasons. Mumia is found amongst a list of natural substances; earlier in this list Maimonides cites Avicenna, whom we know to have used the term mumia to refer to natural bitumen, and from whom Maimonides may have borrowed some of the terms of this list, including mumia; and Maimonides himself acknowledged the medicinal value of asphalt and bitumen elsewhere in his medical works. See Uriel

post-dates Maimonides, and Egyptian mummy was only first prescribed after Maimonides' time. Consequently, Maimonides, like his contemporaries, prescribed natural bitumen. Alternatively, Elmagar pre-dates Maimonides, and Maimonides continued to prescribe the original mumia, either being unaware or disapproving of the Egyptian variety.

If, however, Maimonides refers to Egyptian mummy,[36] then this would represent the earliest primary source on its use, and possibly, depending on the dating of Elmagar, the earliest known prescription of Egyptian mumia.

The next account of the use of mumia is found in the biblical commentary of R. Eliezer Ashkenazi (1513–1586).[37] God commanded Lot and his wife, when they departed from Sodom, not to look behind

---

Barzel, trans., *Maimonides' Medical Writings—The Art of Cure: Extracts from Galen* (Maimonides Research Institute, 1992), 176; Fred Rosner, trans., *Moses Maimonides' Glossary of Drug Names* (American Philosophical Society: Philadelphia, 1979), 99–100 and 121–122. (I thank Dr. Rosner for directing me to these sources.)

On the other hand, in his *Glossary of Drug Names* Maimonides uses the terms *zaft* and *qufr al-Yahud* (bitumen of the Jews) for asphalt and bitumen rather than the term mumia. This may indicate that mumia refers to something other than bitumen (i.e., Egyptian mumia).

36. If Maimonides in fact refers to Egyptian mumia, one might have expected him to deal with, or at least allude to, the halakhic ramifications of the use of parts of a corpse for medicinal purposes. In general, however, Maimonides makes no halakhic pronouncements in his medical works, and largely vice versa. In his *Yad HaHazaka, Hil. Avel*, where he discusses the laws of impurity, as well as the laws regarding deriving benefit from a corpse, he makes no specific reference to mumia. There is likewise no discussion of the use of mumia in his responsa. This may support the view that Maimonides prescribed mumia as bitumen, although it is by no means definitive proof.

R. Yehuda Rosanes (d.1727), in his commentary on Maimonides' *Hil. Avel*, addresses the use of Egyptian mumia from a halakhic perspective. (see below)

37. *Ma'asei Adoshem* (E. Grossman's Publishing House: New York, 1962), sect. *Ma'asei Avot*, chap. 17, 97.

There is also an earlier reference to mumia by a physician of the early fourteenth century named Raymund de Tarrega. Like Maimonides, he mentions mumia in a list of medications. It is, therefore, impossible to tell if he refers to mumia the bitumen, or mumia the embalmed body. However, since the list also includes gum arabic, alum, and another clay-like substance, it is likely de Tarrega was prescribing the bitumen. See Raphael Patai, *The Jewish Alchemists* (Princeton University Press, 1994), 198 and 563. Patai, in his footnote, refers to his own article on the topic of mumia and

them, nor to stand in the plain. R. Ashkenazi postulates the possible reason for the latter warning:

> ...and furthermore, God commanded them not to stand in all the flat plains, for it is known that when snow is blown by the winds, and a man or a tree is standing in its path, the snow will overcome and completely cover them. Such is not the case if a man is running....and until today, in the sand-filled deserts, when a strong wind blows the sands, if a man or a tree is in its path, the sand will cover them and form a mound....and until today it is known that sometimes it occurs that a man is unable to withstand the force of the wind-blown sands and he is completely covered by them. Subsequently, another wind blows, and the body is uncovered. The body, found by desert travelers, is brought to the merchants of medicinal spices. They call it mumia and use the dessicated body for the preparation of medical remedies. This is what happened to Lot's wife... when she stood still, the winds blew the salt over her and she became a mound of salt.

R. Ashkenazi served as rabbi and judge in Egypt for over twenty years.[38] It is likely that R. Ashkenazi became exposed during this period to the use of dessicated bodies in the production of mumia. We know from our above discussion that recently deceased, dessicated, unembalmed bodies were used in the manufacture of mumia. Such practices, at least initially, were considered fraudulent, as only the genuine embalmed Egyptian mummies were considered to be of medicinal value. R. Ashkenazi attests to this practice but casts no aspersions upon it. Furthermore, he makes no mention of the other kinds of mumia or the Jewish involvement in the mummy trade. Neither of these topics is relevant to his biblical commentary. One can therefore make no assumptions based on their omission.

---

assumes de Tarrega refers to Egyptian mumia. Whether or not de Tarrega refers to Egyptian mumia, this reference is relevant for the same reasons discussed in the text regarding the reference of Maimonides.

38. Cecil Roth, ed., *Encyclopedia Judaica* (Keter Publishing House), vol. 3, 725, s. v., "Ashkenazi, Eliezer."

The next two sources date from the late nineteenth century and prove that mumia was still in use at this time.[39] The second source, however, objects to its use, not on halakhic grounds, but for medicinal reasons. Both sources refer to the use of mumia in Israel, reflecting the fact that the use of mumia was not restricted to Egypt.

The first reference is found in the work of R. Moshe Reischer entitled *Sha'arei Yerushalayim* (1870), which details the positive traits of the land of Israel, including the customs of its inhabitants.

> The Sephardim make to this day a remedy, mumia, which is pre-
> pared from the ground dry bones of dead people found in the
> desert in the sand. For along the road leading to Mecca there is
> a big desert, and there is a place full of sand which is called the
> Sand Sea. And when a storm arises, it lifts up the sand to a height
> of more than 20 cubits [about 30 feet] and covers everybody who
> happens to be on the road, for a distance of about a mile. And
> people go there and, searching diligently, they find these pieces in
> human form, black and dry as a stone, for even the biggest man
> who is left lying under the sand dries out and becomes as small
> as a finger. And they sell it to apothecaries, and they put it into
> remedies. And the Sephardim, when they have a patient sick for
> many days, God forbid, take it and grind it well and put a certain
> amount of it into honey-water which the patient drinks from time
> to time during three nights. Before he drinks it, they wash him
> and clothe him in a white robe, and lay him on a bed covered with
> a white sheet. Menstruating women are not allowed to enter the
> house as long as the illness of the patient persists, lest this cause
> harm to the patient and to themselves. The patient lies alone, and
> nobody else is with him in the house, not even a hen. Moreover,
> he must beware of the smell of garlic and onions. The only food
> of the patient throughout the nine days is milk, bread, and butter.[40]

---

39. See also Avraham Ben-Yaakov, op. cit.
40. The translation is by Patai, op. cit., 9. He references the 1870 edition of this work. I consulted the Jerusalem, 1967 edition and was unable to find this passage.

R. Reischer mentions exclusively the mumia consisting of the dessicated bodies found in the desert, especially in the Arabian desert on
the road to Mecca. He makes no mention at all of the mumia derived
from embalmed Egyptian bodies. While R. Ashkenazi had a particular reason to mention only the desert mumia, in order to support his
unique commentary of a biblical passage, R. Reischer had no such
agenda. He is simply listing the customs of the land. We can therefore
assume that the use of desert mumia was the normative practice at this
time, perhaps to the exclusion of Egyptian mumia. This may reflect yet
another form of transference of the term mumia from the embalmed
Egyptian mumia, to the more readily obtainable desert mumia which,
although originally a counterfeit substitute of the former, ultimately
supplanted it entirely.

The second source, likewise referring to practices in late nineteenth century Jerusalem, seems to corroborate the theory of this transference, as only desert mumia is mentioned. This source appears in a
journal edited and mostly written by Abraham Luncz, a man who spent
most of his life working to perfect his geograghical knowledge, especially
of Jerusalem.[41] The passage on mumia appears under the chapter heading *Emunat Hevel*, literally translated as belief in nonsense. In a footnote
to the title he states that the following practices have been adopted by
women and fools. Wise and intelligent men, however, not only themselves refrain from such practices, but castigate others who believe in
such nonsense.[42] We know from historical sources that already in the
sixteenth century people questioned the value of mumia, albeit in reference to Egyptian mumia.[43] But despite proclamations against mumia,
its use continued at least until the end of the nineteenth century, as evidenced by the following passage, which includes the author's footnote.

By this name [mumia] is called in Arabic a piece of bone which
has become completely black. [footnote:] According to what the

---

41. Cecil Roth, ed., *Encyclopedia Judaica* (Keter Publishing House), vol. 11, 564–565.
42. Abraham Moses Luncz, *Yerushalayim* 1 (1882), 20, n. 40.
43. See, for example, Lynn Thorndyke, A *History of Magic and Experimental Science*, 8
     (Columbia University Press, 1958), 414.

children of the land of the east say, this bone can be found in the sandy desert of Arabia, and it is a part of the bodies of people who were buried among the waves of that sea of sand while on their way to Mecca or to the other cities of that country, and from the great and burning heat, their bones hardened, became black and exceedingly small, like the form of embalmed bodies. The mumia is offered for sale in Arab pharmacies of medicine and charms. The price of a dirham [drachma] is about 5 piasters, and those who buy a large quantity of it can see in it the shape of the member from which it is derived [end of footnote]. Its power is such as to heal all illness and disease, and especially sudden and unsual ones.

This drug is prepared in the following manner: a certain quantity of mumia, or a part of the black bone, is pounded in a mortar to thin powder, and sometimes they mix some honey and spices into it, and a handful of it is placed on the roof for the night so that the dew descends upon it, or they put it in a coffee cup, and the patient drinks this balm of Gilead for nine successive nights. On the fifth and ninth day, before he drinks of it they wash his body, wrap him from head to toe in white clothes, and a man or a woman sits next to him all night to watch him, for they believe that the two nights are most dangerous for the patient. The patient's food during this period consists of bread, butter and milk only, and they also take care lest the patient inhale any strong smell, and especially the smell of garlic, onions, and fish. Women who are in their menses must not enter the house throughout that period, lest they cause damage to the patient and to themselves, and in general, very few people visit them.

The neighbors who live in the same courtyard, and who believe this nonsense, are very much afraid lest the power of the mumia affect them adversely, and they therefore leave their houses for several days, or, if they do not care about the state of the patient and the improvement of his health, they will draw on the door of his house the picture of a hand which is a well known amulet, and then the power of the mumia is broken, and it will neither help nor harm the patient. Therefore, if the patient is apprehensive lest his neighbors perform this contrary act, he will do everything in secret, unknown to anybody.[44]

Use of Mumia in Legal Sources

Assuming that Maimonides prescribed bitumen, and that Elmagar lived at the latest possible date, then we find the first prescription of Egyptian mumia around 1300. Despite this apparent early usage of Egyptian mumia, it is not until the sixteenth century that we find the first recorded reference to mumia in rabbinic responsa literature.

R. David Ben Abi Zimra (1479–1573), known as Radbaz, served as leader of the Egyptian community for about forty years, until 1553, when he emigrated to Palestine. He was asked the following question: "On what basis do people use as a medicinal remedy the flesh of corpses called mumia? They use it even in cases where there is no grave danger... and they trade in it as well. This should be forbidden, for as we know, it is forbidden to derive benefit from the flesh of a corpse?"[45]

Radbaz justifies the use of mumia, despite the biblical prohibition of deriving benefit from a corpse, on a number of grounds. Regarding the ingestion of mumia, he states, there is surely no problem, "For mumia is the embalmed flesh that is embalmed with many spices... and it becomes an asphalt-like substance (*k'ein zephet*). Therefore [since it has has lost its original identity], it is permissible to eat." Furthermore, he states, when one eats mumia, one does not derive benefit from the part of mumia that derives from the flesh of the corpse, "for spices are mixed with it [mumia]. It is not from the flesh that one obtains [medicinal] benefit, but rather from the spices that are contained therein. Proof of this is that unembalmed corpses are of no [medicinal] value."

The above logic of Radbaz is employed to permit the eating of mumia for medicinal purposes. In such a case, he argues, there is no benefit derived from the corpse (*shelo kiderekh hana'ato*). With regard to selling mumia, however, no such leniency exists, since the merchant is profiting from the sale of corpses. As a result, Radbaz uses a different line of reasoning to permit the trade of mumia. He concludes that there

---

44. Translation by Patai, op. cit., 9–10.
45. *Teshuvot HaRadbaz* vol. 3, no. 979 (548).

is no halakhic prohibition of deriving benefit from non-Jewish corpses. As mumia clearly derives from non-Jewish bodies, there is therefore no prohibition to engage in the mummy trade.

A number of important points can be gleaned from this responsum. Historical sources indicate that mumia was a commonly prescribed drug in Egypt and that the Jews were involved in its trade. As mumia consisted partially of the flesh of a corpse, its use and trade presented unique halakhic problems. Radbaz, living in Egypt, the center or the mumia trade, appears to be the first to address this problem.[46]

Although mumia was apparently first prescribed by Elmagar, its use did not become widespread until centuries later. This may explain why it is only in the time of Radbaz that the halakhic aspects of the use of mumia were addressed. The wording of the question to Radbaz, however, implies that mumia had already been in use for some time, and the response reflects a de facto approval of a pre-existing practice. It is unclear, however, how long mumia was in use before this responsum was written. In any case, it represents the first in a series of halakhic discussions that span over one hundred years and that address a contemporary halakhic problem.

The resolution of medical halakhic problems requires an understanding of the medical realities. Radbaz's decision was partially dependent on his understanding of that reality, as it related to the drug mumia. He described the nature of mumia as being asphalt-like, and he claimed that the medicinal value of mumia lay in the embalming materials (i.e., the asphalt or bitumen) and not in the body of the deceased. As described above, mumia underwent a gradual transference from bitumen to the embalmed body, for which bitumen was apparently used. Radbaz's understanding reflects a stage in that transference. At this period in history, mumia had already become associated with the embalmed body, but it had not completely lost its original association with bitumen, the true medicinal remedy. While Radbaz actually describes the final product of mumia as like *zephet*, or bitumen, he does not acknowledge, nor was he likely aware, that originally mumia was in fact synonymous

---

46. This is evidenced by the fact that subsequent rabbinic authorities who deal with mumia refer to Radbaz, either concurring or disagreeing with his conclusions.

with *zephet*. He also clearly states that the true medicinal remedy is contained in the embalming materials (i.e., the bitumen or original mumia), and not in the corpse, here also reflecting an intermediate stage of the transference. With the completion of the transference, the corpse acquires the primary medicinal value, independent of the bitumen or other embalming materials.

Mumia is next mentioned in a passing reference by R. Jacob Castro (1525–1610), who permitted the eating and selling of mumia based on the premise of Radbaz, that mumia is mere dust.[47] R. Castro was an Egyptian rabbi and based many of his decisions on his predecessor, Radbaz.[48]

R. Abraham ben Mordechai Halevi (late seventeenth century), also an Egyptian rabbi, treats the topic of mumia more extensively.[49] The question posed to him, however, adds a new element to the halakhic discussion:

> I was asked regarding the mumia in Egypt, whether the laws of *tum'ah* [ritual defilement] apply to it with respect to a *Kohen*, and whether it is permissible to eat it and trade in it.

While Radbaz had alluded to the notion of *tum'ah* peripherally, for R. Abraham Halevi this issue takes prominence. In order to appropriately address the issue of *tum'ah* for mumia, the author displays an intimate knowledge of its composition in his detailed discussion about whether mumia contains

---

47. Patai, op. cit., 11, n. 21 references R. Castro's work, *Erekh Lehem* (Constantinople, 1718), 391:1, as the source for this quote. It should be noted that this is a misprint, as the relevant passage is found at no. 349. R. Abraham ben Mordechai Halevi also cites R. Castro in his *Ginat Veradim* (Constantinople, 1716), Y. D., 1, no. 4.

Yet another incorrect citation of R. Castro appears in R. Abraham Eisenstadt's *Pithei Teshuva*, Y. D., 349:2, where he cites "BH"T shel HaMaharit," as the source of a quote which is, in fact, from the aforementioned work of R. Castro. It appears that it should have read Maharik (Morenu HaRav Yaakov Castro) instead of Maharit. The acronym BH"T also appears to be a misprint, perhaps intended to be BH"K, *BeHilkhot Kria*, which is where the citation is found.

48. R. Castro's work, *Sefer Maharikash HaNikra Erekh Lehem* (Constantinople, 1718) is replete with references to the responsa of Radbaz.

49. *Ginat Veradim*, op. cit.

the requisite volume of a *kezayit* (size of an olive) of the corpse in order to generate *tum'ah* (i.e., convey ritual impurity). Mere volume, however, is not sufficient for the prohibition of *tum'ah*; this *kezayit* must be somewhat solid, so as not to crumble easily. According to R. Abraham Halevi, mumia fulfills both of these criteria and therefore conveys ritual impurity.

> Based on what we have written above… the law of *tum'ah* applies to a *kezayit* of flesh of mumia because it does not crumble unless it is crushed. Even though the mumia only achieves this solid state by virtue of being mixed with spices and salves, without which the mumia would be a pile of dust, still, we are… only concerned with its present state.

Like R. Castro, R. Abraham Halevi then quotes Radbaz. However, in contradistinction to R. Castro, he strongly disagrees with Radbaz's conclusions. He enumerates the premises for Radbaz's permissive ruling, then negates them one by one. What is particularly interesting is that the author questions Radbaz's conclusions not only on halakhic grounds, but on medical grounds as well. Radbaz claimed that the value of mumia lies in the embalming spices and not in the flesh of the corpse; hence, one in essence does not derive benefit from the corpse itself. R. Abraham Halevi had a different medical opinion:

> Regarding [Radbaz's] second reason [for permitting mumia], even though there is great value in these spices and salves… still, there is medicinal value to the limbs of the corpse… the reason why they do not use the flesh of unembalmed corpses is because the flesh decays and therefore loses its value. The spices that are used in mumia, however, prevent decay and preserve the medicinal value of the flesh of the corpse forever.

R. Abraham Halevi, who lived about one century after Radbaz, attributes medicinal value to the corpse itself.[50] This reflects the completion of the

---

50. In the seventeenth century, there were many who prescribed medicines derived from living human beings (e.g., urine, feces or saliva) as well as from human cadavers. See

transference, for now it is the body which becomes the primary mumia, independent of the embalming materials. Moreover, the embalming process is viewed here as effectively preserving the otherwise temporary medicinal value of the flesh of the corpse.

In addition to the different medical understanding, R. Abraham Halevi also disagrees with Radbaz about two major halakhic points. First, he maintains that even if the ingestion of mumia is in a manner not involving clear benefit or enjoyment from the flesh of the corpse (*shelo kederekh hana'ato*), as Radbaz claims is the case, it should still be prohibited on halakhic grounds. Second, he opines, as opposed to Radbaz, that it is prohibited to derive benefit from a corpse, even if the body belongs to a non-Jew. Consequently, R. Abraham Halevi prohibits both the eating of and trading in mumia, for both priest and Israelite alike. He is apparently the first to have so ruled.

Our final primary halakhic reference to mumia is the commentary of R. Yehuda Rosanes (1657–1727) to the *Mishneh Torah* of Maimonides. R. Rosanes is the first of our discussants not to have lived in Egypt, as he he was born and lived his entire life in Turkey. However, at this period in history, Egypt was under Turkish rule, making cultural exchange between these two countries likely.

In three separate places, R. Rosanes addresses the issues related to the use of mumia.[51] While he does not directly refer to the previous responsa of Radbaz or R. Abraham Halevi,[52] he discusses the identical issues of deriving benefit from a corpse, and whether or not mumia constitutes a source of ritual defilement. He addresses these issues with respect to both Jewish and non-Jewish corpses.

Thorndyke, op. cit., vol. 8, 415; Ofir Shemesh, op. cit., 52–104. The use of parts of cadavers in medicine cannot be attributed solely to the transference from the use of mumia, but in this context, it appears to be the case.

51. *Hil. Ma'akhalot Assurot*, chap. 8, no. 18; *Hil. Avel*, chap. 3, no. 1; ibid., chap. 14, no. 21.

52. In R. Rosanes' glosses on *Hil. Avel*, chap. 3, no. 1 there is a note in parentheses referring the reader to the work *Ginat Veradim* of R. Abraham Halevi. It is unclear to me, however, whether this note was written by the author or added by an editor. In either case, the works of Radbaz and R. Abraham Halevi are interestingly not discussed in the body of the text in any of the three references of R. Rosanes to mumia.

Whereas the question to R. Abraham Halevi indicated that priests were somehow involved in the use of mumia, he did not stipulate whether they were consumers or traders. The question to R. Rosanes was less ambiguous: "I was asked about the mumia which is sold by *Kohanim* [priests]. Is it proper for them to do this or not?"

Like his predecessors, R. Rosanes was concerned with the constitution of mumia, as it relates to its status of ritual defilement:

> According to what I have heard, this mumia contains no flesh at all, rather just bones covered by skin. [The bones] are very dry with no residual moisture from the flesh. I asked whether these bones crumble spontaneously, and they told me that not only do they not crumble, but it is difficult to break them. Based on this, there is no doubt whatsoever that [mumia] imparts ritual impurity.[53]

R. Rosanes makes no mention whatsoever of spices or salves mixed in with the mumia. As a result, he does not raise the issue, as R. Abraham Halevi had, of whether the spices mixed with the mumia affect the measuring of the requisite olive's bulk for ritual defilement. It is possible that the mumia that he was told about was the desert mumia, which, in fact, contained no spices. This may reflect the transference from Egyptian mumia to desert mumia.

Unlike his predecessors, R. Rosanes split his decision. Radbaz and R. Abraham Halevi had decided to uniformly either permit or forbid the use of mumia, respectively. R. Rosanes, on the other hand, permitted the use and trade of mumia by an Israelite, as he considered mumia to be as mere dust, like the position of Radbaz.[54] However, with respect to *tum'ah*, he agreed with the position of R. Abraham Halevi that mumia imparts ritual impurity. Consequently, he forbade the handling of mumia by *Kohanim*.[55]

---

53. Ibid.
54. *Hil. Ma'akhalot Assurot*, chap. 9, no. 18 (end).
55. *Hil. Avel*, chap. 3, no. 1 (end).

IV. CONCLUSION

Mumia is a topic in medical halakhic history from the sixteenth to the nineteenth centuries that illustrates how an appreciation of medical history can enlighten one's understanding of the Jewish sources. It can now be understood why the responsa cover this particular period. Prior to the time of Radbaz, mumia was prescribed as the bitumen, but only in the time of Radbaz did the use of mumia derived from embalmed or dessicated bodies become widespread. Living in Egypt, the center of the mumia trade, Radbaz is the first to address this issue.

The last of the halakhic authorities to deal with mumia is R. Rosanes, who died in the early eighteenth century. Historical sources state that the mumia trade, which was dominated by Jews, either significantly decreased or possibly ceased in the seventeenth century. The work of R. Rosanes confirms that the trade of mumia by Jews continued into the late seventeenth and possibly early eighteenth centuries. The absence of any later responsa correlates with the diminution of the mumia trade. The two non-halakhic sources from nineteenth century Jerusalem reflect the residual and peripheral use of mumia, relegated at that stage to folklore, as opposed to mainstream medicine.

All the rabbinic figures who grappled with the halakhic problems of mumia lived in Egypt, or in the Turkish empire, of which Egypt was a part. Given the general history of the mumia trade, and the significant role the Jews played, these responsa, taken collectively, represent a halakhic response to a pressing medical halakhic dilemma. The testimonies from multiple sources indicate that the livelihood of many Jews in the Egyptian community would likely have been affected by a rabbinic decision on the permissibility of trading in mumia.

Despite the fact that each of these rabbinic authorities over a period of roughly two centuries was discussing a drug called mumia, the understanding of the nature and constitution of this drug changed from responsum to responsum, influencing the respective decisions accordingly. An appreciation of the evolution and transference of the term mumia gives us a better appreciation of the details of the halakhic discussions as well as an understanding of the apparent inconsistencies between them. The historical analysis also reveals that each rabbinic authority was well versed with the practice of medicine at his time.

This approach to the history of mumia is but one example of how medical history and medical halakha can be integrated in order to provide a more comprehensive understanding of the medical halakhic decision-making process throughout the ages.

A Tale of Two Stones in the Eighteenth Century

I. INTRODUCTION

A recurring theme throughout this book is that while the principles of halakha are immutable, the corpus of medical and scientific theories has changed considerably with the passage of time. As a result, when analyzing a medical halakhic text from any pre-twentieth century period, it is imperative not only to acknowledge that the medical theories discussed in the text may differ from our own, but also to understand those theories in order to best appreciate and extrapolate from the halakhic nuances of the text. This chapter highlights the need for sensitivity to historical context as it analyzes two rabbinic sources from the eighteenth century that both discuss a particular disease and its treatment. The contemporary history of this disease is presented for the purpose of clarifying the ambiguities of the texts, as well as preventing possible anachronistic interpretations and halakhic misapplications.

II. THE RESPONSUM OF RABBI
YEḤEZKEL LANDAU (1713–1793)

On the topic of autopsies and Jewish law, a responsum authored by R. Yeḥezkel Landau serves as a foundation for legal discussions.[1] In this eighteenth century responsum, the question posed to R. Landau regarded a particular clinical scenario for which an autopsy was requested.

The text of the query reads as follows:

> ... in the matter of the query from London regarding one who fell ill with *"ḥoli ha'even bekiso"* and underwent surgery, as was customary practice for this particular ailment, and subsequently died. The elders of the city were then asked if it was permissible to dissect the corpse in the relevant [anatomical] area for the express purpose of learning how to better deal with a similar surgical case in the future. The results of such a dissection would potentially allow the physicians to minimize the surgical incision for subsequent patients, thereby decreasing the mortality of the procedure. Is such a procedure forbidden because of the desecration to the body, or is it permitted because of the potential future life-saving value of the information?[2]

The Hebrew medical terminology employed by R. Landau may seem ambiguous to the modern reader. The phrase *"even bekiso"* is translated literally as "a stone in his pouch (or bladder)." Taken in its medical context, the term refers to calculi, or stones, found in a hollow organ, the likely possibilities being either gallbladder or urinary bladder. Contemporary authors quoting this reference are often unsure which of the two it is.[3] The term *"kis"* in modern terminology can refer to either the

---

1. *Noda BiYehuda*, Y. D., 210. This chapter does not deal with the halakhic aspects of performing an autopsy. Reviews on this topic can be found in A. Steinberg, *Entzyclopedia Hilkhatit Refuit* 4 (Jerusalem, 1994), 528–599. See also Kalman Kahana, "Autopsy in Halakha—A Bibliography," (in Hebrew), *HaMa'ayan*, 7:2 (1966), 43–72.
2. Loose translation by the author.
3. See I. Jakobovitz, *Jewish Medical Ethics* (New York, 1959), 146, who translates the phrase as a "calculus in the bladder"—a literal translation—without specifying which bladder. F. Rosner, "Autopsy in Jewish Law and the Israeli Autopsy Controversy," in

gallbladder or the urinary bladder, but in either case, the noun is usually followed by an adjective (e.g., *kis hamara*, gallblabber; or *kis hasheten*, urinary bladder). When the term *kis* appears alone, it may be difficult to determine which of the two is being discussed. Only an understanding of medical history, in conjunction with the context, will provide us with a definitive answer.

III. PASSAGE FROM RABBI YAAKOV EMDEN (D. 1776)

In the context of addressing the halakhic aspects of the risks and benefits of certain procedures, R. Emden also discusses a medical condition called *even bekis* for which surgery is indicated:

> ...some choose to risk their lives in order to save themselves from great suffering, such as those who undergo surgery for a stone [*even*] in the *kis*, the penis, or the kidneys, which causes them tremendous pain and anguish. These people undergo the procedure as they wish, without rebuke, for sometimes they are healed thereby. However, they should exercise caution. Anyone who does not suffer harm from the pain should not undergo the procedure, even on a weekday. It is not permitted for a person to enter a situation of potential danger even though many have done so and been saved. Many have also done so [undergone surgery] and hastened their deaths thereby. It is, therefore, not permitted [to undergo surgery for the aforementioned conditions] under any circumstance, even on a weekday.[4]

What is the condition of *"even bekis"* mentioned by R. Emden, and is it the same medical condition mentioned by R. Landau? What is the history of this particular disease, and would it have bearing on the halakhic interpretation of these texts?

F. Rosner and J. D. Bleich, eds., *Jewish Bioethics* (New York, 1979), 333, likewise states that the case refers to a bladder calculus. In a parenthetical note, however, he adds, "probably urinary bladder, but possibly gallbladder."

4. *Mor Uetzia*, n. 328. Translation by the author. For an exposition on the halakhic aspects of experimental procedures, see J. D. Bleich, *Contemporary Halakhic Problems* 4 (Ktav, 1995), 203–217.

IV. MEDICAL HISTORY

As mentioned above, *"even bekis"* could theoretically refer to either urinary bladder stones or gallbladder stones. It is, therefore, essential to discuss the history of the treatment of both conditions in order to help clarify which is being referred to.[5] Furthermore, it is clear from both of the aforementioned sources that surgery was the customary treatment for this disorder.

The existence of gallstones has been known for centuries, the earliest known description being that of Alexander of Tralles (525–605 CE), the Byzantine physician. But despite the knowledge of their existence and association with disease, it was not until the late eighteenth century that a Frenchman named Herlin suggested that the human gallbladder be removed for the treatment of gallstones. The first such surgery was only successfully performed over a century later by Carl Johan August Langenbuch of Berlin, in 1882.[6]

With respect to bladder stones, on the other hand, varying forms of surgery have been performed for their removal since antiquity. In eighteenth century England (the time and place from whence the query to R. Landau originated), there were a number of major advances in the field of bladder stone surgery. In the early part of the century, John Douglas (d. 1743) developed a new procedure called the "high" or suprapubic lithotomy.[7] William Cheselden (1688–1752), although initially an advocate of the "high" lithotomy,[8] pioneered a new variation on the old technique, known as the "lateral" lithotomy.[9] The so-called "high" lithotomy was associated with terrible complications and a very high mortality rate. Only in the hands of the expert stone-cutter William Cheselden, using the modified lateral lithotomy, did the mortality rate of urinary bladder

---

5. I will only address the historical aspects of these diseases that are directly relevant to our discussion. For a comprehensive discussion on the history of the treatment of urinary bladder stones, see H. Ellis, *A History of Bladder Stones* (Oxford, 1970).

6. K. Haeger, *The Illustrated History of Surgery* (New York, 1988), 227.

7. T. Woodward, *Lithotomia Douglassiana; or, An Account of a New Method of Making the High Operation, in order to extract the stone out of the bladder* (London, 1720).

8. Haeger, op. cit., 147.

9. A. Reid, "A Remarkable Case of a Person Cut for the Stone in the New Way, Commonly Called the Lateral; by William Cheselden," *Philosophical Transactions* 44 (1746), 33–35.

stone surgery drop to ten percent, a success rate unheard of until that time.[10] No other surgeon came close to his statistics.

In light of the above, it is quite clear that the query posed to R. Landau was referring to a case of urinary bladder stones.[11] For only in cases of urinary bladder stones, not gallbladder stones, was surgery the customary practice in the late eighteenth century. Although surgery for the treatment of gallstones was theorized at that time, it was not for another century that such surgery was successfully performed.[12] It was, therefore, not necessary for the query to specify which *kis* contained the stones, as it would have been evident to any contemporary reader that only patients with urinary bladder stones undergo surgery.

The use of the phrase *even bekis* by R. Emden is less ambiguous and clearly refers to urinary bladder stones, as it is mentioned in the context of a discussion of stones found in other areas of the urogenital system, such as the kidney and the penile urethra.

V. HALAKHIC RAMIFICATIONS

Having established that R. Landau was referring to a case of urinary bladder stones, what are the possible halakhic ramifications? In his analysis, R. Landau developed a principle that would become the cornerstone of legal discussions on the halakhic permissibility of performing autopsies. The existing prohibitions against performing an autopsy could be waved, he claimed, if there was a "*holeh lefaneinu*," literally translated as "a sick person before us."[13] The interpretation of this key phrase has been a subject of debate.[14]

---

10. Haeger, op. cit., 147.
11. For a review of the rabbinic literature dealing with stones in the urogenital system, see Abraham Ofir Shemesh, "*Holeh HaEven: Avanim BeDarkei HaSheten*," Assia 79–80 (January 2007), 57–76.
12. Samuel James Meltzer (1851–1920) was the first to suggest non-surgical drainage of the gallbladder. See his "The Disturbance of the Law of Contrary Innervation as a Pathogenetic Factor in the Diseases of the Bile Ducts and the Gallbladder," *American Journal of Medical Science* 153 (1917), 469–477.
13. R. Moses Sofer is responsible for coining this phrase in his responsum Y. D., 336.
14. See chapter, "The Anatomy of Halakha." Much has been written on this topic. See, for example, Hazon Ish, *Hil. Avelut*, 208:7; R. Shlomo Goren, "The Study of Anatomy

Interpreted in its narrowest sense, it means that an autopsy is permitted only if there is a designated beneficiary of the resulting information. Alternatively, the interpretation might be broadened to include use of the information for treatment of a prevalent illness, as such an illness might fit the definition of "*ḥoleh lefaneinu*."[15]

To argue the latter interpretation, either as the opinion of R. Landau himself or as an independent extension of R. Landau's principle, one must consider how R. Landau himself ruled, given the prevalence of the disease in question. Here, an understanding of medical history can be helpful. Urinary bladder stones were in fact prevalent in England. It is safe to say that at the time the query was posed, there would have been a number of people currently suffering with urinary bladder stones. Yet, despite this fact, R. Landau still ruled that an autopsy to benefit other potential patients with this disease would be forbidden.[16]

Not only is an understanding of the prevalence of disease important, an awareness of the mortality rate of a disease at a particular time may also impact on the interpretation of halakha, as evidenced by the aforementioned passage from R. Emden. It is interesting to note that R. Emden considered the mortality rate of the surgery for urinary bladder stones to be too high to allow the procedure to be performed routinely. The modern reader may be unaware of the fact that the mortality rates for urinary bladder stone surgery in the eighteenth century were roughly 40–50%. If one were to assume that the mortality rates were similar to

---

in Medical School," (Hebrew), *Meorot* (Spring 1980), 5–17; Yaakov Levi, "*HaHoleh Lefaneinu*," in *Assia* 1 (1989), 202–215. See also R. J. D. Bleich, *Contemporary Halakhic Problems* 4 (Ktav, 1995), 188–192.

15. See Ḥazon Ish, op. cit. However, his remarks expanding the principle of "*ḥoleh lefaneinu*" are restricted to contagious diseases (e.g., plague) where the potential for currently healthy people to contract the disease is great, and the disease is truly "*lefaneinu*," present, albeit not in a specific location. Many have argued that in the modern era, when information is disseminated both widely and rapidly, there can virtually always be found a figurative "*ḥoleh lefaneinu*." See Levi, op. cit.

16. One can speculate that while urinary bladder stones may have been prevalent in England, this may not have been the case in Eastern Europe, the domain of R. Landau. Had R. Landau been aware of the high prevalence of the disease in England, he may have permitted the autopsy.

today, or even, for example, ten times higher than today, roughly 5–10%,[17] then the opinion of R. Emden is considerably strict, completely forbidding routine surgery with a relatively low mortality rate. However, knowing that the rates were roughly 40–50% mortality leads us to a more lenient interpretation. High risk procedures, as defined and prohibited by R. Emden, would involve mortality rates of 40–50%. Procedures with lower mortality rates would be permitted.

VI. CONCLUSION

In this chapter, we have provided some historical context to rabbinic sources that are used frequently in contemporary medical halakhic discussions about autopsy and surgical risk. Many today are unfamiliar with the medical reality and context contemporaneous with these sources. This could possibly lead to misinterpretation. While mistaking the exact disease or condition under discussion may, by itself, be of little consequence, failure to appreciate the statistical realities with which the rabbinic authorities were operating could possibly lead to misapplication of their halakhic conclusions.

---

17. Today, a mortality rate of 10% would be considered very high for such a procedure.

The Use of Anesthesia in Circumcision: A Reevaluation of the Halakhic Sources

I. INTRODUCTION

The application of halakha to medical dilemmas is unique in that medical halakhic decisions require continual reevaluation based on medical advances. A decision at one point in time may not necessarily apply to a later point in time, where medical realities may necessitate a fresh or updated approach.

Such a reevaluation is required for the halakhic sources dealing with the use of anesthesia for circumcision. Given our modern understanding of medicine, as well as the development of new and safer anesthetics, we must re-assess the existing halakhic literature on this topic for contemporary relevance and applicability. It may be that former analyses and conclusions are equally applicable to our modern context, but this conclusion can only be drawn after careful analysis of both medical and halakhic literature. Furthermore, the halakhic sources must be understood in their proper medical historical milieu, as scientific and medical knowledge have evolved over time.

The objective of this chapter is to provide an overview of the halakhic discussions throughout history relating to the use of anesthesia for *mila* (ritual circumcision). The halakhic approaches to the use of both general and local anesthesia are presented, prefaced by a section on the history of anesthesia and a review of the current medical literature on the use of anesthesia for circumcision. After analysis of the halakhic sources, their contemporary applicability is discussed.

II. HISTORY OF ANESTHESIA

Throughout history, efforts have been made to alleviate human suffering that accompanies both naturally occurring illness, as well as surgical interventions.[1] Opium, hashish, mandragora (mandrake) root, and coca leaves have been used as analgesic, soporific, and narcotic agents for thousands of years. The coca leaf was known to numb the tongue and gums when chewed and was used as a crude form of local anesthetic.[2] Alcoholic beverages were used to dull the sensorium of patients to a degree that would allow the tolerance of minor surgical interventions. It was only in the nineteenth century, however, that both general and local anesthesia were perfected and applied routinely in surgical procedures.[3]

By the mid-nineteenth century, general anesthesia was being used to perform major surgical procedures. When general anesthesia was first used for childbirth, in 1846, there was opposition from a minority

---

1. For a general history of anesthesia from antiquity to modern times, see V. Robinson, *Victory over Pain* (Harry Schuman, 1946) and M. H. Armstrong Davison, *The Evolution of Anesthesia* (John Sherratt, 1965). See also, H. Glaser, *The Road to Modern Surgery* (E. P. Dutton and Co., 1962), 11–32; G. Williams, *The Age of Miracles: Medicine and Surgery in the Nineteenth Century* (Academy Chicago Publishers, 1987), 39–56; K. Haeger, *The Illustrated History of Surgery* (Beli Publishing Co., 1988), 184–193; I. M. Rutkow, *Surgery: An Illustrated History* (Mosby Publishers, 1993), 331–339.
2. H. Glaser, op. cit., 25–30.
3. Although ether, nitrous oxide, and chloroform had been discovered by the early nineteenth century, it was not until 1846 that general anesthesia was successfully used for surgical procedures. The new discovery was announced to the world by Dr. Henry Bigelow in an article in the November 18 edition of the *Boston Medical and Surgical Journal*, entitled, "Insensibility During Surgical Operations Produced by Inhalation."

of religious Christians, who maintained that the Bible in Genesis 3:16 mandates that childbirth be painful for all womankind. Alleviation or elimination of the pain of childbirth, it was argued, runs counter to the divine will. In fact, James Young Simpson, the first to apply anesthesia in obstetrics, published a pamphlet entitled *Answer to Religious Objections Advanced Against the Employment of Anaesthetic Agents in Midwifery and Surgery*"[4] While there does not appear to have been any halakhic objections at that time to the use of anesthesia in childbirth (see below), ironically, it is a Jew who was solicited by a medical journal in 1849 to interpret the biblical curse in Genesis. R. Abraham de Sola, then the newly appointed Chief Rabbi of Canada and lecturer in Hebrew language at McGill University, wrote an essay, drawing on rabbinic and early Hebrew grammatical literature, asserting that the biblical curse does not preclude the use of anesthesia for childbirth.[5]

Rudimentary forms of local anesthesia have also been known since antiquity,[6] but chemically synthesized forms, systematically applied in the practice of medicine, were only introduced in the 1880s, after Karl Koller isolated the active ingredient from the coca leaf and called it cocaine.[7] To this day, cocaine and its derivatives are used for local and topical anesthesia.

---

4. (Sutherland and Knox, 1847). See also P. Smith, *Scriptural Authority for the Mitigation of the Pains of Labour by Chloroform and Other Anaesthetic Agents* (S. Highly, 1848). For comments on both the Christian and Jewish approaches to the pain of childbirth, see I. Jakobovits, *Jewish Medical Ethics* (Bloch Publishing Co., 1959), 103–104 and notes. On the general opposition to early obstetric anesthesia, including religious, see A. D. Farr, "Early Opposition to Obstetric Anaesthesia," *Anaesthesia* 35 (1980), 896–907.

5. Abraham De Sola, "Critical Examination of Genesis III, 16, Having Reference to the Employment of Anaesthetics in Cases of Labour," *British American Journal of Medical Science* 5 (1849–1850), 227–229, 259–262, and 290–293. See also J. Cohen, "Doctor James Simpson Young, Rabbi Abraham De Sola, and Genesis Chapter 3, Verse 16," *Obstetrics and Gynecology* 88:5 (1996), 895–898.

6. Robinson, op. cit., 15–22.

7. Robinson, op. cit., "The Beginnings of Local Anesthesia," 237–256, as well as sections in sources cited in note 4, above.

III. USE OF ANESTHESIA FOR CIRCUMCISION—
MEDICAL LITERATURE[8]

Over the past several decades, the American Academy of Pediatrics has published several policy statements on neonatal circumcision of the male infant. Beginning with its manual on the hospital care of newborns in 1971,[9] and in revisions published in 1975[10] and 1983,[11] the Academy clearly stated that there was no absolute medical indication for routine circumcision.

The Academy's 1989 statement cited new research that suggested that circumcised males had fewer urinary tract infections and were also at lower risk of developing sexually transmitted diseases.[12]

At that time, the Academy concluded that newborn male circumcision has potential medical benefits and advantages, as well as disadvantages and risks, and recommended that parents should be told of both to enable them to reach an informed decision about circumcision in their newborn boys. Early in 1999, the Academy published a new circumcision policy statement which concludes that:

> [E]xisting scientific evidence demonstrates potential medical benefits of newborn male circumcision; however, these data are not sufficient to recommend routine neonatal circumcision. In circumstances in which there are potential benefits and risks, yet the procedure is not essential to the child's current well-being, parents should determine what is in the best interest of the child. To make an informed choice, parents of all male infants should be given accurate and unbiased information and be provided the

---

8. Dr. Fred Rosner authored this section.
9. *American Academy of Pediatrics, Committee on Fetus and Newborn. Standards and Recommendations for Hospital Care of Newborn Infants*, 5th ed. (American Academy of Pediatrics, 1971).
10. "American Academy of Pediatrics, Committee on the Fetus and Newborn. Report of the Ad Hoc Task Force on Circumcision," Pediatrics 56:4 (1975), 610–611.
11. *American Academy of Pediatrics, Committee on Fetus and Newborn. Guidelines for Perinatal Care*, 1st ed. (American Academy of Pediatrics, 1983).
12. "American Academy of Pediatrics. Report of the Task Force on Circumcision," *Pediatrics* 84 (1989), 388–391.

opportunity to discuss this decision. If a decision for circumcision is made, procedural analgesia should be provided.[13]

The benefits of circumcision include the virtual absence of penile cancer in circumcised males, the lower frequency of urinary tract infections in circumcised infants and children, and the lower risk of contracting sexually transmitted diseases including HIV infection in circumcised men compared to uncircumcised males. The risks of the procedure, such as infection and/or bleeding, are very rare when circumcision is performed by experienced physicians or *mohelim* (Jewish ritual circumcisers).

The 1999 statement of the American Academy of Pediatrics recommended, for the first time, that pain relief be provided for neonatal circumcision. This recommendation may or may not be acceptable to Jews, Muslims, and others to whom circumcision is a religious commandment and who do not require any medical or social justification for its performance. The Academy recognized this fact when it incorporated into its statement the phrase, "it is legitimate for parents to take into account cultural, religious, and ethnic traditions, in addition to medical factors, when making this decision." While this policy has been revisited and updated as recently as 2017, there has been no change to the recommendations of analgesia.

Pain and Pain Relief for Neonatal Circumcision

There is considerable evidence that newborns experience pain and physiologic stress during circumcision as manifested by crying, changes in heart rate, blood pressure, oxygen saturation, and cortisol levels.[14]

---

13. "American Academy of Pediatrics. Task Force on Circumcision. Circumcision Policy Statement," *Pediatrics* 103 (1999), 686–693.
14. L. M. Talbert, E. N. Kraybill, H. D. Potter, "Adrenal Cortical Response to Circumcision in the Neonate," *Obstetrics and Gynecology* 48 (1976), 208–210; M. R. Gunnar, et al., "The Effects of Circumcision on Serum Cortisol and Behavior," *Psychoneuronendocrinology* 6 (1981), 269–275; D. J. Rawlings, et al., "The Effect of Circumcision on Transcutaneous PO2 in Term Infants," *American Journal of Diseases of Children* 134 (1980), 676–678; P. S. Williamson, M. L. Williamson, "Physiologic Stress Reduction by a Local Anesthetic During Newborn Circumcision," *Pediatrics* 71 (1983), 36–40.

There is wide acceptance in the medical community of the use of analgesia for neonatal circumcision. The three most widely used methods are the topical application of EMLA (acronym for eutectic mixture of local anesthetics) cream,[15] dorsal penile nerve block (DPNB),[16] and subcutaneous ring block.[17] Comparisons of these three methods suggest that ring block is the most effective anesthetic.[18] None of these methods are without rare side effects. Two cases of methemoglobinemia have been reported in infants after EMLA cream application.[19] Furthermore, "there are no studies that adequately address safety or efficacy" of the use of EMLA cream for newborn circumcision.[20] The risks of DPNB and ring block include infection; mechanical, neural, or other tissue damage from the needle; and toxic reactions to anesthetic drug. These complications are rare and usually not serious.[21]

Newborn babies routinely receive intramuscular vitamin K. Newborn screening for a variety of treatable conditions requires heel stick or venipuncture, all painful experiences. Yet, very few physicians recommend topical analgesia for venipuncture.[22]

15. A. Taddio, et al., "Efficacy and Safety of Lidocaine Prilocaine Cream for Pain During Circumcision," *New England Journal of Medicine* 336 (1997), 1197–1201.
16. M. Butler-O'Hara, C. LeMoine, R. Guillet, "Analgesia for Neonatal Circumcision: A Randomized Controlled Trial of EMLA Cream Versus Dorsal Penile Block," *Pediatrics* 10:4 (1998).
17. S. Hardwick-Smith, et al., "Ring Block for Neonatal Circumcision," *Obstetrics and Gynecology* 91 (1998), 930–934.
18. J. Lancier, et al., "Comparison of Ring Block, Dorsal Penile Nerve Block, and Topical Anesthesia for Neonatal Circumcision," *Journal of the American Medical Association* 278 (1997), 2157–2162.
19. B. Jakobson and A. Nilsson, "Methemoglobinemia Associated with Prilocaine-Lidocaine Cream and Trimethoprim -Sulfamethoxazole: A Case Report," *Acta Anaesthesiol Scand.* 29 (1985), 453–455; A. R. Kumar, et al., "Methemoglobinemia Associated with Prilocaine-Lidocaine Cream," *Clinical Pediatrics* 36 (1997), 239–240.
20. T. D., Puthoff, et al., "Use of Emla Prior to Circumcision," *Annals of Pharmacotherapy* 30 1996), 1327–1330.
21. L. W. Snellman and H. J. Stang, "Prospective Evaluation of Complications of Dorsal Penile Nerve Block for Neonatal Circumcision," *Pediatrics* 95 (1995), 705–708.
22. J. Ramet, et al., "Neonatal Circumcision" *Lancet* 349 (1997), 1257.

Other methods to attenuate pain during newborn circumcision include acetaminophen[23] and sucrose (sugar water) pacifiers.[24] The latter are routinely used by Jews during newborn ritual circumcision. Since ritual circumcision takes approximately half the time it takes to administer a dorsal penile nerve block, the argument is made that ritual circumcision is so brief that the risk of local anesthesia exceeds the benefit.[25] The traditional Jewish ritual circumcision is also less traumatic than traditional surgical circumcision. Furthermore, a few drops of wine given to the Jewish newborn baby immediately following ritual circumcision serves as an analgesic and soporific potion.

IV. ANESTHESIA IN BIBLICAL AND TALMUDIC LITERATURE

A number of talmudic passages discuss the use of pain relieving medications.[26] In one passage R. Eleazar was given a *samma deshinta* (soporific potion) prior to undergoing an abdominal operation,[27] and in another, it is mentioned that a convicted criminal should be sedated with wine and frankincense prior to his execution.[28] Anesthesia was also utilized by Jews in the Middle Ages, as evidenced by extant Hebrew medical manuscripts from that time.[29] There are, however, no halakhic discussions about the

---

23. C. R. Howard, et al., "Acetaminophen Analgesia in Neonatal Circumcision: The Effect of Pain," *Pediatrics* 93 (1994), 641–646.
24. M. Herschel, et al., "Neonatal Circumcision: Randomized Trial of Sucrose Pacifier for Pain Control," *Archives of Pediatric and Adolescent Medicine* 152 (1998), 279–284.
25. J. Shechet, et al., "Local Anesthesia for Infants Undergoing Circumcision," *Journal of the American Medical Association* 279 (1998), 1170–1171.
26. See J. Preuss, *Biblical and Talmudic Medicine,* trans. F. Rosner (Jason Aronson, 1993), 238; M. Perlman, *Midrash HaRefua* 2 (Devir Press, 1928), 90–91; F. Rosner, "Anesthesia in the Bible and Talmud," *Anesthesia and Analgesia* 50:2 (March-April, 1971), 298–301.
27. *Bava Metzia* 83b.
28. *Sanhedrin* 43a.
29. See S. Marcus, "Surgical Anesthetics in Two Hebrew Medical Manuscripts," (Hebrew) *Koroth* 3:9–10 (August, 1965), 385–3. See also H. Isaacs, *Medical and Para-Medical Manuscripts in the Cambridge Geniza Collections* (Cambridge University Press, 1994). Therein are mentioned manuscripts that discuss the use of opium and other remedies for the relief of pain. See "opium" and "pain" in the index. Manuscript n. 359 suggests the use of opium to ease the pain of a tooth extraction.

use of either general or local anesthesia until the nineteenth century, when anesthesia gained widespread use in the medical community.

V. ANESTHESIA IN HALAKHIC LITERATURE

The First Stage—General Anesthesia

The first halakhic discussions about the use of anesthesia for *mila* appeared in the journal *Tel Talpiyot* in 1896.[30] The topic was introduced by R. Tzvi Trammer,[31] who queried whether chloroform, a general anesthetic, could be used for the circumcision of a *ger* (convert) or an adult Jewish male.[32] His response stimulated further discussion and exchange in later pages of the journal amongst a number of prominent rabbinic authorities.[33] What ensues is a brief discussion of the major halakhic points raised in this first rabbinic interchange on the use of anesthesia for *mila*.[34]

Insensibility During Mila—A Potential Impediment to the Fulfillment of the Mitzva

R. Trammer's major halakhic concern is whether someone under general anesthesia, rendered insensible by the medication, is halakhically

---

30. Volume 4 (5656). The articles are not titled and will be referenced by page numbers in this volume.

31. *Tel Talpiyot*, 4 (5656), 61.

32. The use of anesthesia for *mila* of a convert involves unique halakhic concerns beyond the scope of this article, although some aspects may be mentioned tangentially. These issues are addressed in the articles in *Tel Talpiyot*, as well as in a series of articles in *HaMe'asef* referenced below. For a summary of the halakhic issues related to the *mila* of conversion, see R. S. Y. Zevin, ed., *Entzyclopedia Talmudit* 6 (Jerusalem, 1990), 431–37.

33. See *Tel Talpiyot*, 4 (5656), 65–66, 76–77, 79–80, 92–93.

34. Most later rabbinic authorities seem to be unaware of this first halakhic discussion on the use of anesthesia for *mila*, making no reference to it. This is perhaps due to its publication in a periodical as opposed to a book. The only authorities who reference this first chapter are R. Y. Schwartz, *She'elot Uteshuvot VaYitzbor Yosef* 12: 5, who merely cites and concurs with the opinion of R. Horowitz (see below), and R. A. M. Israel, "Is it Permissible to Use Local Anesthesia for Adolescents and Adults Undergoing Milah?" (Hebrew) *HaMaor*, v. 27, n. 6, issue 226 (*Tammuz*, 5735), 4.

equivalent to a *shoteh* (an incompetent or insane person), who cannot fulfill the mitzva of *mila*. He circumvents this concern by claiming that the mitzva does not devolve upon the *nimol* (the one circumcised)— neither a *ger*, since he is not yet obligated in mitzvot, nor an adult, whose obligation, like that of an infant, devolves upon others (his father or the rabbinic court).[35] Since neither the *ger* nor the adult Jew are themselves obligated to perform the mitzva of *mila*, their possible status as a *shoteh* is halakhically irrelevant. There is, therefore, no reason to forbid the use of chloroform.

R. Amram Fisher counters that the mitzva of *mila* indeed devolves upon both the *ger* and the adult Jew.[36] As a result, their insensibility during the performance of *mila* presents a potential halakhic problem. Nonetheless, after an analysis of the laws of *shlihut* (messengers), R. Fisher opines that since they each appoint a *shaliah* (messenger) while they are competent, and the *mohel* is a valid *shaliah*, the *mila* is valid for both a *ger* and an adult Jew, despite their insensibilty or unconsciousness during the procedure.[37]

A Violation of the Spirit of the Law (*Hithakmut Neged Hok MeHukei HaTorah*)

In a different vein, not focusing on the halakhic details or particulars of general anesthesia and *mila*, R. Pinchas Levi Horowitz rules stringently and prohibits the use of chloroform, as he considers this a case of *hithakmut neged hok mehukei haTorah*, actions which, although not technically legally prohibited, nevertheless run counter to the intent or spirit of the Torah.[38] He borrows this concept from

---

35. He brings proof to this point from the fact that even an adult does not recite the blessing for his own *mila*. Therefore, R. Trammer maintains, the obligation must not be his.

36. *Tel Talpiyot*, 4 (5656), 76.

37. In subsequent articles in the journal, other rabbinic authorities discuss the details and nuances of the laws of *shelihut* (agency), the question of upon whom the mitzva devolves, and the related issue of whether the performance of a mitzva requires specific intent (*mitzvot tzerikhot kavana*). See essays of R. Yitzhak Karpel and R. Gershon Stern in *Tel Talpiyot*, 4 (5656), 65–66 and 79–80 respectively.

38. *Tel Talpiyot*, 4 (5656), 76–77.

a responsum of Radbaz,[39] who addresses the legality of using certain chemicals to hasten the decomposition of a corpse. It was thought that earlier entrance into the World to Come would be facilitated thereby. While Radbaz does not consider the use of the chemicals to be contrary to halakha, he nevertheless counsels against the practice, considering it to be tampering with nature and running counter to the Torah's intent. Radbaz concludes, "Therefore, I proclaim regarding this and similar matters, 'thou shalt be perfect with the Lord thy God' (*tamim tihiyeh im Hashem Elokekha*)."[40] R. Horowitz adds that since the mitzva of *mila* is itself identified with the notion of being "*tamim*," (perfect)[41] one should refrain from tampering with it as well. The use of chloroform, a general anesthetic, is one example of such tampering.

R. Gershon Stern rejects the application of Radbaz's principle to the case of *mila*.[42] According to our tradition, he argues, the deceased experiences the pain of decomposition and being consumed by worms. This pain, a form of penitence (*kapara*) for the deceased, is a miraculous or supernatural phenomenon. We should, therefore, not tamper with this process and affect the supernatural pain and penitence of the individual. The pain of *mila*, on the other hand, is a natural phenomenon and does not achieve penitence for the *nimol*. The alleviation of this pain is subsumed under the license of physicians to heal and would furthermore not minimize or impact on the child's penitence.[43] Consequently, the use of anesthesia for *mila* is not a case of *hithakmut neged hok mehukei haTorah*.

---

39. See *Radbaz* 1:484.
40. Devarim 18:13.
41. Bereshit 17:1 and Rashi, ad loc.
42. *Tel Talpiyot*, 4 (5656), 79–80.
43. R. Horowitz defends his position in a rejoinder (*Tel Talpiyot*, 4 [5656], 92), where he admits that the analogy to the case of Radbaz is not that strong. He claims that what compelled him to make this analogy was the concluding phrase of Radbaz, "Therefore, I proclaim regarding this and similar matters, '*tamim tihiyeh im Hashem Elokekha*,'" along with he fact that the mitzva of *mila* is also identified with the notion of being "*tamim*."

The Benefit of Pain for *Mila* of a *Ger* (Convert)

Another issue advanced independently by two authorities, is the benefit of pain for *mila* of a *ger* specifically.[44] R. Horowitz asserts that many non-Jews convert for the purpose of marriage, having found attractive or wealthy Jewish women. Such converts, he adds, are not desirable, and perhaps the *mila*, and its attendent pain, serve as a deterent for their conversion. If we remove that deterrent by allowing the use of anesthesia, perhaps even more will convert.

R. Mordechai Leib Winkler offers a novel interpretation of a Midrash that yields a similar conclusion.[45] According to the Midrash, Abraham said to God, "Even before I was circumcised people would come to me [to convert].[46]" R. Winkler interprets God's response in the Midrash to mean that the pain of *mila* deters people from conversion. This insures that people convert for genuine and pure reasons. Based on this Midrash, R. Winkler contemplates refraining from any pain relief for the *mila* of a *ger*.[47]

Subsequent halakhic discussions on the use of general anesthesia address the issues raised in this first interchange in *Tel Talpiyot*, with some variations.[48] These issues include 1) concern that insensibility

---

44. There is no mention of pain as a requirement for all routine circumcisions. See opinion of R. Meir Arik below.
45. Cited by R. Gershon Stern, *Tel Talpiyot*, 4 (5656), 80. R. Winkler is the author of *Levush Mordekhai*.
46. *Bereshit Rabba* (Vilna) n. 9, s. v., "*amar ad*."
47. R. Winkler concludes in his halakhic analysis of the laws of *shelihut* that a general anesthetic would pose no halakhic problem for a *ger*.
48. In 1913–14, a series of articles appeared in the journal *HaMe'asef* on the use of general anesthesia: R. Y. Morgenstern year 18, v. 1, issue 6 (1 Adar, 5673), n. 82; R. Y. Schur, year 18, v. 2, issue 3 (Sivan, 5673), n. 24; R. M. D. Eidelsberg, year 18, v. 2, issue 4 (*Tammuz*, 5673), n. 36; R. Y. Denison, year 19, v. 1, issue 1 (*Tishrei*, 5674), n. 3; R. Y. Morgenstern, year 19, v. 1, issue 5 (*Shevat*, 5674). Similar to the exchange in *Tel Talpiyot*, these articles are infrequently cited by later *poskim*. On the use of general anesthesia in *mila*, in addition to the sources cited below, see R. P. Hornblass, *Pithei She'arim* n. 5; R. S. M. Shvadron, *She'elot UTeshuvot Maharsham* v. 6, Y. D., n. 108; R. Y. Weinberg, *Seridei Esh* 3:96; R. O. Yosef, *Yabia Omer* 5:22, reprinted in *Noam* 12 (5729), 1–10. Two excellent articles deal with the contemporary use of anesthesia for *mila*. See J. D. Bleich, "Circumcision: The Current Controversy," in *Tradition* 33:4 (Summer 1999), 45–69, and A. Steinberg, "*Hardama BeMila*," *Shana BeShana* (5761), 137–144.

during *mila* might preclude fulfillment of the mitzva,[49] 2) the nature of *shlihut*, and 3) the nature of the essence of the mitzva of *mila*.[50]

Responsum of the Imrei Yosher

The halakhic discussions on anesthesia and *mila* changed course with the appearance of a responsum by R. Meir Arik, known by his pseudonym, *Imrei Yosher*. Of all the halakhic literature on this topic, R. Arik's responsum seems to have had the most profound impact, and many subsequent halakhic authorities respond to the ideas expressed therein.[51] There follows a detailed analysis of the responsum and the responses that it evoked.

The question posed to R. Arik was whether it is permissible for a thirty-year-old man undergoing conversion to apply a topical anesthetic prior to the *mila* so as to eliminate the pain of the procedure. The following is a summary of his response:

The existence of local anesthetic was known in the times of *Hazal*, yet *Hazal* never introduced anesthesia into the *mila* ceremony.[52]

---

49. Related to this issue is the debate as to whether mitzvot require specific intent (*tzerikhot kavana*). If so, insensibility during anesthesia would seemingly preclude intent. Some question whether some form of intent is required even for an infant, thus obligating the infant to be conscious during the procedure. The three categories to which an anesthetized person has been likened are a *shoteh*, a *shikor* (alcohol intoxication) and *yashen* (one who is sleeping), each with its own halakhic nuances.

50. Is it the *procedure* of the *mila* which is halakhically significant, in which case attention must be paid to the status of the circumcised child during the procedure; or perhaps, it is only the *end result* of being circumcised which is required, in which case the procedure is halakhically tangential.

51. *Imrei Yosher* v. 2, n. 140, letter *gimmel*.

52. His evidence is from a passage in *Bava Kamma* 85a where mention is made of a chemical (*sam*) that could amputate a hand painlessly. R. Arik assumes that since a substance capable of cutting through flesh painlessly was available in talmudic times, a topical anesthetic must also have existed. While it is true that rudimentary forms of anesthesia were used since antiquity, it was not common practice to use either general or local anesthetic for circumcision, even amongst the other peoples who practiced this ceremony. See P. C. Remondino, *The History of Circumcision from the Earliest Times to the Present* (F. A. Davis, 1891). Remondino does mention one case of a child who was rendered insensible with some narcotic drink prior to circumcision (p. 48), but in this case, the circumcision was performed along with a more extensive surgical intervention. It is noteworthy that R. Arik does not cite

It must therefore be, R. Arik maintains, that Ḥazal consider pain to be an integral part of the *mila*. This is further evidenced by the Midrash, which states that according to R. Abba bar Kahana, Abraham endured the pain of *mila* to increase his reward.[53] Since the first, or prototypical, *mila* of Abraham was specifically associated with pain, without any interventions, we should not introduce any innovations that negate this aspect of *mila*.

Responses to Imrei Yosher

Three arguments can be distilled from the responsum of R. Arik, with the central theme revolving around the requirement for pain as an integral part of the *mila*. While earlier authorities discuss the benefit of pain for the *mila* of a *ger* (see above), R. Arik is the first to introduce the notion that pain is a requirement for all routine circumcisions. This responsum evoked a litany of responses by subsequent authorities, who variously address their remarks to the arguments of R. Arik. Whether concurring or dissenting, subsequent authorities felt compelled to address the role of pain in the mitzva of *mila*. The responses to R. Arik are detailed below, arranged according to R. Arik's original points.

Point 1: The omission of Ḥazal's reference to any anesthetic for *mila* is proof that its use is forbidden.

According to R. Feffer, the fact that (local) anesthesia was not used in earlier generations is no proof of its prohibition.[54] Perhaps it was not used for medical reasons, physicians not having perfected its effectiveness without risk to the infant. If such a local anesthetic would have been safe and effective, it might very well have been permitted.

R. Fromer suggests that in the performance of the child's first mitzva, we strive to do it in an ideal fashion, without pain relief, similar to

---

as support *Bava Metzia* 83b, where R. Eleazar underwent an abdominal operation with the aid of a numbing potion referred to as "*samma deshinta.*" Presumably, as this is an example of general, not local anesthesia, it would not have supported his contention that even local anesthesia was known in antiquity.

53. *Bereshit Rabba*, chap. 47, s. v., "*be'etzem.*"

54. R. A. S. Feffer, *Avnei Zikaron* 3:3.

Abraham.[55] Anesthesia was therefore not mentioned by *Hazal* because it was only rarely used.

In another attempt to justify the practice of withholding local anesthesia from newborns in the time of *Hazal*, R. Fromer claims that even a newborn should not be distracted or preoccupied (*mit'asek*) at the time of the performance of a mitzva (in this case, *mila*), and the endurance of pain precludes distraction. Therefore, local anesthesia, which eliminates the pain and introduces the possibility that the infant will be distracted (*mit'asek*), might preclude fulfillment of the mitzva and was therefore not routinely applied.[56]

Others maintain that since no mitzva in the Torah entails an obligation to endure pain,[57] there is no reason for *Hazal* to state the obvious, i.e., that anesthesia is permitted.[58]

Some draw analogy to the use of anesthesia in childbirth.[59] Despite the biblical pronouncement of the curse of Eve, "*be'etzev teldi banim*, in sorrow thou shalt bring forth children,"[60] implying that women will from then on suffer the pangs of childbirth, women have always been permitted to use all available means to alleviate the pain of labor. If anesthetics were available for *mila*, as R. Arik contends, they surely would have been available for women in labor. Yet, the omission by

---

55. R. T. Fromer, *Eretz Tzvi* 56. According to R. Fromer, to use anesthesia for an adult, especially in the case of fraternal death from *mila*, might be different. First, in such a case, *mila* would not be an adult's first mitzva. Second, pain relief could facilitate the performance of the *mila* despite the previous death of his brother. In the absence of pain relief, the *mila* may not be done at all.

56. For an adult, however, who has the intellectual capacity to concentrate on the mitzva despite local pain relief, a local anesthetic would be permitted.

57. There is a mitzva on Yom Kippur of suffering (*inuy*), but this is a unique obligation in and of itself, not an obligation to endure suffering in the performance of a mitzva. For a comparison of the halakhic differences between the pain of *mila* and the suffering of Yom Kippur, see R. A. M. Israel, op. cit.

58. R. A. L. Baron, "On the Issue of Topical Anesthesia for Milah," (Hebrew) *HaDarom* 58 (Elul, 5749), 13–22; R. E. Oshry, *Mima'amakim* 2:15.

59. R. Baron, op. cit., A. Steinberg, op. cit.

60. Bereshit 3:16.

Ḥazal of discussions on the use of pain relief in labor was not construed as tacit disapproval.[61]

Point 2: The Midrash of Abraham implies that pain is a requirement for *mila*.

The most oft repeated refutation of this proof is based on a careful interpretation of the language of the Midrash itself. The Midrash says that Abraham endured pain so that God would increase or double his reward (*ela hirgish venitzta'er kidei sheyikhpol HaKadosh Barukh Hu sekharo*). The implication is that the pain, in fact, is not an integral part of the mitzva, but rather, an additional, non-integral aspect. While it was laudatory or meritorious for Abraham to endure pain, an act which enhanced his reward, it was not incumbent upon him in order to fulfill the basic mitzva.[62]

R. Baron proposes two other reasons why the Midrash about Abraham's pain is not applicable to the halakhic discussion about the use of anesthesia for *mila*. First, while it is admirable to attempt to emulate Abraham's actions, including his performance of *mila*, technically, we are obligated to perform *mila* not because Abraham did so, but rather because Moses commanded us at Mount Sinai to perform *mila*.[63]

---

61. As mentioned above, anesthesia was introduced into the field of obstetrics by Dr. Simpson in 1846. While Christian theologians raised objections to obstetric anesthesia in the early stages, no such objections were apparently recorded in rabbinic literature. There are, however, halakhic concerns relating to the danger involved in the use of anesthesia in childbirth. See, for example, C. Katan and R. Y. Katan, "Epidural Anesthesia in Childbirth," (Hebrew) *Assia* 65–66 (September, 1999), 72–82.

62. See, for example, *Eretz Tzvi*, op. cit., R. Baron, op. cit., and R. M. D. Tendler, "Pain: Halakhah and Hashkafa," in S. Carmy, ed., *Jewish Perspectives on the Experience of Suffering* (Jason Aronson, 1999), 79–83.

63. Maimonides, Mishna Commentary, *Ḥullin*, chap. 7, s. v., "*noheg*." While R. Baron's point is technically correct, it is possible that Moses commanded us to perform *mila* exactly as Abraham had performed it, pain included. In fact, the language of Maimonides may support this. "… and similarly, we do not perform circumcision because Abraham circumcised himself and his household, but rather, because God commanded us through Moses to perform circumcision as Abraham performed it."

Therefore, since Abraham is not the halakhic paradigm for *mila*, the pain that he endured, which was not a feature of the *mila* taught by Moses, is of no halakhic consequence.

Furthermore, R. Baron suggests that Abraham was rewarded for the pain associated with *mila* since he performed the procedure on himself. It is illogical, however, to say that a father is rewarded for inflicting pain on his son, as the infant surely does not receive additional reward for the pain he suffers.[64]

Some cite other *midrashim* about the *mila* of Abraham that make no reference to pain.[65] As there is no compelling reason to adopt one Midrash over another, it is claimed, there is no reason to accept pain as a requirement of *mila*.

Point 3: Innovations in the procedure of *mila*, such as anesthesia, are prohibited.

Throughout the centuries, a number of innovations into the *mila* process have been proposed, including altering the method of wound sucking or *metzitza* (from oral suction to suction through an instrument) and the use of various devices (clamps) to better facilitate the *mila*. All invariably met with initial resistance, with compromise being reached on some of the innovations.[66] The resistance to innovation in *mila* pervades the halakhic discussions of the use of anesthesia as well. Some authorities, however, feel this concern about innovation is not applicable to this case.

R. Israel[67] concurs with R. Arik that new innovations in the mitzva of *mila* should not be adopted.[68] However, he adds, this applies only to innovations in the very performance of the mitzva itself. As

---

64. R. Baron admits that if one maintains that a proper *mila* is not accomplished in the absence of pain, then we could justify a father inflicting pain on his child. But he counters that the language of the Midrash does not reflect this interpretation. It implies that Abraham endured pain to enhance his reward, not because it was required.
65. Steinberg, op. cit.
66. For a more extensive discussion and references on this topic, see Steinberg, op. cit.
67. See Israel, op. cit.
68. R. Israel considers this argument of R. Arik to be an adaptation or application of Ḥatam Sofer's adage, *"ḥadash asur min haTorah."*

anesthesia has no impact on the performance of the *mila*, it is not considered an objectionable innovation. The use of antiseptics for *mila* has never been questioned, R. Israel argues, as they likewise have no relationship to the *mila* procedure itself.

Pain as a Requirement of Mila

The majority of *poskim* disagree with the assertion of R. Arik and offer independent support that pain is not a requirement for *mila*. Some infer from the halakhic discussions regarding one who is born circumcised (*nolad mahul*) that pain is not a feature of *mila*.[69]

R. Zirelson applies the *argument ex silencio*, similar to R. Arik, only with completely contradictory results.[70] While R. Arik claims that Ḥazal's omission of any reference to the use of anesthesia is proof that pain is a requirement for *mila*, R. Zirelson claims that since previous *poskim* (rabbinic decisors), including the greatest rabbinic scholars who usually elaborate upon the logic of their decisions, make absolutely no mention of pain as a factor in *mila*, it is impossible that it should be a requirement.[71]

---

69. There is a debate in the Talmud as to whether one who is born circumcised requires the additional bloodletting procedure known as *hatafat dam brit*. If pain were a requirement for *mila*, then one born circumcised would surely not have fulfilled this requirement and should be obligated to undergo this lesser, albeit painful, procedure. Therefore, it is argued, all rabbis should agree that one born already circumcised, without a foreskin, requires *hatafat dam brit*. Furthermore, the fact that pain is nowhere mentioned in the debate about the requirement for *hatafat dam brit* is proof that it is not a requirement. On this proof see, for example, R. Y. L. Zirelson, *Me'arkhei Lev*, Y. D., 53 and R. Baron, op. cit. R. Zirelson ultimately refutes the proof from *hatafat dam brit*, but claims, nonetheless, that pain is not required for *mila*. Of note, R. Zirelson does not explicitly refer to the responsum of R. Arik. Although the second volume of *Imrei Yosher* was published in 1925, seven years before the publication of R. Zirelson's *Me'arkhei Lev*, it is unclear whether R. Zirelson was aware of R. Arik's position.

70. R. Y. L. Zirelson, *Me'arkhei Lev*, Y. D., 53. See also R. Y. Weinberg, *Seridei Esh* 3:96.

71. Despite his seemingly permissive approach to anesthesia, R. Zirelson concludes, "As to the final decision in this case [of a five-year-old whose mother would only allow *mila* if a local anesthetic was used], even though, in general, we should not introduce new procedures to eliminate the pain of the circumcised child, we should not be stringent and oppose the request of the mother who is concerned about her precious child." R. Yeḥiel Weinberg, while forbidding general anesthesia for other

Another proof that pain is not required is inferred from the literature of the *Aharonim*, which is replete with responsa prohibiting the use of assorted new instruments for the performance of *mila*, since they increase the suffering of the child.[72]

While the majority of *poskim* disagree with R. Arik,[73] a number of contemporary authorities follow his position in maintaining that pain is, in fact, an integral part of *mila*.[74]

R. E. Y. Waldenberg also accepts the importance of pain in the mitzva of *mila*, forbidding local anesthesia for routine neonatal *mila*.[75] As an additional support, he quotes the author known as *Ollelot Ephraim* that one should pray for one's troubles simultaneously with the cries of the infant who cries from the pain of *mila*. Since the cries of the child undergoing *mila* ascend to heaven unencumbered and unrestrained, one's prayers hopefully accompany the child's cries.[76]

Many of the rabbis who do not consider pain to be an integral part of *mila*, nonetheless, believe it to be preferable, either because of the similarity to the *mila* of Abraham, or because pain relief constitutes a break from tradition. By the same token, many of the rabbis who consider pain to be an integral part of *mila* still allow use of anesthesia in

---

reasons, allows local anesthesia, partially based on the permissive ruling of R. Zirelson. R. Waldenberg, in *Tzitz Eliezer* 20:73, claims that R. Weinberg neglected to read the last few lines of the *Me'arkhei Lev*, which limit the latter's permissive ruling considerably.

72. R. Israel, op. cit. R. Israel mentions as an example, *Teshuvot Maharitz Chajes*, 60.

73. See also R. Tendler, op. cit.

74. R. M. M. Schneerson, *Shi'urei Halakha UMinhag Y. D.*, 97; R. E. Waldenberg, *Tzitz Eliezer* 20:73. R. S. Vozner, in his *Shevet HaLevi* 5:147, letter *bet*, claims that pain has traditionally been a part of *mila*, as it says, "But for your sake we are killed all day long" ("*ki alekha horagnu kol hayom*") [*Tehillim* 44:23]. According to tradition, this statement refers to *mila*. Furthermore, R. Vozner adds, pain is clearly part of the original form of the mitzva as it was given at Mt. Sinai.

75. *Tzitz Eliezer* 20:73.

76. R. Waldenberg assumes that this notion is based on the kabbalistic tradition. Dr. A. S. Abraham, however, cites in the name of R. Yaakov Hillel, head of *Yeshivat haMekubalim*, that there is no reference in the Zohar or other kabbalistic works to any unique powers of the cry of an infant during *mila*. R. Hillel adds that despite the Zohar's statement that the pain of childbirth serves as penitence (*kappara*) for the sin of Ḥavva, no one seems to refrain from easing the pain of childbirth through all available methods. See Abraham S. Abraham, *Nishmat Avraham* 5 (Rimonim, 5757), 82–85.

extenuating circumstances, such as an adult Jew or convert, or where a person's brother died as a result of *mila*.[77]

Medical Reasons to Refrain from Anesthesia

In addition to the aforementioned issues relating to the use of anesthesia, some authors cite medical reasons to refrain from the use of anesthesia for *mila*. Ravaz[78] cites *Milḥamot Ari*[79] that *mohelim* are cautious not to perform *mila* on a sleeping infant as it might induce epilepsy (*nikhfeh*).[80] R. M. Feinstein,[81] R. S. Z. Auerbach, R. Y. S. Elyashiv[82] and R. S. Vozner[83] all include medical concerns as one of the reasons to discourage the use of anesthesia for *mila*.

Local Anesthesia

The earliest halakhic sources concerning anesthesia for *mila* confine their discourse to general anesthesia. In addressing the issue of local anesthesia, many authorities assimilate the permissive or prohibitive approaches of general anesthesia.[84] Given recent medical advances, however, local anesthetics merit their own analysis. While some of the halakhic issues of local anesthesia are analogous to those of general anesthesia, such as whether pain is a requirement of *mila*, other issues, such as whether one can fulfill a mitzva while insensible, are not relevant to local anesthesia, as the individual is awake during the procedure. A number of *poskim* of earlier generations voice concerns unique to local anesthesia.

---

77. Each of these cases has its nuances and is considered separately by the different *poskim*. For a listing of which *poskim* address which cases, see Steinberg, op. cit.
78. R. B. Z. Shafran, *Teshuvot HaRavaz* 1:125.
79. As cited in *Koret HaBrit* n. 262, *Naḥal Brit*, 8.
80. This medical concern applies to infants, not adults.
81. *Iggerot Moshe Y. D.*, 4:40.
82. The opinions of R. Auerbach and R. Elyashiv are cited in A. S. Abraham, *Nishmat Avraham* 5 (Rimonim: Jerusalem: 5757), 84.
83. *Shevet HaLevi* 5:147, letter ḥet.
84. The reverse is also true. For example, both *Lev Arye* 1:11 and *Mima'amakim* 2:15 apply R. Zirelson's permission for local anesthesia to a case of general anesthesia. R. Israel (*HaMaor*, op. cit.) applies R. Winkler's permission in a case of general anesthesia (*Tel Talpiyot*, op. cit., 79–80 and 92–93) to a case of local anesthesia. Although R. Arik's ruling forbidding the use of anesthesia for *mila* was made specifically for a case of local anesthesia, it is generally, and logically, applied to all forms of anesthesia.

R. Y. M. Horowitz[85] cites *Bnei Asher* as being concerned that applying a local anesthetic might be equivalent to deadening the limb, and *mila* on a dead limb (*ever met*) is invalid, since no blood is shed thereby.[86] While *Bnei Asher* concludes that the *metzitza* would result in the emission of blood, thus validating the *mila*, R. Horowitz offers his own analysis from the case of a *metzora* (one stricken with the biblical disease *tzara'at*) who is required to undergo *mila*.[87]

R. Feffer addresses the same concern that local anesthesia might render the limb dead and preclude a valid *mila*.[88] Citing proof from the laws of *Shabbat*, he asserts that a dead piece of flesh attached to a living being is not considered halakhically attached (*mehubar*). Therefore, one is not liable for cutting off such a piece of flesh on *Shabbat*. Similarly, an anesthetized limb no longer receives sustenance from the rest of the body and is, therefore, analogous to a dead limb attached to a living organism. For *mila*, the foreskin (*orla*) must be cut from the living body, as it says, "On the eighth day the flesh of his foreskin (*besar orlato*) shall be circumcised."[89] As one does not fulfill the mitzva by cutting a foreskin that is already detached (*talush*), R. Feffer wonders whether local anesthesia might preclude fulfillment of the mitzva of *mila*.[90]

---

85. *Gedolei Tziyon*, n. 120, p. 298.
86. For a discussion of the halakhic debate about defining a limb of the body to be dead, see D. Malach, "*Evarim SheHaNeshama Teluya Bahem Le'Inyan Keviat Mavet*," *Assia* 65–66 (September, 1999), 112–120, esp. 112–114.
87. A *metzora* who is obligated to perform *mila* presents a halakhic conflict between the obligation to preserve the lesions of *tzara'at* (*shomer nega tzara'at*) and the mitzva of *mila*, which may involve cutting through the lesions. The halakha is that the *mila* supersedes the obligation to preserve the lesions of *tzara'at*. R. Horowitz questions that if *tzara'at* renders a limb dead, as some halakhic authorities contend, then how can you perform a *mila* on a *metzora*? No blood is shed and the mitzva of *mila* is not fulfilled. As a result, there is no legal justification for violating the obligation to preserve the lesions of *tzara'at*. The author answers that either the emission of blood (*dam brit*) is not a requirement for *mila*, or perhaps, it is impossible to perform a *mila*, even on a dead limb, without at least some resultant bleeding.
88. *Avnei Zikaron* 3:3.
89. Vayikra 12:3.
90. Even though R. Feffer notes that the physiological detachment of the foreskin from anesthesia is temporary, and he entertains the notion that this might render

VI. MODERN APPLICATION

The halakhic analysis regarding general anesthesia largely remains unchanged, with modern authorities voicing much the same concerns and invoking the same rabbinic sources as in 1896, when the issue was first addressed in halakhic literature.[91] General anesthesia, despite the great strides in medicine, remains a risky procedure with a percentage of fatalities, albeit far less than in the past. With regard to general anesthesia, the rabbinic concerns about the insensibility of the individual during *mila*, the dangers of the procedure, and complete absence of pain all remain equally applicable today. While the notion that circumcising a sleeping infant may precipitate seizures is without modern medical support,[92] and would not be a reason to refrain from anesthesia today, this notion is only peripheral in the halakhic discussions.

With regard to local anesthesia, recent medical advances may impact on the application of earlier halakhic sources. In light of our modern understanding of the mechanism of anesthesia, as well as cardiac physiology and hematology, the premise that an anesthetized limb is considered halakhically dead would be challenged. Despite the injection or application of anesthesia, the foreskin continues to receive sustenance from the body as before, and there is no interruption of blood flow. Only the local nerve supply to the foreskin is affected, not the circulation. Therefore, any incision, for *mila* or otherwise, produces bleeding as per usual.

The choice of local anesthetic, whether nerve block via injection, or topical application of an ointment, may also have halakhic ramifications. Since the concern about the insensibility of the individual during

---

the cutting valid, as the foreskin is not permanently detached, he nevertheless concludes that since at the time of the cutting the foreskin is "physiologically" detached, the *mila* is invalid.

91. See, for example, *Yabia Omer Y. D.*, 5:22; *Teshuvot VeHanhagot* 1:590; *Shevet HaLevi* 5:147, 2.

92. While I have found no medical corroboration for this specific belief, an association between circumcision and epilepsy is noted in the scientific literature of the late nineteenth century. A number of cases were reported in which phimosis (unretractable foreskin) was thought to be the cause of seizures or other neurological conditions. Relief of the phimosis through circumcision reportedly cured the seizures in these cases. See Remondino, op. cit., 257–67.

mila does not apply to local anesthesia, as the person is conscious during the procedure, there are two potential remaining halakhic concerns that might preclude the use of a local anesthetic for *mila*—the requirement for pain,[93] and the concern for danger. Given these two concerns, nerve blocks remain a halakhic problem, as they entirely eliminate the pain and are accompanied by medical risk. Topical anesthetics, on the other hand, such as EMLA, may significantly diminish the pain, but do not entirely extinguish it. Even with the use of EMLA, an infant will feel at least some pain.[94] Furthermore, the risk with the use of topical anesthetics is negligible.[95] Therefore, a reevaluation of the halakhic literature, coupled with the knowledge of new medical advances, reveals no clear remaining halakhic objection to the use of certain topical local anesthetics for routine neonatal *mila*. Indeed, according to R. Auerbach and R. Elyashiv, if there is no danger with the use of a topical anesthetic, it is permitted, and perhaps even desirable, to use it.[96] R. Tendler implies that it is in fact obligatory to use a topical anesthetic for *mila*.[97]

VII. CONCLUSION

The halakhic discussions on the use of anesthesia for *mila* span more than a century. In addressing this topic today, it is imperative not only to know the issues raised by our predecessors, but also to understand contemporary medicine as it relates to the use of anesthetics for *mila*. The halakhic analysis regarding general anesthesia largely remains unchanged, with modern authorities voicing much the same concerns and invoking the same rabbinic sources as in 1896, when the issue was first addressed in halakhic literature. With respect to local anesthesia, however, a new

---

93. As discussed above, most *poskim* do not require pain in order to fulfill the mitzva of *mila*.

94. Dr. Steinberg differentiates EMLA from other preparations of topical anesthetic, where the pain of *mila* might indeed be completely alleviated. See Steinberg, op. cit.

95. One might argue that further medical studies are needed to verify this beyond doubt.

96. Dr. Abraham, op. cit.

97. R. Tendler, op. cit., concludes his remarks on the use of anesthesia for *mila* by claiming that not only would it be permitted to use a topical anesthetic, "It would be, in my opinion, a violation of the halakha of *lo yosif lehakoto* (causing additional, unnecessary harm) to fail to do so."

medical reality requires a reassessment of the pre-existing halakhic literature. The advent of new forms of topical local anesthetic, which are of minimal risk to the infant, and still allow the feeling of some pain, necessitates a reevaluation of the role of topical anesthesia for routine neonatal *mila*.

Lessons from the First Halakhic Analysis of Vaccination

Vaccination is considered by virtually all scientists to be one of the greatest advances in medical history. Yet, in this generation, some have cast aspersions upon its practice, choosing to abandon vaccination altogether.[1] The objective of this chapter is not to thoroughly address the arguments of the anti-vaxxer movement, nor to delve into the

---

1. The Orthodox Jewish community has been singled out in the recent resurgence of measles in 2019 as being partially responsible for the rapid spread of the disease. For but one example, see S. Maslin Nir and M. Gold, "An Outbreak Spreads Fear: Of Measles, of Ultra-Orthodox Jews, of Anti-Semitism," *New York Times* (March 29, 2019). There is a sad historical irony to this fact. In the Middle Ages, Jews were often blamed for the spread of diseases, such as the Black Plague or Bubonic Plague, being accused of poisoning the wells. On this topic, see, for example, S. K. Cohen, "The Black Death and the Burning of the Jews," *Past and Present* 196 (August, 2007), 3–36; T. Barzilay, *Well Poisoning Accusations in Medieval Europe: 1250–1500* (Ph.D. Dissertation, Columbia University, 2017). Thousands of Jews were murdered, often burned at the stake, as a result. These accusations, however, had no basis in fact, and were simply conjured from anti-Semitic imagination. Today, in the twenty-first century,

contemporary halakhic analysis of vaccination,[2] but rather to enlighten the halakhic and general discussion of vaccination by returning to the original body of halakhic literature regarding the treatment of smallpox in the eighteenth and nineteenth centuries.[3] This will hopefully allay some misconceptions that may have arisen with the passage of time.

I. THE FIRST VACCINATION AND ITS HALAKHIC RESPONSE

Perhaps it is because we live in twenty-first-century America, a country which has largely been immune to the widespread ravages and devastation of infectious disease, at least prior to the Covid-19 pandemic, that we take vaccination for granted and some consider not vaccinating their children. A Jew living in the eighteenth century would have longed for any respite from the relentless onslaught of disease and could only have dreamed of vaccinating his child against so many diseases. The thought of refusing these wonders of medicine would scarcely have entered his mind. A cursory review of the origins of vaccination in medical historical

---

Jews are again being accused of the spread of disease. Only this time, there is regretfully some truth to this assertion. Some Jews actually request a religious exemption from vaccination, a claim that has no basis in halakha.

2. We briefly address some halakhic issues below, but for comprehensive contemporary halakhic discussions on vaccination, see Y. Shafran, "Halakhic Attitudes Towards Immunization," *Tradition* 26:1 (Fall 1991) 4–13; A. Bush, "Vaccination in Halakhah and in Practice in the Orthodox Jewish Community," *Hakirah* 13 (Spring 2012), 185–212; A. Glatt, F. Rosner, Y. Breitowitz, and Z. Schostak, "Compelled to Inoculate: May Parents Refuse Vaccinations for Their Children," *Journal of Halacha and Contemporary Society* 65 (Spring 2013), 55–72; J. D. Bleich, "Vaccination," *Tradition* 48:2–3 (2015), 41–56; D. Eisenberg, "The Ethics of Smallpox Vaccination," at http://www.aish.com/societyWork/sciencenature/ The_Ethics_of_Smallpox_Immunization.asp. This chapter was written prior to the Covid pandemic and the development of new mRNA vaccines. While there are some unique halakkic aspects to this development, the core halakhic analysis about vaccinations is essentially the same. On the Covid pandemic, see chapter, "Precedented Times."

3. On the history of the rabbinic response to smallpox inoculation, see, for example, R. Pinḥas Eliyahu Hurwitz (1765– 1821), *Sefer HaBrit* (Jerusalem, 5750), 247ff.; H. J. Zimmels, *Magicians, Theologians and Doctors* (Edward Goldston and Son, 1952), 107–110; D. Margalit, "Smallpox Inoculation Before Jenner," (Hebrew) in his *Derekh Yisrael BiRefua* (Jerusalem, 5730), 376–379: D. Ruderman, "Some Jewish Responses to Smallpox Prevention in the Late Eighteenth and Early Nineteenth Centuries: A New Perspective on the Modernization of European Jewry," *Aleph* 2 (2002), 111–144.

and rabbinic literature might inform our current discussion and provide a little perspective on this issue.

In the late eighteenth century, smallpox was the scourge of Europe, virtually decimating the population. Millions of people died from the disease, and children were afflicted in high percentages. In the eighteenth century alone, an estimated 400,000 Europeans died *each year* from smallpox. When potential relief from the horrors of the disease came on the horizon in the early eighteenth century, there must have been unabashed excitement. The cure, or more accurately, the mechanism of disease prevention, however, was unique in the history of medicine and posed ethical and halakhic dilemmas. Inoculation, as it was called, required removal of fluid from the pox of an afflicted patient and the subsequent injection of that virulent fluid into the body of a healthy individual. The belief was that the healthy person would develop a mild, non-fatal form of the disease and be spared the likelihood of fatality if afflicted with the spontaneous form. Indeed, this was the case the majority of the time, but the procedure was not without risk; some of those inoculated developed the severe form of the disease and died as a result. In fact, there is a tombstone in Huntington, Long Island with the following epitaph:

> In Memory of Peleg,
> Son of Thomas and Mary Conklin, who died of the smallpox by inoculation
> Jan. 27th, 1788, aged 17 years

The Jewish population was not immune to the ravages of smallpox, and in 1785, R. Abraham Nansich published a small pamphlet entitled *Alei Terufa* detailing the tragic loss of two of his children to smallpox and beseeching the rabbis of his generation to allow inoculation.[4]

However, the treatment was considered controversial at the time, as never in the history of mankind had one taken a healthy individual and injected them with the very cause of an illness, even if the objective was

---

4. Abraham ben Solomon Nansich, *Alei Terufa* (*Aleksander bar Yehuda uveno Yehuda Leib bar Aleksander,* London, 1785).

to prevent more severe disease. This unique treatment posed a dilemma for the Torah observant Jew. The Torah gives license to the physician to heal the sick, but does it give license to the physician to bestow illness upon the healthy, albeit for ultimate cure?

The debate about the medical and theological aspects of smallpox inoculation occupied a significant chapter in eighteenth-nineteenth-century history. Benjamin Franklin reported in the March 1730 issue of his *Pennsylvania Gazette*, that of seventy-two Bostonians who had been inoculated only two had died, while the rest recovered perfect health. He later shared a personal tragic story in his autobiography regarding smallpox and inoculation:

> In 1736, I lost one of my sons, a fine boy of four years old, by the smallpox, taken in the common way. I long regretted bitterly, and still regret, that I had not given it to him by inoculation. This I mention for the sake of parents who omit that operation, on the supposition that they should never forgive themselves if a child died under it.[5]

Rabbis of that generation debated the issues and were well aware of the risks associated with this treatment. R. Israel Lifschutz, author of the *Tiferet Yisrael* commentary on the Mishna, argued in favor of inoculation, despite the known risks.[6]

In his view, the benefits clearly exceeded the risks. Even though one in a thousand may die as a result of the inoculation, he argued, if one contracts the disease spontaneously during an epidemic, the odds of dying are much higher. This logic is reminiscent of that of Benjamin Franklin. Other prominent rabbis advocated vaccination as well, including R. Mordechai Banet (1753–1829), R. Eliezer Fleckeles (1754–1826), and R. Ishmael HaKohen (1723–1811).

There was an additional halakhic issue created by the practical dissemination of the smallpox inoculation. During that period, inoculation was performed by barber surgeons, who traveled from town to town

---

5. B. Franklin, *Autobiography of Benjamin Franklin* (D. C. Heath, 2008), 163.
6. *Tiferet Yisrael, Yoma.*

and spent only a few hours in each location. Halakhic issues arose as to whether one could receive inoculation on Shabbat, if that happened to be the day the inoculation was offered. The discussions related to both the nature of the exact prohibition of the injection (which was subcutaneous, as opposed to intravenous),[7] as well as the status of the patient who received the injection. Shabbat violation was permitted for patients falling into specific halakhic categories of illness. In this case however, the recipient of the inoculation was healthy. Could one be considered in the category of *holeh she'ein bo sakana* (non-life-threatening illness) by virtue of their presence in an epidemic area.[8] A number of *poskim* allowed the inoculation of healthy individuals, which entailed possible Shabbat violation, in order to protect them from potential exposure to infectious disease.

The more crude inoculation for smallpox was soon replaced with the scientifically tested vaccination of Edward Jenner, which inoculated patients with the cowpox virus in order to protect them from smallpox.[9] R. Israel Lifschutz famously lauded Jenner as one of the great sages of the non-Jewish world.[10]

II. THE FIRST JEWISH ANTI-VAXXER

The anti-vaxxer movement is by no means new. Already in the times of Jenner (early 1800's) there was both individual and organized opposition to vaccination.[11] My objective here is to bring attention to what is to my knowledge the first recorded case of a Jew claiming religious exemption from vaccination, in 1896—a little known, yet remarkably prescient, historical incident. This incident is chronicled in a slim volume by J. H.

---

7. This is the first historical instance of halakhic discussions about different types of injections, a topic that is very common in the medical halakhic works of today.

8. See, for example, *Teshuva Me'Ahava* 1:134; *Zekher Yehosaf O. H.*, 104; *Shu"t VeLa'Asher Amar* 15.

9. For further discussion on the rabbinic response to Jenner's vaccination, see R. Pinḥas Eliyahu Hurwitz (1765– 1821), *Sefer HaBrit* (Jerusalem, 5750), 247ff.

10. *Yakhin UBoaz Commentary, Mishna Avot* 3:14. The others on his list were Sir Francis Drake for introducing the potato into the European diet, and Johannes Gutenberg for inventing the printing press.

11. See, for example, E. Watling, "The 200-Year History of the Anti-Vaxxer Movement: From 'Cowpox Face' to Autism Claims," *Newsweek* (March 13, 2019).

Levy.[12] At the top of the cover page appear the words in Hebrew, *"yehi or"* (let there be light). The contents are indeed illuminating, perhaps even more so today than at the time of its printing.

In the late nineteenth century, it was legally required to vaccinate in the United Kingdom. Mr. Henry Levy refused to have his child vaccinated, claiming that his religion (Judaism) was opposed to the procedure. He was subsequently prosecuted by Mr. Harris, also of the Jewish faith, found guilty, and imprisoned for his violation of the law.

Shortly thereafter, Mr. J. H. Levy, the volume's author, spoke at a meeting defending the actions of Mr. Henry Levy (no relation) and sympathizing with the plight of his fellow Jew. His words were quoted by the local press:

> The people of my own race, it seems to me, are specially bound to detest the inoculation mania and all its works. Anything more opposed to the spirit of the ancient Judaism than the insertion of an animal disease in the human body I find it difficult to conceive.

The reference here is to smallpox vaccination, which is derivative from cows afflicted with the disease cowpox. The vaccine was derived from sick cows, which would be prohibited from consumption according to Jewish law. Levy therefore claimed, among other arguments, that injection of material from these diseased cows would likewise be prohibited according to Jewish law.

The quotation prompted Mr. Harris, the prosecutor who was responsible for the imprisonment of Mr. Henry Levy, to petition the R. Herman Adler, Chief Rabbi of England, regarding his opinion on vaccination. He was concerned that if indeed Jewish law rejects vaccination, he would have then jailed his fellow Jew in error.

R. Adler responded:

> (Mr. J. H. Levy) was not justified in making the statements contained in the letter; that the most competent medical authorities

---

12. J. H. Levy, *State Vaccination: With Special Reference to Some Principles of Ancient Judaism* (P. S. King and Son, 1897).

were agreed as to vaccination being a prophylactic against small-pox … and its use was in perfect consonance with the letter and spirit of Judaism.

This response precipitated a subsequent exchange of letters and statements between R. Adler and Mr. J. H. Levy, including the convicted Mr. Henry Levy as well. These exchanges comprise the substance of the volume and are, in essence, the precursor of the contemporary debate between the mainstream Orthodox Jewish community and the Jewish anti-vaxxer movement.

III. VACCINATION TODAY

Over two hundred years have passed since the discovery of Edward Jenner, and the effectiveness of vaccination is beyond question. In fact, the discovery of vaccination is on virtually every top ten list of the greatest discoveries in the history of medicine, appearing as number one on many of them. While there is no way to estimate the lives saved globally as a result of vaccinations for diseases such as smallpox, diphtheria, measles, polio, pneumococcus, and influenza—tens of millions would be a very conservative estimate. Indeed, smallpox, the first disease for which vaccination was used, has been declared eradicated from the face of the earth. The mortality rate of smallpox has gone from some three hundred million deaths in the eighteenth and nineteenth centuries to zero deaths today.

However, vaccinations do have side effects, though rare, that are well documented.[13] Despite these known side effects, scientific research has proven that the risk-benefit analysis weighs very heavily in favor of vaccination. These side effects must be viewed in the context of general medical practice. The general issue of assuming risk and self-endangerment is the substance of many halakhic discussions, but the assumption of some risk in the pursuit of medical treatment is an

---

13. For a comprehensive review of the medical literature on the side effects of vaccines and the medical literature on the association of vaccination and autism, see the Centers for Disease Control website (www.cdc.gov).

accepted fact.[14] There is arguably not a single medication, from Tylenol to vaccinations to chemotherapy, which is free of side effects, many of them serious. Ramban acknowledged this very point in the Middle Ages. Yet, the obligation to seek cure and prevent disease remains in full force, despite the risks. Keep in mind that *poskim* who allowed inoculation in the nineteenth century did so given a mortality rate which today would be considered far beyond unacceptable for a medical treatment. To be sure, each treatment requires its own risk-benefit statistical analysis based on the medical consensus of the time.

There are anecdotal accounts of associations of vaccinations with other conditions, such as autism. The notion of vaccination being associated with autism was first advanced by Andrew Wakefield in an article in the Lancet Journal in 1998.[15] This article was subsequently retracted by the journal in 2010, something rarely done in the medical literature, for research protocol and ethics violations. No additional studies have confirmed this link, and a recent study of over 650,000 patients has put the proverbial nail in the coffin of the theory of an autism-vaccination connection. The study concludes that, "MMR vaccination does not increase the risk for autism, does not trigger autism in susceptible children, and is not associated with clustering of autism cases after vaccination."[16]

Furthermore, unvaccinated individuals expose themselves to additional risk for vaccine-associated diseases. It is often claimed, however, that their risk is low due to the concept of herd immunity, a type of immunity that occurs when the vaccination of a large portion of the population (or herd) provides protection to unvaccinated individuals. Herd immunity theory proposes that, in diseases passed from person-to-person, it is more difficult to maintain a chain of infection when large numbers of a population are immune. The more immune individuals

---

14. On the general risk of medical procedures (including the application of the principle of "*shomer p'taim Hashem*") see J. David Bleich, "Hazardous Medical Procedures," in his *Bioethical Dilemmas* 2 (Targum Press: Southfield, MI, 2006), 239–275; D. Shabtai and R. Sultan, "Metzitzah, b'Peh: Paradigm for Halakhic Risk Taking," *Jewish Medical Ethics* 6:1 (December, 2007), 26–48.

15. A. Wakefield, et al., "Lancet 351:9103 (February 28, 1998), 637–641.

16. A. Hviid, et al., "Measles, Mumps, Rubella Vaccination and Autism: A Nationwide Cohort Study," *Annals of Internal Medicine* 170:8 (April 16, 2019), 513–520.

present in a population, the lower the likelihood that a susceptible person will come into contact with an infected individual. Since most of the people in the community are vaccinated against the disease, it is less likely that the virus or bacteria will flourish in that area and, therefore, less likely for an unvaccinated individual to contract these diseases. This argument is not without some merit, but the fewer people who vaccinate, the less protective herd immunity will be.

However, there is another dimension beyond the individual to consider. Even amongst those who are vaccinated, small percentages do not achieve immunity. If unvaccinated individuals contract a disease, they can spread it to this population. Furthermore, if the number of unvaccinated people rises, the possibility of epidemic outbreaks exists, reminiscent of the pre-Jenner days. The recent outbreak of measles is testimony to this fact. Therefore, it is not only a personal decision to refuse vaccination; it is a decision that impacts the entire community. It is thus within the Jewish community's right to mandate vaccination, for example, as a pre-requisite for day school admission.

One might argue that assumption of risk for treatment of an existing medical condition is different than assuming risk for preventative care, but even preventative care is considered a mitzva.[17] When global epidemics of infectious disease were more prevalent, *poskim* were more willing to allow vaccination on Shabbat, but even today, in unique circumstances, *poskim* have allowed violation of Shabbat for the preventative procedure of vaccination. For example, R. Shlomo Zalman Auerbach allowed for vaccination on Shabbat in a situation where if one did not receive the vaccination on Shabbat, it would be a number of years until they would again be able to receive the vaccine.[18] Rav Eliezer Waldenberg allowed a vaccine for tetanus to be given on Shabbat.[19] While these

---

17. For a discussion on halakhic aspects of preventative medicine, including vaccination, See J. DiPoce and S. Buchbinder, "Preventative Medicine," *Journal of Halacha and Contemporary Society*, 42 (Fall 2001), 70–101.

18. R. S. Z. Auerbach, *Minḥat Shlomo* 2:29, letter *dalet*; *Shmirat Shabbat KeHilkhata*, chapter 32, n. 2.

19. R. Eliezer Waldenberg, "Vaccination for Tetanus on Shabbat," (Hebrew) in *Halakha URefua* 4 (Regensburg Institute, 5745), 179–180. In the next volume of *Halakha URefua*, Dr. David Applebaum, *a"h*, took issue with the permissive ruling of R. Waldenberg and

cases are limited, it reflects the fact that *poskim* considered vaccination, though a preventative measure, still enough of an obligation to consider violating Shabbat. While of course the nature of medicine has evolved since the first smallpox inoculation, this approach is similar to that of R. Eliezer Fleckeles discussed above.

In the exceedingly rare cases of fatality possibly associated with vaccination, *poskim* have addressed the issue of the permissibility of autopsy to clarify the cause of death and perhaps prevent others.[20] R. Dr. Halperin recounts a case in Israel in 1992 of an infant who died shortly after receiving a hepatitis vaccine. The Ministry of Health requested an autopsy and R. Halperin discussed the case with R. Shlomo Zalman Auerbach. R. Auerbach rendered an unambiguous decision that the postmortem should be carried out on account of the dangers, although, and he stressed this, it was clear even to him that the danger was remote. R. Elyashiv prohibited autopsy in a similar case of an infant who died after vaccination, part of the logic being that the odds of association with the vaccine were small, coupled with the fact that the autopsy would likely not produce useful results.

To be sure, there are certain patients for whom vaccinations are medically contraindicated, but these are the rare exceptions that should be discussed with a physician on a case-by-case basis. To forgo vaccination because of anecdotal claims is halakhically irresponsible.

IV. CONCLUSION

In conclusion, the halakhic discussions of vaccination began centuries ago, at the dawn of this novel treatment's invention. Issues of risk, statistical analyses and Shabbat violation were considered and analyzed. While the halakhic discussions of vaccination today have evolved with the advances in medicine, they are clearly an outgrowth of this earlier

---

claimed that since in this case tetanus could be given after Shabbat, and would provide the same immunity, perhaps Shabbat violation would not be necessary. Rabbinic authorities, such as Rav Asher Weiss, *shlit"a*, have allowed the violation of rabbinic prohibitions in order to obtain a Covid-19 vaccine in the midst of the pandemic.

20. For discussion on the permissibility of autopsy after death from vaccination, see M. Halperin, "The Laws of Saving Lives: The Teachings of Rabbi S. Z. Auerbach," *Jewish Medical Ethics* 3:1 (January, 1997), 44–49, esp. 46–47; A. Steinberg, "Autopsy in the Case of Death After Vaccination," (Hebrew) *Assia* 59–60 (June, 1997), 129–132.

historical narrative. Today, mainstream halakhic authorities strongly and unequivocally support vaccination, considering the preservation of health in our community as paramount. Indeed, some poskim maintain that vaccination should be required.[21] They support the accepted view of considered medical opinion that it is incumbent upon the community to vaccinate their children and protect them from the possibility of acquiring infectious diseases. We should therefore expect nothing short of 100% compliance with vaccination in the Jewish community, with the exception of medical contraindications. Regretfully, this is not the case. A vocal minority within our community rejects the proven effectiveness of vaccination, against the overwhelming preponderance of evidence to the contrary. Even this contemporary Jewish anti-vaxxer movement has its antecedent in the late nineteenth century,[22]

I believe that our success with vaccinations is the cause of complacency about their use. We in the twenty-first century may have forgotten the lives of our ancestors, filled with mourning for children dying of smallpox and measles and lamenting the consequences of paralysis from polio. These occurrences are fortunately a thing of the past, with the unfortunate exception of the Covid-19 pandemic, due largely to the success of vaccination. Whether perspectives will change in the post-Covid era remains to be seen. An injection of a bit of historical perspective will hopefully immunize us against the distorted thinking that rejects one of the most extraordinary medical achievements Hashem has guided us to develop.

---

21. For example, R. Elyashiv *zt"l* cited in A. Glatt, op. cit.
22. For example, some antivaxxers today claim that vaccines should be prohibited because they contain non-kosher ingredients. This argument was advanced by Jews in the nineteenth century as well. See J. Levy, op. cit. Even if these claims were true, the halakhic prohibition involves orally ingesting non-kosher food, not intramuscular injections. Likewise there is no prohibition to use porcine insulin or to have a porcine or bovine heart valve implanted. See T. Pager, "'Monkey, Rat and Pig DNA': How Misinformation Is Driving the Measles Outbreak Among Ultra-Orthodox Jews," *New York Times* (April 9, 2019).

Ebola: A New Disease with an Ancient Tradition

I. INTRODUCTION

One routine day while on call in the Emergency Department, an Ebola patient presents with nausea and vomiting. Consistent with his disease, there is extensive hemorrhage from the eyes and mouth. Suddenly his heart stops. A code red is called. I hesitate to tell you what I do next. I hesitate not because I am withholding the truth from you, but rather because I honestly do not know what happens next. This is not a real case, but, as a practitioner of emergency medicine, one that I play out in my mind and that I genuinely fear. Do I initiate CPR and expose myself to significant risk of contracting a fatal disease? Or do I stand idly by as the blood of my patient sheds, knowing that the patient will surely die?[1] What would halakha say in this case?

This article first appeared in *Jewish Action* in 2015. When I first read the e-mail from the editors of *Jewish Action* inviting me to write an article on Ebola, I was literally on the way to my mandatory hospital Ebola preparedness-training seminar. Montefiore Medical Center, where I work, is one of New York City's designated Ebola receiving hospitals.

---

1. For a discussion of this issue from a secular perspective, see L. Altman, "Ethicist Calls CPR Too Risky in Ebola," *New York Times*, October 20, 2014.

As such, the opportunity to place this "Ebola scare" into a Jewish historical and halakhic context is one that I welcome.

How would my research begin? I would ask the same questions as for any medical halakhic issue. Is Ebola mentioned in *Tanakh* or the Talmud? Does Maimonides or *Shulḥan Arukh* mention Ebola? If not, perhaps later responsa deal with the halakhic ramifications of this virulent disease? As the reader will doubtless realize, the answer to all of these questions is negative. The Ebola virus was only identified in 1976. Is there precedent for halakhic analysis of previously unknown diseases? Yes, AIDS is a relatively new disease and has generated a fair amount of halakhic literature.[2] But in truth, the precise identity of the disease is not of particular consequence; rather, it is the issues of contagion,[3] infectious disease,[4] and risk. Is there precedent for these issues in rabbinic literature? The answer is a resounding yes.

---

2. On AIDS in Jewish law, see, for example, A. Steinberg, "AIDS: A Jewish Perspective," in *Medicine and Jewish Law* 2 (Jason Aronson, 1993), 89–102; J. D. Bleich, "AIDS: Jewish Concerns," *Bioethical Dilemmas* (Ktav, 1998), 131–185; G. Freudenthal, ed., *AIDS in Jewish Though and Law* (Ktav, 1998).

3. Notions of contagion are discussed by biblical commentaries on the stories of Lot and Korach. See Naḥmanides on Bereshit 19:17, and *Rabbenu Baḥya* on Bamidbar 16:21.

4. Some have suggested that naturally occurring infectious diseases account for a number of the ten plagues. For a most imaginative example, see H. M. Duncan Hoyte, "The Plagues of Egypt," *Medical Journal of Australia* (May 17, 1993), 706–708, who writes, "In summary, the series of disasters was: a bloom of red dinoflagellates killed the fish in the Nile, dehydration then killed the frogs, the people were attacked first by swarms of culicine mosquitoes then by swarms of stable flies, these flies initiated an epidemic of surra in the farm animals and their bites caused an epidemic of ecthyma in the people, then there was a hail storm, a swarm of locusts and a sand storm and, the last plague of all, an epidemic of typhoid fever that killed, among many others, the Pharoah's eldest child."

The modern Hebrew term for anthrax is *"sheḥin,"* based on the biblical plague, though this identification is not universally agreed upon. See L. Ben Noun, "Characteristics of Anthrax: Its Description and Biblical Name—Shehin," *Harefua* 141:4–6 (May, 2002), 124, and Z. Amar, "Shechin in the Language of Chazal—What is it?" (Hebrew) *Assia* (January, 2005), 65–69. Also, the generic term for plague or epidemic is *"dever,"* derived from the biblical plague.

But why has Ebola specifically received so much attention? We have had recent outbreaks of other infectious diseases, such as mumps, measles, polio and, flu, some of these with an interesting predilection for the Jewish population.[5] So why the exponentially greater response and concern for Ebola? For one, there is no approved therapy. In addition, the mortality rate is very high, and there is no vaccine to prevent the disease. In the previous chapter, we discussed the issue of vaccination. In the opening lines, we noted:

> Perhaps it is because we live in twenty-first-century America, a country largely immune from true epidemics, that we take vaccination for granted and some consider not vaccinating their children. A Jew living in the eighteenth century would have longed for any respite from the relentless onslaught of disease and could only have dreamed of vaccinating his child against so many diseases.

This Ebola scare gives us a tiny glimpse into what life was like prior to vaccinations. Incurable, fatal diseases were rampant; death was ever present for young and old alike; healthcare practitioners often risked their own lives in their care of patients. Given this reality, the halakhic literature already from the pre-modern era is replete with discussions relating to both the treatment and communal response to contagious, fatal diseases.

Special prayers and fasts were instituted in times of plague or epidemic.[6] The *Shulḥan Arukh* codifies exactly what percentage of the population needs to be affected in order to constitute a "halakhic" epidemic, a passage with which modern day epidemiologists would have a

---

5. See A. E. Barskay, et al., "Mumps Outbreak in Orthodox Jewish Communities in the United States," *New England Journal of Medicine* 367:18 (November, 2012), 1704–1713. The authors attribute the rapid spread of the disease amongst the young Jewish population to the close contact during "*ḥevruta*" study. See M. Orbach, "How Failure to Immunize Makes Mumps a Hazard in the Beit Midrash," *Jewish Action* (September 30, 2013). See also, "Notes from the Field: Measles Outbreak Amongst Members of a Religious Community—Brooklyn, New York, March- June 2013," *Morbidity and Mortality Weekly Report* 62:36 (September 13, 2013), 752–753.
6. On saying special prayers for the community during a cholera epidemic, See *Ḥatam Sofer, Likutim BeKovetz Teshuvot* 1. One example of a special prayer composed for recital during an epidemic has been displayed in Jerusalem at a special exhibit at the

field day.[7] R. Moshe Isserles (1520–1572) discusses whether one is permitted to flee the city in times of plague,[8] something he himself did in 1555 when he fled from his home in Cracow due to an epidemic.[9] R. Yisrael Salanter (1810–1883) is reported to have made *kiddush* in synagogue on Yom Kippur in order to illustrate the importance of not fasting during a cholera epidemic.[10] R. Yaakov Reischer (1661–1733) addressed the issue of alternate burial and the use of quicklime to hasten decomposition of the body after death from plague to prevent contagion.[11]

The Bikur Cholim societies of previous generations, branches of the Chevra Kadisha (burial society), often provided medical care and assistance at the patient's home, the primary location of care in those days. Detailed manuals were written which included protocols and guidelines for the members of the society.[12] These often included a discussion about the visitation of patients with contagious diseases

Tower of David entitled, *Jerusalem: A Medical Diagnosis*. For more on cholera and other epidemics throughout history in rabbinic literature, see chapter, "Precedented Times: The Rabbinic Response to Covid-19 and Pandemics Throughout the Ages."

7. *O. Ḥ.,* 576:2.

8. *Y. D.,* 116:5.

9. See the introduction to his *Meḥir Yayin* on *Megillat Esther*, which he composed in exile for his father in lieu of *mishloaḥ manot*, as he had insufficient funds and rations to provide for a celebratory meal or the requisite mitzva of *mishloaḥ manot*.

10. On the variations and historical background of this oft-repeated story, see A. Lvov, "Rabbi Isroel Salanter, the *Haskalah* and the 'Theory of Secularization': An Analysis from a Folkloristic Point of View," at http://lvov.judaica.spb.ru/salanter-en.shtml (accessed December 20, 2014); N. Kamenetsky, *Making of a Gadol* 1 (2004), 1104ff; I. Taub, "The Rabbi Who Ate on Yom Kippur: Rabbi Israel Salanter and the Cholera Epidemic of 1848," *Verapo Yerapei* 1 2009), 295–313. For a recent halakhic analysis of R. Salanter's actions, see R. A. Weiss, "Regarding the Decision of Rav Yisrael Salanter During the Time of Plague," (Hebrew), at http://tvunah.org/2013/09/10/ (Accessed December 21, 2014).

11. *Shevut Yaakov* 2:97. See also *Ḥatam Sofer* v. 2, *Y. D.,* 334. On the topic of burial on Shabbat during an epidemic, see *Iggerot Moshe Y. D.,* 4:55.

12. See, for example, S. Goldberg, *Crossing the Jabbok: Illness and Death in Ashkenazi Judaism in Sixteenth through Nineteenth Century Prague* (University of California Press, 1996); *From this World to the Next: Jewish Approaches to Illness, Death and the Afterlife* (Library of the Jewish Theological Seminary, 1999), which accompanied a library exhibit.

due to the inherent danger to the visitor.[13] While the specific causes and mechanism of transmission of infectious disease were not clarified until modern times, there has always been an appreciation of the concept of contagion. In the 1750 manual for the Berlin Bikur Cholim Society, for example, it says, "We have accepted upon ourselves to visit all those afflicted with illness, except..."[14] It then proceeds to list a number of conditions thought to be contagious and life-threatening, including smallpox and measles.

II. EBOLA IN HALAKHA TODAY

What are the halakhic issues of today? Let us entertain some fictional questions a modern rabbi might encounter regarding Ebola.[15] We of course pray that this remains fictional and would never occur in real life.

Flying

A man is visiting Mali on business and is concerned he may have contracted Ebola. He wants to fly to America where he will receive better treatment. May he board a plane without informing anyone of his possible illness, knowing that he may possibly infect other passengers?[16] R. Yitzchak Zilberstein was asked a similar question during the swine flu epidemic as to whether one who does not yet exhibit clinical symptoms of disease could fly to another city.[17] In this specific case, he permitted the flight, but regarding Ebola, one should consult both a physician and a rabbi before boarding.

---

13. R. David Leiter discusses whether attending to a patient with contagious disease might constitute a violation of self-endangerment and might even be akin to suicide. See his *Beit David* 22:1.

14. Aaron ben Moses Rofeh, *Takanot shel Bnei HaHavura DeBikur Holim* (Berlin, 1750).

15. Each issue merits its own full halakhic treatment, which is beyond the scope of this chapter.

16. See J. Lapook, "2nd Nurse with Ebola Called CDC Before Boarding Flight," *CBS News* (October 15, 2014).

17. "Is a Patient with a Severe Contagious Disease Allowed to Board and Aircraft Where He May Infect Others," in F. Rosner, trans. and ed., *Medical Halachic Responsa by Rav Yitzchak Zilberstein* (Maimonides Research Institute, 2013), 205–207.

Praying in Synagogue

A physician just returned from West Africa after treating Ebola patients and shows up in synagogue the next morning for *Shaḥarit* service, where he promptly sits down right next to you. You immediately approach the rabbi in wonderment, "Should this man be allowed to *daven* in *shul*?" R. Ḥayyim Palachi (1788–1869) was asked by members of a synagogue whether they could prevent a physician treating patients with the plague from praying in the synagogue out of fear that they might contract the disease. While R. Palachi said they indeed could, the modern answer to this question requires dialogue with an infectious disease expert to clarify both the time frame and mechanism of contagion.

Tefillin

The local Chabad rabbi is making rounds in the hospital with *tefillin* in hand, looking for those who have not had an opportunity to perform the mitzva. There happens to be a Jewish patient with Ebola (*raḥmana litzlan*) who is thankfully improving. The nurse informs the rabbi that everything that comes in contact with an Ebola patient has to be incinerated. May the rabbi give the patient *tefillin* knowing that while he will perform a mitzva, the *tefillin* will be incinerated after use? Rav Moshe Feinstein addressed this exact question and maintained that it would be prohibited to provide the *tefillin* when it would lead to the destruction of the name of God, which is sacred.[18]

Financial Transactions

A man learning in the Dallas Kollel supplements his income by renting out apartments. After completing a rental agreement with a tenant, he reads in the paper that this person's sister is a nurse at the local hospital who was diagnosed with Ebola. May he renege on the contract for fear of financial consequences? A similar question was posed to R. Moshe

---

18. *Iggerot Moshe O. Ḥ.*, 1:4. Not only do objects that come into contact with the body require incineration, but even the body itself of patients who succumb to Ebola is cremated to prevent contagion. In Ebola, as opposed to other conditions, the body remains highly contagious after death. Cremation would be halakhically problematic as it is prohibited in Jewish law. See above references to burial issues in times of epidemic.

Isserles (*Rama*) in the sixteenth century, when a landlord discovered that a renter's wife developed a contagious disease[19] and wanted to rescind the contract.[20] Rama, based on an analysis of contract law, ruled that he could not rescind and ends with a remarkable discussion about his theory of contagious diseases.[21]

Circumcision

A pregnant Jewish woman is seen in the emergency room for abdominal pains. Shortly thereafter, she is contacted by the Department of Health and informed that she had exposure to a patient with Ebola. As a result, she is quarantined.[22] A few days later, while still in quarantine, she gives birth to a male child. She calls her family *mohel* to perform the *brit*. Should the *mohel* perform the *brit*?[23] What about performing oral *metzitza*, which is his custom? This issue was addressed by *poskim* during the onset of the AIDS epidemic,[24] and while there are similarities, this case would require a separate medical and halakhic analysis.

---

19. The German term for the disease mentioned by R. Isserles is *gelbsucht*, or jaundice, which refers to hepatitis.
20. *She'elot UTeshuvot Rama* 20.
21. See the annotated edition of Rama's responsa by Dr. Asher Ziv (Feldheim Publishers, 1970) for references and discussion of Rama's notion of contagion, as well as references to other responsa on the financial impact of contagious diseases. See also *Shu"t Maharam MiPadua* 86, regarding whether a tutor can claim payment from a student who fled during the plague.
22. For a discussion about halakhic issues related to quarantine, see F. Rosner, "Involuntary Confinement for Tuberculosis Control: The Jewish View," *Mount Sinai Journal of Medicine* 63:1 (January, 1996), 44–48. R. Josh Flug provides references about the issue of quarantine in his "Ethical Dilemmas Relating to the Swine Flu Epidemic," an unpublished source sheet from a *shiur* delivered in 2009 (reference available upon request). For additional sources on quarantine in Jewish sources, see chapter, "Precedented Times."
23. If the baby was infected, God forbid, and symptomatic with Ebola, a *brit* would be too risky for the baby, let alone the *mohel*.
24. See A. S. Cohen, "*Brit Milah* and the Spector of AIDS," *Journal of Halacha and Contemporary Society* 17 (Spring 1989), 93–115; N. Daniel Korobkin, "*Metzitzah B'peh* Controversy: Rabbinic Polemics and Applying the Lessons of History," *Jewish Action* (Winter 2006). For an account of the position of R. Moshe Feinstein, heard orally from him some two weeks before his passing, see R. Cohen, *Bris Avraham* (self-publication, 1993), section *Migdal Oz* 8:6.

Refusal to Treat

A physician receives word that his hospital is now an Ebola center. He promptly calls his rabbi and asks if he can refuse to treat such patients, or is he halakhically obligated to treat them? How much risk must one accept in order to save the life of another? In halakhic literature, this is addressed in the analysis of the biblical phrase, "Do not stand idly by as the blood of your brother is being shed." Is a healthcare provider halakhically required to endure a higher level of risk than the general population? R. Eliezer Waldenberg answers in the affirmative and provides a number of reasons why, including both halakhic and societal.[25] He adds that when one treats patients with highly contagious diseases, one should say a special prayer, in addition to the prayers a physician should generally recite, that he/she should be the proper instrument or messenger of God to provide the patient's cure.

III. CONCLUSION

We have briefly touched on some halakhic issues related to the treatment of patients with contagious diseases. We have seen that this is not a new problem, though application of the halakha to our present case of Ebola requires a fresh medical analysis and halakhic update. As to whether I would perform CPR on an end-stage Ebola patient? Let us hope that both an effective therapy and vaccine[26] are developed and that I will never need to know the answer to this question. Meanwhile, let us use this "exposure" to Ebola as an opportunity to appreciate how God has graced us with the advances in medicine that protect us from the ravages of infectious disease.

---

25. *Tzitz Eliezer* 9:17, *Kuntres Refua BeShabbat*, chapter 5.
26. R. Kanapathipillai, et al., "Ebola Vaccine—An Urgent International Priority," *New England Journal of Medicine* 371 (December 11, 2014), 2249–2251.

Lehitra'ot Ebola, Goodbye Rubella, Hello Zika

I. INTRODUCTION

In the previous chapter, we explored the unique halakhic issues related to Ebola, a highly contagious and fatal disease. When treating such patients, physicians must wear special protective gear (hazmat suit). As a physician in a designated Ebola center, I had to train in the use of such materials. The procedure of putting on the gear is called to "don," and to remove it (ironically a much more complicated process) is called to "doff." At the height of the Ebola scare, I was doing a "doff" a day. It gradually tapered down to a "doff" a week, and then a "doff" a month. I am happy to report that I am no longer doing the "doff" at all. At least for now, the Ebola scare has dissipated. I am further delighted to report that our halakhic discussion about whether one should perform CPR on an Ebola patient has remained hypothetical. This disease, however, is by no means gone, and it will likely resurface again. To Ebola we bid, unfortunately, *lehitra'ot* (we will see you again).

As Ebola slips to the periphery of our radar screen, another disease has replaced it front and center: Zika. Both Zika and Ebola are part of a long tradition of infectious diseases that have generated halakhic dilemmas, but Zika itself is replacing yet another disease, as we shall see.

II. THE HALAKHIC DISCUSSION OF
RUBELLA (GERMAN MEASLES)

If one was born before approximately 1960, it is very likely that they, or someone they know, would have contracted a case of rubella. In contrast, those born more recently are not only highly unlikely to have contracted the disease; they may even be unaware of its very existence. Rubella is a relatively benign disease that can cause a fever, rash, headaches, and eye redness, and is spread from person to person through coughing or sneezing. While a mere nuisance for most adults, its wrath is unleashed on the unborn fetus. If contracted during pregnancy, rubella can possibly cause deafness, blindness, heart disease, microcephaly (small brain), and, tragically, even death for the fetus. When rubella epidemics were common in the mid- to late-twentieth century, a number of halakhic issues arose.

Abortion

One challenging halakhic issue was whether abortion could be considered for those women who were exposed to or contracted rubella in pregnancy. It is important to note that many of the manifestations of congenital rubella are not anatomical, and while ultrasound did exist at that time, albeit in a less sophisticated form, it would not necessarily have revealed any abnormality.

This discussion needs to be placed in the context of the broader halakhic analysis of the prohibition of abortion.[1] The nature of the prohibition of abortion is a matter of rabbinic debate, with the classic polar extremes represented by R. Moshe Feinstein *zt"l* who forbids abortion for any fetal abnormality, such as Tay Sachs, or as in this case of rubella, and R. Eliezer Waldenberg, who allowed abortion for limited cases of fetal disability, which could include rubella, even up to the seventh month of gestation.

To give us a sense of the magnitude of the epidemic, according to an account from the Rabbinic Court of Rav Shmuel Vozner, over

---

1. For a review of the halakhic issues of abortion, see A. Steinberg, *Encyclopedia of Jewish Medical Ethics*, trans. F. Rosner (Feldheim Publishers, 2003), s. v., "abortion."

one thousand cases were presented to the court requesting abortion. The court prohibited abortion in every single case (consistent with the general approach of R. Feinstein). As a postscript, it is further reported that in all the cases, save one, no harm befell the subsequent children. As this is an anecdotal account, absent any details of the cases, we cannot know whether the women had confirmed cases of rubella, and if so, during which trimester. In any case, it is a remarkable number.[2]

Contraception

A vaccine for rubella was developed in the 1960s. To prevent birth defects, the medical community recommended vaccinations for all women of childbearing years. The vaccine, however, was comprised of a live, attenuated virus (as opposed to a killed virus) and had potential for the transmission of disease to the woman. As such, it was recommended that women practice contraception for three months after receiving the vaccination. This created a halakhic dilemma, as one would be delaying the mitzva of *peru urevu* (be fruitful and multiply). Proper treatment of the halakhic topic of contraception is beyond the scope of this chapter.[3] R. Yitzḥak Zilberstein responded to this specific query with the following nuanced conclusions:[4]

1) If the husband already fulfilled *peru urevu*, the wife can receive the vaccine.
2) If *peru urevu* has not been fulfilled, the woman should not receive the vaccine and "*shomer mitzva lo yada davar ra* (one who preserves and performs a mitzva will not be harmed)."
3) If the woman is extremely fearful/concerned about the risk to the fetus, she can vaccinate and use contraception.
4) The husband may also refrain from the mitzva of *peru urevu* if the wife is extremely afraid of disease transmission to her fetus.

---

2. R. Simcha HaKohen Kook, "Abortion and the Treatment of Handicapped Children," *Beit Hillel* 6:3 (*Tammuz*, 5745) (Hebrew)
3. See A. Steinberg, *Encyclopedia of Jewish Medical Ethics*, trans. F. Rosner (Feldheim Publishers, 2003), s. v., "contraception."
4. *Shiurei Torah LeRofim*, n. 225.

5) One can rely on the *Ezer MiKodesh* that *peru urevu* can be delayed for 6 months to learn a profession. So too in this case.

III. GOODBYE RUBELLA, HELLO ZIKA[5]

In April of 2016, global health officials declared that rubella has officially been eliminated from the Americas.[6] This miraculous feat was accomplished through vaccination (the "R" of the MMR vaccine stands for rubella), and this is why those born in the last few decades have not seen a case of the disease.

Behold the following observation: Just as we are saying goodbye to a disease which, although benign for the adult, wreaks havoc on the fetus, we read the very next day about a new disease called Zika,[7] with a profile remarkably reminiscent of rubella (there are important differences, especially in the mode of transmission). Is God perhaps sending a not so subtle message that while man believes he can claim the eradication of disease, it is perhaps a misplaced arrogance? While this interpretation is purely speculative, the observation nonetheless remains.

---

5. Another halakhic aspect of rubella is the liability for its transmission. One of the most famous American rubella victims was the actress Gene Tierney. In 1943, newly pregnant, she volunteered to be in a show at the Hollywood Canteen, a nightclub for American troops. She purportedly caught the disease that night, and her daughter Daria was born weighing only three pounds, deaf, with cataracts and with brain damage so severe that she never learned to speak.

   According to Ms. Tierney's biography, two years later, at a tennis match, she met a fan, a former member of the Marine Corps Women's Reserve, who said she had slipped out of a rubella quarantine to go see her show at the Canteen that night. See D. G. McNeil, "Rubella Has Been Eliminated from the Americas," *New York Times* (April 29, 2015). For an analysis as to whether this woman would be halakhically liable, see F. Rosner trans. and ed., Y. Zilberstein, *Medical Halachic Responsa* (Maimonides Research Institute, 2013), 211–212.

6. D. G. McNeil, "Rubella has Been Eliminated from the Americas, Health Officials Say," New York Times, April 29, 2015. Smallpox was eradicated from the globe in 1979 and Polio from the Americas in 1994.

7. On the history of the discovery, spread and diagnosis of the Zika virus, see J. Waggoner and B. Pinsky, "Zika Virus: Diagnostics for an Emerging Pandemic Threat," *Journal of Clinical Microbiology* 54:4 (April, 2016), 860–866.

Zika Virus

Zika (not etymologically related to *mazik*, a tortfeasor) is a virus named after the forest where it was first identified in Uganda, a country until now known to the Jewish community for two things: as the location of the legendary raid at Entebbe, and as the place Herzl supported as a Jewish homeland. This mosquito-borne disease has now created an international stir for reasons we shall presently address.

Below are the basics of Zika virus, highlighting aspects of the disease relevant to the halakhic discussion.[8]

- Zika virus is transmitted primarily through the bite of a mosquito. It typically causes a rash, joint pains, fevers, and eye-redness and is usually benign, with rare possible neurological effects.
- It can be transmitted through sexual contact, more commonly from male to female, though recently the reverse has been observed. (I call this *"zikat haba'al,"* not to be confused with the term from *Yevamot*.)
- With the exception of a small area in Florida, almost all of the cases initially identified in the U.S. were of travelers from endemic countries.[9]
- Zika can cause birth defects, typically microcephaly (small brain) in a percentage of pregnant women. The exact percentage remains unknown with recent studies showing a range from 1% to 13%.
- There is no treatment or vaccine for Zika as yet.

IV. ZIKA VIRUS — HALAKHIC ISSUES

Zika shares some of the same halakhic concerns as rubella, with some variations and additions. While a detailed expansive analysis of the halakhic ramifications of Zika is beyond the scope of this chapter, we identify here some of the major issues.[10]

---

8. Further information may be gleaned from the CDC website. Due to the infancy of this disease and the continuing accumulation of data, the information will surely evolve.
9. I have seen less than a handful of cases of Zika, all of which were from endemic countries.
10. There are many aspects of both the medical and halakhic aspects of Zika that will not be addressed in this brief chapter, including details of the viral identification, the nature of the different types of testing, the gender differences of the CDC recommendations,

Contraception (Communal)

In January 2016, in an unprecedented move, El Salvador, an area of Zika prevalence, advised *all* women living in the country not to get pregnant until 2018 for fear of their contracting Zika through a mosquito bite.[11] The CDC has also advised against conception for those living in endemic areas. Even the Pope suggested that contraceptives may be used to prevent the spread of Zika.[12] The Jewish community in Brazil, ground zero for the Zika virus, is struggling with these issues.[13]

There are in fact a number of discussions in rabbinic literature about the concept of communal contraception. When Amram, the father of *Moshe Rabbenu,* saw that Pharaoh decreed to kill all the male children, he said, "We are toiling in vain," and he divorced his wife. All the men of Israel then divorced their wives. However, he subsequently reevaluated his decision, remarried and continued to have children. The others followed suit.[14] In addition, the Talmud learns from Yosef that one should not engage in marital relations in times of famine.[15]

Both of these cases were invoked in the modern era in discussing the propriety of contraception amidst the horrors of the Holocaust and its aftermath. After World War II, R. Hillel Posek convened a congress of rabbis to address the unsanctioned refusal of many women to engage in the mitzva of *peru urevu.*[16]

Contraception (Personal)

The major concern with Zika is the transmission of the disease to the fetus. Depending on the circumstances of travel to infected areas,

---

the statistics of fetal infection in the case of Zika infection for the pregnant woman, the halakhic issues of traveling to endemic countries, the permissibility to kill mosquitos on Shabbat.

11. A. Ahmed, "El Salvador's Advice on Zika Virus: Don't Have Babies," *New York Times* (January 25, 2016).
12. "Pope Suggests Contraceptives Could be Used to Slow Spread of Zika, *New York Times* (February 18, 2016).
13. M. Moreas, "Battling Zika at Ground Zero," JTA (March 7, 2016).
14. *Sota* 12b.
15. *Ta'anit* 11a.
16. See, for example, R. Y. A. Landa, *Shu"t Beit Yisrael E. H.,* 152; R. Hillel Posek, *Ha-Posek* 23:834–837.

suspected or actual infection, and even gender of the exposed person,[17] the recommendations of the Centers for Disease Control differ. There is concern for the transmission of the virus both through mosquito bites and through sexual transmission. There are many variables that are not yet fully understood, and, as a result, the recommendations will surely change over time.

In addition, there are a number of tests for Zika virus, including tests for active infection and exposure. Any halakhic inquiry needs to take into account the current knowledge of the time, and accuracy of the testing as interpreted by medical experts. All questions should be presented to a rabbinic authority for consultation.

Preventing Conception

In situations where one of the married partners has either been possibly exposed to or confirmed infected with Zika, the objective is to prevent conception so as not to risk the birth of a severely diseased child. Issues for consideration:

- Is contraception allowed in general, and if yes, is it allowed in this case?[18]
- Is abstaining preferred to contraception? This will depend on the length of the time involved. If the time period is relatively short, abstaining may be preferred; if the time period is prolonged, contraception may possibly be permitted in consultation with a rabbinic authority.
- Does the type of contraception matter? Most definitely. There are major differences in the types of contraception that are permitted. In this case, a hormonal method (e.g. the pill) may be halakhically least objectionable. However, while a hormonal method may prevent pregnancy, it would not prevent transmission of the virus. Thus, for example, a Zika-infected woman taking hormonal contraception could potentially transmit the disease to her husband through

---

17. The disparate recommendations for men and women derive from medical evidence of the lingering presence of Zika virus, or its remnants, identified in sperm.
18. See A. Steinberg, *Encyclopedia of Jewish Medical Ethics*, trans. F. Rosner (Feldheim Publishers, 2003), s. v., "contraception."

marital relations. If the husband contracts Zika, it may remain in his reproductive seed for a long period and necessitate the need for contraception for a prolonged period.

- Does testing for Zika impact the halakhic discussion? Yes, testing, when done with expert medical consultation, may possibly obviate the need for any form of contraception if it can be reliably confirmed that there has been no exposure to or infection with Zika.

When the Woman is Pregnant

When the woman is pregnant and contracts Zika virus, there is a chance for the disease to be transmitted to the fetus, though the exact percentages remain unclear. A pregnant woman (or one in the age of fertility) should clearly avoid elective travel to endemic areas due to the potential *sakana* (danger) to the fetus.[19]

Due to the concern of sexual transmission, if the man is exposed or has acquired Zika, the CDC recommends that the couple should use a barrier method of contraception throughout the entire pregnancy. All the same issues mentioned above would apply here, except in this case, the only medically effective method of contraception in order to prevent Zika transmission to the fetus is a barrier method. This method is more halakhically problematic than other contraceptive forms. There is halakhic precedent regarding the use of barrier contraception in cases of AIDS, where the concern is likewise the transmission of disease.[20] Rabbinic authorities should be consulted. Here as well, testing may obviate the need for any form of contraception.

---

19. This issue of travel involving danger, either as a result of the journey or the presence of disease at the destination, merits fuller treatment. Travel for the purpose of one's livelihood is another matter. See the classic responsum of *Noda BiYehuda, Mahadura Tinyana Y. D.*, 10. Regarding discussions of fleeing during a plague, see next chapter, "Precedented Times."

20. See *Minḥat Shlomo* 3:103, letter 16; *Shevet Levi* 10:238; *Assia* 61–62, 95ff and 100ff; J. D. Bleich, "AIDS: A Jewish Perspective," *Tradition* 26:3 (1992), 49–80, esp. 68–69; G. Freudenthal, ed., *AIDS in Jewish Thought and Law* (Ktav, 1998), liv, n. 99.

Freezing Reproductive Seed

An option that some participants in the Olympics exercised was to freeze their reproductive seed prior to travel to Rio, a Zika area. This reproductive seed could then be subsequently used for procreation without the fear of Zika transmission.[21] There is much to discuss here from a halakhic perspective. Egg freezing for women has become much more common recently and is permitted, and even encouraged by a number of rabbinic authorities in certain situations. However, this specific case has not been addressed.[22] The different mechanism of transmission for the Zika-infected woman and the required waiting period for conception would need to be considered. Freezing of sperm is halakhically more problematic, especially for the unmarried man.[23] It is unlikely that such a practice would be sanctioned for men traveling to Zika-infested areas.

Abortion

The issue of abortion in cases of Zika would be similar in concept to cases of rubella. The rabbinic authorities, such as Rav Moshe Feinstein, who forbid abortion for any fetal indication, would similarly forbid abortion in this case; those who allow abortion for severe disability of the fetus, such as R. Eliezer Waldenberg would consider the possibility of abortion here. Questions that would need to be addressed for cases of Zika would include:

- Is exposure to the virus enough to consider abortion, or is documented maternal infection required?
- Even if the mother is infected, would anatomical evidence of fetal infection (such as an ultrasound showing microcephaly) be required to entertain the possibility of abortion? This is only possible later in pregnancy.

---

21. J. Branch, "Among Olympians' Zika Precautions: Fewer Guests, Frozen Sperm," *New York Times* (June 15, 2016).
22. See E. Rybak, "Aging Ovaries and the Age-Old Tradition: Elective Egg Freezing in Jewish Law," *Journal of Halacha and Contemporary Society* 63 (Spring 2012), 22–50.
23. J. D. Bleich, "Sperm Banking in Anticipation of Infertility," *Tradition* 29:4 (Summer 1995), 47–60.

- How does the statistical likelihood of fetal Zika infection with maternal disease impact the halakhic equation regarding abortion?
- How will Zika virus testing affect the decision?

May we be *zokheh* (merit) that Zika will not *mazik* us, and that, with God's help, a vaccine should be developed,[24] or a method to genetically modify mosquitos,[25] to render all these halakhic discussions moot.[26] Hopefully, one day soon, when the question is asked, "Have you have seen or heard of a case of Zika?" we will be able to answer in the negative, just as for rubella.

---

24. On the halakhic approach to vaccination, see chapter, "Lessons from the First Halakhic Analysis of Vaccination."
25. J. Achenbach, "Genetically Engineered Bugs to Fight Malaria and Zika? Not So Fast," *Washington Post* (June 8, 2016).
26. There is also a halakhic question as to whether one can kill a mosquito on Shabbat in a Zika-infested area to prevent it from biting a pregnant woman? If we define this as a case of *pikuaḥ nefesh*, then the answer will be yes. Further analysis is required.

Precedented Times: The Rabbinic Response to COVID-19 and Pandemics Throughout the Ages

In November of 2019, a new virus appeared on the world stage. Initially called the Novel Coronavirus, later renamed COVID-19,[1] it initially reared its head in China, though only shortly thereafter swept across the entire globe with reckless abandon. To be sure, there have been plagues throughout the millennia. The Plague of Justinian in 541 CE killed an estimated thirty to fifty million people; the Black Death[2] killed some

---

1. Hereinafter referred to as Covid.
2. For discussion of the Black Death in Jewish sources, see Ron Barkai, "Jewish Treatises on the Black Death (1350–1500): A Preliminary Study," in Roger French, et al., eds., *Medicine from the Black Death to the French Disease* (Ashgate Publishing, 1998), 6–25; Gerrit Bos, "The Black Death in Hebrew Literature: *HaMa'amar be-Qaddahat Ha-Dever* (Treatise on Pestilential Fever)," *European Journal of Jewish Studies* 5:1 (January, 2011), 1–52; Gerrit Bos and Guido Mensching, "The Black Death in Hebrew Literature: Abraham Ben Solomon Hen's *Tractatulus de Pestilentia*," *Jewish Studies Journal* 18

twenty-five million people between 1348–1350; smallpox,[3] yellow fever, and cholera[4] killed untold millions as well. In more recent times, AIDS, swine flu, SARS, Ebola,[5] and MERS have joined the list. Yet, the present pandemic has been repeatedly called "unprecedented," and deservedly so. We in the United States have not seen a disease spread of this magnitude for over a century, since the Spanish Flu Pandemic of 1918.[6] Never before has a plague spread across the globe with such lightning rapidity. At no time in American history has virtually the entire nation been asked/required to cease their normal daily activities and quarantine for a prolonged period of time.

As I write these words, we are still very much in the midst of the Covid pandemic. As an emergency physician in one of New York's largest medical centers, I am experiencing this pandemic in a very intimate fashion. Our facility has seen thousands of Covid patients, and in the emergency room, I am exposed daily to countless patients with the virus. Indeed, I contracted a case of Covid at the end of March 2020 and have, thank God, recovered and returned to full time work.

(2011), 32–63; Susan Einbinder, *After the Black Death: Plague and Commemoration Among Iberian Jews* (University of Pennsylvania Press: Philadelphia, 2018). For discussion of the persecution of Jews and anti-Semitism associated with the Black Death, see Samuel Cohn, "The Black Death and the Burning of the Jews," *Past and Present* 196 (August, 2007), 3–36; Tzafrir Barzilay, *Well-Poisoning Accusations in Medieval Europe: 1250–1500* (Ph.D. Dissertation: Columbia University, 2017); Einbinder, op. cit.

3. On the rabbinic response to smallpox, see chapter, "Lessons from the First Halakhic Analysis of Vaccination."

4. For rabbinic responses to cholera pandemics, see H. J. Zimmels, *Magicians, Theologians and Doctors* (Edward Goldston and Son, 1952), 106–107; E. Reichman, "From Cholera to Coronavirus: Recurrent Pandemics with Recurrent Rabbinic Responses," *Tradition Online* (April 2, 2020) https://traditiononline.org/from-cholera-to-coronavirus-recurring-pandemics-recurring-rabbinic-responses.

5. On the halakhic issues of Ebola, see chapter, "Ebola: A New Disease with an Ancient Tradition."

6. On the history of the Spanish Flu, see Jeremy Brown, *Influenza: The Hundred Year Hunt to Cure the Deadliest Disease in History* (Atria Books, 2018). For an example of the rabbinic response to the Spanish Flu, see lecture of R. Gavriel Bechhofer, with accompanying source booklet, https://www.youtube.com/watch?v=rFFBPFAUwVU&t=16s (accessed July 19, 2020).

There has been much written, and even more to yet be written, about the medical aspects of this disease, many of which are genuinely unprecedented. In this chapter, I focus on the Jewish and rabbinic responses to this pandemic in comparison to the rabbinic responses to plague and disease throughout the centuries. It is actually in the very nature and dissemination of rabbinic responses that this pandemic is truly unprecedented. In past centuries, rabbis most assuredly responded to halakhic issues stemming from the ravages of disease. Yet, when rendered, these decisions were known only to the questioner and perhaps to his or her immediate contacts. On occasion, the rabbis would subsequently commit these decisions to writing, and on rarer occasion, they would ultimately be published. Even then, the responsa would be buried amongst hundreds of others on various halakhic topics. Today, in sharp contrast, decisions rendered are often disseminated in real time to the global Jewish community through a variety of social media. In addition, a number of rabbinic authorities have collected their responsa relating to this pandemic into dedicated volumes.[7] We are, therefore, privy, intrapandemic, to the rabbinic approach to the Covid virus, given a view our predecessors were denied by virtue of circumstance.

In this chapter, we discuss selected categories of response to the contemporary pandemic of Covid. Our primary objective is to highlight the historical precedents to each of these categories.

DEFINITION OF A PANDEMIC

On March 11, 2020, the World Health Organization declared that an outbreak of Covid had officially become an international pandemic. While an epidemic describes a widespread occurrence of an infectious

---

7. Examples include *Piskei Corona* by R. Hershel Schachter and a dedicated Corona volume of *Minḥat Asher* by Rav Asher Weiss. Both of these have already been revised and expanded multiple times. R. Dr. Avraham Steinberg has written an essay on all halakhic matters relating to the pandemic, which includes the responsa of contemporary *poskim*. It has been rendered into English by R. Jason Weiner. For a review of all the current literature relating to Covid, including detailed references to the above, see Eliezer Brodt, "Towards a Bibliography of Coronavirus-related Articles and Seforim written in the past month (updated), Black Weddings and Other Segulot," *Seforimblog.com* (May 4, 2020) (accessed July 7, 2020).

disease in a community at a particular time, a pandemic involves spread beyond a local geographical area, to other countries and noncontiguous geographical regions. In its extreme, as has been the case with Covid, a pandemic can spread across the entire world. Reaching this threshold can impact the mobilization of resources by countries to combat the outbreak.

Historical Precedent

Rabbinic literature also discusses a threshold of sorts for the declaration of widespread disease, as it states in the Mishna of *Ta'anit*:[8]

> And so too, a city which has a plague ... that city fasts and they sound a blast... What constitutes a plague? If, in a city that can supply five hundred foot soldiers, three deaths occurred on three consecutive days, behold this constitutes a plague; less than this is not a plague.

There was a need to define a threshold for the declaration of catastrophic plague. Once this threshold was crossed, the requirement for fasting and *shofar* blowing would be activated. For less than this, it would not.

SHELTERING IN PLACE VS. FLEEING

During the Covid pandemic, many states and countries strongly suggested or mandated that people remain in their homes and significantly limit movement or travel. Many fled the densely populated cities for more remote areas if they were able to do so.

Historical Precedent

The Talmud expresses one suggestion as to one's course of action during a plague: "Our Rabbis taught, if there is plague in the city, gather your feet (*kanes raglekha*) [i.e., shelter in place at home]." It brings scriptural support for this notion. Centuries later, a number of rabbinic authorities seemed to reject the Talmud's recommendation in favor of fleeing the city during plague. R. Moshe Isserles explicitly recommends fleeing,

---

8. 3:4.

citing support from Maharil,[9] though he hastens to add that one should flee at the beginning stages of the plague and not later. He apparently practiced what he preached, as he records in the introduction to his commentary on *Megillat Esther, Meḥir Yayin,* that he fled from Cracow to Shidlov due to plague. In fact, he wrote the book for his father-in-law as a gift in lieu of *mishloaḥ manot,* which was unattainable due to the famine and dearth of resources during the plague. R. Yeshaya Horowitz, known as Shela HaKadosh (1555–1630), likewise strongly advised fleeing the city with one's children during a smallpox outbreak.[10]

Evidence that Jews experiencing plague were aware of both the talmudic advice and its opponents regarding fleeing can be gleaned from the poem of Moshe Catalano regarding the plague in Padua in 1631.[11] The poem begins, "*dever bitokh ha'ir pazer raglekha,*" when plague is within your city, scatter your feet (i.e., flee). While he recommends that ideally one should flee, he adds in his second verse, that if not possible, then,"*dever ba'ir kanes raglekha,*" one should shelter in place. The phrasing is a clear allusion to the talmudic passage above, while heeding the advice of the rabbis of his time to flee if possible.

There is debate as to whether leaders of the community are halakhically permitted to flee during a plague, when, if anything, the need for their services is greater. While many stayed, heeding the advice of the Talmud,[12] other did not. We have record of both rabbis and physicians

9. *Teshuvot Maharil,* n. 35.

10. *Sha'ar HaOtiyot,* n. 4, *Derekh Eretz,* n. 14. For further halakhic discussion on this issue, see M. D. Chechik, "The Prohibition or Obligation to Flee the City in Times of Plague," (Hebrew) *HaMa'ayan* 233 (*Nissan,* 5780), 22–34; T. Morsel-Eisenberg, "Is It Permitted to Flee the City?" *Tablet Magazine* (April 22, 2020), 1–19.

11. This poem appears at the end of *Olam Hafukh* by Abraham Catalano, the father of Moshe. See Cecil Roth, ed., Abraham Catalano, "*Olam Hafukh,*" *Kovetz al Yad* 4:14 (1946), 67–101. This work is discussed below. For more on this poem and other Hebrew poetry associated with plagues, see S. Einbinder, "Poetry, Prose and Pestilence: Joseph Concio and Jewish Responses to the 1630 Italian Plague," in Haviva Yishai, ed., *Shirat Dvora: Essays in Honor of Professor Dvora Bregman* (Ben-Gurion University: Beer Sheva, 2019), 73–101.

12. See, for example, R. Meir Vaknin, *Vayomer Meir* (Tiberius, 5755), chapter one, who writes, "A plague of cholera broke out in Tiberius in 1913, … and many inhabitants fled from the city to the villages around … with God's compassion, I did not want to

fleeing during times of plague. David Loria, one of the Jewish physicians of the Padua ghetto, fled to nearby Montagnana at the onset of the plague in 1630. He left money to support the community upon his departure and continued to provide extensive assistance from exile.[13]

R. Jacob Sasportas, who had arrived in London from Amsterdam in the Summer of 1664 to lead the community, fled shortly thereafter to Germany upon the onset of the Great Plague of London. In July 1666, he wrote from his new abode, "These are the words of him who writes and signs here at Hamburg and who fled from fear of the destroying hand of the Lord which was against our community in London."[14]

WEARING MASKS

During the Covid pandemic, masks have been an essential part of the prevention strategy, being strongly encouraged, if not mandatory.

Historical Precedent

I mention here two precedents in rabbinic literature, one remote, one more recent, for wearing masks to prevent the spread of disease. According to the Torah, one afflicted with the disease *tzara'at*[15] is required to perform the following actions, "As for the person with *tzara'at*, his clothes shall be rent, his head shall be left bare, and he shall cover his lip (*al safam ya'ateh*)."[16]

---

leave; rather, I fulfilled the words of Ḥazal, 'if there is a plague in the city then draw in your legs,' and I established in my house and courtyard '*daled amot* of *halakha*,'" I thank Dr. Ari Greenspan for this reference.

13. Roth, op. cit., 81.

14. Cited in W. S. Samuel, "The Jews of London and the Great Plague," *Miscellanies of the Jewish Historical Society of England* 3 (1937), 11.

15. While often translated as Leprosy, *tzara'at* is a unique disease for which no contemporary clear medical identification has been made. The association with leprosy likely derives from the translation of the word *tzara'at* as "lepros" in the Septuagint, the Greek translation of the Torah from the third century BCE. Lepros at that time meant a generic skin condition. Only later in history was a specific disease called Leprosy (Hanson's disease) which then became inextricably linked, erroneously, with the biblical *tzara'at*.

16. Vayikra 13:45.

Ibn Ezra (1089–1167), in his comments on the phrase, "and he shall cover his lip," reflects a sensitivity to the concept of contagion: "… and the reason [for covering his mouth], so that he should not harm others with the breath of mouth."[17]

More recently, we find a reference to a protective mask of sorts in the writings of the Ḥafetz Ḥayyim. In the laws of Tisha B'Av,[18] regarding the obligation to fast when sick, the Ḥafetz Hayyim cites the work *Pithei Olam* in his *Bi'ur Halakha* that during times of cholera pandemic, if one is otherwise healthy and wishes to fast, it is preferable to stay at home. If one wishes to leave the house, however, he should place around his nose and mouth a piece of camphor, as well as a special type of grass.[19] Camphor was used for centuries as a fumigant for plague.

This passage was interpreted by one of the great contemporary Torah sages, R. Ḥayyim Kanievsky, *shlit"a*, that one should wear a mask in times of plague. According to the written account, a man who came to visit R. Kanievsky noticed he was wearing a mask. He innocently asked, "Are you donning a mask because of the government regulation?" R. Kanievsky replied, "Why do you say that it is a government decree, the Ḥafetz Ḥayyim already ruled that one is required to wear a mask [in times of plague]!"[20]

ISOLATION AND THE LAZZARETTO

Isolation is used to separate people infected with a contagious disease from people who are not infected so as to prevent additional spread. Isolation has been a mainstay of the strategy to control Covid. Its use is

---

17. There is rabbinic debate as to whether *tzara'at* was a unique, divine punishment for the person, or whether it was a naturally occurring disease which could be contagious.
18. *O. Ḥ.,* 554:6.
19. The source for this statement of the *Pithei Olam* is R. Menachem Mendel Schneer-sohn (1789–1866), known as the Tzemaḥ Tzedek. See special insert for *Hamodia* (7 Adar, 5780), 29–30. I thank R. Eliezer Brodt for this reference. See *Tzemaḥ Tzedek, O. Ḥ.,* 110. Here, the grass is spelled with the letter *nun, minta* or *mienta,* and appears to refer to mint grass or mint weed. In the printed *Mishna Berura,* the letter *nun* is missing.
20. Y. Lavi, "The *Sar HaTorah* on Wearing a Mask," (Hebrew) *Shaharit Digital Newspaper* (May 24, 2020), 13, https://shaharit.com/wp-content/uploads/2020/05/24052020. pdf (accessed July 16, 2020).

not restricted to times of pandemic, though it is employed more expansively during such times.

Historical Precedent

For a more remote rabbinic reference, I return to the case of *tzara'at*. Upon diagnosis of *tzara'at*, the afflicted person must leave city confines: "Being unclean, he shall dwell apart (*badad yeshev*); his dwelling shall be outside the camp."[21] The *Da'at Zekeinim* (12th–13th century) on this verse suggests the reason for his isolation is to prevent the spread of disease to those with whom he would come into contact.

A remarkable yet tragic source is a more recent reference to isolation for plague in the Jewish community. In the years 1630–1631, plague descended on Northern Italy, including the city of Padua. The Jewish ghetto coordinated a response which included delegating four people to oversee all plague related matters, including medical, financial, social, and religious.[22] One of these delegates was Abraham Catalano (d. 1642), who, unlike many of his compatriots, survived the ordeal. He wrote a daily diary of his experiences entitled *Olam Hafukh, World in Upheaval.* It remained in manuscript form in a number of libraries across the world, only to be published in the mid-twentieth century by Cecil Roth.[23] We will have cause to refer to this work throughout this chapter. With respect to isolation, Catalano discusses the necessity for Jews to build their own lazaretto.[24] A lazaretto[25] was a house designated

---

21. Vayikra 13:46.
22. For more discussion about the Jewish response to plagues in Italy, see Yaffa Kohen, *The Development of Organizational Structures by the Italian Jewish Communities to Cope with the Plagues of the Sixteenth and Seventeenth Centuries* (Hebrew) (Doctoral Dissertation: Bar-Ilan University, submitted *Tishrei*, 5740). I thank Naomi Abraham, librarian at Bar-Ilan University, for her truly exceptional efforts in making this dissertation available to me in the midst of the Covid pandemic.
23. Roth, op. cit.
24. Roth, op. cit., 80.
25. The etymology of this term remains in question. Some associate it with Lazarus, the patron saint of lepers. The Order of St. Lazarus cared for lepers, who required isolation. Others suggest it is an alteration of the name Nazaretto. Nazaretto took its name from the church of Santa Maria di Nazareth, a location of isolation on an island in Venice.

for isolation of those afflicted with plague and intended to limit disease spread. Without their own facility, Jews would be required to isolate in the general lazaretto, where religious accommodations, such as kosher food and possibly prayer services, would not likely be forthcoming. The term lazaretto was used for centuries in many European countries to refer to houses of both isolation and quarantine.

QUARANTINE

Quarantine is technically different than isolation, though the terms are often used interchangeably. Quarantine is used to keep someone who might have been exposed to a disease away from others. This serves to prevent spread of disease before a person is aware of their symptoms or if they are asymptomatic carriers. The word quarantine comes from the Italian *quarantena*, meaning "forty days," used in the fourteenth and fifteenth centuries and designating the period that all ships were required to be isolated before passengers and crew could go ashore during epidemics such as the Black Death and others. This exact procedure has been employed by many countries during the Covid pandemic that quarantine visitors from abroad, though for a lesser time period.

Historical Precedent

The concept of quarantine, as reflected by the very etymology of the word, is an old practice. Catalano mentions its use many times during the 1631 Padua plague. For example, "Then Immanuel Bono fell ill and bubos [the typical skin lesions of the Bubonic Plague] were seen near his ear. Eliyahu Francisi attended to him, and Bono subsequently died. Francisi was then quarantined. Then the wife of Menachem Minkin died, and her entire household was quarantined."

The prominent Jewish physician of the early eighteenth century, David de Silva, records his unique experience of being quarantined for the required forty days in the Italian port city of Livorno upon his arrival from the island of Malta.[26] His neighbor in the lazaretto had a

---

26. Z. Amar, *Pri Megadim by R. David de Silva Physician of Jerusalem* (Yad Ben-Zvi Press, 2003), 73.

pet monkey who kept escaping and wreaking havoc, not to mention possibly spreading disease.

The great Jewish philanthropist, Moses Montefiore (1784–1885), endured quarantine multiple times during his world travels, especially during his journeys to Israel.[27] Cholera was widespread during those times in the Holy Land.[28] In fact, Montefiore's personal physician, Thomas Hodgkin (of Hodgkin's disease) died in Israel on a trip accompanying Montefiore, likely from cholera.[29]

PRAYER

Prayer is an essential and integral part of the Jewish response to tragedy, including times of plague. Special prayers were written and recited across the world for the Covid pandemic. An element found in many of these prayers is the recitation of *Pitum HaKetoret*, a detailed description of the preparation of the incense burned daily in the Beit HaMikdash.

Historical Precedent

The liturgy of past centuries is replete with specific prayers recited during times of plague. While these prayers are sometimes labeled for a specific disease, the content is not disease specific. For example, the National Library of Israel lists some thirty prayers for cholera.[30] Many of these prayers include the recitation of *Pitum HaKetoret*. In fact, the addition of the *Ketoret* passage to contemporary pandemic prayers is by no means a modern concoction. It is, rather, simply a continuation of a

---

27. See Sally Style, "Montefiore Risked Cholera, Quarantine for 19th-Century Holy Land Jews," *Times of Israel* (July 18, 2020).
28. There were other prevalent diseases in the Holy Land at that time as well. See Rachel Neiman, "Pandemics and Plagues in the Holy land," *Israel21c* (March 23, 2020), https://www.israel21c.org/pandemics-and-plagues-in-the-holy-land (accessed July 19, 2020).
29. See S. J. Plaschkes, "The Cholera Epidemic in Palestine in 1866: With Remarks about the Cause of the Death of Thomas Hodgkin," *Acta Medica Orientalis* 16:5–6 (May-June, 1957), 136–138.
30. On saying special prayers for the community during a cholera epidemic, see *Ḥatam Sofer, Likutim BeKovetz Teshuvot*, 1.

centuries-old tradition of invoking the *ketoret* in times of plague.[31] This practice traces back to the episode that follows the rebellion of Koraḥ, when God unleashes an unrestrained *magefa* (plague) upon the people of Israel. Moshe instructs Aharon to take *ketoret* from the Temple and to wave it amongst the sufferers of the plague.[32] This rapidly brings about the cessation of the plague, *"vate'atzar hamagefa."* This may be the only direct effective treatment for plague mentioned in the Torah.

Abraham Yagel, a sixteenth-century physician, mentions the story of Aharon and the *ketoret* and supports the recitation of *Ma'aseh Ketoret* in times of plague.[33] He also cites R. Judah Muscato who adds that by delving into the *ketoret*, the infestation will stop by natural means and the air will be purified.[34] The Ari *z"l* likewise recommends the recitation of *Pitum HaKetoret* in times of plague.[35] Catalano also mentions the value of the recitation of the *Ketoret* passage during the Padua plague of 1631.

In the early twentieth century, David Macht performed experiments which identified antiseptic properties of the ingredients of the

---

31. See, for example, Susan L. Einbinder, "Prayer and Plague: Jewish Plague Liturgy from Medieval and Early Modern Italy," in Lori Jones and Nükhet Varlik, eds., *Death and Disease in the Medieval and Early Modern World: Perspectives from Across the Mediterranean and Beyond* (York Medieval Press, 2021), forthcoming.
    Einbinder devotes an entire section to the *ketoret* prayer. For more on *ketoret* and plague, see E. Reichman, "Incensed by Coronavirus: Prayer and *Ketoret* in Times of Epidemic," *Lehrhaus* (March 15, 2020) https://thelehrhaus.com/timely-thoughts/ incensed-by-coronavirus-prayer-and-ketoret-in-times-of-epidemic.
32. Burning the *ketoret* outside the *Mishkan* was generally prohibited, though an exception was made for the sake of saving human life. On the implication of this episode for contemporary medical halakha, see Yosef Aryeh Lawrence, *Mishnat Pikuaḥ Nefesh* (Bnei Brak, 5763), chapter 62.
33. See Abraham Yagel's plague tract, *Moshia Hosim* (di Gara: Venice, 1587), 63 and 66. On Yagel, see David B. Ruderman, *Kabbalah, Magic and Science: The Cultural Universe of a Sixteenth-Century Jewish Physician* (Harvard University Press, 1988), esp. 32–34 and 181 at n. 45.
34. See Andrew Berns, "Judah Moscato, Abraham Portaleone, and Biblical Incense in Late Renaissance Mantua," in Giuseppe Veltri and Gianfranco Miletto, eds., *Studies in Jewish History and Culture, Volume 35, Rabbi Judah Moscato and the Jewish Intellectual World of Mantua in the 16 –17th Centuries* (Brill, 2012), 119–133.
35. *Sha'ar HaKavanot, Derush Tefillat Shaḥarit.*

ketoret.[36] Indeed, he penned an entire volume dedicated to identifying the exact ingredients of the Temple incense.[37]

LIMITATION OF PUBLIC GATHERINGS

During the course of this pandemic, large social gatherings have been variously restricted or cancelled, depending on the stage of the outbreak.

Historical Precedent

Ḥatam Sofer also faced concerns in Pressburg regarding limiting social gatherings in the midst of a cholera pandemic. In the year 1831 physicians banned public gatherings to limit the spread of disease. The secretary of the Chevra Kadisha planned to cancel the annual dinner, which was scheduled, according to tradition, for seventh of Adar. Ḥatam Sofer instructed that under no circumstances should the *seuda* (festive meal) be canceled.[38]

CLOSING HOUSES OF WORSHIP

The limitation of large social gatherings has impacted houses of worship, which have been prevented from opening their doors. As I write these words, synagogues have begun to open, but only with restrictions. At one point, virtually all synagogues across the globe where simultaneously closed, with very few exceptions. This is truly unprecedented.

Historical Precedent

Synagogue closures in times of plague are not new to the twenty-first century. R. Shmuel Yehuda Katzenellenbogen (1521–1597), also known as Mahari Mintz, son of famed Meir Katzenellenbogen (Maharam MiPadua), published a book of twelve sermons and eulogies, which included eulogies for R. Moshe Isserles, who died in 1572, and R. Yosef

---

36. David Macht and William Kunkel, "Concerning the Antiseptic Action of Some Aromatic Fumes," *Experimental Biology Medicine* (1920), 68–70.

37. David Macht, *The Holy Incense* (Baltimore, 1928). For the previous attempt by Abraham Portaleone to identify the ingredients of the *ketorot*, see Berns, op. cit.

38. As per the testimony of R. Shmuel Reinitz, heard from the students of Ḥatam Sofer. See B. Schwartz, "Customs of the Seventh of Adar" (Hebrew) *BeNetivei Ḥesed veEmet* (5761), 125–129, esp. 128.

Karo, who died in 1575. The introduction to the eleventh published essay, a eulogy for R. Zalman Katz of Mantua reads, "This eulogy I delivered in the courtyard of the Ghetto [of Venice] ... because all the synagogues were closed as a result of the plague."[39] While no date is given, this eulogy follows that of R. Karo. I thus assume he is referring to the Venetian plague of 1576–1577, which killed an estimated 50, 0000 people, almost a third of the population of Venice.

Another reference to synagogue closures, again in Italy, is found, surprisingly, in a medical work of Yaakov Zahalon (1630–1693),[40] *Otzar HaḤayyim*. Zahalon was both a rabbi and physician in Rome, and in his chapter on pestilential fevers he digresses to give an account of the plague that afflicted Rome in 1655–1656. In addition to his account of the community organization to address different aspects of the plague, he records how it affected his rabbinic practice:[41] "As the community was unable to attend synagogue, on Shabbat *Parashat Toldot, 2 Kislev,* 5417 (November 18, 1656), I, Yaakov Zahalon, delivered a sermon at the corner of Via Catalani, from the window of the home of David Gotini, and the congregation stood in the street below to listen. On another occasion, I delivered a sermon on Via Tuscani from the window of the home of Yehuda Gotini."[42] These sermons must have been delivered in the early stages of the plague, as Zahalon himself reports that public gatherings were prohibited. Furthermore, he writes that a gallows was erected at the entrance to the ghetto to be used as punishment for violators of this decree.

---

39. Shmuel Yehuda Mintz, *Shneim Asar Derashot* (Warsaw, 1875), 59. I thank R. Daniel Kramer for bringing this source to my attention.
40. On Zahalon, see, for example, Harry A. Savitz, "Jacob Zahalon, and His Book, 'The Treasure of Life,'" *New England Journal of Medicine* 213:4 (July, 1935), 167–176; Harry Friedenwald, "Jacob Zahalon of Rome: Rabbi, Physician, Author and Moralist," in his *The Jews and Medicine* 1 (Ktav, 1967), 268–279; Jonathan Jarashow, "Yakov Zahalon and the Jewish Attitude Towards Medicine," *Koroth* 9:9–10 (1989), 725–736.
41. On Zahalon's abilities and reputation as an orator, see Henry A. Sosland, *A Guide for Preachers: The Or HaDarshan of Jacob Zahalon—A Seventeenth Century Italian Preacher's Manual* (Jewish Theological Seminary, 1987).
42. Y. Zahalon, *Otzar HaḤayyim* (Venice, 1683), 21b. This work of Zahalon is also mentioned in our chapter on the doctrine of the seven-chamber uterus.

THE BALCONY MINYAN—CREATING A MODIFIED
MINYAN DURING TIMES OF PLAGUE

Despite the ban on congregational gatherings, including prayer, the desire of Jews to pray together in a *minyan* (a quorum of ten men over the age of Bar Mitzva) has led to creative applications of the concept of a minyan. For example, Jews in multi-level apartment buildings are praying outside on their balconies together with at least nine other neighbors to form a minyan. This would potentially allow them to say the communal prayers such as the repetition of the silent *Amida*, *Kaddish*, Torah reading, and other prayers that could not otherwise be recited. The halakhic propriety of these so-called "balcony *minyanim*" has occupied virtually all the major rabbinic authorities of our day, with no current consensus on the matter.[43]

Historical Precedent

There is evidence that Jews of former generations likewise longed for communal prayer in restricted times of plague. R. Ḥayyim Yosef David Azulai (Ḥida, 1724–1806) was asked about the halakhic permissibility of creating a *minyan* with two groups of people who resided in separate houses, four in one house and six in another.[44] One group of six lived in a private residence. The other group of four lived in the adjoining house. This adjoining house, however, was a lazaretto, and the four residents were legally confined to the premises, thus precluding their ability to physically join the other group. Ḥida ruled that since it was effectively impossible for them to physically join, as long as they could visually see each other, the group would be considered halakhically connected and could be considered a legal *minyan*.

SOCIAL DISTANCING IN SYNAGOGUE

One of the compromise approaches to praying in synagogues during the pandemic, utilized both in the early stages, prior to full closure, and in

---

43. For example, the Israeli journal *Teḥumin* 40 (5780) contains six entries devoted to this topic, including articles by R. Asher Weiss, R. Hershel Schachter and the Sephardi Chief Rabbi Yitzḥak Yosef.

44. *Maḥazik Berakha O. Ḥ.*, 55.

the gradual re-opening phases, is to hold prayers in the synagogue with social distancing. The requisite distance to prevent contagion between people has been determined to be six feet, though masks are nonetheless recommended as well. Hundreds of synagogues across the world are presently in this phase. All communities have faced the challenge of how to navigate the High Holidays—given the current restrictions, there was not enough space inside synagogues to accommodate the men, let alone the women.

Historical Precedent

The concept of increasing distance between congregants in synagogue during a plague to minimize contagion is not at all new. There have been examples of both informal and formal forms of social distancing in synagogues in the past.

Catalano records that at one point in the 1631 Padua plague, the community decreed that in order to maintain distance between the people during prayer, the unmarried men should leave the main sanctuary and pray in the courtyard of the Ashkenazi Synagogue. Furthermore, the members of the Italian rite synagogue, who had joined the Ashkenazi Synagogue during the plague, would be assigned to the women's section.[45] Parenthetically, this very synagogue about which Catalano writes has been recently converted into the Jewish Museum of Padua. The Italian Synagogue, which is still in use, is a few yards down the street.

There came a time later in the plague, when illness and fatalities had increased, when even this informal social distancing was not necessary. Catalano writes at that stage that it was a synagogue of few, and desolate (*vayehi lemikdash me'at mibli ba'ei mo'ed*). There was only an occasional *minyan*, and even then, through great effort, though the prayers were haphazard in structure and custom.[46]

On September 23, 1857, R. Yaakov Tzvi Mecklenburg, a prominent German rabbi, author of *HaKetav VeHaKabbala*, penned a letter during a cholera pandemic recommending that the women of the community should refrain from attending services for Yom Kippur and should pray

---

45. Roth, op. cit., 78.
46. Roth, op. cit., 85.

at home.[47] Though not explicitly stated, this may have served a dual purpose of allowing the men to socially distance by expanding the seating to the women's section.

There is a remarkable example of formal social distancing in a nineteenth century Polish synagogue. R. Akiva Eiger (1761–1837) was the rabbi of Posen during the second cholera pandemic (1829–1837). He penned a number of letters between 1830 and 1831 regarding multiple aspects of the disease and its impact.[48] The first of these letters addresses in part the impact of contagion concerns on the daily prayer services, which by nature congregated large groups of people in relatively small spaces. The letter is written to R. Eliyahu Guttmacher, the rabbi of the nearby community of Pleschen:

> Regarding prayer in the synagogue, in my view, it is true that gathering in a small space is inappropriate, but it is possible to pray in groups, each one very small, about fifteen people. Prayer should begin at first light, with the next group following after. Furthermore, each one should have a designated time to come pray there. The same for *Minḥa*... And they should be careful that people beyond the aforementioned quota not push their way into the synagogue. Perhaps a guard from the police should oversee this. Once they have reached the number [15], they should not allow others to enter until that group is finished.[49]

This letter is remarkable for its sensitivity to the notion of contagion and crowding, as well as the consideration of involvement of the secular authorities to enforce compliance. Consistent with his earlier letter about crowd limitation in the synagogue, in 1831 R. Eiger and the members of the rabbinic court of Posen issued a decree, paraphrased below,

---

47. I was unable to view the complete document, which was auctioned by Legacy Judaica, and my account is based solely on the catalogue entry. See http://www. legacyjudaica.net/product/lot-197-r-yaakov-tzvi-mecklenburg-ksav-vkabbolah-konigsberg-1857-כתב- מקלנבורג- צבי- יעקב- ר (accessed July 19, 2020).
48. *Iggerot Rabbi Akiva Eiger* (*Makhon Da'at Sofer*, 5754), letters 71–73.
49. Adapted from the translation by R. Mordechai Torczyner, whom I thank for his permission.

providing guidance in advance of the High Holidays in the midst of the cholera pandemic:[50]

> All synagogues, including both the men's and women's section, should fill to only half of their seating capacity such that every other seat is empty. To allow for equal access during the High Holidays, half the congregants will attend for the two days of Rosh Hashana while the other half will attend for Yom Kippur, with the specific holiday being determined by lottery.[51] A military guard should be posted at the synagogue entrance to maintain orderly seating. The length of the service for Rosh Hashana should not exceed five hours, *piyyutim* should be omitted, and the cantor should not prolong the prayers with melodies or musical flourishes.[52]

MEZUZA AND PLAGUE

One of the earliest responsa from the Chief Rabbinate in Israel regarding the Covid pandemic was on the issue of *mezuza*. In a letter dated March 1, 2020, R. Lau wrote that there is no obligation to kiss the *mezuza* and that this custom evolved only recently. Given the possibility of contagion during the Covid pandemic, this practice should be abandoned, and it should be prohibited to kiss or even touch the *mezuza*.

Historical Precedent

In previous centuries, rabbis likewise cautioned against kissing the *mezuza* during times of epidemics.[53] However, there was another more halakhically pressing issue regarding *mezuza* that surfaced as a result of

---

50. See Natan Gestetner, *Pesakim VeTakanot Rabbi Akiva Eiger* (Jerusalem, 5731), letter 20, 70ff.
51. A lottery was used to determine who would be able to attend services at the Kotel for Shavuot this year (5780).
52. Similar guidelines were provided for Yom Kippur. The assumption, addressed in the decree, was that the people designated by lottery to not attend synagogue would pray in private house minyanim. Provisions for contagion precautions were set forth for these situations as well.
53. R. Lau mentions in his letter that one prominent Hassidic rebbe of the nineteenth century cautioned against kissing the *mezuza* in times of disease, though he does not mention a name or reference.

plague. Ḥida considered the question of whether one is required to place a *mezuza* on the doorpost of a lazaretto.[54] He concluded that since by its very nature a lazaretto is a temporary residence, even if one dwells there more than the requisite thirty days, one would not be required to erect a *mezuza*.

MENTAL HEALTH DURING A PANDEMIC

During the Covid pandemic a number of rabbis have invoked the psychological impact of the disease as an integral part of their halakhic response to topics including listening to music during *sefira*, driving one's laboring wife to the hospital, issues of *mikvah*, and communicating with family members suffering from mental illness via phone or internet on Yom Tov.[55]

Historical Precedent

While the field of mental health has developed exponentially in the last century, rabbinic authorities in previous centuries nonetheless showed sensitivity to the psychological dimension and its impact on halakha. For example, R. Shaul Landau, the Chief Rabbinic Judge of Cracow, asked Ḥatam Sofer about the following incident in his community.[56] During a cholera outbreak, the people greatly desired to recite *Kiddush Levana* (the blessing over the new moon). However, the moon was not visible during the halakhically allowed time for recitation. The community was greatly distressed and fearful that this was a bad omen. In light of the medically accepted fact that emotional distress and worry can have negative implications for one's health, R. Landau declared that there would still be an opportunity to bless the new moon on the 16th of the month (past the usual time for the blessing) if the skies were clear. As it happened, the skies were cloudless, and hundreds gathered to recite the prayer.

---

54. *Ḥayyim She'al*, n. 22
55. For discussion of these topics, as well as a general discussion about mental health and halakha, see Sharon Galper Grossman and Shamai Grossman, "Coping Under Corona: A Review of Halakhic Approaches to Mental Health and Covid-19," *Lehrhaus* (June 18, 2020), thelehrhaus.com/scholarship/coping-under-corona-a-review-of-halakhic-approaches-to-mentalhealth-and-covid-19/ (accessed July 19, 2020).
56. *Ḥatam Sofer, O. Ḥ.*, 102.

R. Ḥayyim Palachi (1788–1868) made special allowance for behavior during times of pandemic that he vehemently objected to otherwise:

> I decree that any man who is called by the term wise man [*talmid ḥakham*] should never play dice or any game, any time. Not on Purim, or *Ḥol HaMo'ed*, or at weddings, and not in the small villages, never and no place at all. Except if he is sick or a sickness abounds in his city, like the sickness of cholera and the like… If he is very fearful and his heart is worried about it, and by playing he will find calm and it will distract him from fear, specifically this is permitted to do.[57]

VISITING THE ILL AND RISK TO THE VISITOR

With our heightened sensitivity in the modern era to virology, bacteriology and the nature of contagion, contemporary authorities discuss the nature of risk versus the obligation to heal during this pandemic for all forms of health care providers, ranging from physicians[58] to those visiting the sick. A number have authorities have prohibited visiting those in isolation due to the clear risk involved, preferring alternatives such as phone or video conferencing.[59]

Historical Precedent

Bikur Ḥolim societies of old provided more than just food and emotional support, they often provided needed medical and physical support as well. Concern for contagion was reflected in the society manuals providing guidelines to its members. In one such manual from

---

57. *Sefer Ḥayyim* (Salonica, 5628), 94b. I thank Dr. Ari Greenspan for this reference. This unique decision may not have been appropriate for all, as we find in the autobiography of R. Yehuda Arye Modena, who was a known compulsive gambler, that he relapsed into his gambling habit during a pandemic. See Mark Cohen, trans. and ed., *The Autobiography of a Seventeenth Century Venetian Rabbi: Leon Modena's Life of Judah* (Princeton University Press, 1988), 34ff.

58. On the topic of whether a physician or health care provider is expected to tolerate a higher threshold of risk than others in the care of patients with contagious disease, see, for example, *Tzitz Eliezer* 9:17, chapter 5, as well as the works of Rabbis Weiss and Steinberg on Covid cited above.

59. See, for example, R. Avishai Tahareini, *Yadber Amim* (Jerusalem, 5780), 238.

mid-eighteenth-century Berlin, we read: "We have accepted upon ourselves to visit all those afflicted with illness, except if they are afflicted with certain [contagious] illnesses, God forbid, from which one must distance oneself."[60] Examples of such illnesses included diarrheal maladies (such as cholera), smallpox, and measles.

R. Ḥayyim Soloveitchik (1853–1918) personally attended to those afflicted with cholera despite the potential risk of contracting the contagious disease. He did, however, differentiate between levels of risk, stipulating that if the risk of contagion were close to certain, one would not be permitted to incur such risk. One is not required to expose oneself to certain danger, he argued, even if he is aiding one who is in certain danger.[61]

BURIAL AND *TAHARA*

During the present outbreak the Ministry of Health in Israel initially suggested that no *tahara* (religious preparation for burial) should be performed for patients with Covid, and that no shrouds (*takhrikhim*) should be used. They quickly reversed this decision and allowed a limited *tahara* performed by specially trained individuals.[62] The American based National Association of Chevra Kadisha, under the guidance of R. Elchanan Zohn, and in consultation with infectious disease experts, issued guidelines for the *tahara* of those infected with Covid or other contagious diseases.[63]

Some countries mandated cremation for those who died of Covid. Rabbis allowed burial on Shabbat in such circumstances, albeit with the assistance of a non-Jew, if it would preclude cremation.[64]

---

60. Aaron ben Moses Rofeh, *Takanot shel Bnei HaḤavura DeBikur Ḥolim* (Berlin, 1750).
61. R. Yosef Dov Soloveitchik, *Reshimot Shiurim, Bava Metzia* 30b. R. Eliyahu Ḥayyim Meisels (1821–1912), rabbi of Lodz, likewise assisted those in need during an epidemic despite the possible danger. See R. Moshe Sternbuch, *Teshuvot VeHanhagot* 5:390.
62. David Israel, "Health Ministry Reverses Guidelines to Permit Cleansing the Coronavirus Dead," *Jewish Press* (March 18, 2020).
63. For further halakhic discussion see Yehoshua Veisinger, "Tahara in Cases of Contagious Disease" (Hebrew) *Teḥumin* 36 (5776), 234–247.
64. Marcy Oster, "Bucharest Jews Can Bury Coronavirus Dead on Shabbat to Avoid Cremation," *Jerusalem Post* (March 31, 2020). R. Kenneth Brander considered cremation a "posthumous mitzva" if it were required by the government. See Nathan Jeffay, "State-Mandated Cremation is a Posthumous Mitzvah Says One Leading Orthodox Rabbi," *Times of Israel* (March 29, 2020).

Historical Precedent

Burial practices were similarly altered during earlier epidemics due to the concern for contagion of the body even after death. In the times of the Ḥazon Ish, there was a cholera pandemic and the physicians cautioned against touching the bodies of those who had died. The Chevra Kadisha initially heeded the medical recommendations, and as a result, many Jewish bodies remained unburied in a state of disgrace. So it remained until Ḥazon Ish personally picked up one of the bodies and attended to his burial. The Chevra Kadisha was profoundly impacted by this act and returned to performing their customary burials (presumably with modifications to prevent contagion).[65]

The issue of Shabbat burial was also discussed during previous pandemics.[66]

TEMPORARY BURIAL AND REINTERMENT

Many people who reside in the United States or other countries of the Diaspora choose to be buried in Israel upon their demise. Due to the travel restrictions during the Covid pandemic, transport of the body after death to Israel has not been possible. As a result, families were forced to bury relatives in local cemeteries, unable to fulfill their loved one's wishes. The question has arisen as to the permissibility of exhuming and reinterring a body when it becomes possible. R. Herschel Schachter has noted that this very issue is explicitly discussed in *Shulḥan Arukh*,[67] and

---

65. See Moshe Yosef Raziel, "Endangering Oneself to Save Others," (Hebrew) *Vaḥai Bahem* 1 (5752), 37–45.

66. On the topic of burial on Shabbat during an epidemic, see *Iggerot Moshe, Y. D.,* 4:55; *Ḥatam Sofer* II, *Y. D.,* 334. R. Ḥayyim Palachi discussed the permissibility of asking a non-Jew to dig graves on Shabbat during a cholera pandemic in 1865. See *Ruaḥ Ḥayyim, O. Ḥ.,* 325:4 (he was hesitant to permit). R. Yaakov Reischer (1661–1733) addressed the use of quicklime to hasten decomposition of the body after death from plague to prevent contagion. See *Shevut Yaakov* 2:97. This practice is also mentioned by the Malbim in his commentary to *Amos* 6:10. Burial procedures during the Covid pandemic have also included chemical treatment of the body to reduce contagion, but contemporary rabbinic authorities have not addressed this issue.

67. *Y. D.,* 363.

while reburial is generally prohibited, one exception is if the reburial takes place in Israel.[68]

Historical Precedent

In premodern times, there was also concern for contagion of the body after death.

In Bialystok, Poland, for example, a designated "cholera" cemetery was established in 1840 to house the graves of contagious disease victims.[69] Similar plague cemeteries were established throughout Europe. Ḥatam Sofer addressed the halakhic issue of exhumation and reburial in these cases in light of the fact that the government would in any case exhume the bodies after a few years to repurpose the land.[70]

MOURNING AND *SHIVA*

The Covid pandemic has radically altered the observance of *shiva* (the seven-day mourning practice after burial). Restrictions on public gathering preclude visitation. The traditional visit with a mourner in a room of their home has been replaced by a Zoom room, a form of videoconferencing *shiva*. The primary, if not sole, reason for curtailing *shiva* practices today is the fear of contagion.

Historical Precedent

In previous centuries, *shiva* was also curtailed due to fear, but the nature of the perceived fear was different. It explicitly states in *Shulḥan Arukh*:[71] "Some say that in times of plague, one does not observe mourning rites *out of fear*, and I have heard that some have adopted this practice."[72] The

---

68. https://www.yutorah.org/sidebar/lecture.cfm/951535/rabbi-hershel-schachter/piskei-corona-23–temporary-burial-in-chu-l-and-issues-of-aveilus (accessed July 21, 2020).

69. The cemetery closed in 1892. The "cholera" cemetery is now located under the ZUS (Poland's Social Security Administration) Building and its parking lot. As recent as 2001, the ZUS building was expanded unearthing many Jewish graves.

70. *Ḥatam Sofer, Y. D.,* 2:334.

71. *Y. D.,* 374

72. R. Shaul Nathenson attests that it was indeed the practice to cancel the *shiva* observance during times of plague. See his *Sho'el UMeishiv, Mahadura Kama* 1:78; *Yad*

concern for increased fear and worry during plague is an idea prevalent in rabbinic literature.[73] During a late nineteenth-century cholera pandemic, R. Malkiel Tannenbaum (1847–1910) offered two possible explanations for the phrase of the *Shulḥan Arukh*, "out of fear."[74] One possibility is the concern for the fear that will descend upon the entire community if they are notified of so many deaths associated with a plague. An alternate explanation offered by R. Malkiel is that the mourners themselves may develop fear and anxiety when they remain closed in their homes, and this may endanger their health. While R. Malkiel preferred the first explanation, neither is raised in contemporary discussions where the focus is exclusively medical.[75]

KADDISH RECITATION

One of the lesser appreciated repercussions of the Covid pandemic and the closure of synagogues is the inability to say *Kaddish* for those who are in mourning or are commemorating the anniversary of a death of a loved one (*yahrzeit*). Mourner's *Kaddish* can only be recited in the presence of a *minyan*. The *Kaddish* prayer is imbued with great significance and for many its absence creates a spiritual void and emotional distress. I myself experienced this when deprived of the opportunity to say *Kaddish* for my deceased parents, *a"h*. There is a custom to enlist others to say *Kaddish* on your behalf if, for some reason, you cannot. There are organizations that address this need. But even this solution was not forthcoming as most synagogues across the globe were closed or severely restricted in operation.

Historical Precedent

The impact of a cholera pandemic on the recitation of Mourner's *Kaddish* is reflected in the writings of R. Eiger. The custom of R. Eiger's community

---

Shaul, Y. D., 375. The question also arose as to whether the *shiva* should be observed if the government restrictions were lifted prior to the completion of the shloshim period. See *Rav Pe'alim* III, *Y. D.,* 28; *Yalkut Yosef, Y. D.,* 374:1 notes.

73. See, for example, Meir Katzenellenbogen, *Shu"t Maharam Padua,* 86; *Ḥatam Sofer, O. Ḥ.,* 102.

74. *Divrei Malkiel,* 2:90.

75. If these earlier notions of fear were considered today, then even a Zoom *shiva* might not be permitted.

was for only one person to recite *Kaddish* at a time, and the mourners would rotate. The death toll was so vast that each person could not even recite *Kaddish* once a month. R. Eiger, therefore, ruled that for the *Kaddish* after the *Aleinu* prayer, all the mourners could recite *Kaddish* together.[76]

CONCLUSION

One inescapable conclusion from the Covid pandemic is that we in the twenty-first century need to restore our humility. Perhaps the following passage will inject a little perspective:

> Plagues are sent from God from time to time due to our sins. They result in widespread death of young and old, women and children, for no discernible reason. These illnesses confuse and befuddle the physicians, and none amongst them can discern which [treatment] is good and which is bad. They offer a good prognosis for a patient, yet only one or two hours later, the patient dies.[77]

Remarkably, this was written some five hundred years ago by Eliyahu di Vidas,[78] and is no less true today than it was then. Despite our astounding achievements in the world of science and medicine, we must always appreciate, and perhaps sometimes need to be reminded, that God is the ultimate healer.

As I write this conclusion, the Covid-19 pandemic still lingers. Tragically, we have lost many precious souls to this disease. Many new radical rabbinic decisions have been rendered and more are sure to follow. Appreciating what our predecessors faced in times of pandemic will hopefully provide perspective, inspiration, and guidance on how to cope with our present predicament, as well as those in the future. Some of the parallels are striking, and it is humbling that despite our remarkable, divinely guided advances in both the understanding and treatment of disease, in many ways, little has changed.

---

76. *Piskei Teshuvot, He'arot* 132, n. 106.
77. Eliyahu di Vidas, *Reshit Ḥokhma, Sha'ar Ahava,* chapter 6. Cited in Y. Y. Buksbaum, *Ne'emnu Me'od* (Makhon Yerushalayim, 5780), 51.
78. Di Vidas was a student of R. Moshe Cordovero and the Ar"i.

Perhaps the talmudic suggestion to gather your feet in times of plague (*kanes raglekha*) has an alternate interpretation. In such unprecedented times, one must take stock, regroup, recalibrate, or in modern parlance, reboot. With God's help, and with continued prayer and enhanced religious observance, Klal Yisrael has survived all previous pandemics. God willing, we will one day share the religious and halakhic lessons learned from our current reality with our own descendants.

Death and Resuscitation

The Halakhic Definition of Death in Light of Medical History

I. INTRODUCTION

There has been much debate over the last few decades regarding the halakhic status of brain death. When this debate is ultimately consigned to history, it will be noted that the issue only became relevant in the late twentieth century, when the use of artificial respirators was commonplace; when, for the first time in medical history, brain death was temporally dissociated from cardiac death; when there was widespread confusion as to the differentiation between cortical and brain stem death; when the universal medical community underwent a major reassessment of the definition of death and decided to accept brain death criteria as valid. It will be important for one who confronts the large corpus of halakhic responsa literature generated on this issue to appreciate that a full understanding of each responsum can only be possible by taking into consideration its author's level of medical and scientific knowledge. In addition, for the reader of each responsum to clearly understand the discussion, he or she must also be fully conversant with the concepts and terminology used by the author as he or she [the reader] understands them. One is often guilty of superimposing current medical knowledge onto the words of predecessors, a practice that will inevitably lead to faulty interpretation. It is only by placing the responsum into its proper historical context that the reader will best be able to interpret it in its own right, as well as apply its ideas and conclusions to other contexts.

It is this principle of seeing a medical halakhic text in its own historical context that I wish to apply to the pre-twentieth century halakhic sources that deal with the definition of death.[1] It is not my intention to address the halakhic ramifications of such an analysis, nor will I address the basic halakhic discussion of the determination of death. Discussion of the latter can be found in contemporary Jewish literature.[2]

The foundation and chronological starting point for any halakhic discussions is the Torah. While there are multiple biblical references to death,[3] and even resuscitation,[4] there is no clear statement of the halakhic determination of death. We, therefore, turn to the text of the Talmud

---

1. According to the Ḥazon Ish, the halakha with respect to *treifot* was established based on the medical knowledge of the rabbis of the Talmud. Therefore, even if our medical understanding should change, we are·legally bound by the decision of our predecessors. See *Ḥazon Ish, Y. D.,* 5:3; *Hil. Nashim* 27:3. R. Hershel Schachter applies this principle to the determination of death as well and claims that we should be bound by how the rabbis of the Talmud defined death. See his *"BeDinei Met VeGavra Ketilla,"* Beit Yitzḥak 21 (1989), 121. This is a legal principle, yet it impacts on the value of studying medical history. According to this position, while changes in medical understanding may be acknowledged throughout history, they bear little relevance to the process of deciding halakha. According to this position, therefore, the content of this chapter is purely academic.

2. See, for example, J. D. Bleich, *Time of Death* (Z. Berman, 1991); M. D. Tendler, *Responsa of Rav Moshe Feinstein,* Volume 1 (Ktav, 1996); Abraham S. Abraham, *Nishmat Avraham* 2 (Mesorah Publications, 2003); A. Steinberg, *Encyclopedia of Jewish Medical Ethics* 2, trans. F. Rosner (Feldheim Publishers, 2003), s. v., "Moment of Death"; D. Shabtai, *Defining the Moment: Understanding Brain Death in Halakhah* (Shoresh Press, 2012).

3. See Samuel Weiss, *"Kevi'at Rega HaMavet BeRefua UVeHalakha"* (M.D. thesis; The Hebrew University/ Hadassah Medical School; July, 1983), 1–4 for biblical descriptions of death.

4. John A. Parashos, "Biblical Accounts of Resuscitation," *Journal of the History of Medicine* 47 (July, 1992), 310–321. See also Abraham S. Abraham, *"Hanshama Melakhutit BeTanakh,"* HaMa'ayan 28:3 (1988), 72–76. See chapter, "The Resuscitation of Halakha."

as our historical point of departure for this issue, which we shall follow until pre-modern times.

In many places, the Talmud discusses medical issues.[5] Both the Jerusalem and Babylonian Talmuds were compiled while the Jews lived in the Greco-Roman empire, the world's center of medical practice and teaching. Galen, the forefather of western medicine until modern times, whose often erroneous teachings remained undisputed for well over a thousand years, was roughly contemporary with R. Yehuda HaNasi, the compiler of the Mishna. The question arises as to the extent of cross-cultural borrowing. Were the rabbis of the Talmud, in fact, familiar with the Greco-Roman sources?[6] This can be determined either by explicit direct references to Greco-Roman

---

5. For some of the major works which deal exclusively with this topic, see M. Perlman, *Midrash HaRefua* (Tel Aviv, 1926); Y. L. Katznelson, *HaTalmud VeHokhmat HaRefua* (Berlin, 1928); J. Snowman, *A Short History of Talmudic Medicine* (London, 1933); Charles Brim, *Medicine in the Bible* (New York, 1936); Solomon Kagan, "Talmudic Medicine," *Medical Leaves* 3:1 (1940), 164–173; Maurice Bear Gordon, "Medicine Among the Ancient Hebrews," *Isis* 33 (1941), 454–485; Benjamin Lee Gordon, "Ancient Hebrew Medicine," in his *Medicine Throughout Antiquity* (Philadelphia, 1949), 251–294; Jacob Glenn, *The Bible and Modern Medicine* (New York, 1959); Edward Neufeld, "Hygiene Conditions in Ancient Israel," *Journal of the History of Medicine and Allied Sciences* 35:4 (October 1970), 414–437; Fred Rosner, *Medicine in the Bible and the Talmud* (New York, 1977); Julius Preuss, *Biblical and Talmudic Medicine* (New York, 1978). See chapter, "Biblical and Talmudic Medicine."

6. For previous studies on the interface between talmudic and Greco-Roman medicine see, for example, Stephen Newmyer, "The Concept of Climate and National Superiority in the Talmud and its Classical Parallels," *Transactions and Studies of the College of Physicians of Philadelphia*, Medicine and History Series 5: 1 (March, 1983), 1–12; idem, "Talmudic Medicine and Greek Sources," *Koroth* 9:1–2 (1985), 34–57; idem, "Talmudic Medicine: A Classicist's Perspective," *Judaism* 29 (1980), 360–367; J. Preuss, op. cit.

   For information regarding the familiarity of Greek authors with Jews and Jewish medicine see, for example, R. Walzer, *Galen on Jews and Christians* (Oxford, 1949); Menachem Stern, *Greek and Latin Authors on Jews and Judaism* (Jerusalem, 1980), 307–328.

   For evidence that the Jews of the Middle Ages and Renaissance were familiar with Galen, see Elinor Lieber, "Galen in Hebrew" in Vivian Nuttun, ed., *Galen: Problems and Prospects* (London, 1981), 167–186; H. Isaacs, *Medical and Para-Medical Manuscripts in the Cambridge Genizah Collections* (Cambridge University Press, 1994) (see index for manuscripts of Galen in Hebrew). In addition, Maimonides wrote a commentary on the works of Galen.

authors or implicitly, by unattributed references to contemporaneous Greco-Roman theory and practice. I will analyze both of these possibilities and, in the process, will attempt to provide a general medical historical overview of some of the issues discussed in the halakhic literature on brain death.

It is important to note that the medical topics addressed in rabbinic literature are only mentioned secondarily, in the course of halakhic or midrashic discussions. There are no primary Jewish or rabbinic medical treatises extant from the talmudic period.[7] In addition, although the influence of the Greco-Roman medical tradition on the Talmud has been debated, it is abundantly clear, as will be partially evidenced in this chapter, that Galenic medicine had a strong influence on post-talmudic halakhic and Jewish medical literature.[8] As Galenic theories dominated western medical thinking well into the seventeenth century,[9] spanning the period of the *Rishonim* and early *Aharonim*, a basic outline of Greco-Roman principles of anatomy and physiology will be helpful for interpreting medical halakhic discussions of this period in general, and of our topic in particular.

---

7. The earliest Hebrew medical manuscript is generally believed to be that of the "Book of Remedies" attributed to Asaph the physician. Regarding the dating of Asaph, see Suessman Muntner, "The Antiquity of Asaph the Physician and His Editorship of the Earliest Hebrew Book of Medicine," *Bulletin of the History of Medicine* 25 (1951), 103–131; Elinor Lieber, "Asaf's Book of Medicines: A Hebrew Encyclopedia of Greek and Jewish Medicine, Possibly Compiled in Byzantium on an Indian Model," *Dumbarton Oaks Paper* 38 (1984), 233–249; Joseph Shatzmiller, "Doctors and Medical Practices in Germany Around the Year 1200: The Evidence of Sefer Asaph," *Proceedings of the American Academy for Jewish Research* 50 (1983), 149–164; Stephen T. Newmyer, "Asaph's 'Book of Remedies': Greek Science and Jewish Apologetics," *Sudhoffs Archiv* 76:1 (1992), 28–36.

   However, Professor James Charlesworth published the translation of a small medical fragment discovered amongst the Dead Sea Scrolls, which dates back to pre-Mishnaic times. See J. H. Charlesworth, *The Discovery of a Dead Sea Scroll (4Q Theropeia): Its Importance in the History of Medicine and Jesus Research* (Lubbock, Texas, 1985).

8. See E. Lieber, op. cit. Galen is quoted extensively by Asaph, by Maimonides in the twelfth century, and by Tobias Cohn in the eighteenth century.

9. See Everett Mendelsohn, *Heat and Life: The Development of the Theory of Animal Heat* (Cambridge, 1964), 17.

II. PRINCIPLES OF GRECO-ROMAN/ GALENIC PHYSIOLOGY[10]

1. *The Doctrine of the Four Elements, Qualities, and Humors*

Galen accepted the doctrine of the four elements—fire, earth, air, and water—embodying the four qualities—hot, cold, dry, and wet—and corresponding to the four essential humors of the body—blood, black bile, yellow bile, and phlegm.[11] Proper health, according to Galen, was dependent upon a delicate balance between and combination of these four elements, qualities, and humors.

2. *Three Souls*

Galen perpetuated the Platonic idea of the three souls that rule and serve the body. These are the rational, irascible, and concupiscible souls, situated in the brain, heart, and liver respectively. "The first presides over reasoning and thought and provides sensation and motion; the second controls the passion and is the vital force; and the third, also known as the vegetative soul, is in charge of nutrition."[12]

---

10. The terms Galenic medicine and Greco-Roman medicine are used here interchangeably. Galen's theories are largely derived from and are variations on the ideas of his predecessors, primarily Hippocrates, Empedocles, Aristotle, and Erasitratus. Some major differences between them exist, and they will be noted as relevant to our topic. Generally speaking, however, Galen was the last and perhaps the greatest of the Greek men of medicine, and his works represent the culmination of Greco-Roman medicine and physiology. See George Sarton, *Galen of Pergamon* (Lawrence, Kansas, 1954).

11. The doctrine of the four humors is as old as Empedocles (500–430 BCE), but Galen refined the doctrine by also incorporating the ideas of Hippocrates (b. 460 BCE) and Aristotle (384–322 BCE). See Margaret Tallmadge May, *Galen: On the Usefulness of the Parts of the Body* (Ithaca, 1968), 44–45, and n. 191. Whether the rabbis of the Talmud accepted the doctrine of the four humors is a matter of debate. Some talmudic passages can be interpreted in light of this doctrine. It is clear, however, that later Jewish authors did accept it. See H. J. Zimmels, *Magicians, Theologians and Doctors* (London, 1952), 78–80; 217, n. 5; 219, n. 13.

12. See May, op. cit., 45. The concept of the soul or a soul being associated with an organ or limb is found in Jewish sources. The phrase used is *"ever shehanesham teluya bo."* See *Entzyclopedia Talmudit* 1 (1990), 109. Following Galen, Maimonides states that the organs associated with the soul are the heart, brain and liver. R. Hershel Schachter's article on the definition of death, op. cit., is based on this notion.

3. *Innate Heat*

The theory of an "innate" body heat was first suggested by early Greek medical writers. This innate heat became the "single most important motive power in the animal system."[13] It was responsible for growth, digestion, movement, sensation, and thought. The maintenance of "innate heat" coincided with life; its destruction coincided with death. The source of this innate heat was the heart, more precisely the left ventricle of the heart.[14] Galen, too, granted paramount importance to this principle.[15]

4. *Purpose of Respiration*

The primary function of respiration according to Galenic physiology was to cool and conserve the innate heat of the heart. It was felt that this "heat" must be refrigerated by respiration and kept under control if life is to persist. If refrigeration is not provided, the heat will consume itself and the body will die.[16]

5. *Pneumas or Spirits*

The basic principle of life according to Galen was a spirit or pneuma drawn from the air into the body through the act of breathing. The idea of the pneumas or spirits probably originated with Erasistratus, but the theory underwent significant alteration by Galen. This nondescript air travels to

---

13. Mendelsohn, op. cit., 8. For the appearance of the idea of innate heat in Jewish sources, see chapter, "The Incorporation of Pre-Modern Scientific Theories into Rabbinic Literature: The Case of Innate Heat."

14. See E. Mendelsohn, op. cit., 8. The idea of innate animal heat continued in different forms into the late eighteenth century. See Max Neuburger, *The Historical Development of Experimental Brain and Spinal Cord Physiology Before Flourens* (Baltimore, 1981), 231–236. The belief that the heart had a higher temperature than the rest of the body persisted until the seventeenth century, when Giovanni Alfonso Borelli disproved it with the use of a thermometer. See May, op. cit., 53, n. 231.

15. See May, op. cit., 50–53; Mendelsohn, op. cit., 17–22. The principle of innate heat was accepted by rabbinic scholars as well. See the sources quoted by Ḥakham Tzvi, cited below. See chapter, "Innate Heat."

16. This idea originated with Hippocrates and Aristotle. See May, op. cit., 51 and Mendelsohn, op. cit., 20–21. See also David J. Furley and J. S. Wilkie, *Galen on Respiration and the Arteries* (Princeton, 1984), 14–17. Oxygen was only discovered in 1771 by Joseph Priestley. See Fielding Garrison, *History of Medicine* (Philadelphia, 1960), 328–330.

the heart where it meets the innate heat.[17] At this stage, it becomes the "vital" spirit and serves to cool the innate heat. From the heart, the spirit travels to the brain where it undergoes further cooling and subsequent conversion into the "psychic" spirit, the source of intellect.[18]

It is important for our purposes to note that there is a direct relationship between respiration and cardiac function. The air inhaled ultimately reaches the heart itself.[19] Furthermore, the heart appears to initiate respiration by the following mechanism: "The heart expands through increasing heat, and thus causes expansion in the lungs and the air is drawn into the lungs and the heart." In sum, "the idea that the heart is an organ of respiration was established early in the history of Greek physiology and was still strongly entrenched in Galen's theory."[20]

6. Functions of the Heart and Brain

Aristotle, who wrote before the discovery of nerves, considered the heart as the center of the natural heat of the body. As a result, he considered it to be the primary cause of nutrition (i.e., transforming food into blood) and, more importantly, the controlling center of all sensation and movement in the body.[21] The brain was relegated to secondary significance.

---

17. The exact anatomical pathway of the air was believed to be as follows: "It enters the body through the windpipe or trachea and so passes to the lung and thence, through the 'arteria venalis'—which we call the pulmonary vein—to the left ventricle of the heart, where it encounters the blood." See Charles Singer, *A Short History of Medicine* (Oxford, 1928), 56.

18. The pneuma travels from the heart to the brain via the carotid arteries. However, according to Galen, before the carotid arteries bring the blood to the brain, they divide at the base of the brain to form a marvelous network of vessels. This so-called "rete mirabile" is found in ungulates but not in man and is one of the gross errors in human anatomy that was perpetuated by Galenic teachings. See May, op. cit., 47; Henry Karplus, "Cooling of the Blood and the Rete Mirabile of Herophilus," *Koroth* 8:9–10 (August 1984), 436–440; Charles Singer, "Some Galenic and Animal Sources of Vesalius," *Journal of the History of Medicine and Allied Sciences* 1:1 (January 1946), 18–19.

19. As to the pathway the air takes to reach the heart, see above, n. 16. Galen believed that the inspired air could not proceed directly to the heart for distribution to the whole body. It was required to undergo preliminary preparation before becoming the vital spirit. See May, op. cit., 47.

20. See Furley and Wilkie, op. cit., 17–18.

21. See Furley and Wilkie, op. cit., 17–20, n. 17. For a comprehensive study of ancient Greek notions of cardiovascular physiology, see C. R. S. Harris, *The Heart and the Vascular System in Ancient Greek Medicine* (Oxford, 1973).

Galen disagreed with Aristotle and proved experimentally that the brain, not the heart, is the source of sensation, respiration, and movement.[22] He did, however, agree with Aristotle that the heart is the seat of passion and the source of innate heat.[23] It is important to remember that the notion of the circulation of the blood through the body was only discovered in the 1600s by William Harvey.[24]

7. Content of the Vessels[25]

Galen proved experimentally that the vessels contain blood.[26] Many, however, maintained that the vessels contained air.[27]

---

22. Galen designed an intelligent experiment to ascertain the function of the brain and spinal cord. After dissecting the spinal cords of animals at different levels, he observed the attendant neurological deficits. When he cut the section between the skull and the first vertebra, the animal was deprived of sensation, respiration, and motion. See W. L. H. Duckworth, *Galen on Anatomical Procedures: The Later Books* (Cambridge, 1962), 17–26. For Hippocrates' view of the brain, see G. E. R. Lloyd, ed., *Hippocratic Writings* (New York, 1978), "On the Sacred Disease," esp. 249–251.
23. See Charles Singer, trans., *Galen on Anatomical Procedures* (London, 1956), 181–184.
24. Although the discovery of the systemic circulation of the blood is generally attributed to Harvey, the pulmonary circulation was recognized much earlier. See M. Meyerhof, "Ibn An-Nafis and his Theory of the Lesser Circulation," *Isis* 23 (1935), 100–120; L. G. Wilson, "The Problem of the Discovery of the Pulmonary Circulation," *Journal of the History of Medicine* 17 (April, 1962), 229–244. Some scholars have claimed that the idea of the circulation of the blood appears in Hebrew sources that antedate Harvey. See David Margalit, "*Nitzanei HaRa'ayon al Maḥzor HaDam BiMekorotenu HaAtikim*," *HaRofeh Ha'Ivri* 2 (1957), 79–88; Joshua Leibowitz, "*Smukhim Harveyaniyim BiRefua HaIvrit*," idem, 74–79; E. Lieber, "A Medieval Hebrew Presage of the Circulation of the Blood, Based on Biblical and Talmudic Concepts," *Koroth* 9:1–2 (1985), 157–163.
25. The term "vessel" refers to both arteries and veins. The anatomical difference between them was known before Galen's time, but the functional difference was not. The valves of the veins were described by Fabricius of Aquapendente (sixteenth century), and the connection between the arteries and veins, i.e., the capillaries, was first described by Marcello Malpighi (seventeenth century). See Garrison, op. cit., 222–223, 255–256.
26. See Charles Singer, trans., "Against the View that Arteries are Empty," *Galen on Anatomical Procedures* (London, 1956), 197–200. However, this does not preclude the notion that the arteries contained pneuma as well. See Rupert Hall, "Studies on the History of the Cardiovascular System," *Bulletin of the History of Medicine* 34 (1960), 391–413, esp. 410.
27. Some have interpreted a talmudic passage based on the debate as to whether arteries contain air or blood. According to Rav (*Ḥullin* 45b), even a small perforation of the

8. Embryology

Just as there was a debate regarding the organ responsible for movement and sensation (see section 6, above), there was, likewise, controversy about which organ appeared first in the developing fetus. Aristotle, as expected, believed that the heart formed first[28] while others thought that the head developed first.[29] Still others maintained that the fetus began growth from the navel, as it was attached to the umbilical cord,[30] from which all the other organs and limbs branched out. Galen, however, was alone in maintaining that the liver was the first organ to appear.[31]

9. Pulse

Although Hippocrates does mention tangentially the observation of the apex beat,[32] it was Praxagoras of Cos (300 BCE) who first restricted the pulse to a distinct group of vessels and recognized its use as an indicator of disease.[33] Galen wrote on the pulse in several of his treatises and

---

aorta (*"kaneh halev"*) is considered a *treifa*, whereas according to Shmuel, a larger tear is required. *See* J. Preuss, op. cit., 103; David Margalit, *"Pirkei Anatomia Lifnim BiYisrael VeHayom,"* Koroth 1:11–12 (June-July, 1957), 379–380.

28. See A. L. Peck, trans., *Aristotle: The Generation of Animals* (Cambridge, 1953), 193.
29. This was the position of Lactantius of Nicomedia (325 CE). See J. Needham, *A History of Embryology* (New York, 1959), 78.
30. This was the position of Alcmaeon (sixth century BCE). See Needham, ibid.
31. For an overview of the history of embryology, see J. Needham, op. cit.; Howard Adelmann, "A Brief Sketch of the History of Embryology before Fabricius," in his trans. of *The Embryological Treatises of Hieronymous Fabricius of Aquapendente* I (Ithaca, 1967), 36–70. For references to embryology in Jewish sources, see Samuel Kottek, "Embryology in Talmudic and Midrashic Literature," *Journal of the History of Biology* 14:2 (Fall 1981), 299–315; David I. Macht, "Embryology and Obstetrics in Ancient Hebrew Literature," *Johns Hopkins Hospital Bulletin* 22: 242 (May, 1911), 1–8; W. M. Feldman, "Ancient Jewish Eugenics," *Medical Leaves* 2 (1939), 28–37; D. Schapiro, *Obstetrique des Anciens Hebreus* (Paris, 1904); W. M. Feldman, *The Jewish Child* (London, 1917), 120–44; H. J. Zimmels, *Magicians, Theologians and Doctors,* 62–64; Needham, op. cit., 77–82; J. Preuss, op. cit., 41–138. For discussion on reproductive anatomy and physiology in Jewish sources, see chapter, "The Rabbinic Conception of Conception."
32. The apex beat is usually palpable on the left anterior chest in the fifth intercostal space. See G. E. R. Lloyd, ed., *Hippocratic Writings,* 348.
33. Ibid., 31. Herophilus, a student of Praxagorus, developed a complex system of mea-

discussed the value of palpating the pulse in the extremities and, in particular, in the wrists where it is easily felt.[34]

III. PASSAGE IN TRACTATE *YOMA*

With this understanding of some of the elementary principles of Greco-Roman medicine, we can begin our analysis of the rabbinic sources on the determination of death. *Talmud Yerushalmi* (*Yoma* 8:5) states:

> Rav Zera and Rav Ḥiyya said in the name of Rav Yoḥanan: If one Jew lives in an area [enclosure] that is inhabited by non-Jews and a house collapses [there on the Sabbath], one is permitted to uncover the rubble. How far can one dig [before determining the death of the victim]? There are two opinions. One says until the nostrils [*ad ḥotmo*] because these are the source of life, and *ḥurna* [the other opinion] says until the navel [*ad tiburo*] because from here the body grows.[35]

On one level, this discussion is simply medical in nature, the point of contention being how to assess if the person is still alive. Checking the nostrils for respiration is one alternative. One opinion, however, recommends examining the navel. However, how can inspection of this area be helpful from a medical perspective and what diagnostic information can be gleaned from such an examination? I propose two possibilities. First, one could theoretically be searching for pulsations of the abdominal aorta, which is a reflection of heartbeat and simply another way of measuring the pulse. It is important to note, however, that although Galen and his peers may have routinely measured the pulse, nowhere in the Talmud, to the best of my knowledge, is there any mention of

---

suring the pulse based on musical rhythms. Because of the intricacy of this method, it could not be applied in clinical medical practice. See Karl Zurbach, "Early Ideas and Theories on the Motion of the Blood," *Ciba Symposium* (1939), 71–77, esp. 71–72.

34. See Logan Clandening, *Sourcebook of Medical History* (New York, 1960), 42–45. Asaph the Physician also discusses the value of palpating the peripheral pulses, (see Lieber, op. cit.) though this may have been borrowed from Galen.

35. The two phrases *behu dehava kayam* and *behu dehava ribon* are subject to interpretation. I have provided a loose translation.

the taking of the pulse.[36] In addition, if one wished to take a pulse, the abdomen is not the ideal place to check, for the abdominal pulse will only easily be felt in an emaciated person; Galen was aware of this fact. To examine the pulse, one should better palpate the arteries of the extremities where the absence of fat or muscle allows for easier, more direct palpation. And, if searching for the direct beat of the heart was the intent of the proponent of the second opinion in the *Yerushalmi*, he perhaps should have stated so explicitly.

Secondly, it is possible to examine the abdomen for movement during respiration. With normal respiration, the diaphragm descends, and the abdominal wall protrudes. Although this can be altered in pathological states, in a normal individual it can be easily observed, without the need for palpation. Although the Rabbis may not have understood the physiology of respiration, diaphragmatic excursion, or abdominal wall motion, this would have been an easy way to search for movement.

This discussion can also be understood in a philosophical sense. Although, admittedly, the issue being decided is of pragmatic concern regarding the violation of the Sabbath, there may be strong philosophical overtones that impact that decision. Which area of the body is considered to be the origin or the source of life? One *Ammora* claims that breath is the source of life, although no medical or biblical support for this notion is cited in the text of the *Yerushalmi*.[37] Consequently, it is this element for which we must search in the man underneath the rubble. This position may have its analogue in Greco-Roman physiology as an example of the prime importance of the pneuma/spirit/breath in Galen's system mentioned above (#4 and #5). The other *Ammora* counters that one must uncover up to the navel, because it is from there that the body originates and gives forth the remaining organs and limbs.[38]

---

36. There is an allusion to palpation of the pulse in *Midrash Tehillim* 73:1, quoted by Preuss, op. cit., 143.

37. The *Korban HaEdah* on *Talmud Yerushalmi, Yoma* 8:5 cites the scriptural verse, "All in whose nostrils was the breath of life" (Bereshit 7:22), as does the *Talmud Bavli* discussed below.

38. See *Korban HaEdah*, loc. cit.

This position of the other *Ammora* may have its basis in embryological notions of antiquity and is consistent with the position of Alcomaeon.[39]

Other talmudic passages present opposing embryological views. In discussing where the point of measurement should be on the body of the deceased in the case of the *egla arufa*, the Talmud (*Sota* 45a) mentions a debate about the embryological origins of the fetus.[40] One position, buttressed by scriptural proof, maintains that the head is formed first. Abba Shaul, identifying with the other opinion in the *Yerushalmi*, believes the navel to be the origin of the fetus. This passage, however, as opposed to the *Yerushalmi*, clearly differentiates between embryology and physiology. Abba Shaul may argue and maintain that the navel is the embryological origin of the fetus, but regarding the determination of the presence of life, even he would agree, the Talmud says, that the examination of the nostrils is the determinant. This latter notion is also supported by a biblical verse, "All in whose nostrils was the breath of life" (Bereshit 7:22).

These embryological views have analogues in the contemporaneous Greco-Roman world (see #8, above). In addition, the value of air, spirit or pneuma was paramount in the Galenic system of physiology, as mentioned above (#5). The air, which was ultimately converted to different pneumas, was breathed in through the nostrils.

However, the very enterprise of interpreting these rabbinic opinions in light of concurrent medical history is clouded by the citation of biblical verses as support for these opinions. Are these verses quoted as a reflection of a particular tradition about the definition of life or of man's embryological origins, or are they perhaps examples of *asmakhta* (literary association of a rabbinic idea with a biblical text), in which case they do not reflect a specifically unique tradition, and the verses are merely used to support positions consistent with contemporaneous medical knowledge? This is a truly crucial question, for if the former is true, then it not only renders our discussion futile, but any discussion revolving around changes in medical/scientific understanding between our generation

---

39. See J. Needham, op. cit., 78.
40. The author of *Ein Ya'akov* 2 (Jerusalem, 1961) 37a actually juxtaposes the two passages from *Yoma* and *Sota*. Cf. *Nidda* 25b where Abba Shaul maintains that the head is formed first, a seeming contradiction to his position in *Sota*.

and that of the Talmud is out of place. We would be dealing not with talmudic medicine, but with biblical assumptions which clearly are not subject to the same type of historical analysis.[41] I appreciate the gravity and volatility of this issue. I refrain here from addressing the theological implications and will confine myself solely to the historical aspects.

We now turn to the Babylonian Talmud's version of the passage (*Yoma* 85a). The Mishna states:

> If debris falls on someone, and it is doubtful whether or not he is there, or whether he is alive or dead, or whether he be an Israelite or a heathen, one should open [even on the Sabbath] the heap of debris for his sake. If one finds him alive one should remove the debris, and if he be dead one should leave him there [until the Sabbath day is over].

The Talmud then elaborates:

> Our Rabbis taught: How far does one search? Until [one reaches] his nose. Some say: Up to his heart. If one searches and finds those above to be dead, one must not assume those below are surely dead. Once it happened that those above were dead and those below were found to be alive. Are we to

---

41. For the issue of the integration of scientific knowledge into halakha, and the conflict between the opinion of the sages and that of modern science see, for example, D. Frimer, "*Kevi'at Avhut al yedei Bedukat Dam beMishpat haYisraeli ubemishpat haIvri,*" in M. Halperin, ed., *Sefer Assia* 5 (Jerusalem, 1986), 185–209; D. Cohen, "*Shinuy Hateva*: An Analysis of the Halachic Process," *Journal of Halacha and Contemporary Society* 31 (Spring 1996); S. Sprecher, "*Divrei Ḥazal VeYedi'ot Mada'iyot,*" B.D.D. 2 (Winter 1996), 2–39; S. Z. Leiman, "R. Israel Lipshutz and the Mouse that is Half Flesh and Half Earth: A Note on Torah U-Madda in the Nineteenth Century," in *Ḥazon Nachum* (Yeshiva University Press, 1997), 449–458; N. Gutal, *Sefer Hishtanut HaTeva'im BeHalakha* (Makhon Yaḥdav, 5758); A. Steinberg, *Encyclopedia of Jewish Medical Ethics*, trans. F. Rosner (Feldheim Publishers, 2003), s. v., "change in nature"; N. Slifkin, *Mysterious Creatures* (Targum Press, 2003), 17–41; M. Halperin, "Science and Medicine in the Talmud: *Kabbalah o Actualia,*" *Assia* 71–72 (January, 2003), 90–102 (Hebrew); Yehuda Levi, *The Science in Torah: The Scientific Knowledge of the Sages* (Feldheim Publishers, 2004); M. Meiselman, *Torah, Chazal and Science* (Israel Bookshop, 2013).

say that these *Tannaim* dispute the same as the following *Tannaim*? For it was taught: From where does the formation of the embryo commence? From its head, as it is said "Thou are he that took me (*gozi*) out of my mother's womb," and it is also said: "Cut off (*gozi*) thy hair and cast it away." Abba Saul said: From the navel which sends its roots into every direction? You may even say that [the first view is in agreement with] Abba Saul, inasmuch as Abba Saul holds his view only touching the first formation, because "everything develops from its core (middle)" but regarding the saving of life he would agree that life manifests itself through the nose especially, as it is written: "In whose nostrils was the breath of the spirit of life." R. Papa said: The dispute arises only as to from below upwards, but if from above downwards, once one had searched up to the nose, one need not search any farther, as it is said: "In whose nostrils was the breath of life."[42]

There are some fundamental differences between the *Bavli* and *Yerushalmi* versions, but for our discussion it is noteworthy that the *Bavli* substitutes the word *libo* (heart) for *tiburo* (navel).[43] We must, therefore, again wonder what is being examined when one uncovers "up to the heart." Unlike the examination of the navel, there is no room for interpretation here. It is clearly the heartbeat that is either being palpated or listened for. We have mentioned that Hippocrates noted the apex beat (section 9, above). However, similar to the abdomen, this is not the most reliable place to examine the heartbeat. The apex beat cannot always be seen or palpated even in the presence of a normally functioning heart. The ribs and muscle prevent deep palpation. As was stated earlier, examination of the extremities, or perhaps the carotid arteries in the neck, is more reliable. In any case, checking for heartbeat is clearly what is being advocated.

The *Bavli* also attempts to parallel the debate as to whether one should search for life in the nares or the heart with the debate whether

---

42. Translation by Leo Jung, *Soncino Talmud* (London, 1984).
43. The Rif, Ran, and Rosh all preserve the text of the *Talmud Yerushalmi* of "*ad tiburo.*" The Meiri says "*tiburo o lev.*"

the head or the navel are of the earliest embryological origin. We have stated that these positions have antecedents in medical history. Implicit in this attempted parallelism, however, is the identification of the "navel" with the "heart." Applying the hermeneutic circle of analysis, we can perhaps reinterpret the *Yerushalmi* position and suggest that the examination of the navel is actually a reflection of heartbeat, one of the alternatives we had suggested. The *Bavli*, however, subsequently rejects the parallel and clearly differentiates between embryology and physiology.[44]

Position of Rashi

Rashi, like most *Rishonim*, explains the positions in the Talmud without explicit recourse to known medical theories or medical works. However, in his elucidation of the position requiring examination of the heart, Rashi makes a statement whose interpretation may be aided by an understanding of both medical history, in general, and of Rashi's unique anatomical understanding, in particular. He states:

> One says to examine the heart for presence of life *(ḥiyut)* "*shen-ishmato dofeket sham*," and one says to examine up to the nostrils because sometimes life is not observed in the heart, yet is observed in the nostrils.[45]

A proper understanding of this Rashi hinges on the interpretation of the phrase "*nishmato dofeket sham*." The word *nishmato* can mean either "his soul," a derivative of *neshama*, or "his breath," a derivative of *neshima*. Elsewhere, Rashi adopts the latter usage,[46] and I believe this usage to be contextually appropriate here as well.

Further support for the notion that *nishmato* refers to breathing is provided by the use of the term *dofeket*. This term, meaning "pulsates" or "beats," most likely refers to a physiological process. To associate the term *dofeket* with the soul would be awkward. In

---

44. See above regarding the passage from *Sota 45a*.
45. Rashi, *Yoma* 85a, s. v., "*hakhi garsinan*."
46. *Keritut* 22a. Rashi, ad loc., s. v., "*mishratz sharitz*."

light of the above, Rashi claims that the heart is checked because the breath pulsates or is transmitted there. Therefore, when the heart is examined, its movement is a reflection of breathing; its *ḥiyut* a manifestation of respiration.

It follows that the heart is a respiratory organ and that Rashi subscribed to the notion that the inspired air ultimately reached the heart, ideas widely held throughout antiquity and the Middle Ages (see sections 4 and 6, above). While Galen and his followers had postulated an indirect route for the inspired air to reach the heart (above, n. 16), it appears that Rashi believed that there was a direct connection between the trachea and the heart. This is evident from his commentary on *Ḥullin* 45b: "Amemar said in the name of Rav Naḥman: There are three vessels, one to the heart, one to the lung, and one to the liver." The three "vessels" mentioned could possibly refer to the vessels attached to the four-chambered heart, i.e., the aorta, the pulmonary artery, and the inferior vena cava. Rashi, however, does not adopt this approach. He states: "There are three vessels; after the trachea enters the thorax, it divides into three."[47] Once the trachea enters the thorax, according to Rashi, it branches into three parts, one leading to the heart, one to the lung and one to the liver. The inspired air can reach the heart directly via one of the tracheal branches.[48] Rashi

---

47. Rashi, ad loc., s. v., "*telata kanei.*"

48. Admittedly, this Rashi and the ones later mentioned refer to animal anatomy. However, it is unlikely that so fundamental an anatomical notion should vary, according to Rashi, between humans and animals. Indeed, *Tosafot* (*Ḥullin* 42b, s. v., "*ve'amer*") states regarding *treifot* that one should differentiate between man and animal, but only in matters where their anatomy differs. The Talmud, however, does explicitly prohibit the extrapolation from animal to human anatomy. See *Ḥullin* 68a, "*adam mibehema lo yalif*" and *Tosafot*, ad loc., s. v., "*shilya.*"

As human dissection was frowned upon during most of antiquity, the great scientists almost uniformly extrapolated from animal anatomy. Aristotle states that the inner parts of the body are unknown, especially those of man; consequently, one must refer to the parts of animals which have a nature similar to the nature humans possess and examine them. See Jonathan Barns, ed., *Complete Works of Aristotle* (Princeton, 1985), 788. Galen is notorious for having extrapolated his anatomy from animals, leading to many erroneous conclusions. See, for example, Charles Singer, "Some Galenic and Animal Sources of Vesalius," op. cit., 6–24.

reiterates this anatomical understanding in other passages in his commentary on *Ḥullin*.[49]

Rashi's anatomical approach does not correlate with contemporary understanding of anatomy, nor is there, to the best of my knowledge, any school in the history of anatomy that described the trachea as directly connecting to the heart.[50] In addition, anatomical dissection

---

49. In *Ḥullin* 49a, the Talmud discusses a case where a needle was found in the large vessel of the liver of an animal and presents a debate as to whether or not the animal is kosher. Rashi, however, addresses the question of how the needle reached its location. In doing so, he details the relevant anatomy and concludes that the needle must have been ingested by way of the trachea. It reached the large vessel of the liver by passing through the branch of the trachea that leads to the liver. In passing, Rashi also mentions the branches of the trachea that lead to the heart and lungs.

Another such example appears in *Ḥullin* 111a. In the context of a discussion on the necessary preparations for eating liver, the Talmud mentions a case where a particular dish was brought before Yanai, the son of Rebbe Ami. The dish was called *kanya bikufya* and Rashi explains it to consist of the trachea and all that is attached to it, namely the lung, heart and liver. All these organs were cooked together. For reasons related to that passage, the Talmud constructs a scenario whereby the blood of the liver can flow directly out of the pot and not be cooked with the other organs. In explaining this unique circumstance, Rashi (s. v., "*dilma*") elaborates on the anatomy of these organs and postulates a pathway for the blood. He states, "The small vessels of the liver drain into the tube (*kaneh*) of the lung (i.e., trachea). From here the blood traverses through the hollow (of the trachea) to the outside of the pot." Here, again, it is quite clear that Rashi believed that the three major organs, including the heart, are directly connected to the trachea.

50. Preuss, op. cit., 103, claims that this position of Rashi is consistent with the teaching of Aristotle. I have been unable to verify this assertion. Aristotle believed that the air ultimately reached the heart, but it is unclear whether he believed that the trachea connected directly to it. Leonardo da Vinci postulated a more direct route for the air to reach the heart than did Galen, but it was not as direct as it would be according to Rashi. See J. Playfair McMurrich, *Leonardo da Vinci, the Anatomist* (Baltimore, 1930), 195. Da Vinci obviously post-dates Rashi by some 400 years. For further discussion of Rashi's unique anatomical position, see, E. Reichman, "The Life and Work of Dr. Menachem Mendel Yehuda Leib Sergei: A Torah U'Madda Titan of the Early Twentieth Century," *Hakirah* 27 (Fall 2019), 119–146.

was not routinely performed during this period in history.[51] One can only fruitlessly speculate as to the source of Rashi's anatomical ideas.[52] This particular inaccuracy of Rashi has been pointed out in the seventeenth century by R. Yitzhak Lampronti.[53] However, the notion

---

51. There are no clearly documented human dissections from the time of Rashi, although scattered references to autopsies and dissections appear in the thirteenth and fourteenth centuries. Mundinus (1270–1326) is recognized to have been the first to incorporate human anatomical dissection into the medical curriculum. See, for example, C. D. O'Malley, *Andreas Vesalius of Brussels* (Berkeley, 1964), 1–20; Ludwig Edelstein, "The History of Anatomy in Antiquity," in *Ancient Medicine* (Baltimore, 1967), 247–302; Charles Singer, *A Short History of Anatomy and Physiology From the Greeks to Harvey* (New York, 1957); Mary Niven Alston, "The Attitude of the Church Towards Dissection Before 1500," *Bulletin of the History of Medicine* 16:3 (October 1944), 221–238; Nancy Siraisi, *Taddeo Alderotti and His Pupils* (Princeton, 1981), 66–69. On the history of anatomy in rabbinic literature, see chapter, "The Anatomy of Halakha."

52. Regarding Rashi's relationship with a Jewish physician named Meshulam, and regarding his general medical knowledge, see John R. W. Dunbar, trans., *History of the Jewish Physicians: From the French of E. Carmoly* (Baltimore, 1845), 42–43. Note, however, that Carmoly quotes no sources. The veracity of his assertions is in question, and I have seen no other source that corroborates his claims.

53. See his *Pahad Yizhak* 10 (Bnei Brak, 1980), 53–54, s. v., "*telata kanei.*" R. Lampronti was himself a physician who graduated from the University of Padua. See Abdelkader Modena, *Medici E Chirurghi Ebrei Dottorati E. Licenziati Nell Universita Di Padova Dal 1617 al 1816* (Bologna, 1967), 55–57. It is worth quoting R. Lampronti's critique of Rashi:

> "I, the young author, question the position of Rashi. For it appears that he believed that the trachea enters into the liver and heart. Any scholar with knowledge of anatomy can see with his own eyes ... that this is not so."

Y. L. Katznelson makes a similar comment in his book, *HaTalmud VeHokhmat HaRefua* (Berlin, 1928), 131. He defends Rashi by claiming that this statement must have been inserted by a student of Rashi, as Rashi knew too much about anatomy to make such a gross error. David Margalit likewise defends Rashi against R. Lampronti and claims that Rashi was actually referring to the major heart vessels, i. e., the aorta, etc. See his "*Erkhim Refui'im SheBiEntzyclopedia HaHilkhatit 'Pahad Yitzhak' le-R. Y. Lampronti,*" *Koroth* 2: 1–2 (April 1958), 59. In my humble opinion, however, had Dr. Katznelson and D. Margalit seen the other two passages of Rashi in *Hullin* discussed above, it is doubtful whether they still could have maintained their defenses. For further discussion of Rashi's position, see M. M. Sergui, *Meishiv Nefesh* (Rosenkrantz Publishers: Vilna, 5666), 22a–23a (Hebrew); A. Ben David, *Sihat Hullin al Masekhet Hullin* (*Midrash Bekhorei Yosef*: Jerusalem, 5755), 162–163 (includes diagrams) (Hebrew). For further discussion on the three "vessels" see

of *Rishonim,* and Rashi in particular, espousing erroneous anatomical beliefs is not without precedent. Ḥatam Sofer, in discussing the identification of the terms used by the Rabbis to refer to the female anatomy,[54] makes the following comment:

> After searching through anatomy books and speaking with experts in anatomy, it is impossible to deny that the reality is not like the explanation of Rashi and *Tosafot*.... But after begging forgiveness from our holy Rabbis, they were incorrect in this matter. The truth is with the position of Maimonides,[55] as proven by experimentation by anatomists and as found in the anatomy books from expert physicians... I have also asked physicians...[56]

Position of Rabbi Yehuda Aryeh of Modena

Until this point, I have attempted to place the talmudic passages in *Yoma* and *Sota* into their medical historical milieu and to align, in a general way, the embryological and physiological beliefs of the Rabbis with contemporaneous Greco-Roman theories. In addition, I have suggested that the *Talmud Bavli* in *Yoma* and *Sota* differentiates between embryology and physiology.

S. Sternberg, "Book Review of I. M. Levinger's *Guide to Masekhet Ḥullin and Masekhet Bekhorot,*" *B. D. D.* 4 (Winter, 1997), 81–102, esp., 88–91; P. Roth, "Responsum of R. Yitzḥak Kimḥi on the Law of a Needle Found in the Liver," (Hebrew), *Yeshurun* 29 (*Elul,* 5773), 28–32.

54. I refer here to the terms used in Mishna, *Nidda* 2:5. For further discussion about the identification of these terms, see, for example, Preuss, op. cit., 115–119; Abraham S. Abraham, *Nishmat Avraham,* Y. D., 76–79; I. M. Levinger, "HaMivneh HaAnatomi shel Evarei HaMin BeIsha UVeBa'alei Ḥayyim," *Koroth* 4: 8–10 (June, 1968), 611–615; Tirzah Z. Meachum, "Mishna Tractate Nidda with Introduction: A Critical Edition with Notes on Variants, Commentary, Redaction and Chapters in Legal History and Realia" (unpublished doctoral dissertation: Hebrew University, 1989), 224–231.

55. Even Maimonides' anatomical description is difficult to understand today. He discusses this matter extensively in his *Commentary on the Mishna, Nidda* 2:5, and, more succinctly, in his *Mishneh Torah, Hil. Issurei Bi'ah,* chapter 5. It is difficult to identify the structure called the *"lul"* according to the interpretation of Maimonides. For a comprehensive discussion on this topic, see M. Halperin, *Realia and Medicine in Seder Nashim* (Schlesinger Institute, 2011), 3–40 (Hebrew).

56. See *She'elot UTeshuvot Ḥatam Sofer,* Y. D., n. 167.

R. Yehudah Aryeh of Modena, who lived in the seventeenth century, also engages in the same method of analysis. In his eyes, however,
the Rabbis are clearly and directly addressing the heart-brain debate
of medical antiquity (see above, # 6 and # 8), both in terms of which
has embryological precedence and in terms of which has greater physiological significance. Through this approach, his interpretation of the
conclusion of the *Yoma* passage is quite remarkable, and is worthy of
being cited in toto:[57]

"From where is the fetus created, etc." Next to this passage [in
Yoma], the author of *Ein Yaakov* juxtaposes a passage from Tractate *Sota*. I will address the reason for this juxtaposition. There
are varying opinions amongst the [natural] philosophers regarding which organ of a developing fetus is created first. Some [i.e.,
Aristotle] say the heart, some say the liver,[58] and some say both
of these together, [simultaneous] with the brain. And regarding
the source of life (*mishkan haḥiyut*), some say it is in the heart,[59]
which is, therefore, called the king of all organs, and some [i.e.,
Galen] say it is the brain. The brain is in close proximity to the
nostrils and a tube connects the two for the purpose of evacu-
ating the phlegm, breath and pneuma from the brain.[60]That is
why the brain has continuous motion[61] similar to the heart. . . .

Now, understand from this passage how the *Tannaim*
engage in a similar argument. Regarding embryology, one says the
fetus grows from the head, i.e., the brain, and one says from the
navel, meaning to say the heart and liver. And, regarding the seat

---

57. A small excerpt of this passage was quoted by F. Rosner and M. Tendler, op. cit.
58. See May, op. cit., 58. This is the position of Galen. See also Adelmann, op. cit., 41, 43.
59. May and Adelmann, ibid.
60. For discussion on the importance of the evacuation of the phlegm, one of the four
humors, from the brain, see Lloyd, *Hippocratic Writings*, op. cit., 241–247. For a
discussion on the anatomy and physiology of the canal that connects the brain to
the nostrils, see May, op. cit., 428–430.
61. Maimonides, in his medical aphorisms, mentions that the brain undergoes constant
pulsatile motion which contributes to the expulsion of waste from the brain. See F.
Rosner, *Maimonides' Medical Writings: The Medical Aphorisms of Moses Maimonides*
(Haifa, 1989), 14–15.

of life, one says from the nostrils, meaning to say the brain, and one says the heart. It is in this context that the *Tannaim* debated how one checks to see if a person has died. If respirations are absent, one *Tanna* says check up to the nostrils, and the other says check up to the heart. Rav Papa, however, says that everyone agrees that the source of life (*ḥiyut*) is in the brain. Therefore, if one first checks the nostrils, which are functionally connected to the brain [as stated above], and there is no breath, everyone would agree that the brain is no longer functioning and the person is dead .... When do they argue? In a case when one reaches the heart first. In this case, one authority maintains that if the heart has stopped beating, surely this is a reflection that brain function has ceased as well, and the person is considered dead. The other authority claims that it is possible for pulsations of the heart not to be appreciated, yet the brain may still be functioning, as evidenced by the breath from the nostrils. [Therefore, one must check the nostrils even if he starts from the bottom up.]

The Torah, the source of truth, supports this position of Rav Papa with the verse, "all in whose nostrils is the breath of life," revealing that the presence of breath in the nostrils indicates the presence of life.[62] We see from here how the knowledge of the Rabbis covers all domains.

R. Yehuda Aryeh of Modena interprets the discussion in *Yoma* to be about the best method to determine brain death, albeit not the way we understand this phrase. According to one opinion, the absence of a heartbeat is an adequate assessment of brain death, while the other contends that the brain may still be functioning even in the absence of a discernible heartbeat. Therefore, according to the latter, the function of the brain must be assessed directly, by checking for respiration.[63]

---

62. Most contemporary halakhic sources have viewed the checking of the nostrils as a means of assessing respiration, but not necessarily specific organ function; the issue being whether the absence of respiration itself is a sign or a definition of death. R. Modena, however, views the checking of the nostrils to be a direct assessment of brain function.
63. Although R. Modena himself had no formal medical training, he was friendly with a number of medical students at the nearby University of Padua. See Howard E.

What is important from R. Modena's words is not so much the details of his discussion as the methodology of his approach. He frames the talmudic discussion within the context of contemporary medical theory, thereby reaching a conclusion different from other rabbinic authorities.

IV. THE MISHNA IN *OHALOT* AND POST-DECAPITATION MOVEMENT

The halakhic debate about the determination of death has also included discussion of rabbinic sources dealing with decapitation and postmortem body movements. Brain death has been termed "physiological decapitation " and has therefore been argued to be analogous to the passages discussing physical decapitation.[64]

The starting point for this approach is a Mishna in *Ohalot* (1:6):

> Man does not spread impurity until his soul departs. Likewise, for animals. If they are decapitated, even if they are "moving" they can spread impurity, similar to the tail of a lizard that "moves" independently.[65]

Here the Mishna discusses the halakhic relevance of postmortem movement. It does not, however, detail the physiology of movement, nor does it reveal the origin or center that controls bodily movement. The Talmud (*Ḥullin* 20b-21a) elaborates on the case of "severance of the spine" in defining a "*neveila*." The issue raised is whether that state is sufficient to constitute a *neveila* or whether severance of a majority of flesh in the

---

Adelman, "Leon Modena: The Autobiography and the Man," in *The Autobiography of a Seventeenth-Century Venetian Rabbi,* trans. and ed. by Mark R. Cohen (Princeton, 1988), 30, and n. 76.

64. See the articles by M. Tendler, op. cit.

65. The assumption is that the latter half of the Mishna ("If they are decapitated ...") refers to man as well as animals. This appears to be the opinion of Maimonides (*Hil. Tum'at Met* 1:15). According to the *Gilyon HaRosh* on the Mishna in *Ohalot,* however, both Rashi and *Tosafot* in *Ḥullin* maintain that this phrase excludes man. The *Ḥidushei Rashash* on *Ohalot* adjusts the text of *Tosafot* to include man. See also *Tiferet Yisrael,* ad loc.

neck area is also required (*"rov basar imo"*). Again, the discussion is halakhic and not physiological.

Maimonides, however, alludes to a coordinating center of movement whose control is lost with limb or tail amputation:

> This creature moves its tail a great deal after it is severed. However, this occurs to a number of "species" whose source of movement is not localized and coordinated from a central source but is rather spread throughout the body.[66]

Although Maimonides refers to a central origin of movement, he does not reveal whether this origin is the brain, or the heart, or perhaps some other organ. From Maimonides' medical writings, however, it is clear what he believed to be the source of movement.[67]

We have mentioned above (section 6) the debate between Aristotle and Galen regarding whether the heart or the brain is the controlling center of sensation and movement. Maimonides explicitly addresses this controversy and supports the position of Aristotle:

> I have prefaced [my remarks] with this introduction in order to stimulate you to [critically appraise even] a statement of the great sage Galen. You already know that his opinion is that there are three major organs, the heart, the brain, and the liver, and that not one of these can receive its power from another organ under any circumstances. The opinion of Aristotle and his followers is, as you know, that there is a single main organ, namely, the heart, and the heart sends powers to each of the other organs and, with this power, the other organs perform their specific functions. Therefore, according to the view of Aristotle, the heart sends powers to the brain and with this power the brain performs its function,

---

66. Maimonides, *Commentary on Mishna, Ohalot,* ad loc.
67. In Maimonides' medical writings, there are virtually no references to religious or halakhic matters, and, in general, rabbinic authorities do not consult them at all. In this discussion, however, I believe a deviation from the norm is indicated, as will be evident.

and it [in turn] gives sensation and movement to other organs. So too the powers of imagination, thought, and memory are powers that are brought into existence in the brain through the principle that the brain receives from the heart. Similarly, all other organs in the body contain the powers with which they perform their special functions. This [thesis of Aristotle] is correct and logical because the brain performs its functions, and likewise every organ performs its functions, and all [together] they constitute the total life situation of an individual. However, the heart sends the specific power of life to each organ.[68]

Another rabbinic figure roughly contemporary with Maimonides also addresses the Galen-Aristotle controversy. The thirteenth century Rabbenu Gershon b. Shlomo, father of the Ralbag and son-in-law of Naḥmanides, cites multiple proofs for both sides of the controversy:

Galen claims that the source of movement is the brain, and he brings the following proof: He [i.e., Galen] once removed the heart from a monkey, and the monkey continued to move for twelve hours. It [therefore] appears that the source of movement is the brain.... There is also support for the position of Aristotle: After a man is decapitated, the remaining body can walk a few steps. So I was told by a scholar who claimed to have seen with his own eyes that when a man was sentenced by the king to decapitation, he stated that after his head is severed, his body

---

68. See F. Rosner, op. cit., 446, treatise n. 25, item n. 70. This section is devoted exclusively to criticism of Galen. This item, as well as the following two items, deal extensively with the issue of whether the heart or brain is the source of movement, and Maimonides here, as in the remainder of this treatise, severely criticizes Galen's view. These items comprise the concluding section of the book of aphorisms, which may reflect their relative significance. Although Maimonides believes the heart to be the primary organ providing the power or energy which ultimately is responsible for movement, he clearly acknowledges a major role of the brain in movement. See ibid., 16. Regarding Maimonides' view of the heart, see also Maimonides' *Guide* 1:38, 72. Regarding Maimonides' criticism of Galen, see Max Meyerhof, "Maimonides Criticizes Galen," *Medical Leaves* 3:1 (1940), 141–146. See also works by Gerrit Bos.

will walk to a designated spot. And so it was, the body walked to this spot and there it fell.[69]

The post-decapitation movement mentioned in support of Aristotle is likely a reference to the Lazarus reflex which was first described for guillotine victims and later found to occur in brain-dead patients as well.[70]

The quote from Galen is also of historic and halakhic import. Whether the body can function without a heart or whether a heart can function without a body has long preoccupied the minds of anatomist and halakhist alike. Already in the second century, Galen observed that "the heart, removed from the thorax, can be seen to move for a considerable time."[71] In the sixteenth century, Andreas Vesalius, the premier anatomist of the Renaissance, described dogs and cats running around after their hearts had been excised.[72] One century later, William Harvey, the discoverer of circulation, "proved by the frequent dissection of living animals . . . that when the animal was already dying and no longer breathing, the heart continued to pulsate for a while and kept some life in itself."[73]

V. THE ḤAKHAM TZVI AND THE "HEARTLESS" CHICKEN

The discussion of whether an animal could live without a heart has occupied a prominent place in halakhic responsa literature as it relates to the status of an animal as *treifa* or *neveila*.[74] A case in the year 1709

---

69. See H. Y. D. Azulai, *Shem HaGedolim* (Jerusalem, 1954), "Sha'ar HaShamayim," 68b. This work is largely a compilation of other sources and apparently includes excerpts from Maimonides' *Sefer HaNefesh*. The Ḥakham Tzvi disputes this latter notion. See *She'elot UTeshuvot Ḥakham Tzvi*, 77.

70. Rabbenu Gershon makes no reference here to the Mishna in *Ohalot*, but if we applied the position of Aristotle to the Mishna, then a decapitated man or animal, if it is moving, should still be considered alive and should not convey impurity.

71. See C. Singer, *Galen: On Anatomical Procedures*, op. cit., 184.

72. See Samuel W. Lambert, trans., *Andreas Vesaliius: De Fabrica Corporis Humanis* in L. Clandening, *Source Book of Medical History*, op. cit., 149.

73. See Gweneth Whitteridge, trans., *William Harvey, Disputations Touching the Generation of Animals* (Oxford, 1981), 243.

74. See sources quoted in H. J. Zimmels, op. cit., 39–41, 196–197. See *Shulḥan Arukh, Y. D.*, 40:5. The question the later rabbinic authorities address is if an animal cannot survive at

caused a great sensation when a young girl, preparing a hen for dinner, was unable to locate its heart. There was some suspicion that a nearby cat may have eaten it. The case was brought before the Ḥakham Tzvi to decide if the hen was kosher. During the course of his discussion, the Ḥakham Tzvi took the opportunity to elaborate on the importance of the heart, both from a halakhic as well as a physiological perspective.[75] His famous responsa on this subject have already been incorporated into the halakhic discussions of brain death, but I wish only to highlight a few of the medical historical elements.

It is interesting to note that this responsum was written after the discovery of the circulation of the blood, generally credited to William Harvey, yet no mention of this revolutionary discovery is found there.[76] The notion of the heart being the center of the circulation perhaps could have further buttressed the Ḥakham Tzvi's argument of the importance of that organ.

It is clear that the Ḥakham Tzvi subscribed to the position of Aristotle. He writes, "All the life and power of the body are dependent upon it [i.e., the heart] It is the first created and [life] is inconceivable without it." In addition, he quotes R. Gershon b. Shlomo's opinion, discussed above, regarding the case of the monkey whose movement was observed twelve hours after the heart was removed: "Anyone who is the least bit familiar with science will realize that the words of the *Sha'ar HaShamayim* are the opinion of Galen." Aside from the fact that

---

all without a heart, then such an animal should be considered a *neveila* and not a *treifa*. For further discussion of this halakhic episode, see Maoz Kahana, *A Heartless Chicken: Religion and Science in Early Modern Rabbinic Culture* (Bialik Institute: Jerusalem, 2021); chapter, "A Letter from a Torah Sage of the Eighteenth Century."

75. *She'elot UTeshuvot Ḥakham Tzvi, n. 77.*

76. Harvey's famous work, *De Motu Cordis,* first appeared in 1628. However, Harvey earlier alluded to the idea of systemic circulation in his lectures on anatomy. See C. D. O'Malley, et al., annotated translation, *William Harvey: Lectures on the Whole of Anatomy* (Berkeley, 1961), 191–92.

Although Harvey's work appeared in 1628, it is not clear when his notions of circulation became universally accepted by the medical world. On the delayed transmission of Harvey's work in Spain, see J. J. Izquierdo, "On Spanish Neglect of Harvey's 'De Motu Cordis' for Three Centuries, and How it was Finally Made Known to Spain and Spanish Speaking Countries," *Journal of the History of Medicine* (Winter 1948), 105–124.

R. Gershon b. Shlomo explicitly attributed this position to Galen (see quote earlier in this article), it seems that the Ḥakham Tzvi considered himself to have had at least minimal medical scientific knowledge which obviously included the teachings of Galen.

In discussing the talmudic passage in *Yoma*, the Ḥakham Tzvi cites Rashi as support for his position.

> Rashi *z"l* agrees with our words that the *neshama*[77] dwells in the heart. However, there are times when even if the *neshama* is still within the heart, the pulse may not be palpable on the chest [over the heart]. This may be secondary to the weakness of the pulsations, or because the heart is hidden underneath the chest wall, which prevents transmission of the pulse. But the *neshama* that exits the heart, by way of the lungs, can be observed as long as the heart is functioning. It is quite clear that there can be no *neshama* unless there is life in the heart. For *neshama* exists because of and for the purpose of the heart.

A number of important points can be gleaned from this last passage.

1) The Ḥakham Tzvi acknowledges that the chest is not the best place to examine for heartbeat secondary to the interference of the ribs and muscle. As already indicated, this is consistent with medical teachings since antiquity and is equally true today as well.
2) He believes that the heart is a respiratory organ, also perfectly consistent with the medical understanding of his time. He, therefore, discusses the exhalation of air from the heart, via the lungs, to the outside. We have mentioned above that it was an accepted fact that the inspired air ultimately reached the heart.
3) It seems evident that the Ḥakham Tzvi understands the Rashi as it was explained above, i.e., we check the heart because the breath pulsates or is transmitted there ("*nishmato dofeket sham*").

---

77. Since the term "*neshama*" can be translated as either "soul" or "breath," I preserve the original Hebrew. I believe it is clear from later in the passage, however, that it refers to "breath."

In mustering further support for his position, the Ḥakham Tzvi quotes a series of sources from the Middle Ages including Ibn Ezra, *Kuzari*,[78] *Sha'ar HaShamayim* and *Shevilei Emuna*.[79] The quotes from these authors all discuss variations on the theme of "innate heat" (*ḥom hativ'i*). Without a fundamental understanding of the contemporaneous notions of cardio-respiratory physiology, these passages can easily be misinterpreted.[80] The heart was thought to contain the source of the body's heat and this "innate heat" was thought to be the source of life. (See discussion of Greek physiology, section 3, above.) The purpose of respiration was to cool the flames of the heart, and the inability to cool these flames would lead to excess heat and, ultimately, to death. The notion of the "innate heat" of the heart was only disproved in the seventeenth century by Giovanni Alfonse Borelli when he actually measured the temperature of the heart with a thermometer.[81]

In sum, the Ḥakham Tzvi subscribes to the Aristotelian ideas of the embryological and physiological significance of the heart. His physiological discussion is largely consistent with accepted medical teachings of his time, except for the omission of the notion of the circulation of the blood. In addition, his proofs are firmly rooted in theories of Greco-Roman and Renaissance medicine.

R. Yonatan Eybeschuetz also addressed the question of the heartless chicken and took issue with the decision of the Ḥakham Tzvi.[82] Whereas the Ḥakham Tzvi quoted older sources discussing medical

---

78. 2:26. In this passage, Yehuda Halevi likens the innate heat in the heart to a flame on a candle stick. This candle analogy is strikingly similar to that mentioned by Galen. See May, op. cit., 52. See also Y. Muscato, *Kol Yehuda*, commentary on Kuzari, ad loc., which details the physiology of heat and pneumas.

79. This book was written by Meir ibn Aldabi, the grandson of R. Asher b. Yeḥiel, in 1360. It was reprinted many times, the last of which was in Jerusalem, 1990. I was able to identify one of the Cairo Geniza fragments in Cambridge as being an excerpt from *Shevilei Emuna*. See Cairo Geniza fragment T-S NS 222.71 (folios 3–4) which is an excerpt from *Shevilei Emuna, netiv 5, shevil 7.*

80. For further discussion of the idea of innate heat in Jewish sources, see chapter, "The Incorporation of Pre-Modern Scientific Theories into Rabbinic Literature: The Case of Innate Heat."

81. See May, op. cit., 53, and n. 231.

82. See his *Kreti UPleti, Y. D.,* 40:4.

theory, R. Eybeschuetz wished to settle the matter by sending a letter to the medical faculty of the University of Halle in Germany.[83] The question he posed to the physicians was whether an animal could live without a heart or some other organ serving a similar function. He quotes their response verbatim in his work. He also stresses that the discussion of the Ḥakham Tzvi is based on medical theories which often change with time:

> Regarding scientific principles based on experimentation, today the hypothesis is one way, and when others observe the opposite phenomenon, they retract the initial hypothesis and replace it with another. And such is always the case. Even now, based on experimentation, [scientists] have actually retracted all the assumptions and conclusions of Galen and Aristotle.[84]

In addition, R. Eybeschuetz notes that while certain aspects of Jewish law have a specific *mesora*, such as which animals are considered a *treifa*,[85] there is no such *mesora* for the understanding of the function of the heart. This is perhaps why he felt free to consult contemporary physicians as opposed to quoting from earlier rabbinic sources.

VI. POSTMORTEM CAESAREAN SECTION AND THE PASSAGE IN TRACTATE *ERKHIN*

A medico-legal case in Israel some years ago involving a pregnant brain-dead woman led the brain death controversy into another area of interface between rabbinic and medical knowledge. The question presented before an Israeli court was whether a caesarean section could or should

---

83. For reference to this letter in the University of Halle archives, see chapter, "A Letter from a Torah Sage of the Eighteenth Century."

84. R. Yaakov Emden, the son of the Ḥakham Tzvi, also mentions the fact that the scientists of his times had rebelled against Aristotle and Galen, a trend which he seems to view in a negative light. See his *Iggeret Bikkoret* (Zhitomer, 1867), 47b. The Ḥakham Tzvi himself did not mention this trend either because it had not yet taken place in his day, or because he was unaware of it. Further research will be necessary to clarify this. R. A. Y. Kook invokes the same idea about the changing nature of medical trends in his discussion about *metzitza* and the trustworthiness of doctors. See his *Da'at Kohen* (Jerusalem, 1985), n. 140.

85. See, for example, *She'elot UTeshuvot HaRashba*, 1:98.

be performed on a brain-dead woman in order to deliver the fetus. Although the court decided, as per the husband's wishes, that a caesarian section not be performed, the case sparked discussion amongst halakhic authorities as to the permissibility of performing such a procedure.[86]

The Talmud (*Erkhin* 7a) states that if a pregnant woman dies a natural death, the fetus dies first, but if she is killed (i.e., a traumatic death), the fetus outlives the mother. If the aforementioned brain-dead woman was halakhically dead and died a natural death, how is it possible for her to give birth to a live child? This would seemingly run counter to the teaching of the Talmud that states that the fetus dies first in such a case.

In addition, the Talmud seems to contradict itself. A later passage, in the name of Samuel, states that if a woman dies during labor on the Sabbath, one can carry a knife through a public domain, cut open her abdomen, and remove the child. Once again, if the fetus cannot outlive the mother, why should it be permissible to violate the Sabbath to attempt to remove it?

Both above contradictions can be resolved if one assumes that the statement of the Talmud that the fetus dies first in a natural death was not categorical, but rather only meant to describe the majority of cases.[87] These two circumstances, therefore, can be understood as representing the minority. Alternatively, the Talmud's statement may be categorical, but both of the above cases represent circumstances not addressed by it. In the contemporary legal case, the mother was receiving artificial respiration, a circumstance not accounted for in the talmudic statement.[88] And in the Talmud's own case regarding carrying the knife on Shabbat,

---

86. My thanks to Dr. Abraham Steinberg and R. Yigal Shafran for clarifying the details of the case for me. R. Shafran has compiled a medical ethics teaching manual based on this case, *"She'ela Al Samkhut": Ha'Im LeYeled Ubar HaMazuy BeGufa Shel Nifteret?* (Jerusalem, 1991). For an expansive discussion of this historical and halakhic topic, see chapter, "A Matter of Life 'in' Death: Postmortem Cesarean Section in Jewish Law."

87. This is the position of Rashi, ad loc., s. v., *"umekarin,"* sometimes it occurs [in a natural death] that the mother dies first." See also sources quoted by the *Magen Avraham*, commentary on *Shulḥan Arukh, O. Ḥ.,* 330:10.

88. To prove, in fact, that the statement of the Talmud does not apply to a case when the mother received artificial respiration, a sensational experiment was performed in 1992 involving the decapitation of a pregnant sheep and the subsequent birth, by caesarean section, of a healthy baby lamb. A video was taken of this experiment and it has been

if the woman is in labor, the child may have already begun to exert his physiological independence. As a result, in such a case, the child may outlive the mother.[89] Whatever the case may be, I concern myself here only with the medical historical aspects of a caesarean section.

In addition to this passage, there are multiple passages in Tractates *Nidda* and *Bekhorot* that discuss both live and postmortem caesarean section for both humans and animals.[90] These passages have fueled multiple debates in the medical historical literature regarding the antiquity of caesarean section with maternal survival.[91] Do the passages that discuss live caesarean section (i.e., caesarian section with maternal survival) reflect actual cases or simply theoretical constructs?

While the answer to this question is entirely irrelevant to the halakhist, the medical historian has found the question irresistible. Postmortem caesarian section is well documented from before the Common Era, but the performance of caesarean section with maternal survival is not believed to have occurred before the Middle Ages.[92] The references to live caesarian section in talmudic times, if actual occurrences, would obviously supplant this notion.

A comment should also be made regarding postmortem caesarian section. As we have stated, according to the talmudic passage in *Erkhin*,

---

widely shown at medical halakha conferences. The relevance and details of this experiment can be found in the halakhic literature. See Abraham S. Abraham, *Nishmat Avraham* (Jerusalem, 1992), 175, addendum to Y. D., 339. See also Y. Shafran, op. cit.

89. A number of authorities maintain this position. See, for example, *She'elot U Teshuvot HaRadbaz*, n. 695; the position of R. Isaac Stein quoted by R. Moshe Isserles in his *She'elot U Teshuvot HaRama*, n. 40; *Maḥazit HaShekel* commentary to *Shulḥan Arukh*, O. Ḥ., 330:10.

90. For these passages, see *Sefer HaTashbetz*, 1:10.

91. See J. Preuss, *op. cit.*, 420–426; Jeffrey Boss, "The Antiquity of Caesarean Section with Maternal Survival: The Jewish Tradition," *Medical History* 5 (1961), 117–131. Boss provides an excellent discussion of the Jewish source material on this topic. See also Yehoshua Leibovitz, "*Mavo Histori Refu'i LeSeder Taharot*," *Torah SheBa'al Peh* 6 (1964): 33–39; idem, "*LeToledot HaRefua BiSifrutenu*," *Yavneh* 3:7–12 (1949), 187–189.

92. For general references on the history of caesarean section, see, for example, J. P. Boley, "The History of Caesarean Section," *Canadian Medical Association Journal* 145:4 (1991), 319–322; M. Pierce Rucker, "A Librarian Looks at Caesarean Section," *Bulletin of the History of Medicine* 25 (1951): 132–148 and references.

if a pregnant woman dies of natural causes, the fetus dies first. Such is not the case, however, for a traumatic death of a pregnant woman. There is extensive literature on postmortem caesarean section that dates back to Roman antiquity. Indeed, laws were instituted in the Roman Empire requiring the opening of dead bodies of pregnant women shortly after death.[93] Since these laws were perpetuated and publicized in the times of Julius Caesar, the procedure became known as a caesarean section.[94] It seems obvious that there must have been at least a small percentage of fetal survival; otherwise, the procedure would not have been mandated. Do these cases contradict the Talmud? Unfortunately, it is impossible to know whether the cases of fetal survival were associated with the natural or traumatic death of the mother. In addition, some authorities claim that it is possible for the fetus to survive in a minority of cases, as stated above.

As recently as the late nineteenth century, there are multiple references in the medical literature to the delivery of live infants after postmortem caesarean section. Infant survival was even documented after a child was extracted as much as two hours after the death of its mother.[95] Again, there is no differentiation in this medical literature between natural and traumatic death of the mother. It is also possible that the determination of death was inaccurate, and in fact, the mothers were not dead, neither according to halakhic criteria, however one wishes to define them, nor according to contemporary medical standards. To quote contemporary medical literature about postmortem caesarean section is irrelevant as the intervention of artificial respiration eliminates the equation of these cases to those of the Talmud.[96]

---

93. The first such law was instituted by Numa Pompilia in about 600 BC and was called the Lex Regia.

94. There is little historical foundation for the notion that Caesar, himself, was born by a so-called caesarian section.

95. See George M. Gould and Walter L. Pyle, *Anomalies and Curiosities of Medicine* (New York, 1896), 134–137.

96. See "Brain Dead Woman Miscarries," *London Times* (November 22, 1992). An article appeared that week in the *London Jewish Chronicle* (November 27, 1992) regarding the Jewish view of this case entitled, "Why Not 'Play God'?" For reviews of cases of pregnancy associated with maternal brain death, see M. Esmaaeilzadeh, et al., "One Life Ends, Another Begins: Management of a Brain-Dead Pregnant Mother—A

While the practice of postmortem caesarean section was universally accepted in the secular world throughout history, it seems that such
was not always the case in the Jewish world. As early as the period of the
Geonim there was a ban placed on performing postmortem caesarean
sections.[97] This ban was continued by the author of the *Issur VeHeter*[98]
and reiterated by R. Moshe Isserles.[99] The reason invoked by the latter
two authorities is that "we are not qualified " to determine the death of
the mother.[100] Since one must wait a significant period of time before
declaring her death, a caesarean section is no longer indicated. By that
time, the fetus would surely have died.

Today, however, given our enhanced ability to both determine the
death of the mother, cardiac death as well as brain death, and sustain the life
of the fetus, some authorities would allow a postmortem caesarean section.[101]

VII. CONCLUSION

I have provided a medical historical overview and analysis of some of the
rabbinic sources quoted in contemporary discussions of brain death, a
current issue in the world of medical halakha. Understanding the scientific
theories contemporary with the rabbinic positions expressed enables us
to appreciate their medical frame of reference, their allusions to medical
theory and their quotations of prominent figures in the history of science. In addition, otherwise cryptic rabbinic passages can be clarified.

Systematic Review," *BMC Medicine* 8 (2010), 74; L. R. Erlinger, "Guidelines for
Supporting a Pregnant Patient with Brain Death: A Case Discussion and Literature
Review," Journal of Nursing Education and Ethics 7:8 (2017), 86–92.

97. This ban is quoted by R. Yaakov Reischer (1670–1734) in his *Shevut Yaakov*, 1:13
and seems to contradict the Talmud in *Erkhin*. R. Reischer attempts to answer the
contradictions. For further discussion, and other answers to the question, see R.
Moses Feinstein, *Iggerot Moshe, Y. D.,* Vol. 2, n. 174, section 2.

98. 59:11. Regarding the author of this work, see H. Y. D. Azulai, *Shem HaGedolim,
Ma'arekhet Sefarim* 6, n. 125. See also Menachem Kasher and Yaakov Mandelbaum,
Sarei HaEleph (New York, 1959), 257.

99. See Rama, *Shulḥan Arukh, O. Ḥ.,* 330:5. Cf. *She'elot UTeshuvot HaRama,* n. 40.

100. See the excellent article by H. J. Zimmels, "The Significance of the Statement 'We
are Not Acquainted Anymore' as Echoed in Rabbinic Literature," in the *Leo Jung
Jubilee Volume* (New York, 1962), 223–235.

101. Y. Shafran, op. cit., 50, n. 7 quotes this position in the name of R. Ovadiah Yosef.

The Resuscitation of Halakha: An Animated Discussion

I. INTRODUCTION

In the *haftara* of *Parashat Vayera* we find the story of the Shunamite woman whose kindness towards the prophet Elisha is rewarded with a son.[1] When this son, however, falls ill and dies, the Shunamite woman frantically runs to Elisha for assistance. The ensuing events—Elisha prostrating himself on top of the boy, placing his mouth, eyes and palms on the corresponding parts of the boy, and the boy's subsequent awakening—are reminiscent of modern-day cardio-pulmonary resuscitation. There is a very similar episode of resuscitation performed by the prophet Eliyahu, Elisha's predecessor,[2] who revived the son of the Tzarfatit woman.

The literature relating to the resuscitation episodes in *Tanakh* performed by Eliyahu and Elisha is rich and varied. These passages have received ample treatment in the medical literature,[3] in the medical historical

---

1. II Melakhim 4:1–37.
2. II Melakhim 1:17.
3. The medical literature addresses two distinct, though related issues—the nature of the resuscitation and its relationship to modern day cardio-pulmonary resuscitation;

literature,[4] and in the Bible studies literature.[5] They are also part of broader discussions including other incidents of resuscitation from death or near death in rabbinic literature.[6] One area that has not been fully explored,

and the specific medical cause of death of the young children, specifically the Shunamite child, as more information is provided about his condition in the text. See H. Karplus, "Suspended Animation and Resuscitation: A Historical Review in Light of Experimental Hypothermia," *Journal of Forensic Medicine* 13 (1966), 68–74; F. Rosner, "Artificial Respiration in Biblical Times," *New York State Journal of Medicine* 69:8 (April 15, 1969), 1104–1105; Z. Rosen, "Resuscitation in the Bible," *Harefuah* 79 (1970), 27–28 (Hebrew); Z. Rosen, "Rhinological Aspects of Biblical Resuscitation," *Archives of Otolaryngology* 95:5 (May, 1972), 488–489; L. J. Hurwitz, "A Neurologist's Anecdotes and the Bible," *Practitioner* 206 (1971), 287–292; Z. Rosen and J. Davidson, "Respiratory Resuscitation in Ancient Hebrew Sources," *Anesthesia and Analgesia* 51:4 (July-August, 1972), 502–05; L. Wislicki, "A Biblical Case of Hypothermia-Resuscitation by Rewarming (Elisha's Method)," *Clio Medica* 9:3 (September, 1974), 213–214; R. B. Howard, "... And There is Nothing New Under the Sun," *Postgraduate Medicine* 65:3 (March, 1979), 25; J. H. Comroe, Jr., "... In Comes the Good Air," *American Review of Respiratory Diseases* 119:6 (June, 1979), 1025–31; S. Abraham, "Artificial Respiration in *Tanakh*," (Hebrew) *Ha-Ma'ayan* 28:3 (*Nisan*, 5748), 72–76; J. M. Fisher, "The Resuscitation Greats: The Earliest Records," *Resuscitation* 44 (2000), 79–80.

The proposed medical diagnoses for the Shunamite child have included hypothermia, heat stroke and subarachnoid hemorrhage. Of note, a passage in the *Talmud Yerushalmi*, chapter 15, 14:4, suggests the cause of death to be heat stroke. See *Korban HaEdah*, ad loc.

4. See A. Barrington Baker, "Artificial Respiration: The History of an Idea," *Medical History* 15 (1971), 336–351; J. A. Paraskos, "Biblical Accounts of Resuscitation," *Journal of the History of Medicine and Allied Sciences* 47:3 (July, 1992), 310–321, who discusses episodes of resuscitation in other ancient literatures, in addition to the episodes of Eliyahu and Elisha. See also chapter, "The Incorporation of Pre-Modern Scientific Theories into Rabbinic Literature: The Case of Innate Heat."

5. E. Samet, "'The Double Embrace'—The Story of Elisha and the Shunamite Woman," *Megadim* 13 (5751), 73–95 (Hebrew). M. Sabato takes issue with Samet's approach in his, "The Story of the Shunamite," *Megadim* 15 (5752), 45–52 (Hebrew). See also A. O. Shemesh, "The Resuscitation of Children by Eliyahu and Elisha—Medical Treatment or Miracles?" (Hebrew) *Beit Mikra* 46:3 (5761), 248–260. Shemesh introduces the possibility that ancient magical practices may have influenced the resuscitation methods. See also Nachman Levine, "Twice as Much as Your Spirit: Pattern, Parallel and Paronomasia in the Miracles of Elijah and Elisha," *Journal for the Study of the Old Testament* 85 (1999), 25–46.

6. There are a number of instances in rabbinic literature of explicit or implied resuscitation after death or near death. Some are explicitly mentioned in the text of *Tanakh* or the Talmud, others are found in *midrashim* or biblical commentaries.

however, is the use of these episodes in contemporary medical halakhic discussions.[7] As with all areas of halakha, medical halakha uses the Torah as its starting point for any discussions.[8] Sometimes, however, in the absence of clear precedent, sources are marshaled from *Tanakh* or *midrashim*.[9]

The following is a non-exhaustive list of these references, excluding the episodes of Eliyahu and Elisha discussed in the present article: 1) Yeḥezkel and the resurrection of the dry bones (*Yeḥezkel* 37:1–14). 2) The resuscitation of Yaakov after he fainted upon hearing the news of Yosef's survival. (See Ramban on Bereshit 45:26, s. v., "*vayafag libo*," and further elaboration see chapter " The Incorporation of Pre-Modern Scientific Theories into Rabbinic Literature: The Case of Innate Heat." 3) The resuscitation of R. Zeira after he was decapitated by Rava at the festive Purim meal (*Megilla* 7b). 4) The resuscitation of the babies born in Egypt by Shifra and Puah (*Midrash Rabba Shemot* 1: 17). The *Ba'al HaTurim* on Shemot 1:15 claims that the etymology of Shifra is linked to *shefoferet* and that the midwives placed a reed in the throats of the babies to resuscitate them. This has been mentioned by some as a precursor to tracheal intubation. See E. Tratner, "Intubation Mentioned in the Talmud and by Jacob ben Asher," *Koroth* 8:7–8 (August, 1983), 333–338. See also M. Weinberger, "An Ancient Source on Neonatal Resuscitation," *Koroth* 10 (1993–1994), 63–64, who asserts that the source cited by Tratner as the *Ba'al HaTurim* is actually from the *Maharam MeRotenberg*. 5) The wife of R. Ḥanina b. Ḥakhinai fainted when her husband returned home unannounced after twelve years in yeshiva. R. Ḥanina prayed for her and she was revived. (*Ketubot* 62b and *Vayikra Rabba* 21:7). 6) The spies seemed to collapse and were revived, apparently through some form of mouth-to-mouth resuscitation. See *Yalkut Shimoni, Shlaḥ* chapter 13, s. v., "*Vayishlaḥ otam Moshe*." and *Zayit Ra'anan*, ad loc. 7) The souls of all the people of Israel transiently departed at the giving of the Torah upon hearing the first commandments directly from God. Resuscitation was required to revive them. For discussion see *Ḥatam Sofer Y. D.*, 337. 8) The Talmud discusses some form of resuscitation for infants by breathing air through their nostrils. (*Shabbat* 128b) 9) The Talmud mentions the case of a sheep, with a tracheal perforation, that was resuscitated by placing a tube directly into the tracheal opening (*Ḥullin* 57b).

7. For previous treatment of the halakhic issues, see, for example, A. Rosenfeld, "Refrigeration, Resuscitation and Resurrection," *Tradition* 9 (1967), 82–94; Abraham S. Abraham, "Artificial Respiration in *Tanakh*," (Hebrew) *HaMa'ayan* 28:3 (*Nisan*, 5748), 72–76.

8. See Avraham Steinberg, *Entzyclopedia Hilkhatit Refuit* (2nd edition) for medical halakhic discussions based on or extracted from *parashat hashavua*.

9. In *Tanakh*, for example, the story of the four lepers, the *haftara* of *Parashat Metzora*, is used as a basis for the halakhic discussions about sacrificing a limited life span (*ḥayyei sha'a*) for the potential to gain a longer life span (*ḥayyei olam*). This relates to both end of life issues and to assessing surgical risk. For midrashim, see for example, chapter, "Midrash, Miracles, and Motherhood: The Birth of Dinah and the Definition of Maternity—*Tzarikh Iyun LeDinah*."

There are extensive pre-modern halakhic discussions that relate to a number of aspects of the resuscitation episodes performed by Eliyahu and Elisha. These discussions are complex, creative, and legally brilliant.[10]

One of the more oft quoted passages is in *Nidda* 70b:

> Does the son of the Shunamite convey *tum'ah*? He replied: A corpse conveys *tum'ah* but a living person does not convey *tum'ah*. Will the dead in the hereafter require to be sprinkled upon on the third and the seventh day or will they not require it? He replied: When they will be resurrected we shall go into the matter. Others say: When our Master Moses will come with them.

For centuries, rabbinic commentators analyzed this passage, and other aspects of the resuscitation episodes of Eliyahu and Elisha, but these discussions remained purely theoretical.[11] With the medical advances of the mid-twentieth century, however, including the development of cardio-pulmonary resuscitation, the introduction of brain

---

10. See, for example, *Teshuvot Radbaz*, n. 2203, *Maharsha* on *Nidda* 70b, R. Betzalel Ransburg, *Ḥokhmat Betzalel: Pitḥei Nidda* (Mosad HaRav Kook, 5717), 714–719; *Netziv, Ha'amek She'ela* to *She'iltot* 167:17; R. Shalom Klein, "The Violation of Shabbat or Other Mitzvot in a case of *Pikuaḥ Nefesh*," (Hebrew) *Olat HaHodesh* 3:12 (Elul, 5739), 563–567; R. Shlomo Zalman Graditz in his introduction to R. Shlomo Luria's *Yam Shel Shlomo* on *Yevamot* (Altona, 1740); R. Ḥayyim Yosef David Azulai, *Ḥayyim Sh'al*, n. 43; R. Yosef Shaul Nathanson, *Divrei Shaul* on *Aggadah, Bava Metzia* 114 and *Nidda* 70b; Leib Baron, "Is Miraculous Life Considered Life?" (Hebrew) *HaPardes* 59:2 (October 1984), 14–17.

11. There are two main questions on this passage that have been addressed by commentaries throughout the ages. First, why does the Talmud ask the question about *tum'ah* from the Shunamite boy revived by Elisha? The episode of Eliyahu chronologically preceded that of Elisha. The question of residual *tum'ah* should therefore have been asked about the son of the Tzarfatit woman? Second, the Talmud asks whether sprinkling of water to purify from *tum'at met* (corpse *tum'ah*) will be required for those who are resurrected in the times of *teḥiyat hametim*. As the previous statement discusses the resuscitation of the Shunamite boy from death, why is the question of sprinkling the water not asked about this boy? As he was also resurrected, the question should equally apply to him!

death criteria, and organ transplantation, these previously theoretical discussions were resuscitated. The hypothetical constructs suddenly took on new relevance, were incorporated into practical halakhic discussions and used to render decisions on contemporary medical halakhic dilemmas. This essay explores the contemporary medical halakhic issues for which the resuscitation episodes of *Tanakh* have been invoked.

II. THE DEFINITION OF DEATH

The first example of the invocation of the episodes of resuscitation from *Tanakh* in the context of practical halakhic discussions was in the early nineteenth century. In that period the ability of physicians to accurately diagnose death was called into question and the fear of premature burial was widespread. Many countries legally required the preservation of the body above ground for three days, after the initial declaration of death, in order to unequivocally confirm the diagnosis.[12] Ḥatam Sofer was one of many prominent *poskim* in that generation to weigh in on this debate and to clarify the halakhic time and definition of death.[13] In the course of his discussion about the determination of death, he mentions the resuscitation episodes. While Ḥatam Sofer appears to be the first historically to mention these episodes in the context of a contemporary halakhic discussion, the stories are only mentioned peripherally and do not serve as the basis of *pesak*.

In the twentieth century, the halakhic definition of death again came into focus with the new diagnostic criteria for the determination of brain death. The three-day burial controversy of nineteenth century Europe was the pre-modern precursor to this subject. This topic is one of the modern era's most debated and contentious issues. Well known to the readers of this book, the "brain death debate" has occupied ample space in the contemporary halakhic journals and periodicals. The

---

12. See R. Moshe Samet, "Delaying Burial: The History of the Polemic on the Determination of the Time of Death," (Hebrew) *Asufot* 3 (1989/1990), 613–665, for the most expansive study of this halakhic chapter.

13. *Ḥatam Sofer, Yoreh De'ah*, n. 338.

resuscitation episodes are occasionally referenced, though they do not figure prominently, in these discussions.[14]

III. IS THERE WIFE AFTER DEATH? CARDIO-PULMONARY RESUSCITATION, CORONARY BYPASS AND ARTIFICIAL HEART TRANSPLANTATION

As cited above, a number of miraculous resuscitations are mentioned in rabbinic literature. These cases spawned discussions throughout the centuries about the halakhic consequences of miraculous resuscitation, including whether *tum'ah* is conveyed by one who is revived in such a fashion, or whether one who is resurrected from the dead may legally return to his wife, since death generally dissolves the marital bond. The resuscitation episodes were raised in these halakhic discussions.[15]

These discussions become more than theoretical with the new realities of the twentieth century, and the possibility of complete cardiac cessation followed by reanimation. This scenario became possible in a number of situations, the most common being with cardio-pulmonary resuscitation. It also was intentionally performed in cases of cardiac surgery, when the heart was stopped, and the blood circulated through a machine (cardiac bypass). The heart was then restarted at the completion of the surgery. The introduction of artificial heart transplants created a similar scenario. The innate heart was removed, only to be replaced with an artificial or mechanical heart.

The common denominator in all these cases is the cessation of innate cardiac activity for prolonged periods of time, followed by the return of cardiac function. The hypothetical question of marriage dissolution with miraculous resuscitation now was assimilated to cases of physiological resuscitation. The main halakhic question considered by the *poskim* in these cases was whether a person undergoing these procedures is considered to have been legally dead during the period

---

14. See, for example, R. J. David Bleich, *HaPardes* 51:4 (January, 1977), 15.

15. See *Birkei Yosef, Even HaEzer*, 17; *Otzar HaPoskim, Even HaEzer* 1:1. For an interesting treatise on how Eliyahu's wife was able to remarry, see R. A. M. Friedland, *BiTzror HaHayyim* (*Nahalat Har Chabad*: Israel, 5767).

of cessation of innate cardiac function such that he would be required to remarry his "previous" wife.[16] Furthermore, it was debated whether the reanimation of the heart was considered a form of *teḥiyat hametim*. The resuscitation episodes of Eliyahu and Elisha figure prominently in these halakhic discussions.[17]

IV. CORNEAL TRANSPLANTATION

The first modern rabbinic authority to invoke the resuscitation episodes of *Tanakh*, in conjunction with the passage in *Nidda*, as a clear and direct source for *pesak* appears to be R. Ḥayyim Regensberg,[18] a prominent Chicago *posek* in the mid-twentieth century, who addressed the issue of cadaveric corneal transplantation in an article in the Torah journal *HaPardes* in 1945.[19] The first successful cornea transplant occurred in 1905, but it took decades until the procedure was fully developed.[20] After raising concerns about the prohibitions of *nivul hamet* (desecration of a dead body) and *hana'at hamet* (deriving benefit from a dead body), R. Regensberg explores a permissive approach:

---

16. According to *Matzav.com*, R. Yeḥezkel Roth, the Kalsburger Rov apparently remarried his wife after a near-fatal cardiac illness. See, "Rav Roth, After Release from Hospital, is Mekadeish His Rebbetzin a Second Time," *Matzav.com* (April, 26, 2016). This was apparently later found not to be true. Rav Dovid Feinstein maintains that one is not required to perform a new marriage ceremony in such a case. See his *VeDibarta Bam* 2 (2016), 306.

17. On the case of cardio-pulmonary resuscitation see R. Pinḥas Zevichi, *Ateret Paz* 1:3, *E. H.*, 9; on cardiothoracic surgery and cardiac bypass, see *Tzitz Eliezer* 17:24; on artificial heart transplants see, J. D. Bleich, "Artificial Heart Implantation," in his *Contemporary Halakhic Problems* (Ktav, 1989), 160–193. See also, Rosenfeld, op. cit.; L. Y. Halperin, "Laws Relating to One Who Dies and is Resuscitated," (Hebrew) in his *Ma'aseh Ḥoshev* 4 (Institute of Technology and Halakhah, 5757), 48–51.

18. The five-volume series on medical halakha entitled *Halakha URefua*, published from 1980–1987 by the Regensberg Institute, was dedicated to his memory.

19. "The Transplantation of a Cornea from a Cadaver to a Living Recipient," (Hebrew) *HaPardes* 19:4 (July, 1945), 24–28.

20. On the history of corneal transplantation, see S. L. Moffatt, et al., "Centennial Review of Corneal Transplantation," *Clinical and Experimental Ophthalmology* 33:6 (December, 2005), 642–657.

The cornea recipient derives benefit from the cadaveric cornea only after the cornea becomes fully integrated into his body and after the cornea returns to life or becomes reanimated. Once the cornea becomes reanimated, all the previous prohibitions that applied when the tissue was dead, no longer apply. Just as the laws of *tum'ah* no longer apply to the living tissue, as it states in *Nidda* 70b in the case of the son of the Shunamite that was resuscitated by Elisha, "the dead generate *tum'ah*, the living do not generate *tum'ah*."

R. Isser Yehuda Unterman independently addressed the issue of corneal transplantation, in his *Shevet MiYehuda*. On the permissibility of receiving a cornea transplant, R. Unterman writes:

I wish to state a novel idea that on first glance may seem somewhat strange, but on further analysis appears to be a source of permissibility with solid foundation. The reason it is not mentioned previously in rabbinic writings is likely due to the fact that this surgical procedure was not possible in previous times. However, based on halakhic principles, it appears that there are grounds for a permissive ruling, and I have not found any contradictory ruling in the Talmud or *poskim*.

The essence of the permissive ruling is that the flesh of a corpse is prohibited so long as it is dead. However, once the flesh becomes reanimated, the prohibition dissipates. And just as it is inconceivable to think that regarding the episodes of miraculous resuscitation in *Tanakh*, such as the son of the Tzarfatit, the son of the Shunamite, or the resurrection of the dry bones of Yeḥezkel, that these people were *asur behana'a* (after their resuscitation); so too a portion of a corpse that returns to life after transplantation should not generate a prohibition of *hana'a*.

The reason for this ruling is that the basis for the prohibition of benefit from corpse flesh is *not* that the soul had previously departed therefrom, but rather that it is *presently* dead flesh. When the flesh is reanimated, the prohibition disappears. It is the dead flesh that the Torah prohibited, not the living flesh.

The fact that the body from which the flesh was derived is still dead is irrelevant.

R. Unterman argued that just as *tum'ah* applies only to dead flesh, so too the prohibition of benefit only applies to dead flesh.[21] In analyzing the passage in *Nidda*, R. Unterman points out that the questions focus exclusively on whether *tum'ah* is generated and *not* on whether there is any prohibition of deriving benefit from those revived from death. He explains the reason for this omission to be that there is no thought as to the prohibition of benefit once the people are actually alive. The prohibition only applies *while they are dead.*[22]

R. Unterman comments on the essay of R. Ḥayyim Regensberg, who had also invoked the episode of the Shunamite boy as a source to allow corneal transplants. However, R. Unterman maintains that his interpretation and application of this episode are highly novel and not similar to the interpretation of R. Regensberg.[23] Clearly both authorities arrived at this novel thesis independently, though R. Unterman has generally been credited with the *"ḥidush"* in the medical halakhic literature.[24]

R. Unterman subsequently defended his position against criticism. For example, R. Yeḥiel Weinberg rejected R. Unterman's novel thesis claiming that a detached piece of flesh is *asur behana'a*, irrespective

---

21. R. Unterman points out that there is not always parity between *tum'ah* and the *issur hana'a*, as in the case of corpse flesh that becomes powder, which is not *tamei*, yet is still *assur behana'a*. However, he maintains that parity should apply in this case.

22. My emphasis.

23. R. Don Well, in a brief biographical essay of R. Regensberg, recounts how R. Unterman and R. Regensberg met, and that "R. Unterman was enthralled with the courage and incisive scholarship demonstrated in a landmark Regensberg *teshuva*." While R. Well omits the topic of the *teshuva*, in a personal communication he confirmed it was indeed this very one. See M. Hershler, ed., *Halakha URefua* (Regensberg Institute: Jerusalem, 1980), IX-XV.

24. R. Mikhael Forshleger advances the identical "reanimation" theory, based on the passage in *Nidda*, in his *Torat Mikhael*, 56, but makes no mention of either Rabbis Regensberg or Unterman's writings. R. Forshleger died in 1958, and his individual responsa are not dated. It is therefore impossible to determine if he could have seen the opinions of the aforementioned authorities when he penned his responsum.

of its subsequent reanimation, as one is still benefitting from the corpse, which remains dead.[25] Despite its rejection by some, R. Unterman's analysis served as a basis for many subsequent halakhic discussions on corneal transplants[26] and on organ transplants in general.[27]

V. A *KOHEN* ORGAN RECIPIENT

The burgeoning field of transplantation medicine also presents unique problems for the *Kohen*. Since the organs are often transplanted from a cadaver, may a *Kohen*, who is proscribed from contacting a corpse, receive an organ transplant? Of course, the prohibition is waived in a case of *pikuah nefesh*, but a cornea transplant, for example, does not fall into this category. In this case, as well, the "reanimation" theory, as advanced by Rabbis Regensberg and Unterman, was invoked to resolve the issue.[28]

R. Lau, former Chief Rabbi of Israel, devotes a number of responsa to the question of the *Kohen* as an organ recipient.[29] Therein, he brings the opinion of R. Unterman to support the permissibility of a *Kohen*

---

25. See R. Yeḥiel Weinberg, *Seridei Eish* 2:120. For other critiques of R. Unterman, see R. Y. M. Erenberg in *Kol Torah* (*Sivan-Elul* 5714); R. Dov Borstein, "Plastic Surgery From the Dead to the Living," (Hebrew) *HaPardes* 28:3 (*Kislev*, 5714), 5–7; idem, response to R. Erenberg in *Kol Torah* 11:1 (*Tishrei*, 5717), 11–12.

26. See, for example, R. Yitzḥak Isaac HaLevi Herzog, *Ketavim UPesakim* 5:157; R. Shmuel Hibner, "The Use of Eyes From a Cadaver to Treat Blindness," (Hebrew) *HaDarom* 13 (*Nisan*, 5721), 54–64; S. L. Levine, *Minḥat Shlomo* 1 (Bashon Printers: Brooklyn, 1963), n. 26; R. Simcha Levy, "The Use of Eyes From a Cadaver to Treat Blindness," (Hebrew) *HaDarom* 14 (*Elul*, 5721), 31–34, with rejoinder by R. Shmuel Hibner; R. Ovadia Yosef, *Yabia Omer*, C. M., 8:11.

27. References to the novel thesis of R. Unterman can be found in the contemporary works of Drs. Abraham Abraham, Fred Rosner and Avraham Steinberg.

28. The issue of exposure to *tum'ah* by a *Kohen* is also discussed extensively with respect to the resuscitation episode of Eliyahu. According to tradition, Eliyahu was the embodiment or incarnation of Pinḥas HaKohen. As such, it would have been prohibited for him to come into direct contact with a corpse. See, for example, Radbaz, n. 2203; Netziv, *Ha'amek She'ela*, *She'iltot* 167:17; Shalom Klein, "The Violation of Shabbat or Other Mitzvot in a Case of *Pikuakh Nefesh*," (Hebrew) *Olat HaChodesh* 3:12 (*Elul*, 5739), 563–567; Ḥayyim Yosef Dovid Azulai, *Ḥayyim Sh'al*, n. 43; A. S. Abraham, "Artificial Respiration in *Tanakh*," (Hebrew) *HaMa'ayan* 28:3 (*Nisan*, 5748), 72–76.

29. *Yaḥel Yisrael*, 2:81 and 2:83.

receiving an organ. Once the organ becomes reanimated in the *Kohen* recipient, he argues, there is no longer any *tum'ah* associated with it. R. Lau further posits that R. Weinberg's objection to R. Unterman's position would not apply in this case, as R. Weinberg took issue only with the prohibition of deriving benefit (which, according to him, would apply even if the body part was reanimated). Even R. Weinberg should agree, R. Lau argued, that with respect to *tum'ah* alone, the body part would no longer convey *tum'ah* once incorporated into the recipient's body.[30]

R. Waldenberg addresses a more common question related to *Kohanim* and transplantation—whether a *Kohen* who suffers an amputation may have his own limb or digit reimplanted.[31] Once amputated, even a *Kohen's* own digit will generate *tum'ah*. He cites the *Noda BiYehuda* who maintains that one's own limb conveys *tum'ah* just as a foreign limb. In addition, and directly relevant to R. Waldenberg's question, the *Noda BiYehuda* understands the passage in *Nidda* regarding whether the Shunamite boy was *metameh*, to refer specifically to *after* he was again alive. If one were in direct contact with the boy at any time before his resuscitation, even immediately before, he would, of course, contract *tum'ah*. Thus, in the case of reimplanting the digit, while once the finger is reanimated, the *tum'ah* may dissipate; it would nonetheless be prohibited to reconnect the digit, as at that precise moment of reconnection, the *Kohen* would be coming into direct contact with the "dead" body part.[32]

VI. THE SELLING OF HUMAN ORGANS

Since the beginnings of organ transplantation in the twentieth century, there have been rapid and extraordinary advances in transplantation

---

30. R. Moshe Feinstein argued a similar notion of the possibility of the *tum'ah* no longer applying to the transplanted organ, but it is not based on the passage in *Nidda* and the story of the Elisha and the Shunamite boy. See *Iggerot Moshe Y. D.*, 1:230.

31. *Tzitz Eliezer*, 13:90.

32. While acknowledging that there would be a prohibition in reconnecting the digit, R. Waldenberg nonetheless permits the reimplantation. While most *poskim* maintain that Shabbat cannot be violated for the saving of a limb, R. Waldenberg argues that other prohibitions, such as exposure to *tum'ah* for a *Kohen*, may indeed be violated in order to save a limb. For further discussion of the application of R. Unterman's novel approach to organ donation in general and to the case of a *Kohen's* amputated digit, see *Binyan Av*, 3:53.

medicine. The transplantation of hearts, livers, and kidneys are now commonplace. These successes have spawned other dilemmas, including the limited supply of organs. One suggestion to increase the donor pool that is being reevaluated is to offer compensation to the donors (in the case of living donation) or their families (in the case of cadaveric donation). This issue has received extensive treatment in the halakhic literature.[33]

A major impediment to a family's receiving compensation for agreeing to cadaveric donation is the issue of *hana'at hamet*, the prohibition of deriving benefit from the corpse. For many *poskim*, this prohibition is insurmountable and thus compensation is prohibited. R. Waldenberg, however, suggests a permissive approach to allow the families to receive compensation.[34] In conjunction with his permissive stance, he adds an additional suggestion to minimize the potential prohibition. He suggests that the transfer of money to the family take place only after the transplanted organ has been integrated or animated within the recipient. At this point, he argues, based on the story of the Shunamite boy and the talmudic passage in *Nidda*, the organ is no longer "dead," but has been reanimated. There is, therefore, no prohibition of *hana'at hamet*, as the organ is not in fact *met*.

---

33. For discussions in the English language, see R. B. Grazi and J. B. Wolowelsky, "Non-altruistic Kidney Donations in Contemporary Jewish Law and Ethics," *Transplantation Forum* 75:2 (January 27, 2003), 250–252; J. D. Kunin, "The Search for Organs: Halakhic Perspectives on Altruistic Giving and the Selling of Organs," *Journal of Medical Ethics* 31 (2005), 269–272; S. Resnicoff, "Supplying Human Body Parts: A Jewish Law Perspective," *DePaul Law Review* 55 (2005–2006), 851–874; A. Cohen, "Sale or Donation of Human Organs," *Journal of Halacha and Contemporary Society* 52 (Fall 2006), 37–64; R. Warburg, "Renal Transplantation: Living Donors and Markets for Body Parts—Halakhah in Concert with Halakhic Policy or Public Policy?" *Tradition* 40:2 (Summer 2007), 14–48; R. Steinbuch, "Kidneys, Cash and Kashrut: A Legal, Economic, and Religious Analysis of Selling Kidneys," *Houston Law Review* 45 (2009), 1529–1607. For a review of the halakhic literature on selling organs, see F. Rosner and E. Reichman, "Payment for Organ Donation in Jewish Law," in A. Levine, ed., *Oxford Handbook of Judaism and Economics* (Oxford University Press, 2010), 324–339.
34. *Tzitz Eliezer*, 19:53.

VII. POSTHUMOUS INSEMINATION

A unique example of the application of the idea of reanimation is found in an article by R. Levi Yitzḥak Halperin on the issue of posthumous insemination.[35] The particular case involved an Israeli soldier who fell in battle *al kiddush Hashem* and whose widow requested to harvest his reproductive seed postmortem to produce progeny. In addressing the concern that there might be a prohibition of *hana'at hamet* by using the reproductive seed from a corpse, he posits that just as many have permitted cadaveric transplants based on the notion that the organ becomes reanimated, so too it should be permitted in this case when the sole purpose of the endeavor is to animate or create an entire life (human being) from the seed.

VIII. CONCLUSION

This essay reflects the evolving process of contemporary medical halakha. New discoveries and advances create novel dilemmas that necessitate a reevaluation of the existing corpus of halakha. One may find relevant pre-modern theoretical discussions that now take on practical halakhic relevance in light of new realities. We have illustrated this through the resuscitation episodes of Eliyahu and Elisha. These episodes, which generated significant halakhic analyses in pre-modern times, were revisited and adapted to modern medical halakhic dilemmas. I suspect we will see other areas of previously "theoretical" halakha resuscitated and applied to modern circumstances as science continues to venture into new and uncharted territories.

---

35. "Harvesting Sperm from a Soldier Postmortem in Order to Inseminate his Widow," (Hebrew) *HaBerakha* 1 (*Tammuz*, 5769), 13–16.

A Matter of Life "in" Death: Postmortem Caesarean Section in Jewish Law

I. INTRODUCTION

Today, the term caesarean section refers exclusively to a surgical procedure performed on living pregnant women, either electively or emergently, in order to deliver a living baby (henceforth referred to as living caesarean section). For the majority of human history, however, this was not the case. In fact, according to medical historians, until roughly 1500, caesarean sections were only performed exclusively postmortem (henceforth referred to as postmortem caesarean section). Caesarean sections on living women, with maternal survival, were unheard of until the Middle Ages. Despite its antiquity, postmortem caesarean section has been, and remains, one of the most infrequently performed procedures in the history of medicine. In a case report in the *Journal of the American Medical Society* in 1957, the authors write, "only 113 successful postmortem sections have been reported in the world literature of the last 250 years."[1] As to how the

---

1. H. DeKruif, et al., "Postmortem Cesarean Section with Survival of Infant," *Journal of the American Medical Society* 163:11 (March 16, 1957), 938–939.

procedure arrived at its unique name, there have been more than a few conjectures.[2]

The performance of the postmortem caesarean section has been documented since antiquity.[3] The Catholic Church prescribed such caesarean sections primarily for the sake of baptizing the newborn child, though they did debate whether the baby or mother takes precedence if

---

2. Pliny the Elder suggests that the name Caesar comes from the word *caesum*, "cut out," because the first Caesar was cut from his mother's womb. Many illustrations throughout the centuries depict this supposed birth of Caesar. However, according to most historians, Julius Caesar himself could not have been so delivered, because this dangerous operation was normally done only upon a dead woman, and his mother Aurelia was known to have lived for many years after his birth. There is a tradition that Caesar's mother indeed did not survive the operation. This version is found in *Tosafot* (*Avoda Zara* 10b s. v., "*kol*"), who cites Yosippon as the source of this tradition. Some suggest that the term derives from the fact that during the time of the Caesars (not a specific Caesar), the law, Lex Regis (or Lex Caesaria) (715–672 BCE), forbade the burial of a pregnant woman before the fetus had been excised. One who does otherwise, the law stated, clearly causes the promise of life to perish with the mother. For a lengthy discussion on the etymology of the term, see "Creative Etymology: 'Caesarean Section' from Pliny to Rousset," in R. Blumenfeld-Kosinski, *Not of Woman Born: Representations of Caesarean Birth in Medieval and Renaissance Culture* (Cornell University Press, 1990), 143–153. This work also discusses artistic depictions of caesarean section, as well as the general history of this topic. See also T. N. Raju, "The Birth of Caesar and the Cesarean Misnomer," *American Journal of Perinatology* 24:10 (November, 2007), 567–568.

For general works on the history of caesarean section, see, for example, J. H. Young, *Caesarean Section: The History and Development of the Operation from Early Times* (H. K. Lewis and Company, 1944); R. M. Pierce and E. M. Rucker, "A Librarian Looks at Cesarean Section," *Bulletin of the History of Medicine* 25 (March, 1951), 132–148; H. A. Gabert, "History and Development of Cesarean Section," *Obstetrics and Gynecology Clinics of North America* 15:4 (1988), 591–605. A recent contribution appeared in the Hebrew medical literature, A. Zilberlicht, et al., "The Incredible Story About the Cesarean Section rom Ancient Times Till Nowadays," (Hebrew) *HaRefua* 153:8 (August, 2014), 471–474 and 497.

3. G. M. Gould and W. L. Pyle, *Anomalies and Curiosities of Medicine* (W. B. Saunders, 1896), 134–137. E. M. Hillan, "Caesarean Section: Historical Background," *Scottish Medical Journal* 36:5 (October, 1991), 150–154; Q. Warraich and U. Esen, "Perimortem Caesarean Section," *Journal of Obstetrics and Gynaecology* 29:8 (November, 2009), 690–693. M. do Sameiro Barroso, "Post-Mortem Cesarean Section and Embryotomy: Myth, Medicine and Gender in Greco-Roman Culture," *Acta Medico-historica Adriatica* 11:1 (2013), 75–88.

only one can be saved.[4] When Henry VIII's third wife, Jane Seymour, was in labor and her life was at risk, he is purported to have proclaimed, "Save the child by all means, for it is easier to get wives than children."[5] There is evidence in the sixteenth century that postmortem caesarean section was still a well-known and widely accepted procedure, which may have been motivated by financial, legal, or religious concerns, relating to the dowry of the mother and the desire to baptize the progeny.[6]

Many historians record the first living caesarean section as having been performed in 1500 by Jakob Nufer, a Swiss pig-gelder, on his wife, who is reported to have survived until the age of 77 after bearing additional children thereafter. The first physician known to have recommended the performance of a living caesarean section was Francois Rousset (1535–1590), in his *Traitte Nouveau de l'Hysterotomotokie ov Enfantement Caesarien.*

In this chapter, we will briefly address living caesarean section; in particular, the rabbinic sources that reflect its possible performance in antiquity. We will then explore the history and halakha of postmortem caesarean section.

II. EVIDENCE OF LIVING CAESAREAN SECTION FROM THE TALMUD

While the conventional literature of medical history records the first living caesarean section around 1500 CE, there are some historians who have cited the Talmud as evidence of the practice over a millennium earlier, based on multiple passages in the Talmud and its commentaries that imply the performance of a living caesarean section. The discussions revolve around the interpretation of the phrase *"yotzei dofen,"* which is used in rabbinic literature to describe a form of non-natural birth whereby the fetus exits outside the birth canal. There are two distinct issues addressed by scholars: Does the phrase *"yotzei dofen"* refer to a

---

4. R. Blumenfeld-Kosinski, op. cit., 26–27.
5. Ibid., 27.
6. See K. Park, "The Death of Isabella Della Volpe: Four Eyewitness Accounts of a Postmortem Caesarean Section in 1545," *Bulletin of the History of Medicine* 82 (2008), 169–187.

caesarean section or to some other surgical or obstetrical procedure? If indeed it refers to caesarean section, is this a reflection of actual clinical practice or merely hypothetical legal analysis?[7] I will not revisit the details here but will add a few comments about and additions to the existing literature on this topic.

In his classic work *Ma'aseh Tuvia* (1708)[8], Tobias Cohen, a graduate of the famed University of Padua Medical School, devotes a chapter to the procedure described in the Talmud as *"yotzei dofen."* He clearly assumes that it refers to living caesarean section and writes, "how strange this chapter must appear to the 'modern' reader as the procedure is so exceedingly rare (*reḥoka*) and is not performed on the daughters of Israel. However, since the rabbis discuss it in the Talmud, I will explain their words." He gives detailed instructions how such a procedure should be performed.[9]

---

7. See *Arukh HaShalem*, s. v., *"dofen."* The *Arukh* assumes *yotzei dofen* refers to postmortem only. *Tashbetz* 1:110 accepts the possibility of living caesarean section and disagrees with the interpretation of the *Arukh*, struggling to reinterpret him as referring to a case of a deathly ill women, although still alive. Alexander Kohut, in his explanatory notes on the *Arukh*, likewise finds difficulty with the latter's position that caesarean section is only performed on a deceased woman.

8. Section *Gan Na'ul*, chapter 18. On Cohen and his work, see D. Ruderman, "On the Diffusion of Scientific Knowledge Within the Jewish Community: The Medical Textbook of Tobias Cohen," in his *Jewish Thought and Scientific Discovery in Early Modern Europe* (Yale University Press, 1995); *Koroth* 20 (2009–2010), where five articles are devoted to Tobias Cohen and his work *Ma'aseh Tuvia*.

9. Though living caesarean section was first recommended by a physician in the sixteenth century, it took many years, in fact centuries in many places, for it to become part of accepted medical practice.

   Cohen's citation of an interpretation in the name of a "R. Heschel," linking caesarean section with the requirement for a woman to bring a postpartum sacrifice, is worth recording. The students of R. Shimon bar Yoḥai asked why a woman has to bring a sacrifice after childbirth. According to the Talmud, when a woman is in the throes of labor, she takes an oath not to cohabitate again with her husband, lest it lead to another painful labor. For this inappropriate oath, she brings a sacrifice. R. Heschel explained it in the following way: According to the Talmud, if a woman undergoes a living caesarean section, she will not be able to give birth again. When a woman is in labor, she does not yet know whether she will deliver naturally or through caesarean section, but the pain leads her to take an oath not to cohabitate again with her husband. If she delivers via caesarean section, she would not have

Abraham Hartog Israels[10] was one of the first to seriously entertain the possibility that the Jews were performing living caesarean sections long before medical historians believed it was done. His medical school dissertation in 1845, upon graduation from Groningen, Netherlands, was on the subject of obstetrics and gynecology in the Talmud.[11] He devotes a lengthy chapter to caesarean section.[12]

In a letter to Dr. Simeon Abrahams[13] in 1857 about the permissibility of postmortem examinations, R. Dr. Bernard Ilowy writes that even the great operations in obstetrics were not unknown to the Talmudists. He enumerates caesarean section amongst them, but claims it was mainly performed on a corpse.[14] R. Yekutiel Kamelhar, in his work on scientific matters in the Talmud, likewise lauds the rabbis for their great knowledge of obstetrical procedures, including caesarean section, though he hedges as to whether the knowledge was theoretical or actual.[15]

---

had to take an oath, as in any case she would not be able to have another child. She, therefore, brings the sacrifice because she could have prevented a false oath by waiting. While clearly a novel interpretation, it is based on the fact that if a woman delivers by caesarean section, she cannot bear children subsequently. It is unclear to me how R. Heschel infers this from the Talmud, when in fact it appears quite the opposite, that the Talmud discusses the legal ramifications of a second child born to a woman whose firstborn was delivered by caesarean section. (*"yotzei dofen vehaba aharav"*)

10. On Israels, see H. S. Hes-Swartenberg, "Abraham Hartog Israels, M. D., 1822–1883: Netherlands' First Professor in the History of Medicine," *New York State Journal of Medicine* 79:9 (August, 1979), 1445–1447; idem, *Jewish Physicians in the Netherlands 1600–1940* (Van Gorcum: Assen, 1980), 80–81.

11. *Dissertatio Historico—Medica Inauguralis Exhibens Collectanea Gynaecologica ex Talmude Babylonico*, defended in Groningen, March 15, 1845.

12. See full text at http://babel.hathitrust.org/cgi/pt?id=nnc1.cu58942270;view=2up; seq=104, pp. 160–184.

13. On Dr. Abrahams, see Y. Levine, "Dr. Simeon Abrahams: More than a Footnote," *Jewish Press* (September 28, 2010).

14. http://www.jewish-history.com/Illoway/letter11.html (accessed November 9, 2014). Ilowy cites *Tosafot, Avoda Zara* 10a, who mention the story of Caesar's death. He mistakenly attributes the source of *Tosafot* to Josephus, instead of Yosippon, which was a work of different authorship often confused with Josephus. In addition to this letter, Ilowy addressed issues of science and Jewish law in a remarkable letter entitled "The Science of the Talmudists," *The Occident* 14 (1857), available at http://www.jewish-history.com/Illoway/letter03.html.

15. *HaTalmud UMada'ei HaTevel* (Lvov, 1928), 51.

Preuss, in his classic *Biblical and Talmudic Medicine* published in 1911 visits this issue as well, briefly addressing Israels and a few other scholars who had subsequently taken up the issue, and concludes:[16]

> It is certain that the Talmud mentions a type of birth other than by way of the normal birth canal, with a happy outcome for both mother and child (i.e., both remain alive). It is likely that laparotomy for an abdominal pregnancy, and perhaps also caesarean section on a living woman, is what the Talmud is referring to. There is no conclusive evidence however that either of these two operations was ever actually carried out during the time of the Talmud.

Jeffrey Boss picked up the issue again in the mid-twentieth century, adding to the core work of Israels.[17] Boss' excellent article includes a more expansive analysis of rabbinic commentaries, but is perhaps more remarkable for his omission of the work of Preuss. He concludes that living caesarean section was indeed performed in talmudic times, based on the assumption that halakhic discussions are always rooted in observed fact.

> On internal evidence, it appears very unlikely indeed that the operation existed only in Tannaitic imagination. Rabbinical teaching contained halakha and *hagada*, the former being precepts of conduct and the latter including discussion of theology, ethical principles, history and other branches of learning; on *hagada* speculation was common, but fantasy was never a feature of halakha, and the passages to be discussed in this paper are all halakhic.[18]

Boss' statement, "fantasy was never a feature of halakha," is simply not true. In a number of cases, the Talmud construes imaginary or fantastical

---

16. J. Preuss, *Biblical and Talmudic Medicine*, trans. F. Rosner (Hebrew Publishing Company, 1978), 421–426, esp. 426.

17. J. Boss, "The Antiquity of Caesarean Section with Maternal Survival: The Jewish Tradition," *Medical History* 5 (1961), 117–131.

18. Ibid., 120.

cases for the purposes of legal clarification.[19] Even if it is agreed upon that the talmudic passages indeed refer to living caesarean section, this, in and of itself, does not attest to the actual performance of this procedure. It is possible that these are merely hypotheticals to clarify the nuances of the law.

Unbeknownst to Boss, this same idea, that caesarean was performed then later forgotten, was espoused by none other than Ḥazon Ish, in the context of a discussion about the superior knowledge of Ḥazal.[20] If indeed living caesarean section was performed in talmudic times, as some would have us believe, we would then require an explanation as to why and when it fell into disuse, and why any trace of this practice was effectively erased from classic historical sources.

Furthermore, Boss invokes geopolitics to explain a debate between Rashi and Maimonides about the performance of living caesarean section. Rashi clearly assumes that the Talmud refers to living caesarean section and he describes the procedure. Maimonides, however, is explicitly dismissive of the medical possibility of living caesarean section, even devising a creative scenario to explain the case of the Mishna.[21] Boss asserts that Maimonides, living in an Islamic country, was averse to interpreting the Mishnaic texts as referring to a living caesarean section due to the Islamic approach to this procedure. According to Islamic tradition during that period, caesarean section was associated with the devil, and any child born of caesarean section was to be slain.[22]

---

19. See for example the many cases discussed in *Ḥullin* 70a. *Tosafot, Ketubot* 4b, s. v., "*ad*," explicitly states that we find a number of purely hypothetical cases in the Talmud that never did or could occur. It is possible, as Preuss notes, that there is a distinction between mishnaic and talmudic cases and that the Mishna, a guide to practical halakha, does not venture into the hypothetical. If we accept this distinction, then we must perforce conclude that postmortem caesarean section (if identified with "*yotzei dofen*"), which is described in the Mishna, is indeed describing an actual case.

20. *Emuna UBitaḥon*, chapter 5.

21. See his commentary to *Bekhorot* 8:2.

22. See H. E. Fadel, "Postmortem and Perimortem Cesarean Section: Historical, Religious and Ethical Considerations," *Journal of the Islamic Medical Association of North America* 43:3 (December, 2011), 194–200. While Fadel does not address the Islamic approach to caesarean section in the times of Maimonides, he does contend that postmortem caesarean section is fully consonant with Islamic law and teachings.

Boss argues, "It would clearly have been dangerous for the Jews to have been known as the practitioners of such an unholy art, and the greatest centers of Jewish learning… came under the rule of the Caliphate of Baghdad." However, such an act of self-censorship, at the expense of the plain meaning of the text, would have been highly uncharacteristic of Maimonides, whose allegiance to the rational explanation of rabbinic texts is unparalleled.

Professor Yehoshua Leibowitz, the great modern Jewish medical historian, summarizes the literature on caesarean section,[23] and Lurie contributes the most recent addition to the literature, though he appears to be unaware of the work of his predecessors.[24]

Toldot Yeshu—An Unexpected Reference to the Performance of Living Caesarean Section in Antiquity

As Preuss astutely points out, the Talmud never prefaces its discussions of cases of living caesarean section with a phrase such as, *ma'aseh she-haya* ("there was a specific case"). As there is no testimony of any actual case, there is therefore no conclusive evidence from the Talmud that living caesarean section was actually performed. There is, however, an interesting source which may support the theory of Israels, Boss and others that the Jews were indeed performing living caesarean section in antiquity and the medieval period. The work *Toldot Yeshu* (The History of Jesus) is a medieval parody of the Christian gospel. Its authorship and date are unknown, and scholars have dated it anywhere from the sixth

---

23. See Y. Leibowitz, *"Mavo Histori Refui le-Seder Taharot,"* Torah She-Ba'al Peh (5724), 33–39. See also his *"Le-Toldot ha-Refuah bi-Yisrael,"* in Yavneh 3:7–12 (5709), 184–200, esp. 187–189. Leibowitz mentions Theophile Reynaud's 1637 work as the first medical treatise on caesarean section. This was in fact preceded by the work of Francois Rousset in 1581.

24. See S. Lurie, "Vaginal Delivery after Caesarean Delivery in the Days of the Talmud," *Vesalius* 12:1 (2006), 23–24. There is no mention of the expansive analyses of Israels, Preuss or Boss, and the rabbinic citations are scant. As opposed to Boss, he realizes that "it is possible that these passages are of theoretical nature, due to the known tendency of the Jewish writings to provide commentaries for even the most unlikely cases." He argues, however, that the terminology used is of a "concrete category," reflecting that these were actual cases. He cites no specifics, and it is unclear to me how one would infer from the language whether these cases were real or imagined.

to the tenth centuries.[25] There is one line in one of the earliest recensions of this work that bears on our discussion.[26]

Yeshu claimed that he was the son of God and that he was able, through divine powers, to make a virgin pregnant in the absence of a human male partner. The king challenged him to perform this feat with a woman in the kingdom. After nine months of sequestration, the woman had not yet borne a child. The king asked of Yeshu as to why she had not produced issue. Yeshu replied that sometimes the pregnancy can be prolonged. He then asked the king to allow him to tear open the abdomen to remove the baby in order to prove the success of his endeavor, adding that "there are those amongst the Jews who do similar to this." This seems to imply that Jews were performing caesarean sections on living women in the medieval period.[27]

Potential Halakhic Ramification of Living Caesarean Section Debate

Aside from the interesting historical aspect of the above debate, there may be one halakhic implication. The Talmud in *Erkhin* 7a discusses a case of postmortem caesarean section, a case we will discuss in detail presently. One halakhic issue of performing a postmortem caesarean section is the prohibition of desecration of the corpse, *nivul hamet*. R. Yaakov Ettlinger (1798–1871) suggests one possibility as to why there would be no desecration in the performance of this specific procedure. A procedure that is performed on the living, such as caesarean section, he

---

25. J. Dan, "*Toldot Yeshu*," in M. Berenbaum and F. Skolnik, eds., *Encyclopaedia Judaica* 20 (Gale Virtual Reference Library, 2006), 28–29.

26. See Y. Deutch, "An Ancient Version of *Toldot Yeshu*," (Hebrew) *Tarbitz* 69:2 (5760), 177–197, esp. 190–191. I thank my dear friend, Jay Zachter, for drawing my attention to this source.

27. The other versions of *Toldot Yeshu* either do not contain this section or cannot be read this way, and while they preserve the phrase "there are those amongst the Jews who do similar to this," it is used in a different context. See Deutch, op. cit. Upon completion of this essay, I fortuitously discovered an article that identifies and elaborates upon the passage in *Toldot Yeshu* as a possible reference to living caesarean section. See M. Meerson, "Yeshu the Physician and the Child of Stone: A Glimpse of Progressive Medicine in Jewish-Christian Polemics," *Jewish Studies Quarterly* 20:4 (December, 2013), 297–314.

argues, would not constitute desecration when performed on the dead.[28] This proof is predicated on the discussion in the Gemara of "*yotzeh dofen*," which he assumes are accounts of actual cases of living caesarean section. If, however, the talmudic cases were purely hypothetical, and not accounts of actual cases, then this proof would be invalid.[29]

III. POSTMORTEM CAESAREAN SECTION
TO RESCUE A LIVING FETUS

While the aforementioned discussion addresses living caesarean section, for the remainder of this chapter, I will focus on postmortem caesarean section, performed after the death of the mother for the purpose of rescuing a living fetus.[30] We will trace this procedure from antiquity to modern times with particular emphasis on its treatment in rabbinic literature.

Akin to the gestation of the fetus itself, the procedure of postmortem caesarean section has undergone a number of developmental stages in rabbinic literature. However, quite apart from normal gestation, there have been significant periods of regression, as we will elaborate. Our research reveals four distinct stages in the rabbinic response to postmortem caesarean section throughout history. Our discussion begins in the talmudic period, with the literary and historical stage of infancy for postmortem caesarean section.

STAGE 1—THE ERA OF CERTAINTY IN THE
PERFORMANCE OF POSTMORTEM CAESAREAN SECTION

Talmudic and Post-Talmudic Era

In the context of a discussion about capital punishment, the Talmud (*Erkhin* 7a) addresses the case of a pregnant female criminal and the question of whether we delay execution till the birth of the child. Based on textual interpretation the Talmud concludes that we do not

---

28. *Binyan Tzion*, 171.

29. Regarding the criterion of R. Ettlinger with respect to *nivul hamet*, see R. J. David Bleich, "*Nivul Ha-Met*," communication in *Tradition* 37:3 (Fall 2003).

30. The topic of postmortem caesarean section in rabbinic literature has received brief treatment in the works of Preuss, Zimmels, and Jakobovits.

delay, and the fetus is executed along with its mother. Furthermore, prior to the execution, fetal demise is to be induced by striking the woman's abdomen. The purpose of this act is to prevent *nivul* or disgrace lest a living baby be delivered after execution.[31] This concern assumes that the mother predeceases the baby, a fact which is contested by the Talmud.

This debate about when and if the mother can predecease the baby is critical to our discussion about postmortem caesarean section and requires further clarification. The Talmud states as undisputed doctrine that the fetus predeceases the mother and offers what appears to be a physiological explanation. Since the vitality or viability of the unborn fetus is fragile, when the "poison" of the Angel of Death enters the woman, it will exert its fatal effect first on the fragile fetus. If true that the fetus always predeceases the mother, the Talmud queries, our concern that the fetus may survive the execution of its mother is unfounded. This contradiction is resolved by distinguishing between traumatic versus natural death. For a traumatic death, such as by execution, which occurs both rapidly and through external, non-natural means, it is indeed possible for the fetus to survive after the mother's death, hence the concern for *nivul*. In a case of natural death, however, the fetus predeceases the mother.

The question remains, however, as to whether the statement that the fetus predeceases the mother in a case of natural death is absolute or not. This very issue is a matter of debate in the subsequent talmudic passage, which bears directly on our discussion.

> Rav Naḥman said in the name of Shmuel. Regarding a pregnant woman who sat on the birth stool and died on Shabbat during childbirth, we bring a knife, incise her abdomen and remove the child.[32]

---

31. The exact nature of the *nivul* is a matter of debate. See Y. Mitnick, *Avoda Berura, Erkhin* 7a (Brooklyn, 5764), 136. He mentions other opinions including postmortem bleeding, and the public observance of the event. Some suggest that the *nivul* would result from the birth of a dead fetus.

32. *Erkhin* 7a.

This unambiguous reference to postmortem caesarean section is the *locus classicus* of our discussion. The Talmud elaborates upon this pronouncement and concludes that one may violate biblical prohibitions of Shabbat, such as carrying a knife through a public domain, in order to perform the procedure.

How is this statement to be interpreted, in light of the unequivocal pronouncement mentioned above, that in the case of natural death, the fetus predeceases the mother? If the fetus will not survive after the death of mother, what is the purpose of performing a postmortem caesarean section? Rashi maintains that this pronouncement is not absolute and merely describes the majority of cases. It is indeed possible, albeit in a minority of cases, for the fetus to outlive the mother in a case of natural death. In this case of *pikuaḥ nefesh* (saving a life), we would perform the postmortem caesarean section for even a small possibility that the fetus survived. *Tosafot*, however, are of the opinion that the talmudic statement, that in the case of natural death the fetus predeceases the mother, is absolute and unexceptionable. What justifies the postmortem caesarean section in this case is the fact that the woman is on the birth stool, and the fetus has begun to separate from its mother. In this situation only, is it possible for the fetus to survive the mother's natural death.[33]

---

33. This interpretation of the debate between Rashi and *Tosafot* is as per *Rema* in his responsa (n. 40) and many others. According to R. Yaakov Reischer, in his Shevut Yaakov, for example, Rashi concurs with *Tosafot* that the baby predeceases the mother in a case of natural death unless she is on the birth stool. For further discussion of the Rashi-*Tosafot* debate, see R. E. Oshry, *She'elot UTeshuvot MiMa'amakim* 2:10; S. Schneider, "Is It Permitted to Operate on a Pregnant Woman Who Died in Order to Save the Fetus?" (Hebrew) *HaMaor* 222 (*Kislev-Tevet*, 5735), 10–12, republished in his *Divrei Shlomo* 3:362 with additions.

According to the *Kaf HaḤayyim*, Maimonides would agree with Rashi that one always performs a postmortem caesarean section, even if not in labor and is a natural death. The *Livyat Ḥen* cites the *Shita Mekubetzet* who found a manuscript version of Rashi that seems to be more in line with the position of *Tosafot*. For discussion of these sources, see S. Magnus, *Adnei Shlomo O. Ḥ.*, v. 6, *siman* 330, n. 32. *Ba'al Halakhot Gedolot* (*Shabbat*, chapter 18) appears to follow *Tosafot* and simply states as a matter of fact, without dissent, that when a pregnant woman dies of natural causes her child predeceases her, while if the death is traumatic the child may survive.

See T. H. Zablodover, *Beit Shmuel* v. 1, n. 5 (5697), 20–24, who provides a novel interpretation of the position of the Vilna Gaon on this talmudic passage. He addresses

An important distinction between these two opinions is whether one may perform a postmortem caesarean section if the woman is at an earlier stage of pregnancy. According to Rashi, it may indeed be permitted, as the fetus may be alive, whereas according to *Tosafot*, as there is no chance whatsoever for the fetus to survive prior to parturition, there would be no halakhic justification for performing a postmortem caesarean section at any pre-parturition stage.[34]

The conclusion of the Talmud, that one can violate biblical prohibitions to perform a postmortem caesarean section on a pregnant woman who dies on the birthing stool, remains without dissent.

The Period of the Geonim

In the period of the *Geonim*, we find a number of passages that discuss the postmortem caesarean section. We will address three passages that appear to yield three different conclusions. Our first passage is clearly in synchrony with the talmudic dictum.

> If a woman dies on the birth stool and the fetus is moving within her, we cut open the abdomen on Shabbat, for in all cases of *pikuah nefesh* we violate Shabbat.[35]

Furthermore, the agreement with the talmudic dictum is evidenced by the fact that the reference above concludes with a quote directly from the relevant passage in Talmud *Erkhin*.

Our second passage from the *Geonim* states:

---

the issue of whether a pregnant woman who dies during childbirth, on the birth stool, is considered as a natural death, or as a murder/traumatic death. If the latter, this would lead to a different understanding of Rashi. R. Zablodover proudly writes that he discussed his interpretation of the Vilna Gaon with R. Ḥayyim Ozer Grodzinsky, who accepted his analysis. R. Shlomo Zalman Auerbach appears to have agreed with this position. See Y. Gefen, *Deliyat HaKerem* 1 (5767), 240.

34. There are some who expand on *Tosafot*'s permission to perform postmortem caesarean section to include not only the case of sitting on the birth stool, but also a case where the fetus is completely developed (*kalu lo ḥadashav*), as in this case as well the fetus is independent. See for example, Y. Kohen, *Zera Emet* 2:50.

35. S. Asaph, *Teshuvot HaGeonim* (*Mekitzei Nirdamim*: Jerusalem, 5702), 85, n. 76.

> If a woman dies pregnant there is no need to incise the abdomen as the fetus dies before her.[36]

This appears to be contrary to the above statement of the *Geonim*, and to the talmudic passage that explicitly requires a caesarean section for a deceased pregnant woman. However, closer analysis reveals a key difference in this statement. In this statement of the *Geonim*, the woman is pregnant upon death, but no mention is made of the stage of pregnancy. It could very well be an early stage of pregnancy. The Talmud's case, as well as that of the geonic passage above, is specifically of a woman who dies on the birth stool. In this latter case all agree that a postmortem caesarean section should be performed, though they may disagree as to the reason. There is a debate between Rashi and *Tosafot* (according to some interpretations) as to whether the pronouncement allowing postmortem caesarean section is limited to a woman on the birthing stool (*Tosafot*) or whether the permissibility to perform the procedure applies to earlier stages of pregnancy as well (Rashi). It is possible that the geonic author of this passage espouses the position of *Tosafot*.

> It is our third passage from the *Geonim* which is the most remarkable:
> Question: If a pregnant woman dies on the birthing stool and the fetus is noted to be moving within her abdomen, may we open the abdomen to extract the fetus or not?
> Answer: We do not incise [the abdomen]; rather we wait. We place a stone on the abdomen until the fetus dies, then we bury her.[37]

Given the undisputed passage in the Talmud allowing for postmortem caesarean section in this very circumstance, this excerpt from the *Geonim* seems especially enigmatic, especially since movement of the fetus is observed. Even the publisher of this passage could not refrain

---

36. A. A. Harkavy, *Zikhron LeRishonim VeGam LeAḥaronim* (*Teshuvot HaGeonim*) (Berlin, 5647), n. 508, p. 339.

37. T. Moscowitz, ed., *She'elot UTeshuvot HaGeonim* (Jerusalem, 5720), p. 74, n. 248. As per the editor, this paragraph was censored in the Vilna edition and restored in this work based on the Mantua edition.

from noting the inconsistency and offering a possible solution. The bla-
tant asynchrony led one modern scholar to declare, "This response does
not appear to have been written by any sage of Israel, neither *Rishon*
nor *Aharon*. I recall that some have written that these responsa require
further investigation [as to their veracity]."[38]

R. Yaakov Reischer suggests that perhaps at the time of the
Geonim there was a concern for the misdiagnosis of the death of the
pregnant woman. As such, one should not incise the abdomen lest this
hasten or cause the death of the mother.[39] This concern, while inferred
by R. Reischer from the passage of the *Geonim*, is explicitly stated by
Rema and will be explored presently. This assumption may explain why
one should not perform a caesarean section, but it does not explain why
one should actively cause fetal demise.[40]

This geonic directive to induce fetal demise may perhaps be the
origin of the custom addressed by R. David ben Zimra in Egypt some
centuries later, which is remarkably reminiscent of this case.[41]

> I was asked to render my opinion on a common practice in Egypt
> that when pregnant women die in childbirth, and there is fetal
> movement within the abdomen, women strike the abdomen with
> a broom to hasten the death of the fetus. Is there a concern for
> the prohibition of murder [*netilat neshama*], and if it occurs on
> Shabbat, is there also a violation of Shabbat?

While Radbaz does not mention the passage from the *Geonim*, he does
vehemently reject this practice and reports that many times he urged

---

38. See R. David Avitan's notes to his edition of *Birkei Yosef, O. H.,* 330. See also, *Knesset
    HaGedola* on *O. H.,* 330. For an alternative interpretation of the *Geonim,* see *Shu"t
    Zera Emet* 2:50.
39. *Shevut Yaakov* 1:13. See Y. Fischer, *She'elot UTeshuvot Even Yisrael* 8:33, who questions
    this interpretation based on the position of *Shita Mekubetzet* in *Erkhin*
7a. For another explanation of this passage, see Y. Weinberg, *Seridei Aish* 1, p. 316.
40. The editor of the Mantua edition cited by Moscowitz, op. cit., suggests that the rock
    was placed on the abdomen of the pregnant woman to prevent dehiscence of bodily
    contents, and not to hasten the death of the fetus.
41. *Radbaz* 2:695.

these very women to perform a postmortem caesarean section to save the child based on the explicit talmudic passage in *Erkhin*.[42] This responsum is also clear evidence that the unambiguous decision of the Talmud, that a postmortem caesarean section should be performed, albeit limited to certain cases, was in force during this period, which coincides with the writing of the *Shulḥan Arukh* and *Rema*.[43]

This custom may have even lasted into the modern period, as evidenced by this passage discussing the custom of the Jews of Beirut:

> When the corpse [of a woman who had died in pregnancy] has been washed and dressed in the shroud, the women who lay out corpses watch with eye and ear whether the young life in the dead woman stirs. If so, they rain blows on the abdomen of the corpse until all is still in it. For it would be a dishonor for the dead woman and her family if they ventured to open the corpse and it would be a sin to bury the living child alive.[44]

The third of our passages from the *Geonim* appears to be a deviation from the talmudic tradition and is not consonant with the other two geonic passages. The talmudic tradition, permitting the performance of postmortem caesarean section, is clearly accepted in the mainstream halakhic literature and is codified into law by both Maimonides[45] and *Shulḥan Arukh*.[46]

---

42. Radbaz adds that a postmortem caesarean section would only be allowed if the woman was on the birth stool (i.e., died during childbirth), as only in this case, and for traumatic death, would the fetus still survive. It appears Radbaz held like *Tosafot*.

43. This may be an indication that there were differences in the Ashkenzic and Sefardic practices. *Rema*, as we shall see, was not in favor of the practice of postmortem caesarean section. Radbaz may have followed the tradition of R. Yosef Karo. Some contend, however, that *Rema* is not arguing on the *Shulḥan Arukh*, but rather elaborating upon his statement.

44. H. H. Ploss, M. Bartels and P. Bartels, *Woman: An Historical, Gynecological and Anthropological Compendium* (William Heinemann Ltd., 1935), 412. H. J. Zimmels, in his *Magicians, Theologians and Doctors* (Edward Goldston and Son, 1952), 90, quoting the same source, mentions this as a custom among non-Jews. I was unable to find the original source from Ludwig Frankel.

45. *Hil. Shabbat* 2:15.

46. *O. Ḥ.*, 330:5.

In concluding our discussion of stage one, it appears that the talmudic permission to perform a postmortem caesarean section remained in force up to the sixteenth century, the inexplicable, lone third responsum of the *Geonim* notwithstanding. We have every reason to believe that the talmudic statement allowing postmortem caesarean section was religiously followed as normative practice. The fact that we have no record of postmortem caesarean sections in rabbinic literature during this time period is likely more a reflection of the dearth or paucity of literature, combined with the rarity of the procedure, rather than of the lack of its performance.[47]

STAGE 2—*REMA* AND THE ERA OF DOUBT

It is the brief gloss of *Rema* on the *Shulḥan Arukh* which introduces our next stage.

> As to why we do not practice it [postmortem caesarean section] today, even during the weekdays, it is because we no longer have expertise in diagnosing the death of the mother within enough time for the fetus to still survive.[48]

The *Magen Avraham*[49] explains this to mean that we may err in the determination of the death of the mother. By the time we wait to confirm the diagnosis, the fetus will surely not have survived, and there will be no justification to perform a caesarean section.

If one reads the *Rema* carefully, it appears that he is placing a halakhic imprimatur on a pre-existing practice of refraining from the

---

47. See K. Park, "The Death of Isabella Della Volpe: Four Eyewitness Accounts of a Postmortem Caesarean Section in 1545," *Bulletin of the History of Medicine* 82:1 (Spring 2008), 169–187.
48. *Shulḥan Arukh*, O. Ḥ., 330:5. *Rema's* comment is based on an earlier source, the *Issur VeHetter* (59:11) by R. Yonah Kalman Babad HaAshkenazi (1470–1550), but this source only slightly predates *Rema*. H. J. Zimmels lists this statement of *Rema* among a number of examples of lost knowledge or expertise discussed in rabbinic literature. See his, "The Significance of the Statement 'we are not acquainted any more' as Echoed in Rabbinic Literature," *Leo Jung Jubilee Volume* (1962), 223–235.
49. Ad loc.

performance of postmortem caesarean section rather than making a new halakhic pronouncement.[50]

From the words of *Rema*, we have no idea how long prior to this statement the practice of postmortem caesarean section had fallen into disuse. It is theoretically possible that as early as the time of the *Geonim*, it was already not being performed, as R. Reischer suggests, though we have no other sources to corroborate this theory. We do know, however, that moving forward from this point, given the imprimatur of the *Rema*, it became halakhically sanctioned to generally refrain from postmortem caesarean sections, as we shall see.

Consistency in the Cases of Postmortem Caesarean Section v. the Standard Determination of Death

It is noteworthy that while *Rema* is concerned with the misdiagnosis of death in the unique case of postmortem caesarean section, he did not voice the same concern in the section of *Shulhan Arukh* which deals directly with the diagnosis of death.[51] Is *Rema* consistent in these two cases? It could be argued that in this case, as a procedure will be performed on the recently deceased, it is essential to delay until the confirmation of death, which presumably would be a relatively short period of time. In a standard case of declaration of death, there is typically built in time for preparations for burial, which would preclude the necessity for adding additional delay.[52]

The attempt to achieve halakhic consistency between the diagnosis of death in a standard case versus in the case of the pregnant woman is also relevant to the position of Maimonides.[53] In this case, however,

---

50. R. E. Posek, *Koret HaBrit*, O. H., 310, n. 15 ascertains from the fact that *Rema* does not use a more legalistic formulation (such as, "and there are those who say it is prohibited to cut, and so is our practice") that he is not disagreeing with R. Karo, but rather commenting based on the present medical reality. See also *Tzitz Eliezer* 10:25 Chap. 6.

51. O. H., 329. In *Rema*'s gloss to E. H., 145:9 he also comments that *"ein anu beki'in bizman hazeh"* (we are not experts today) with regard to medical diagnoses and the cause of death, but this does not refer to the actual determination of death.

52. *Rema* also addresses the issue of postmortem caesarean section in his responsa, n. 40.

53. See Y. Weiss, *Minhat Yitzhak* 5:7 and Y. Fischer, *She'elot UTeshuvot Even Yisrael* 8:33.

while Maimonides is concerned about hasty diagnosis of death in a standard case and cautions against even closing the eyes in the peri-mortem period lest one accidentally hasten death, he raises no such concern in codifying the obligation to perform postmortem caesarean section. One would think that the time delay necessary for confirming the diagnosis of death would preclude the utility of the performance of a postmortem caesarean section, as the fetus would be dead, exactly as the *Magen Avraham* interpreted the *Rema*. Maimonides' required delay, however, seems to be momentary and perhaps not long enough for the fetus to demise. R. Y. Fischer suggests another novel explanation. He limits Maimonides' permission of postmortem caesarean section to a case of "sitting on the birth stool."[54] In this case, the baby has already "separated" from the mother and is somewhat independent. As such, the required delay to confirm death would not be harmful to the fetus, and one could then proceed with the postmortem caesarean section.

Validation of Rema's Concern

That the *Rema's* concern for the misdiagnosis of death with respect to postmortem caesarean section was well founded can be inferred from the following passage which, perhaps not coincidentally, is drawn from a work which would ultimately set the stage for one of the most remark-able and protracted debates in medical halakhic history—the halakhic definition of death.[55]

---

54. This assumes that Maimonides holds like *Tosafot*. See Y. Fischer, *She'elot UTeshuvot Even Yisrael* 8:33.
55. For a discussion of this topic in Jewish sources, see. M. Samet, "*Halanat HaMet*," *Asupot* 3 (5749), 413–465; S. Kottek, "The Controversy Concerning Early Burial," *Assia: Jewish Medical Ethics* 1:1 (May, 1988), 31–33; F. Wiesemann, "Jewish Burials in Germany—Between Tradition, the Enlightenment and the Authorities," *Leo Baeck Institute Yearbook* 37 (1992), 17–31; J. M. Efron, "Images of the Jewish Body: Three Medical Views from the Jewish Enlightenment," *Bulletin of the History of Medicine* 69 (1995), 349–66; S. Goldberg, *Crossing the Jabbok: Illness and Death in Ashkenazi Judaism in Sixteenth through Nineteenth Century Prague* (University of California Press, 1996), 195–200. An excellent recent addition to the literature on the rabbinic response to the delayed burial controversy has been written by R. Yeḥiel Goldhaber and is as yet unpublished. For discussion of this topic in the general historical literature, see J. Bondeson, *Buried Alive* (W. W. Norton, 2001); G. K. Behlmer, "Grave Doubts:

Philip Peu (17th century), a successful surgeon and man-midwife in Paris, with a degree of candour no less uncommon than laudable, (in his *Prax. Obstetr.* II. C. ii. 2) relates an unlucky accident which happened in his own hands; for being warmly solicited to perform a caesarean section on a pregnant woman, whom he thought perfectly dead because he perceived no pulsation in the sides of the breast, and because a mirror applied to her mouth was not tarnished by her breath, he did not hesitate to begin the operation. But he had hardly plunged the point of his instrument into the integuments, when the trepidation or trembling of the patient's body, the grinding of her teeth, and the motion of her legs, convinced him, though too late, of his rashness. This blunder filled his mind with such terror, that he bound himself by an oath never for the future to attempt the same operation, till he was thoroughly satisfied with respect to the death of the pregnant woman.[56]

The possibility of misdiagnosis of death was not restricted to cases of postmortem caesarean section. There is also an account of Vesalius, the father of modern anatomy and a contemporary of *Rema*, attempting a routine dissection only to realize that the woman was actually still alive.[57]

Why the Regression?

The *Rema* is historically the first to introduce legal ambiguity into a practice long held to be on solid legal ground.[58] To what can we attribute this regression? It appears to be an early reflection of the belief that

---

Victorian Medicine, Moral Panic, and the Signs of Death," *Journal of British Studies* 42:2 (April, 2003), 206–235. For a superb discussion on the evolution of the definition of death throughout history, including the early burial controversy, see M. S. Pernick, "Back from the Grave: Recurring Controversies over the Defining and Diagnosing Death in History," in R. M. Zaner, ed., *Death Beyond Whole-Brain Criteria* (Kluwer Academic Publishers, 1988), 17–74.

56. J. J. Bruhier D'Ablaincourt, *The Uncertainty of the Signs of Death* (1746), 5.

57. J. Snart, *Thesaurus of Horror* (1817), 79.

58. According to R. Reischer above, the ambiguity may have begun earlier, in the geonic period.

physicians were incapable of accurately diagnosing death. While the misdiagnosis of death is as old as death itself, the organized and public belief that it was a systemic problem requiring intervention evolved over a period of time, reaching its zenith with the publication, translation, annotation and dissemination of the book, *The Uncertainty of the Signs of Death*. The account above of Phillip Peu is found within the pages of this work. With this book and others like it, a widespread fear was instilled within every individual that they might be buried alive. This ultimately led to legislation in many European countries requiring delay of burial after initial pronouncement of death until such time as death could be confirmed with certainty, often a period of two to three days.

Given the halakhic requirement of immediate burial after pronouncement of death, this presented a serious challenge for contemporary rabbinic authorities. This so-called three-day burial controversy involved virtually every major rabbinic authority of that period and has received ample treatment in halakhic and academic literature. I do not revisit it here except to highlight some aspects of this historical topic that bear relevance to our present discussion. Further research will surely reveal additional connections.

There is evidence that the legislators of the new laws requiring delay of burial specifically singled out the case of a pregnant woman. If the diagnosis of death was in doubt, this should clearly impact the advisability of performing a caesarean section, lest we find a recurrence of the incident mentioned by Peu above. Despite this concern, some countries specifically legislated that a postmortem caesarean section should be performed if a woman died in a state of advanced pregnancy.[59]

According to one contemporary rabbinic scholar, the three-day burial controversy had an unexpected impact on a Jewish practice related to our discussion.[60] It was a custom to delay burial of a pregnant woman

---

59. See, for example, the article in Belgian law which states that, "When a woman has died in a state of advanced pregnancy, they shall direct the artificial extraction of the infant, supposed to be yet living; and, in the lack of an attending doctor, shall perform it themselves when necessary." See W. Tebb and E. P. Vollum, *Premature Burial and How It Can Be Prevented* (Swan Sonnenschein, 1905), 295.
60. What follows derives from personal correspondence with R. Yeḥiel Goldhaber.

who died in order to facilitate the delivery or spontaneous passage of the fetus. It is possible that this practice was an outgrowth of postmortem caesarean section, and while delayed burial was originally intended to deliver a living fetus, it evolved into the delivery of a deceased fetus.[61] In light of the halakhic opposition to the delay of burial, at least one prominent rabbinic authority, R. Isaiah Berlin, suspended this albeit unsubstantiated practice and required burial of all pregnant women without significant delay, similar to all deaths, lest one think that delay of burial would be permitted in other cases as well. R. Yeḥiel Goldhaber asserts that R. Berlin was responding to the recent dictates requiring delay of burial and specifically did not want the Jewish community to delay the burial of a pregnant woman, a common practice up to that point, lest it be misconstrued as a tacit approval of delay of burial in all cases, something to which R. Berlin was clearly opposed.

Cases of Postmortem Caesarean Section in the Post-Rema Era

As opposed to the historical period preceding the *Rema*, for which we have no recorded actual cases in rabbinic literature of postmortem caesarean section, in the ensuing centuries we find a number of such cases. Through these reports we can see the impact of the *Rema's* pronouncement on the subsequent halakhic landscape. Was the *Rema's* concern universally accepted or was postmortem caesarean section still performed? As mentioned above, Radbaz, a rough contemporary of *Rema*, advocated for the performance of postmortem caesarean section, and makes no mention of the concern for the misdiagnosis of death. It is unclear, however, if he would have known of *Rema's* position. We focus on later responsa, after the dissemination of the *Shulḥan Arukh* with the *Rema's* glosses. Perhaps the most oft quoted responsum on postmortem caesarean section is that of the tragic case presented to R. Yaakov Reischer (1661–1773).[62] His response not only reflects the

---

61. See E. Reichman, "Postmortem Fetal Extraction Before Burial of a Pregnant Woman: A Forgotten Custom That Should Remain Buried," *Korot* 24 (2017–2018), 19–43.

62. *Shevut Yaakov* 1:13. A. Buczacz (1770–1840), in his glosses *Eshel Avraham* to *Shulḥan Arukh*, *O. Ḥ.*, 330, briefly cites virtually the identical case. *Sha'arei Teshuva O. Ḥ.*, 330:5 asserts that he is referring to the very case of R. Reischer.

acceptance of the comments of Rema, it also gives insight into its application.

> Regarding a case, which should never occur again in Israel, of a pregnant woman who was decapitated with a sword on Shabbat, and her fetus was observed to be moving. A man incised the abdomen to save the fetus and after the procedure found that the fetus had died. He asked if he needs penitance (*kappara*) for the accidental violation of Shabbat.

In R. Reischer's response, he clearly follows the position of *Rema* that we do not perform a postmortem caesarean section "today," as we are no longer experts in determining death. He limits this to cases of natural death. However, in this case, as it is a traumatic death, and furthermore, decapitation renders the diagnosis irrefutable, the concern of the *Rema* is irrelevant, and it is clearly permissible to perform the postmortem caesarean section. We may infer that if it would have been a case of natural death, the position of *Rema* would have been in force and R. Reischer would have prohibited a postmortem caesarean section. Of note, R. Reischer is of the opinion that Rashi and *Tosafot* do not argue regarding the accepted fact that in a natural death the fetus *always* dies first. As such, according to R. Reischer, in the case of a natural death, all authorities agree that one is only permitted to perform a caesarean section if the woman is on the birth stool.

The acceptance of the decision of *Rema* is reflected in a responsum of another prominent rabbinic authority, R. Moshe Teitelbaum (1759–1841), progenitor of the Satmar chassidic dynasty. In dealing with a related issue about the burial of a pregnant woman with her fetus, and whether a caesarean section should be performed to remove the deceased fetus in order to provide a separate burial,[63] he states that there are rabbinic discussions about postmortem caesarean section to save a living fetus, "something that is not possible in our time, as explained in *Rema* ..."[64]

---

63. The custom of attempting to extract or deliver a deceased fetus after the death of its mother was widespread in Jewish communities in Europe in the Middle Ages.
64. *Heshiv Moshe*, O. Ḥ., 13.

While the tragic case presented to R. Reischer above was straight-forward from a legal perspective,[65] the case presented to R. Avrohom Ḥayyim Oppenheim (1796–1894) was not.

> Regarding an incident that occurred in a nearby village: A preg-nant woman died, and according to her previous testimony, at the day of her death she was exactly 8 months and 1 day pregnant. In her village there is a physician who is expert in the determination of death, and no villager is buried until he confirms the diagnosis of death. When this physician examined the woman, he declared that she was definitively dead, and that her fetus was still alive.
>
> Is one permitted to desecrate the body and remove the fetus from her? The reason we are not accustomed to incise the abdomen and remove the fetus is because we are not expert in determining death, and perhaps the woman merely fainted. The fetus would die first (if we wait for the definitive diagnosis), as it states in *Shulḥan Arukh* … Such is not the case here where the physician, who is an acclaimed expert, affirms that both the fetus is still alive and that the mother is definitely dead. Do we say that the permission to remove the fetus is only if the baby is completely formed, as in the talmudic passage where the woman is on the birth stool, and that if not (as in this case) it is better not to desecrate unnecessarily?[66]

There are two variables here that require analysis. The first is the accuracy of the medical diagnosis for both the mother and fetus. If this were the only issue, the decision would likely be clear. *Rema* was concerned about the misdiagnosis of death; once this factor is corrected for, as in this case, we can invoke the talmudic permission to perform a caesarean section.

---

65. R. Akiva Eiger, in his glosses on the *Shulḥan Arukh*, states that if the woman is decapitated, it is obvious that the statement of *Rema* does not apply. He cites the *Shevut Yaakov*.

66. *Har Evel*, p. 20. This case is usually quoted from the responsa of R. Moshe Kunitz, who received the question from R. Oppenheim, but the latter's analysis is important for our discussion as well.

The other variable is the gestational age of the fetus. Above we discussed the debate between Rashi and *Tosafot* as to whether the postmortem caesarean section can be performed only for a woman on the birth stool, or whose fetus is fully developed, or even at an earlier gestational age.

In his halakhic analysis, R. Oppenheim initially leans against performing the caesarean section because of the early gestational age.[67] In this case, he argues, the fetus would predecease the mother (agrees with *Tosafot*). As to the observation of the physician regarding fetal movement, he likens it to the talmudic comment that it is like the movement of the tail of a lizard (i.e., the movement is reflex, or perhaps artifact, and not an indication of the presence of life). He ultimately allows the procedure based on an analysis of the laws of desecration of the dead (*nivul*).

His final comment and conclusion, however, are of particular interest regarding the interface of the history of postmortem caesarean section and the three-day burial controversy.

> I am inclined to allow the desecration [*nivul*] in this case … for as explained in your question, it appears that the deceased will not be buried immediately [in any case] due to the decree of the government. If so, even if you do not desecrate now [to perform the postmortem caesarean section] there will ultimately be desecration when the fetus exits after death, as Rashi interprets in *Masekhet Erkhin*…

We see how the decree regarding delaying burial could potentially have halakhic impact on our case of postmortem caesarean section.

The young R. Oppenheim forwarded his response to the prominent rabbinic authority, R. Moshe Kunitz (1774–1834), for validation.[68] Of note, he omitted the final comment regarding delayed burial in his letter. While R. Kunitz took the young rabbi to task for some of his

---

67. R. Oppenheim also discusses the legal status of the fetus at different gestational ages, and the prohibition of murder, as they impact on this case.

68. *Sefer HaMetzaref*, n. 101. R. Kunitz explicitly comments that he thought the question so significant that he includes it verbatim in his work.

misguided analyses, he ultimately concurred that it would be appropriate to perform the postmortem caesarean section. R. Kunitz does not specifically address the fear of *Rema* regarding the misdiagnosis of death, assumedly being satisfied with the oversight of the expert physician. This decision of R. Kunitz, allowing postmortem caesarean section if a physician pronounced the death, was incorporated into other legal texts.[69]

What is clear from these cases is that they interpreted *Rema*'s statement as situational, and if circumstances reveal a clear diagnosis of death, whether through decapitation or by expert physician examination, the original talmudic permission to perform a postmortem caesarean section would remain in force.

In his Holocaust responsa, R. Ephraim Oshry describes a profoundly tragic case of postmortem caesarean section.[70] On May 7, 1942, the Germans decreed that any Jewish woman found to be pregnant would be shot on sight. That very day an innocent woman, not knowing of the decree, was walking in the street. When a Nazi soldier noticed her, he immediately shot her in the chest. The woman was brought to the local hospital where she was pronounced dead, and the physicians thought they could possibly save the fetus. R. Oshry himself witnessed the event and was consulted by a Jewish physician as to the permissibility of performing a postmortem caesarean section. The physician raised the issue of *nivul hamet*, desecration of the dead, as well as the possibility that the woman was still alive.

R. Oshry ruled at the bedside that the procedure was permitted. In his later published discussion, he based his analysis on the passage in *Erkhin*, addressing the debate between Rashi and *Tosafot*, as well as the position of *Rema*. He also invokes the similar case of traumatic death in pregnancy discussed by R. Reischer above. The procedure was technically a success, and the baby was delivered alive.[71]

---

69. See, for example, Avraham ben Naḥman HaKohen, *Taharat HaMayim*, p. 36b, n. 45; *Bikur Ḥolim Landshuta* (5626).

70. *She'elot UTeshuvot MiMa'amakim* 2:10.

71. R. Oshry records the even more tragic postscript at the end of his responsum.

In conclusion of our analysis of stage two, the rabbinic authorities in the post-*Rema* era appear to have accepted *Rema*'s ruling as normative,[72] and postmortem caesarean sections were generally not performed. There are a number of specific cases of postmortem caesarean section recorded during this period, all of which are justified by the rabbinic authorities as being consistent with the position of *Rema*, as the death of the pregnant mother was ascertained with certainty.

STAGE 3—THE RETURN OF CERTAINTY AND RESTORATION OF THE TALMUDIC RULING

While the likelihood of a definitive diagnosis of death was less likely in the pre-modern era, in the modern era, this is no longer the case, and it is far easier to definitively diagnose both the death of the mother as well as the remaining life of the fetus. The advances in modern medicine led to the revisiting of the question of postmortem caesarean section by both medical and rabbinic authors.

Dr. Yaakov Levi, writing in *HaMa'ayan* in 1971, interprets the statement of *Rema* similar to his predecessors, Rabbis Reischer and Kunitz, though he updates the medical reality for his time.[73] He advocates, given the advances in medicine, for the restoration of the original ruling of the Talmud and codified by the *Shulḥan Arukh*. R. Shlomo Schneider, writing in the journal *HaMaor* in 1974, in essence makes the same argument, though he buttresses it with other halakhic analyses.[74] R. Shmuel Vozner echoes the same sentiment that today, given our enhanced ability to both diagnose the death of the mother and the life of the fetus, we should restore the practice of postmortem caesarean section.[75] It was also brought to his attention that R. Isser Zalman Meltzer was of the

---

72. For another source on the acceptance of *Rema*'s position in postmortem caesarean section see, *Minḥat Elazar* 4:28.

73. 11:4 (*Tammuz*, 5731), 218–225. See the review of Levy's essay by R. J. D. Bleich in his *Contemporary Halakhic Problems* 1 (Ktav, 1977), 123–125.

74. S. Schneider, "Is It Permitted to Operate on a Pregnant Woman who Died in Order to Save the Fetus?" (Hebrew) *HaMaor* 222 (*Kislev-Tevet*, 5735), 10–12, republished in his *Divrei Shlomo* 3:362 with additions; a version was also published in *Kobetz Ohel Moshe* 7 (5755), 71–74.

75. *Shevet Levi* 6:27. See also 8:89.

same opinion. Rav Vozner hastens to add, however, that one should not rely on his decision until there is concurrence from other Torah sages.

STAGE 4—THE ERA OF BRAIN DEATH
AND THE RETURN OF DOUBT

In the late twentieth century, there evolved a new and alternate diagnosis of death that has reintroduced ambiguity into the procedure of postmortem caesarean section. In 1968, a Harvard committee published an article defining a clinical condition called irreversible coma.[76] This ultimately became known as brain death and was eventually accepted by the Western world as an alternate definition of death. The status of brain death in halakha has become one of the most complex subjects in modern medical halakhic history, and we shall address it here only inasmuch as it interfaces with our topic.

The Impact of the Case of Postmortem Caesarean Section on the Halakhic Literature on the Definition of Death

The case of postmortem caesarean section, and the talmudic passage of *Erkhin* above, plays a critical role in the halakhic analysis of the legal status of the brain-dead patient. While a number of rabbinic authorities invoke the case of postmortem caesarean section in their analyses of the case of brain death, we will focus specifically on the position of R. Shlomo Zalman Auerbach, for whom this case played a central role in his discussions.

As a major rabbinic authority in the late twentieth century, R. Auerbach was asked to render his opinion as to whether brain death is considered halakhic death. Apparently, he was seriously considering acceptance of brain death when he was made aware of cases where pregnant women were diagnosed with brain death, yet able to deliver healthy babies via caesarean section.[77]

---

76. "A Definition of Irreversible Coma," *JAMA* 205:6 (August, 1968).

77. A specific tragic case transpired in Israel of a young pregnant woman who was diagnosed with brain death. According to physicians, the fetus was still viable and there were discussions with the family and legal experts as to whether the fetus should be delivered. This case, and its halakhic ramifications, is discussed in a lengthy monograph by R. Y. Shafran, "A Lack of Authority: On the Borders of Life and Death,"

The key aspect of this case for R. Auerbach was the medical fact that the fetus was able to survive despite the fact that the mother was brain-dead. According to *Masekhet Erkhin*, in the case of a natural death, unless the woman is on the birth stool, the fetus always predeceases the mother.[78] If indeed brain death is halakhic death, it should simply not be possible for the fetus to outlive the mother. It must therefore be, he reasoned, that brain death cannot be halakhic death.

The counter argument, advanced by R. Dr. Steinberg, among others, was that modern science has created a new reality and that the artificial delivery of oxygen to the body via a respirator, and the preservation of blood flow and blood pressure supplying all the required sustenance for the fetus, can allow a corpse to serve as an incubator despite the legal and halakhic death of the brain-dead patient. To demonstrate this point, the following animal experiment was proposed. A pregnant sheep would be decapitated and then sustained through artificial means long enough to deliver the fetus. If this were possible it would lead to the following conclusion. All would agree that a decapitated sheep is legally dead, based upon the Mishna in *Ohalot* (1:6). It is only through modern interventions that the fetus can still be delivered even after the legal status of death. It is therefore possible that brain death is halakhic death, yet it is still possible, through modern technology, to deliver a living baby after its determination. This experiment was performed on 17 *Shevat*, 5752.[79] While the experiment may have led to a reinterpretation

---

(Jerusalem, 5753); idem, "Saving a Fetus from the Mother Postmortem: Halakhic Analysis," (Hebrew) *Sefer Assia* 9 (5764), 274–300, including a letter exchange with R. Yaakov Ovadia. R. Shafran also created a short film based on this case.

78. R. Auerbach apparently held like *Tosafot*. Regarding his interpretation of Rashi, see *Beit Shmuel*, op. cit., and Y. Gefen, *Deliyat HaKerem* 1 (5767), 240.

79. On the sheep experiment, see A. Steinberg and M. Hersch, "Decapitation of a Pregnant Sheep: A Contribution to the Brain Death Controversy," *Transplantation Proceedings* 27:2 (April, 1995), 1886–1887; A. Steinberg, *"Keviat Rega HaMavet,"* *Assia* 53–54 (August, 1994), 5–16; *Minhat Shlomo* 83, chapter 12; A. S. Abraham, *Nishmat Avraham* (2nd ed.) Y. D., 339, p. 465. For a detailed discussion of the impact of the sheep experiment on the positions on brain death of Rabbis Auerbach and Elyashiv, see M. Halperin, *Refua, Metziut VeHalakha* (Schlesinger Institute, 2011), 143–151. Y. Gefen has a lengthy and detailed section in his *Deliyat HaKerem* 1 (5767), 238ff.

of the talmudic passage by R. Auerbach, it did not completely assuage his concerns about accepting brain death as halakhic death.

Of historical interest, contrary to popular belief, this is not the first time this type of experiment was performed. In fact, in 1627, William Harvey, who first described the circulation of the blood, decapitated a rooster and preserved the circulation and respiration with a bellows. It could be argued that that was the first case of "brain death" to be maintained on a "respirator."[80]

Impact of Brain Death on the Performance of Postmortem Caesarean Section

In the modern era, since the acceptance of the brain death criteria, there have been a number of cases of pregnant women diagnosed with brain death. In some of these cases attempts were made, with varying success, to sustain the mother in order to deliver the fetus.[81] The halakhic approach to this unique case is linked to the position one maintains about brain death.

If one considers the brain-dead patient to be alive, then this is no longer a discussion about postmortem caesarean section, but of living caesarean section.[82] According to this position, as the mother is halakhically alive, one is clearly obligated to sustain her life, and by extension, the fetus' as well. The issue now becomes the assessment of danger and risk to the pregnant mother. There is debate as to whether a brain-dead patient has the status of a *gosses* (moribund) or *safek gosses* (possibly moribund). This status carries halakhic ramifications, such as the prohibition of even moving a *gosses*, lest it hasten death. While it may be

---

80. See Pernick, op. cit., who mentions the case of Harvey, as well as others who performed similar experiments in the eighteenth and nineteenth centuries.

81. M. Esmaeilzadeh, et al., "One Life Ends, Another Begins: Management of a Brain Dead Pregnant Mother—A Systematic Review," *Biomed Central* 8:74 (2010). They report 30 cases found in the medical literature from 1982–2010. These cases involve other variables and ethical issues, such as the wishes of the husband and family, and the health status of the fetus.

82. For a discussion of how the rabbinic authorities who do not accept brain death address this case, see Shafran, op. cit. The position of R. Eliezer Waldenberg (*Tzitz Eliezer* 18:31) in this case is somewhat enigmatic. On his position, see Y. Sasson, *Ruaḥ Yaakov* (Jerusalem, 5770), 64–65.

theoretically possible to deliver a child from a brain-dead patient naturally, with external abdominal compression, given the lack of consciousness of the woman, this would be challenging. Would the performance of
a caesarean section to deliver the fetus be considered a violation of the
prohibition of moving the *gosses*? What if the health status of the brain-
dead patient was compromised by the pregnancy? Would we perform
an abortion to prolong the life of the brain-dead patient, or would it be
preferable to deliver the fetus, which is a potential life? It is quite possible that the performance of caesarean section on a brain-dead woman
would cause undue physiological stress and possibly hasten her death.
Ironically, while it would be obligatory to sustain the pregnant mother,
who is halakhically alive according to this position, it may possibly be
prohibited to deliver the baby through caesarean section, lest it hasten
the mother's death.

If one considers the brain-dead patient as halakhically dead, we can
then invoke our discussion about postmortem caesarean section. Would
the talmudic pronouncement codified by the *Shulḥan Arukh* allowing for
postmortem caesarean section apply here? Or, would the *Rema's* doubt
about the diagnosis of death apply? In either case, the unique status of the
brain-dead pregnant patient creates a scenario that was simply unimagi-
nable previously in the history of medicine—a clinically dead woman
with a living child in utero who can be sustained for weeks to months.
All the previous halakhic discussions relate to sustaining the woman for
minutes, perhaps a few days at most, in order to possibly deliver the child.
What if the woman is only a few weeks pregnant? Will we sustain the
body as a human incubator for months, or is this halakhically untenable?

The case of the Talmud and Codes clearly refers to the performance of a caesarean section immediately upon determination of death,
without delay. For this case there is some discussion of desecration of
the corpse, *nivul hamet*, for the procedure. In the brain death case, however, in addition to the issue of *nivul hamet*, there is also the concern for
halanat hamet, abrogation of the mitzva of timely burial, as burial would
be delayed until the delivery of the baby, which could be months. One
could compare this to a situation of organ donation from a brain-dead
patient, which is permitted by a number of rabbinic authorities who
accept the brain death criteria as halakhically valid. In this case, burial is

delayed sometimes for days until organ harvest occurs and is permitted based on the *pikuah nefesh* for the organ recipient. Would we apply the same logic to delaying burial of the deceased woman for *pikuah nefesh* for the fetus? Does the fetus have the same status as a living person in the eyes of halakha with respect to *pikuah nefesh*? We do allow violation of Shabbat in order to save the life of a fetus. Does it matter that the delay could be months instead of days? These issues clearly merit a more expansive halakhic analysis, which is beyond the scope of this article.[83]

IV. CONCLUSION

This chapter discusses one of the rarest performed surgical procedures in the history of medicine, the postmortem caesarean section, from historical and halakhic perspectives. The halakhic approach to this procedure has evolved since antiquity and has undergone a number of distinct stages. In the initial stage, the medical determination of death was unquestioned, and rabbinic authorities universally advocated the performance of the postmortem caesarean section. In the second stage, the accuracy of the medical determination of death was called into question, and the rabbinic authorities generally withheld consent for the procedure, with some notable exceptions. In the third stage, the medical diagnosis of death was again restored to a state of accepted accuracy, and the rabbinic authorities again advocated for the performance of the procedure. In the final and present stage, the medical community has adopted a new and alternative determination of death, so-called "brain death." While the medical accuracy of this diagnosis is accepted, it is now the halakhic status of this diagnosis that is in question and that has generated renewed halakhic ambiguity in the performance of the postmortem caesarean section. This chapter illustrates the complex relationship between medical history and medical halakha, and the responsiveness of rabbinic authorities throughout the centuries to contemporary medical developments.

---

83. Regarding delay of burial for a pregnant woman, there is a corollary analysis to the topic of postmortem caesarean section which may possibly be assimilated to this issue. There is extensive discussion in halakhic literature about whether the burial of a pregnant woman should be delayed in order to allow efforts, either through physical or spiritual means, to induce the delivery of the deceased fetus before burial. See E. Reichman, "Postmortem Fetal Extraction," op. cit.

Medicine and
Rabbinic Literature

Biblical and Talmudic Medicine: A Bibliographical Essay

As you pick up this book and begin to leaf through its pages, you are sharing a centuries-old fascination with the study of medicine in relation to rabbinic literature with quite an eclectic group of people. Since the first systematic treatises on medicine in the Bible were published in the seventeenth century, a great number of people—Jews and non-Jews, physicians, scientists, historians, clergy, and lay people—have contributed, in varying degrees, to this field.

While this book analyzes the medical aspects of rabbinic literature throughout the ages, my objective in this brief essay is to provide an overview, through a narrative bibliography, specifically of the study of biblical and talmudic medicine. It is this endeavor that occupies a fair percentage of the pre-modern discussion of the relationship of Judaism and medicine.

Studies of the eighteenth century were devoted primarily to the medicine in the Bible, one of the earliest of these works being that of the prominent seventeenth-century physician Thomas Bartholin.[1] Dealing with topics such as Jacob's limp, Moses' withering hand, leprosy, and King Asa's arthritis, Bartholin applied the then current understanding of medicine as a means of textual interpretation. For example, in claiming that Jacob suffered from a dislocation of the hip, he marshals support from the works of Celsus and Galen.

The earliest work on biblical medicine written by a Jewish physician is that of Benjamin Mussaphia.[2] This 173-page work, published in 1640, lists all the verses from the Bible that relate, in the broadest sense, to medicine. Each of the roughly 650 verses cited is followed by a brief explanation.

The earliest treatise to include talmudic medicine was that of Wolff Gintzburger, whose dissertation on talmudic medicine completed in 1743 fulfilled his requirement for graduation from the medical school of the University of Gottingen.[3] Gintzburger attempted to place the medicine of the Talmud into an historical context, stating that a small portion of the Talmud precedes the time of Galen, while the remainder is either coeval or of a later date. That is why, he claims, much of the Talmud agrees with the Galenic tradition.

Gintzburger was a religious student who encountered conflict between his religious obligations and his medical training, as evidenced by a question he posed to one of the leading rabbinic figures in Germany of his time, R. Yaakov Emden. The query, published in R. Emden's collected responsa, regards the permissibility of performing dog dissection on the Sabbath. R. Emden's response, addressing both

---

1. J. Willis, trans., *Thomas Bartholin On the Diseases of the Bible: A Medical Miscellany, 1672* (Danish National Library of Science and Medicine, 1994).

2. See H. Friedenwald, "Bibliography of Ancient Hebrew Medicine" in his *The Jews and Medicine* (Johns Hopkins Press, 1944), 112; D. Margalit, "Rav Binyamin Mussaphia," *Koroth* 2:7–8 (1960), 307–318.

3. F. Schiller, "Benjamin Wolff Gintzburger's Dissertation on Talmudic Medicine," *Koroth* 9:7–8 (Fall 1988), 579–600. For additional biographical notes on Gintzburger, see N. M. Gelber, "History of Jewish Physicians in Poland in the Eighteenth Century," (Hebrew) in Y. Tirosh, ed., *Shai LeYeshayahu: Sefer Yovel LeRav Yehoshua Wolfsberg* (*HaMercaz LeTarbut shel HaPoel HaMizrachi*; Tel Aviv, 5716), 347–371, esp. 356; *Koroth* 9 (Special Issue, 1988) [Proceedings of the Third Symposium on Medicine in the Bible and Talmud], 255–261; J. Efron, *Medicine and the German Jews: A History* (Yale University Press, 2001), 190–197.

human and animal dissection, serves as a basis for modern discussions on autopsy and anatomical dissection in Jewish law.[4]

Gintzburger concludes his dissertation with the following comment:

> Here I will stop. I could further diverge in this enormous field, entered by few, and collect scattered opinions by using a less unsystematic method, also compare them more precisely with the medicine of a more recent kind. But as this would require more work, reading and contemplation, I rest for now with this first outline of talmudic medicine.[5]

It was not long before Benzion Raphael Kohen (Benedetto) Frizzi contributed to the field with his *Dissertazione di Polizia Medica sul Pentateuco* (Pavia, 1787–1790), a thematic analysis of medicine and public health in the Torah and Jewish tradition. He subsequently expanded his research to produce a multivolume work in Hebrew of over a thousand pages addressing the medical and scientific aspects of the Talmud, *P'tah Einayim.*[6]

The nineteenth century saw more extensive contributions to the field of biblical and talmudic medicine. Eliakim Carmoly's *Histoire des Medicins Juifs Anciens et Modernes*, published in 1844, is one such work. However, despite its breadth and chronological precedence to the works of Wunderbar and Ebstein (see below), it is of little consequence in the history of the study of biblical and talmudic medicine, as Carmoly's theories are considered by many to be baseless and fantastical.[7]

---

4. *She'ilat Yavetz*, n. 41.
5. Schiller, op. cit., 600.
6. On Frizzi, see S. Simonsohn, *History of the Jews in the Duchy of Mantua* (Kiryat Sefer, 1977), 649, n. 226; Friedenwald, op. cit., 115. On his work, see B. Dinaburg, "Ben Tzion Hakohen Frizzi and His Work *Petah Einayim*," (Hebrew) *Tarbitz* 20(1948/49), 241–64; L. Dubin, "Medicine as Enlightenment Cure: Benedetto Frizzi, Physician to Eighteenth-Century Italian Jewish Society," *Jewish History* 26(2012), 201–221.
7. See S. Muntner, "*Yulius Preuss. Miholel HaMehkar BeToldot HaRefua HaIvrit HaKeduma*," *Koroth* 2:9–10 (May, 1961), 410. Carmoly only merits citation by Preuss for purposes of refutation. See J. Preuss, *Biblical and Talmudic Medicine*, trans. F. Rosner (Hebrew Publishing Company, 1978), 42 and 162.

The Dutch medical historian Abraham Hartog Israels, wrote his dissertation on talmudic gynecology upon completing his medical training at the University of Groningen, Netherlands in 1845. However, R. J. Wunderbar's *Biblisch-Talmudische Medicin*, completed in 1860, is the first systematic and comprehensive modern treatise of biblical and talmudic medicine. I. M. Rabbinowicz followed Gintzburger in composing a treatise restricted to talmudic medicine. Published in Paris in 1880, *La Medicine du Thalmud* is organized according to the tractates of the Talmud, with the tractate of *Ḥullin* occupying a disproportionately large part. Rabbinowicz later included a section on talmudic medicine in his introduction to the Talmud.[8] Wilhelm Ebstein also produced an important two-volume work; *Die Medizin im Alten Testament* (Stuttgart, 1901), devoted to biblical medicine, and *Die Medizin im Neuen Testament und im Talmud* (1903), devoted to talmudic medicine.

Despite the aforementioned ventures into the world of biblical and talmudic medicine, it is Julius Preuss who truly accomplished what Gintzburger only contemplated doing. His *Biblisch-Talmudische Medizin*, first published in 1911, remains the definitive reference work in this field. Arranged topically, it covers all organ systems and diseases mentioned in the Bible and Talmud with accompanying medical and historical commentary. Although others had endeavored to cover the entire field of biblical-talmudic medicine before him, Preuss considered his work to be a first for two reasons: it is the first composed by a physician, and the first derived from the study of the original sources.[9] Wunderbar was a layman, and Ebstein relied on translations to compile his work. All work subsequent to this *magnum opus* can only be considered supplemental in nature.

Despite the comprehensiveness of Preuss' work, there have been a number of noteworthy contributions thereafter. Dr. Judah Loeb Katznelson, a Russian-Jewish physician, poet and novelist wrote extensively on biblical and talmudic medicine.[10] After completing his medical

---

8. *Mavo HaTalmud* (1894).
9. J. Preuss, *Biblical and Talmudic Medicine*, trans. F. Rosner (Hebrew Publishing Company, 1978), 1.
10. See H. A. Savitz, "Judah Loeb Katznelson (1847–1916): Physician to the Soul of His People," in his *Profiles of Erudite Jewish Physicians and Scholars* (Spertus College Press, 1973), 56–61.

training, Katznelson opted to write a dissertation and take special exams in order to practice academic hospital-based medicine. The topic of his dissertation in Russian was normal and abnormal anatomy in ancient Hebrew literature in relation to ancient Greco-Roman medicine. This was followed by the publication of a small volume in Hebrew on talmudic anatomy in 1886 entitled *Remaḥ Evarim*, wherein Katznelson posits a creative physiological explanation to account for the rabbinic description and enumeration of 248 limbs in the body. This anatomical essay, in a revised form, was later incorporated into his *magnum opus, HaTalmud VeHokhmat HaRefua*," which was written in Hebrew and published posthumously in 1928 by his family. This work contains essays on hemophilia as described in the Talmud, the dermatological conditions of the Bible, including *tzara'at*, from a medical perspective, a dictionary of medical terminology translated into Greek, Russian and Hebrew, and a commentary on the section of the Talmud that deals with the laws of *kashrut*.

In 1926, Moshe Pearlman published *Midrash HaRefua*, a compilation and brief commentary of all passages relating to medicine and health found in the Babylonian and Jerusalem Talmuds and *midrashim*. Pearlman relates that he sent a copy of the third draft of his completed manuscript to Dr. Katznelson, and it was the latter who first informed him that others before had ventured into the field of biblical and talmudic medicine.[11] Aside from sharing his own works with Pearlman, Katznelson informed him of the works of Rabinowicz, Ebstein, and Preuss, none of which Pearlman had seen. In Pearlman's introduction, he says, "Had I known then that others had already done research in this field, I clearly would not have continued this work. However, I did not know... that voluminous works had been written by scholars versed in these topics... and I thought myself to be the redeemer of this long-forgotten discipline."[12] While, admittedly, there is significant overlap with earlier works, *Midrash HaRefua*, published with the notes of Dr. Katznelson, is still a novel and valuable contribution.

---

11. M. Pearlman, *Midrash HaRefua* (Devir Publishers, 1926), IX–XI.
12. Ibid.

In 1936, a novel contribution made its way into the field of biblical medicine by Charles Brim, a New York physician.[13] Victor Robinson best describes the nature of Brim's work:

> In method and interpretation, it does not follow any predecessor. It follows only the Hebrew text of the Torah and the commentary of Rashi (R. Shlomo Yitzhaki, eleventh-century biblical commentator). With the original text before him, the author brings to the subject a rare clinical insight, an unusual diagnostic ability. He perceives symptoms hidden from previous investigators and determines conditions not told in contemporary Gath or published in the streets of modern Ashkelon.

Much of the literature since the 1930s has appeared either in periodicals or as book chapters. Between 1937 and 1943, five volumes of the journal *Medical Leaves* were published. This journal of Jewish medical history contains many articles on biblical and talmudic medicine. Examples include R. Isaacs, "Hematology in the Bible and Talmud,"[14] S. R. Kagen, "Talmudic Medicine,"[15] D. I. Macht, "The Bible as a Source of Subjects for Scientific Research,"[16] and S. Boorstein, "Orthopedic Passages in the Bible and Talmud."[17]

The contributions of Dr. David Macht merit special mention. Born in Moscow in 1882, he emigrated to the United States where he completed his medical training at Johns Hopkins University in 1906. Macht was a prolific writer, publishing three books and over nine hundred original articles in the fields of science and medical/scientific history. Of the roughly one hundred works he wrote on medical history, many are devoted to biblical and talmudic medicine, with special emphasis on the pharmacological and physiological interpretations of biblical and rabbinic passages.[18]

---

13. C. J. Brim, *Medicine in the Bible* (Froben Press, 1936).

14. *Medical Leaves* 1 (1937), 76–80.

15. *Medical Leaves* 3:1 (1940), 164–173.

16. *Medical Leaves* 3 (1940), 174–184.

17. *Medical Leaves* 5 (1943), 49–55.

18. David Wilk composed a brief bio-bibliography of Macht's medical historical contributions which was published in *Koroth* 8:7–8 (August 1983), 305–317.

Other medical historians who devoted articles or chapters to biblical or talmudic medicine include M. B. Gordon,[19] B. L. Gordon,[20] and S. R. Kagan.[21]

Koroth, first published in April 1952, is a journal devoted entirely to Jewish medical history. For the first twenty years, the journal was edited by a triad consisting of Professor J. O. Leibowitz, Dr. S. Muntner, and Dr. David Margalit, all of whom contributed significantly to the field of Jewish medical history. Dr. Margalit devoted some of his efforts to biblical and talmudic medicine,[22] as did Professor Leibowitz, although to a lesser extent.[23] Professor S. Kottek joined the editorial staff of *Koroth* in the 1980s and, after the passing of the founding editors, assumed the editorial mantle, a position he maintains until this day. Professor Kottek has written more extensively on biblical and talmudic medicine than his predecessors and authored a serial column in the *Israel Journal of Medicine and Science* entitled "Gems from the Talmud."[24]

Throughout the years of its publication, *Koroth* has included numerous articles relating to biblical and talmudic medicine. Authors with multiple contributions in this field in the pages of *Koroth* include A. Shoshan, H. Kook, and M. Michael. Volume 8:7–8 (Fall 1982) is devoted entirely to biblical medicine, and a special issue of volume 9 (1988) contains the Proceedings of the Third International Symposium on Medicine in Bible and Talmud.

Another important journal in the field of Jewish medical history was the French language *Revue d'Histoire de la Medicine Hebraique*. Spanning almost forty years (1948–1985), it covered a broad range of

---

19. "Medicine Among the Ancient Hebrews," *ISIS* 33 (1941), 454–485.
20. "Ancient Hebrew Medicine," in his *Medicine Throughout Antiquity* (F. A. Davis, 1949), 25–294.
21. "Ancient Jewish Medicine," in his *Jewish Medicine* (Medico-Historical Press, 1952), 27–63.
22. See bibliography of his works until 1973 in *Koroth* 6:5–6 (November, 1973), 367–372.
23. See bibliography of his works in *Koroth* 8:11–12 (Summer 1985), 7–23.
24. See bibliography of his works until 1991 in *Koroth* 9:11–12 (Summer 1991), 755–766.

topics including those related to biblical and talmudic medicine. Selections from the journal were recently republished in a separate volume.[25]

For the past thirty years, the contributions to this field can largely be found in the periodical literature of three disciplines: medical history, Judaic studies, and medicine. The topic of artificial respiration in the Bible is illustrative, as articles on this topic have appeared in every one of the aforementioned literatures, as listed by discipline below:

Medical Literature

F. Rosner, "Artificial Respiration in Biblical Times," *New York State Journal of Medicine* 69:8 (April 15, 1969): 1104–1105; Z. Rosen, "Rhinological Aspects of Biblical Resuscitation," *Archives of Otolaryngology* 95:5 (May, 1972): 488–489; Z. Rosen and J. Davidson, "Respiratory Resuscitation in Ancient Hebrew Sources," *Anesthesia and Analgesia* 51:4 (July-August, 1972): 502–505; L. Wislicki, "A Biblical Case of Hypothermia-Resuscitation by Rewarming (Elisha's Method)," *Clio Medica* 9:3 (September, 1974): 213–214; R. B. Howard, "… And There is Nothing New Under the Sun," *Postgraduate Medicine* 65:3 (March, 1979): 25; J. H. Comroe, jr., "…In Comes the Good Air," *American Review of Respiratory Diseases* 119:6 (June, 1979): 1025–1031.

Judaic Studies Literature

A. S. Abraham, *"Hanshama Melakhutit BeTanakh,"* *HaMa'ayan* 28:3 (*Nisan*, 5748): 72–76.

Medical History Literature

E. Tratner, "Intubation Mentioned in the Talmud and by Jacob ben Asher," *Koroth* 8:7–8 (August, 1983), 333–338; J. A. Paraskos, "Biblical Accounts of Resuscitation," *Journal of the History of Medicine and Allied Sciences* 47:3 (July, 1992): 310–321.

Access to this vast and diverse literature is no longer restricted only to the expert of any particular field, nor does it require visitation to obscure libraries. Computer databases now make this material easily

---

25. G. Freudenthal and S. Kottek, *Etudes Choisies de la Revue d'Histoire de la Medicine Hebraique* (Brill, 2003).

accessible to any interested researcher, and the searches can be performed on the Internet. A search on Histline, the National Library of Medicine's (NLM) database on medical history, will yield roughly five hundred items relating to biblical and talmudic medicine; a search on NLM's Medline, which includes hundreds of contemporary medical journals in its database, will likewise yield hundreds of entries on these topics. My objective is not to provide a list of these works, which can be easily accessed by the reader, but I should like to point out a few trends that can be found in the literature.

Determining the medical diagnosis of biblical or talmudic personalities still occupies a significant part of the research, and articles of this nature can be found in the literature of varied disciplines. Not dissimilar to Bartholin's essay some three hundred years ago, one author has endeavored to provide a modern medical explanation for Jacob's limp.[26] Many others have applied the same diagnostic principles to other biblical personalities.[27]

The identification of biblical diseases—in particular, the skin disease *tzaraʼat*—continues to maintain the interest of physicians and historians, with enough material being produced so as to necessitate bibliographical articles restricted exclusively to this topic.[28]

Another common trend is to interpret biblical and talmudic cases as being "the first reported case" of a particular disease. While it is true that the Bible and the Talmud, by virtue of their antiquity, often contain early descriptions of certain diseases, many of these articles

---

26. L. J. Hoenig, "Jacob's Limp," *Seminars in Arthritis and Rheumatism* 26:4 (February, 1997), 684–688.

27. See, for example, A. de Vries and A. Weinberger, "King Asaʼa Presumed Gout," *Koroth* 6:9–10 (December, 1974), 561–567; A. Shoshan, "The Illness of Rabbi Judah the Patriarch," *Koroth* 7:5–6 (November, 1977), 521–524; S. Levin, "Isaac's Blindness: A Medical Diagnosis," *Judaism* 38:1 (Winter 1988), 81–83.

28. See, for example, A. D. Rabinowitz and Bezalel Naor, "The Medical Aspects of Zaraʼat: Selected Bibliography," *Orot* 1 (1991): 30–32; G. Milgram, "On Zaraʼat: A Bibliographical Overview," *Koroth* 9:11–12 (Summer 1992), 818–825. Some have utilized medicine to interpret biblical passages in a new light. See, for example, E. V. Hulce, "Joshua's Curse and the Abandonment of Ancient Jericho: Schistosomiasis as a Possible Medical Explanation." *Medical History* 15:4 (October, 1971), 376–386.

involve reinterpretation of passages based on modern understanding of medicine.[29]

These are just three trends found in the literature, but the evolution of the study of biblical and talmudic medicine parallels the evolution of medicine itself. As new discoveries continue to affect our understanding of medicine and human disease, there will always be those who will apply this new knowledge to the interpretation of the medical passages in the Bible and Talmud. One author employs a modern understanding of the transmission of infectious diseases to advance the theory that the requirement to eliminate the storage houses of grain for Passover served in the Middle Ages to effectively prevent the spread of plague amongst the Jewish people by eliminating the rodents' vectors.[30] The veracity of this theory notwithstanding, it could not have been advanced until but a few decades ago. What does the future hold for the field of biblical-talmudic medicine? I suspect we will have to follow the developments in medicine in order to find out.

ADDENDUM: BIBLIOGRAPHICAL LITERATURE ON BIBLICAL AND TALMUDIC MEDICINE

The earliest bibliography of ancient medicine was published in the *Dictionare des Sciences Medicales* in Paris, 1819, listing twenty-six items. In 1842, J. L. Choulant included many entries about biblical and talmudic medicine in his classic *Bibliotheca Medico-Historica*.[31] As part of his monumental contribution to Jewish bibliography in general, Moritz Steinschneider published, in 1886, *Schriften uber Medicin in Bibel und*

---

29. S. Leons, " The First Reported Case of Radial Nerve Palsy," *Southern Medical Journal* 86:7 (July, 1993) 808–811; M. A. Goldenhersh, "Rapid Whitening of the Hair First Reported in the Talmud: Possible Mechanisms of This Intriguing Phenomenon," *Americal Journal of Dermatopathology* 14:4 (1992), 367–368; H. Decher, "Brachio-cervical Syndrome: First Case Report Over 3,000 Years Ago," Laryngorhinootologie 75:4 (April, 1996), 255–6; I. Schiff and M. Schiff, "The Biblical Diagnostician and the Anorexic Bride," *Fertility and Sterility* 69:1 (January, 1998), 8–10.

30. M. J. Blaser, "Passover and Plague," *Perspectives in Biology and Medicine* 41:2 (Winter 1998), 243–256.

31. See H. Friedenwald, *The Jews and Medicine* (Johns Hopkins Press, 1944), 109–110; S. R. Kagan, "The Bibliography of Ancient Jewish Medicine," *Bulletin of the History of Medicine* 22 (1948), 480–485.

Talmud.[32] Wunderbar and Ebstein both included bibliographies in their works. Preuss wrote an extensive bibliography covering the literature up to his time. However, it was not comprehensive and was apparently completed by Adolph Levinger, who circulated this supplement in stencil form.[33] In 1935, Friedenwald, like Preuss before him, compiled an extensive bibliography of the works that had appeared until his day.[34] S. R. Kagan supplemented and updated Friedenwald's bibliography in 1948.[35] A bibliography of Jewish bibliographies, including those relating to biblical-talmudic medicine, was compiled by S. Shunami.[36] Nahum Rakover's *Bibliography of Jewish Law*, first published in Hebrew in 1975, with second editions in both Hebrew and English published in 1990, contains a section on medical Jewish law (halakha), wherein numerous entries are devoted to biblical and talmudic medicine. Finally, the contemporary bibliographical periodical *Current Works in the History of Medicine*, published by the Wellcome Institute of the History of Medicine, contains entries on Bible and Talmud.

In the spirit of Gintzburger, cited above, here I will stop. I could further diverge in this enormous field, entered by many. But, alas, I rest for now with this outline of the bibliography of biblical and talmudic medicine.

---

32. In *Wiener Klinische Rundschau* 10 (1896), 433–435 and 452–453.
33. The supplement was apparently not published. See Muntner, op. cit., 412.
34. H. Friedenwald, *The Jews and Medicine* (Johns Hopkins Press, 1944), 99–145.
35. S. R. Kagan, "The Bibliography of Ancient Jewish Medicine," *Bulletin of the History of Medicine* 22 (1948), 480–485.
36. S. Shunami, *Bibliography of Jewish Bibliographies* (Magnes Press, 1965), 313–318.

A Letter from a Torah Sage of the Eighteenth Century to the Faculty of a Medical School: The Selective Deference of Rabbi Yonatan Eybeschuetz to Medical Expertise

I. INTRODUCTION

The study of medical halakha today is the most complex it has ever been in history. The literature of medicine is so vast that its mastery has long been out the grasp of any one individual. The halakhic dilemmas increase exponentially in tandem with the science. As always, good halakhic decisions require good facts. It is impossible to be a *posek* in all areas of medical halakha today without a cadre of medical experts in your contacts list. The notion of consulting medical experts to adjudicate areas of halakha is by no means a new one, though perhaps its need has become more acute. The Talmud already records such cases, as we shall see. The exact nature of the acceptance of medical testimony into the halakhic process, however, has been a matter of continued debate. The discussions fall under the heading of "*ne'emanut harofim*," the reliability or trustworthiness of physicians. While this topic has been amply covered elsewhere,[1] we focus here on the writings of one rabbinic authority. This brief entry represents a small contribution to this evolving literature.

In this chapter, I focus on the relationship of one great Torah sage of the eighteenth century, R. Yonatan Eybeschuetz[2] (1690–1764), to contemporaneous medical knowledge. While his name has surfaced a number of times in this book in the course of halakhic discussions on various topics, here we shift our focus to the individual, in an attempt to glean R. Eybeschuetz's unique approach to integrated medical knowledge into his halakhic decisions. R. Eybeschuetz was a Talmudist and Halakhist of the highest order, an internationally recognized Torah giant who held positions as the *dayan* (rabbinic judge) of Prague, and later as the rabbi of the "Three Communities" (Altona, Hamburg and Wandsbek). He authored halakhic works on the *Shulḥan Arukh and* Maimonides' *Mishneh Torah*, as well as a variety of homiletic works. He is famously known as the protagonist in the protracted Emden-Eybeschuetz controversy, to which we will refer below.[3]

---

1. See A. Steinberg, *Entzyclopedia Hilkhatit Refuit* (2nd ed.) 5 (Schlesinger Institute, 5766), s. v., "*Ne'emanut HaRofeh*." This general topic includes both the reliability of physician testimony, as well as the reliability of medical knowledge, such as blood typing, HLA testing, and DNA testing. See also, Rav Kook, *Da'at Kohen*, n. 140 (re: *metzitza*), and S. T. Rubenstein, "The Reliability of Physicians in Matters of Halakha," (Hebrew) *Torah Sheba'al Peh* 33 (5752), 47–51. For a list of cases where rabbis consulted physicians, see H. J. Zimmels, *Magicians, Theologians and Doctors* (Edward Goldston and Son, 1952), 177, note 59.

2. There are variant spellings for the name: Eybeschütz, Eybeschutz, Eibeschutz, Eyebeschutz, Eyebeschuetz.

3. This essay represents a small contribution about the writings of R. Eybeschuetz on medicine, a topic about which little has been written. R. Yaakov Emden, however, addressed medicine more explicitly and frequently in his writings, especially relating to alchemy. For more on this topic, see the excellent work of Maoz Kahana, "An Esoteric Path to Modernity: Rabbi Jacob Emden's Alchemical Quest," *Journal of*

R. Eybeschuetz cultivated relationships with non-Jews as well; for example, collaborating with the Jesuit, Father Franciscus Haselbauer, and other Catholic clergy, to publish editions of the Torah and Talmud.[4] He also taught Hebrew to Christians, such as Olaf Gerhard Tychsen,[5] who later became professor at the University of Butzow.[6] Tychsen is infamous in Jewish medical history for instigating the Duke of Mecklenberg to legislate delay of burial for three days to confirm death, targeting the Jewish population specifically. This law precipitated worldwide halakhic debates of the definition of death and delayed burial.[7]

R. Eybeschuetz was also conversant in the sciences, such as astronomy, as reflected in his comments on the theories of Copernicus, with whom he disagreed, and about which he debated with Christian theologians.[8]

In this chapter, we address the approach of R. Eybeschuetz to medical issues.[9] The first example in our discussion, to which the title refers, is one that I had initially intended to address independently in

Modern Jewish Studies 12:2 (July, 2013), 253–275; idem, "The Scientific Revolution and the Encoding of Sources of Knowledge: Medicine, Halakha, and Alchemy in Hamburg-Altona, 1736," (Hebrew) *Tarbitz* 82:1 (*Tishrei-Kislev* 5774), 165–212.

4. See P. Maciejko, "The Rabbi and the Jesuit: On Rabbi Jonathan Eibeschutz and Father Franciscus Haselbauer Editing the Talmud," *Jewish Social Studies* 20:2 (Winter 2014), 147–184. I thank R. Dr. J. J. Schacter for directing me to this reference, as well as for other helpful suggestions.

5. S. Z. Leiman, "Two Cases of Non-Jews with Rabbinic Ordination," http://seforim. blogspot.com/2006/11/dr-leimans-post-two-cases-of-non-jews.html (November 16, 2006), accessed October 22, 2015. For more on Tychsen, see E. Reichman,"What Became of Tychsen? The Non-Jewish 'Rabbi' and his 'Congregation' of Jewish Medical Students," Seforim Blog (https://seforimblog.com), November 1, 2020.

6. In that capacity, Tychsen mentored Markus Moses, a Jewish medical student who completed a number of medical research papers on Jewish topics under his tutelage. See D. Wilk, "Markus Moses' Doctoral Dissertation or Who Remembers Butzow," *Koroth* 9:3–4 (1986), 408–426.

7. R. Yaakov Emden would play a key role in the discussion of this halakhic issue.

8. See Jeremy Brown's recent definitive work on the Jewish approach to the work of Copernicus, *New Heavens and a New Earth* (Oxford University Press: 2013), 155–161.

9. While R. Eybeschuetz is perhaps best known for his prescription of amulets, these were not in the realm of conventional medical practice. As such, we refrain from addressing this topic here and restrict ourselves to conventional medical matters. See S. Z. Leiman and S. Schwarzfuchs, "New Evidence on the Emden Eibescheutz Controversy: The Amulets from Metz," *Revue des Etudes Juives* 165:1–2 (January-June 2006), 229–249.

order to highlight a new discovery. This source stands at the interface of two of Jewish history's most storied and contentious episodes. On further reflection, however, I deemed it necessary to place this passage in the context of other references of R. Eybeschuetz to medical knowledge. Following our historical discussion of the first reference, we will analyze a number of other medical passages culled from his different works in order to flesh out his approach to medicine.

II. THE CASE OF THE HEARTLESS CHICKEN

Background

In his commentary on *Yoreh Deʾah*, R. Eybeschuetz comments on the halakhic status of an animal whose heart has been removed.[10] Is such an animal considered a *treifa*, a term applied to animals with terminal pathological conditions that limit their longevity; or perhaps, it is considered a *neveila*, a term restricted to a dead animal, as it is impossible for an animal to live without a heart for even a moment? There are legal ramifications to this definitional distinction. While R. Karo codifies an animal whose heart has been removed as a *treifa*, Maimonides famously omits this law from his code. This glaring omission spawned much conjecture over the centuries. R. Eybeschuetz postulates that while Maimonides was medically convinced that a "heartless" animal would indeed be a *neveila*, as it could not possibly live at all in such a state, his inability to find clear halakhic support for this scientifically based position forced him to omit this law altogether.

It is in this context that he cites a related responsum. In 1709, a housewife asked a simple question of R. Tzvi Ashkenazi, known as Ḥakham Tzvi, the answer to which would reverberate for centuries. In preparing a chicken for dinner, the woman was unable to locate the heart. Is such a chicken kosher, she asked?[11] R. Ashkenazi used this question as a springboard to discuss the importance of the heart in general.[12] Regarding the matter at hand, he concluded that the chicken

---

10. *Kreti UPleti*, Y. D., 40:5. On this case, see Maoz Kahana, *A Heartless Chicken: Religion and Science in Early Modern Rabbinic Culture* (Bialik Institute, 2021).
11. *Teshuvot Ḥakham Tzvi*, 74 and 77.
12. In other chapters of this book, we have placed the theories of R. Ashkenazi on cardiac and respiratory physiology into a medical historical context. See chapters, "The

was kosher because it is impossible for the chicken to have been born and to have survived to the point of slaughter without a heart. It must therefore be that the chicken was never in fact heartless, rather, simply appeared so, as a cat had likely eaten or removed the heart. R. Ashkenazi went even further and added that if two upstanding witnesses opened a chicken and claimed they found no heart, we would declare them false witnesses,[13] and the chicken would be considered kosher. This controversial statement was subsequently addressed by a number of rabbinic authorities.[14] Amongst them was R. Eybeschuetz, who while agreeing with R. Ashkenazi's ruling in this specific case, took particular exception to his additional statement, which he militantly refuted.[15]

The Letter of R. Eybeschuetz to the Medical Faculty of the University of Halle

R. Eybeschuetz argued that perhaps animals can have structures that serve the function of the heart but do not externally appear to have a "normal" heart. Such animals would be considered a *treifa* due to the abnormal anatomy. It could, therefore, possibly appear to witnesses that an animal was "heartless," when in fact it possesses a heart substitute and is a *treifa* (as opposed to a *neveila*) and thus not halakhically permitted. To support this novel scientific theory and clarify the facts, R. Eybeschuetz wrote a letter to the University of Halle medical faculty to obtain the definitive medical opinion on this issue. He enlisted the assistance of R. Henoch Halle to personally deliver an inquiry "that they call responsa" to the university. He records their response in its entirety:

Halakhic Definition of Death in Light of Medical History," and "The Incorporation of Pre-Modern Scientific Theories into Rabbinic Literature: The Case of Innate Heat."

13. Based on Rashba 1:98.

14. *Ḥakham Tzvi im Likutei He'arot*, 2nd ed. (Makhon Dovev Meisharim, 5765), 409–413. I thank Professor Shnayer Leiman for directing me to this reference.

15. Rashba had ruled that if witnesses testify that an animal designated by Ḥazal as a *treifa* actually lived longer than twelve months we would consider them false witnesses and uphold the words of Ḥazal. According to R. Eybeschuetz, this decision was applied to render a stricter decision, but could not be applied to render a lenient decision, as R. Ashkenazi is doing in this case (by considering the chicken kosher and allowing it to be eaten).

We have received two questions for which we do not know the reason. It has been requested of us to provide our expert medical opinion from this institution based on the principles of medicine and anatomy. We convened together and after analysis and discussion we agreed upon the following response, which we present before you. The substance of the first question: Is it possible for an animal to live for any period of time after the heart has been removed either through sickness or through any other means? First of all, you should know that there is no possibility whatsoever for a heart to disintegrate through sickness. It is true that there are illnesses that affect the heart directly and experience has shown that these can weaken and diminish the heart's function. One may also find a growth (in the heart) in the shape of an insect, called the polypus... however in all these cases the heart remains anchored in the chest cavity and does not move from its place, nor does it disintegrate or disappear completely, something which is impossible. The animal stricken with this cardiac illness will struggle to survive as long as the disease does not overcome him and the heart, the source of life, does not cease to beat entirely. But if the disease progresses to the extent that cardiac motion ceases, then certainly the creature stricken with this disease will die. It is evident from this that if it was conceivable for the heart to somehow be completely removed (through disease) surely the creature would succumb. For it is impossible for a creature to live even one moment, just as it is impossible for any being to live if the heart is physically removed or cut out. Such a creature would die immediately or within a brief time once the heart is removed...

Regarding your second query: If a chicken or similar bird is opened and no heart is found, is it possible that there is another structure that serves the function of the heart? We preface our response with this principle: It is physiologically impossible for any living creature, whether bird or animal, to live without a heart or some analogous structure which serves the same function. Such a structure must have a cavity with connected vessels, which serve to transmit and circulate the blood to the rest of the body.

Therefore, if there is such an analogous organ with the required specifications for the physiological function usually required for the heart, it is certainly possible for a bird to live for a prolonged period of time, even if the organ does not bear external resemblance to the heart, even if the organ is found in a different anatomical location than the heart, either above or below.

All this we have agreed upon

A Newly Discovered Corroboration of the Letter

In my research on the history of Jewish medical students,[16] I came across a slim volume that documents the Jewish physicians of the eighteenth and nineteenth centuries at the University of Halle as reflected in the holdings of the university archives.[17] The University of Halle opened its doors to Jewish students at that period, which was a rarity in Europe. In addition to documenting the Jewish medical students at this time, this volume *inter alia* mentions correspondence between the Jewish community and the medical faculty, mostly related to specific medical consultations. It occurred to me that perhaps the archives might have a record of the question posed by R. Eybeschuetz regarding the heartless chicken. I contacted the University of Halle archivist,[18] noting the aforementioned volume, and provided suggested dates and context, using the date of the publication of the *Kreti U'Pleti*, 1763, as a rough chronological guideline. Remarkably, my inquiry was soon met with a positive response.[19]

---

16. E. Reichman, "The History of the Jewish Medical Student Dissertation: An Evolving Jewish Tradition," in J. Karp and M. Schaikewitz, eds., *Sacred Training: A Halakhic Guidebook for Medical Students and Residents* (Ammud Press, 2018), xvii- xxxvii.

17. W. Kaiser and A Volker, *Judaica Medica des 18 und des Fruhen 19 Jahrhunderts in den Bestanden des Halleschen Univeritatsarchivs* (Wisseschaftliche Beitrage der Martin Luther Universitat Halle-Wittenberg, 1979).

18. The authors of the aforementioned book are no longer affiliated with the University of Halle.

19. In retrospect, I realized that the archival section referring to the question of R. Eybeschuetz had actually been pictured in the book of Kaiser and Volker all along, though it was barely legible and not identified. The line above it, regarding a medical consultation from the Jewish community, was noted in the accompanying caption.

Mr. Stefan Fink, whom I thank for his assistance, sent me a copy of a handwritten entry, which though scant on details, clearly refers to the question of R. Eybeschuetz. Below is the text, followed by his translation.

> *1763 den 8. Januar ist ein Responsum auf 2 von der Judenschaft übergebene Fragen, wegen einiger bey ihren Schächten vorkommenden Umstände, ertheilt worden.*[20]
> January 8, 1763: A Responsum to two questions from the Jewish community concerning the circumstances of Jewish kosher slaughter has been issued.

The following reasons lead me to the definitive conclusion that this entry refers to our letter. R. Eybeschuetz used the word "responsum" as the term for the inquiry, which is identical to the term in the text from the archives; the topic of discussion was ritual slaughter; two questions were asked; and the date is appropriate, as the *Kreti U'Pleti* was published later in 1763. Unfortunately, the text of the faculty's response is not included in the archival record. However, as the text of the entire response is included in the work of R. Eybeschuetz (see above), its absence from the archive is of limited consequence.

In addition to highlighting the importance of this one letter as a reflection of the nature of the rabbi-doctor/medical expert relationship, I wish to broaden our scope and fill in some historical context to this letter. This letter was part of a halakhic exchange that would ultimately be co-opted for a contemporary medical halakhic debate, one of medical halakhic history's most famous. In addition, here we describe for the first time a historical corroboration to the letter, with its dating having possible ramifications for another fascinating chapter in Jewish history.

After completion of this article, I found that R. H. J. Zimmels (1900–1974) had also written to the University of Halle to see if the case of R. Eybeschuetz was kept in their records, though he received a negative response. See Zimmels, op. cit., 178.

20. "Tagebuch der Medizinischen Fakultät" 1744–1801, Universitätsarchiv der Universität Halle-Wittenberg, Rep. 29/F/VII, Nr. 1, Bd. 1, Blatt 173r.

Historical Relevance of the Letter

The date of the query, January 1763, may have some historical consequence relating to the famous dispute involving R. Eybeschuetz and
R. Yaakov Emden. Indeed, it may place the final nail in the coffin of an
already long discredited theory about the very origins of their prolonged
embittered battle.[21]

The lifelong bitter rivalry between these two towering Torah
giants of the eighteenth century has provided sustenance for many a
Jewish historian. One of the subsections of this discussion focuses on
the origins of the rivalry. Most trace the beginning of the rivalry to the
discovery of amulets penned by R. Eybeschuetz intended for the protection and safety of pregnant women and their fetuses. These amulets
were found to contain possible veiled references to the false messiah,
Shabbtai Tzvi, which invoked the ire of R. Yaakov Emden.

R. Reuven Margulies suggests that the controversy began when
R. Eybeschuetz disagreed with the *pesak* of the Ḥakham Tzvi, R. Emden's
father, regarding this very case of the heartless chicken.[22] This theory is
predicated on the assumption that R. Eybeschuetz sent the query to the
University of Halle when he was a young man, shortly after the original
responsum of the Ḥakham Tzvi was written. The archival dating of the
question clearly proves otherwise, confirming that in fact the query was
submitted much later, just one year before R. Eybeschuetz' demise. Thus,
as has already been agreed upon by scholars, though now with definitive
chronological evidence, this could not possibly have initiated the feud.[23]

---

21. I thank Professor Shnayer Leiman and R. Dr. J. J. Schacter and for their assistance
and guidance for the content of this section.

22. R. Margulies, *Sibat Hitnagduto shel Rabbenu Yaakov MeiEmden LeRabbeinu Yehonatan
Eybeschuetz* (Tel-Aviv, 1941). I thank Professor Leiman for graciously furnishing me
with this reference.

23. Dr. Leiman has drawn my attention to the fact that there are many substantive reasons why this theory is baseless, including the fact that R. Eybeschuetz in principle
agreed with R. Emden regarding the analysis of the heartless chicken case. In fact,
in R. Emden's personal copy of the *Kreti UPleti*, which contains his handwritten
marginalia, he even accuses R. Eybeschuetz of plagiarizing his writings on this topic.
See Y. Raphael, "The Notes of Rabbi Yaakov Emden to the *Kreti UPleti* of Rabbi
Yonatan Eybeschuetz," (Hebrew) *Sinai* 74 (1974), 37–41.

The University of Halle and the Jews

It is noteworthy that R. Eybeschuetz specifically chose the University of Halle as the destination for his query. There were other prominent medical schools in Germany. Perhaps because in addition to being one of the premier medical schools in the eighteenth century, it was particularly open to Jewish students, similar to the University of Padua in Italy, and was the address for many Jewish students of this period. This would explain perhaps why his esteemed colleague R. Henoch Halle had entrée into the halls of the university.

At the same time as R. Halle was delivering R. Eybeshuetz's letter to the University of Halle, likely sitting in a classroom a few yards away was Leon Elias Hirschel, a Jewish medical student in his final year. Hirschel graduated in 1763, writing his dissertation on manic depression.[24] Many of the dissertations of the Jewish students in Halle have been documented,[25] and of note, in over a span of some 100 years, two of the Jewish students wrote their dissertations on uniquely Jewish topics.[26]

The Heartless Chicken and the Modern-Day Debate on the Definition of Death

While there was debate as to how long the heartless chicken itself could survive, the halakhic debate surrounding it remains very much alive. For millennia, death had always been defined exclusively as cessation of heartbeat, though, to be sure, the ability of physicians to accurately diagnose death was often challenged. In the late twentieth century, a new and alternate diagnosis of death was advanced, known as brain death. This new medical condition generated an array of profound halakhic

---

24. Leon Elias Hirschel, *De Morbis Melancholico-Maniacis*, University of Halle medical dissertation (1763).
25. See, Kaiser and Volker, op. cit.
26. Salomon Bernard Wolffsheimer wrote on gynecology and fertility in rabbinic literature in 1742, and Meyer Levin wrote on the history of the Jews and medicine in 1798. Both of these dissertations were written in Latin, as was the convention for dissertations of that time. For further discussion of Jewish medical student dissertations on Jewish topics, see E. Reichman, "The History of the Jewish Medical Student Dissertation: An Evolving Jewish Tradition," in J. Karp and M. Schaikewitz, eds., *Sacred Training: A Halakhic Guidebook for Medical Students and Residents* (Ammud Press, 2018), xvii–xxxvii.

ramifications for a patient carrying this diagnosis, as any modern reader with a modicum of interest in medical halakha will attest. The discussion of the acceptance of cessation of brain function as a legal definition of death is known as the brain death debate.[27] This debate remains one of the most prolonged animated and contentious debates in medical halakhic history.

In seeking halakhic precedent for this novel dilemma, *poskim* resuscitated the halakhic narrative of the heartless chicken, launched by the responsum of the Ḥakham Tzvi.[28] In that responsum, R Ashkenazi devoted a lengthy discussion to the primacy of the heart in the definition of life. The authorities that required cardiac cessation to define death turned to this responsum as support.[29] The subsequent responses to the Ḥakham Tzvi, including the passage from R. Eybeschuetz have also been incorporated into the contemporary halakhic discussions.

For example, R. Levi Yitzḥak Halperin, on the topic of organ donation and the determination of death in halakha, devotes an entire chapter to the reliability of physicians regarding the determination of death,[30] focusing on the case of the heartless chicken and the responses of Rabbis Ashkenazi and Eybeschuetz. He asserts that both of them invoked and relied upon medical opinion in the formulation of their halakhic responses.[31]

Regarding the approach of R. Eybeschuetz to medical knowledge, the above discussion leaves the impression that he was respectful and deferential to the knowledge of physicians, even actively pursuing their consultation to assist in halakhic analysis. Was this consistently his approach? We now turn our attention to other passages from his works

---

27. For an overview of the brain death debate, see A. Steinberg, *Entzyclopedia Hilkhatit Refuit* (2nd ed.) 6 (Schlesinger Institute, 5766), s. v., "*rega hamavet*."

28. See, for example, *Iggerot Moshe Y. D.*, 2:146.

29. See, for example, J. D. Bleich, "Of Cerebral, Respiratory and Cardiac Death," *Tradition* 24:3 (Spring, 1989), 44–66.

30. *Ma'aseh Ḥoshev* 4:23, chapter 14.

31. R. Halperin specifically emphasizes that R. Eybeschuetz relied upon the physicians when they do not contradict the received tradition (*kabbala*) of Ḥazal. See below for further discussion on this issue.

that relate to medical matters in the hopes of garnering a more complete and nuanced view of his integration of medical knowledge.

III. THE REMARRIAGE OF WIDOWED NURSING MOTHERS

R. Eybeschuetz solicited and referred to medical experts in other cases as well, such as in the case of the widowed nursing woman. In addressing a number of different cases on this topic he provides valuable insights into his approach to medical knowledge.

As this area of halakha is lesser known, a basic overview of the principles of this topic, known as *meineket ḥavero* (the nursing woman/ wife of one's friend) is presented below.[32]

The *Shulḥan Arukh*[33] rules that if a woman is widowed or divorced at the time when she is pregnant, or while she is nursing an infant, she may not remarry until the infant reaches the age of twenty-four months. The sages enacted this prohibition out of concern that the woman, in her desire to remarry, and realizing that her options are more limited while she nurses an infant, may try to wean the child to raise the chances of finding a husband. Twenty-four months is the age when babies would generally stop nursing, and the sages feared that a child would be endangered if the mother discontinued breastfeeding before that age. They therefore enacted that a woman who is divorced or widowed while she is pregnant or nursing should not get married, or even accept *kiddushin* (halakhic betrothal), until the child is twenty-four months old. This ensures that she will continue nursing the child until he or she reaches the age of twenty-four months.[34]

---

32. For a comprehensive review of halakhic issues related to nursing, see S. Kohen, *Torat HaMeineket* (Self-Publication, Jerusalem, 5772). Regarding the application of the decree to delay remarriage today, when ample milk substitutes are readily available, see pp. 120 ff.

33. *Even Ha'ezer* 13.

34. http://www.dailyhalacha.com/m/halacha.aspx?id=2086. If, in a situation where this prohibition does apply, the woman remarried in violation of halakha, then the rabbinic court uses its authority to coerce the new husband to divorce the woman. It places the husband under *nidui* (excommunication) until he agrees to give the wife a divorce, and he pays her *Ketubah*. Assuming he is not a *Kohen* (in which case he is forbidden from marrying a divorcee), he may remarry the woman after the child

In one circumstance, the Elder R. Akiva Eiger,[35] author of *Mishnat Rabbi Akiva Eiger*, penned a permissive ruling to a question regarding the remarrying of a widowed nursing woman. He forwarded his responsum to R. Eybeschuetz for analysis and corroboration of his conclusion, a common practice in responsa literature.[36]

The question to R. Eiger involved a woman who refrained from nursing for a medical reason.[37] R. Eiger ruled that the law of *meineket ḥavero* did not apply to this woman, as the medical situation anyway precluded her nursing, and that she would be free to marry without delay. However, due to the gravity of the situation and ambiguity of the nature of the medical condition, he forwarded the query to R. Eybeschuetz for consideration as well.

R. Eybeschuetz introduces his response with an endorsement of R. Eiger's conclusion and declares *"halakha keRabbi Akiva,"* playing off the talmudic principle that the law follows the position of R. Akiva, though in this case referring to R. Akiva Eiger. From this lengthy responsum we focus primarily on the medical comments. R. Eybeschuetz references a responsum of R. Yaakov Reischer[38] regarding the application

---

reaches the age of twenty-four months, and, of course, he must write a new *Ketubah*. There are a number of exceptions to this law, such as if the child dies, of if the woman stopped nursing even before the husband dies.

35. Grandfather of the better-known R. Akiva Eiger, author of *Ḥidushei R. Akiva Eiger*.

36. See *Bnei Ahuva* 1 (Zikhron Aharon—Weinreb Edition: Jerusalem, 5767), section *She'elot UTeshuvot, siman aleph*, 283–298.

37. The facts of the case are as follows: A physician had married a woman who died of tuberculosis (Schwindsucht is the term mentioned in the responsum), which the physician attributed to her breast-feeding. He subsequently married his first wife's sister and adamantly forbade her from nursing out of fear she would succumb to the same condition. They had ten children, none of whom she nursed. Upon the death of the physician husband, the woman was pregnant. The community suggested she marry another physician, who would practice in the town. Timing was a factor in the marriage arrangements, and there was concern that the physician would not agree to marry her if there was delay. However, the normative halakha required waiting 24 months after the birth of the child of the widowed woman. The question to R. Eiger was whether this case represented a possible exception to the rule of *meineket ḥavero*, as she had not nursed any of her previous children and would dare not nurse any subsequent children due to a medical concern.

38. *Shevut Yaakov, E. H.,* 97. This responsum includes the full text of a rabbinic authority who ruled strictly in the case and forbade the woman from remarrying early. While this author remains anonymous in the published *Shevut Yaakov*, R. Eybeschuetz,

of the law of *meineket havero*.[39] In that case, the physicians determined, after the death of nursed children, that the woman's milk was poisonous, and that she should refrain from nursing any subsequent children lest the same fate befall them. The rabbis who ruled permissively based their ruling on the fact that since the woman's milk was deemed poisonous, there was no fear whatsoever that she would ever nurse, thus the decree of *meineket havero* would be rendered moot.

R. Eybeschuetz cast aspersion on the permissive ruling, though he ultimately accepted it, based on his medical analysis. The doctors had testified that the woman's milk was poisonous. According to R. Eybeschuetz, based on the research of scientists, the woman's milk is a composite derivative from the vessels of the body that come from the heart.[40] Thus, if the milk of a woman were poisonous enough to cause fatal harm to her children, surely she herself would manifest serious signs of illness. However, this woman was known to be quite healthy and well-nourished.[41] He thought the woman's physician to be incompetent.

He consulted with a certain Zalman the physician[42] as to whether a woman with poisonous milk could appear so healthy, and Zalman concurred it was impossible. In addition, as with the case of the heartless chicken, he presented the case to a medical faculty, in this instance the

---

in discussing the case, reveals the author's identity as R. Avraham Brode, who had been involved in a disagreement with Ḥakham Tzvi. R. Brode devotes a section of his response to the reliability of physicians.

39. In that case the woman nursed her first three children, all of whom died during the period of nursing. She went on to have additional children all of whom were nursed by a hired nursemaid. Her husband then died while she was pregnant with an additional child, and she hired a nursemaid for that child as well. The question was whether she could remarry immediately as there was no fear that she would nurse her child.

40. The Talmud states that breast milk derives from blood, presumably menstrual blood. See, for example, *Nidda* 9a. This was not a uniquely rabbinic notion and was espoused by many scientists and cultures from antiquity to pre-modern times.

41. R. Eybeschuetz also happened to have personal knowledge of the facts in this case. The woman was a distant relative of his and later came to visit his wife in Prague, when he was able to confirm the nature of her health.

42. Zimmels identifies him as Zalman Gomperz, though I am not sure on what basis. See Zimmels, op. cit., p. 28. The Gomperz family was a famous European Jewish family dating from the sixteenth century. I found brief reference to a Salman

University of Prague,[43] whose members concurred with his analysis and added that there are but a few cases where the mother's milk can cause harm to the child, and they are both rare and eminently treatable. The halakhic nuances of the case of R. Reischer notwithstanding, R. Eybeschuetz again solicited expert opinion as part of his halakhic analysis.[44]

As a side note in this responsum, he comments on another medical aspect of nursing and its impact on the halakhic analysis. R. Eybeschuetz takes issue with the position held by some rabbinic authorities[45] that if a woman's breasts had "shriveled" (i.e., she had not been able to nurse/produce milk during a previous pregnancy or pregnancies) and is now pregnant when her husband dies, she would not be required to wait the 24 months after the birth of the child to remarry. He questions the assumption that previous lack of milk production portends a future of the same. He argues that according to the scientists each pregnancy is unique and it is completely possible for a woman to be "dry" for one pregnancy yet nurse normally subsequently, "as the matter is explained in all the books of *ḥakhmei nituaḥ*, that they call anatomy in their language."[46]

In a related exchange with R. Aryeh Epstein on another case of a nursing mother,[47] R. Eybeschuetz clarified his criteria for invoking and incorporating medical expertise into his halakhic decisions. This passage

---

Gumperz (d. 1728), who was a physician, with no accompanying biographical information. If this is the correct Zalman, then this passage would have been written by R. Eybeschuetz before the age of thirty-eight.

43. I made no effort to find archival evidence for this consultation as it appears from the language, as well as the absence of any recorded written response, to have been a verbal inquiry. R. Zimmels also wrote, in vain, to the University of Prague to identify reference to this query. See Zimmels, op. cit., 178.

44. While this analysis would clearly impugn the validity of the decision rendered by the rabbis to permit this woman to remarry, R. Eybeschuetz contends that God does not allow legal miscalculations or mistakes to befall the righteous ones (referring to the sages who permitted the woman to marry). Therefore, he argues that there must have been other valid reasons to render a permissive ruling.

45. *Maharik, Yam Shel Shlomo* and *Beit Shmuel*.

46. He repeats the same notion in his response to R. Epstein (addition to *siman aleph*, p. 306)

47. *Bnei Ahuva* 1 (*Zikhron Aharon*—Weinreb Edition: Jerusalem, 5767), section *She'elot UTeshuvot*, appendix to *siman aleph*, 299–306. This *teshuva* of R. Eybeschuetz was

provides specific parameters for the integration of medical information into the halakhic process.

R. Eybescheutz asserts that the permissive ruling allowing the woman to remarry in that case is based exclusively on the physicians' testimony that her milk had caused the death of one child and grave harm to a second. Furthermore, he affirms that this is an appropriate incorporation of medical knowledge into an halakhic decision. He adds the following general rule, "We do not rely on physicians in rendering a lenient decision, but to render a strict decision we can surely rely upon them." He clarifies another dimension of the use of physicians' opinion regarding a case of potential medical risk (*pikuaḥ nefesh*). In such cases we most certainly accept the opinion of physicians to create doubt (*safek*) as to whether a condition is life threatening, and the halakha is unequivocal that we would violate Shabbat based on such a doubt.

IV. BATHHOUSE INSEMINATION

In another passage in his *Bnei Ahuva*, R. Eybeschuetz's approach to contemporary medical knowledge appears at first blush to be utterly inconsistent with the cases above, where he took initiative to enlist medical expertise.[48] In discussing the notion of bathhouse insemination and whether one fulfills the mitzva of *peru urevu* thereby, he cites the Ḥelkak Meḥokek, who answers in the affirmative.[49] In the course of the analysis he takes particular issue with the position of the *Mishneh LeMelekh*, who entirely rejects the physiological possibility of bathhouse insemination.[50] While R. Eybeschuetz refutes his position based on a textual analysis of his sources, he nonetheless wonders how an authority of such stature

---

published in the work of R. Aryeh Leib Epstein and was not originally included in *Bnei Ahuva*. The editors of this edition added it as an appendix as it relates to the same subject matter.

48. On Maimonides, *Hil. Ishut* 15:6.

49. *Even Ha'Ezer* 1:8.

50. This is based on a passage in *Tosafot*, according to which pregnancy can only be achieved through the completion of the act of coition. Conception could, therefore, not be achieved through the waters of a bathhouse. For further discussion of bathhouse insemination in rabbinic literature, see S. Emanuel, "Pregnancy Without Sexual Relations in Medieval Thought," *Journal of Jewish Thought* 62:1 (Spring 2011), 105–120; chapter, "The Rabbinic Conception of Conception: An Exercise in Fertility."

could reject an accepted medical supposition of the Talmud, especially as the Talmud mentions no dissenting opinions. His treatment of this medical issue is quite different than the cases cited above. He writes that:

> Bathhouse insemination is surely possible, as the ancient physicians have written. And do not pay heed to the later physicians … who deny the possibility. They simply reject notions of which their imaginations are incapable of understanding. Their grasp of the realities of nature is as the dog laps from the ocean. There are many examples where they have attempted to supersede their predecessors only to have fallen short. Their practice reflects that they struggle to treat even minor ailments effectively, while their predecessors could successfully and completely cure major diseases.

This would not appear to have been written by the same person who seems so deferential to the expert wisdom of contemporary physicians. This apparent contradiction however is easily explained by one essential fact. Bathhouse insemination, the possibility of which could realistically have engendered a lively debate amongst reproductive physiologists of his time (or ours for that matter), was an accepted rabbinic tradition (*kabbala*) dating back to the Talmud. According to R. Eybeschuetz (and others) such matters, while medical in nature, are not subject to analysis or reinterpretation by even the best of contemporary physicians. It is therefore not inconsistent that R. Eybeschuetz elicited medical consultation in the cases of the heartless chicken and the nursing woman, where no tradition exists.

V. LAWS OF *NIDDA*

The *locus classicus* for the topic of reliability of physicians is a passage in *Nidda* (62b), where medical opinion is explicitly elicited by the rabbis in order to resolve a halakhic issue. This passage has received expansive treatment elsewhere,[51] but our concern presently is restricted to the approach of R. Eybeschuetz.[52]

---

51. See Steinberg and Rubinstein, op. cit., n. 1.
52. I thank R. Mordechai Dinerman for drawing my attention to this passage.

The discussion revolves around the case of a woman who was passing particulate matter. In general, any natural uterine bleeding confers the status of *nidda*. However, if there is an abnormal uterine lesion or wound, which is the source of the bleeding, then this blood flow does not render the woman a *nidda*. How does a rabbi make such a determination, and is medical consultation considered or required in such cases? The Talmud records such a case where the sages consulted the physicians, who determined that the woman had an internal lesion that was the source of her discharge. Upon hearing the medical opinion, the sages declared that a scientific test should be performed on the particulate matter and that the material should be placed in water—if it dissolves, the woman is rendered impure (an indication that it is menstrual blood); if not, she is pure (indicating that it is tissue from a pathological lesion).

The fundamental question addressed by R. Eybeschuetz is the purpose of the medical consultation. If the sages required the water test, it appears on the surface that either they did not trust, or did not rely upon, the medical opinion. Tissue that is determined to be from a pathological lesion is considered pure and does not convey *nidda* status. The testimony of the physicians about the presence of such a pathological lesion should have been sufficient to resolve the matter. Furthermore, if the medical opinion is completely discounted and has no bearing on the halakhic conclusion, then its recording in the Talmud seems superfluous. After citing his predecessors (including the Ḥakham Tzvi, who had debated this precise point) and attempting to clarify their respective positions, R. Eybeschuetz offers his own novel resolution. Indeed, the Rabbis required verification of the medical opinion through the use of the water test. However, once the water test would be performed three times with the discharge not dissolving, thus confirming the medical opinion by virtue of *ḥazaka* (legally established pattern), there would be no need to test any further episodes of discharge. In the absence of medical testimony, he argues, it would be required to test every single discharge of this woman in perpetuity to clarify its halakhic status. Therefore, the medical testimony is indeed an essential component of the halakhic decision and merits inclusion in the talmudic passage. Evident from this analysis is a respect for medical opinion, though not an unqualified blind acceptance.

In a tangent he gives further insight into the limitations placed on the acceptance of medical consultation.

> Our Rabbis taught: The best of physicians are destined for *Gehinom*, even though the Torah states "and heal you shall heal," giving license for the physician to practice medicine. However, the Torah only speaks of the treatment of external conditions, such as a fractured hand or a skin lesion or wound, as this is visible to the naked eye and readily perceivable… In such case, the physician can fully comprehend the condition. Such is not the case, however, for ailments of the internal organs, over which the eye (i.e., perception) of the physician has no rule. In such situations, the physicians merely judge according their intellect… such that many have died as a result…

This internal-external distinction is not unique to R. Eybeschuetz, though he does find himself in a distinct minority.[53]

VI. FORMATION OF TWINS

Our final source derives from the homiletic works[54] of R. Eybeschuetz and is, perhaps, more noteworthy for the absence of medical consultation. R. Eybeschuetz invokes a medical notion in the service of a homiletic idea, though his medical comments, not verified by specific medical consultation, nearly produced disastrous results for one innocent man.

In the context of a homily in his *Ya'arot Devash*, R. Eybeschuetz addresses the origins of King David and the ultimate Messiah.[55] In

---

53. Ibn Ezra is most famous for espousing this notion, though the Karaites believed it as well. See his commentary on Shemot 21:19. For a novel interpretation of the position of Ibn Ezra, see M. M. Sergui, *Meishiv Nefesh* (Vilna, 1908), 20a–21a. For other authorities who specifically link the reliability of physicians to the internal-external distinction, see H. J. Zimmels, *Magicians, Theologians and Doctors* (Edward Goldston and Son, 1952), 24 and n. 99 at p. 181. Zimmels does not mention this passage from R. Eybeschuetz.

54. See also *Ya'arot Devash* n. 14 on *teshuva*, which refers to Hazal as expert physicians in their understanding of spiritual and mental health and in their guidance on how to perform *teshuva*.

55. *Ya'arot Devash* (Lvov, 5623), 100a. For an expanded discussion of this source and topic, see chapter, "Is There Life After Life: Superfetation in Medical, Historical and Rabbinic Literature."

discussing the lineage of King David, R. Eybeschuetz queries why the progeny of the union of Yehuda and Tamar should be considered tainted. After all, prior to *matan Torah*, the obligation of *yibum* devolved upon the father as well as on the brother. Therefore, Yehuda was fulfilling a mitzva through his union with Tamar, and the resulting progeny should not only be free of stain, they should be considered superior.

To answer this question, R. Eybeschuetz posits that only the first coition fulfills the mitzva of *yibum*, while any subsequent coition is merely a product of human desire, not for the sake of the mitzva. Furthermore, he asserts, twins cannot be born of one coition, but rather require two. As a result, only the first of the twins (Zerah), who was conceived through the process of a mitzva, is associated with royalty. The second twin (Peretz), however, would be susceptible to stain.

It is this notion of the requirement of two coitions to produce twins that was read and integrated by an eighteenth-century European businessman. Prior to his departure on a long journey, this man engaged in marital relations with his wife. Upon his return some months later, his wife gave birth to twins. Remembering the homily of R. Eybeschuetz, he assumed his wife must have been unfaithful and approached R. Yehezkel Landau for rabbinic advice.[56] R. Landau roundly criticizes the questioner and dismisses out of hand the scientific ideas discussed in R. Eybeschuetz's essay.[57]

VII. CONCLUSION

We began with a discussion of the letter of R. Eybeschuetz to the medical faculty of the University of Halle, addressing both its historical importance, aided by an archival discovery, as well as its role in understanding the approach of R. Eybeschuetz to medical and scientific information. It

---

56. *Nodah BiYehuda Tinyana E. H.*, 81.

57. He further adds that not only are two coitions not required to produce twins—in fact, sequential coitions could not even produce two viable twins, as one would invariably become a sandal. Here, R. Landau invokes the talmudic dictum that superfetation (with the subsequent birth of two viable children) is not possible. According to contemporary medicine, while superfetation is debated, the possibility of superfecundation is universally accepted. Twins could indeed be produced through sequential coitions as long as they occur within one ovulatory cycle.

should now be clear that had I elected to present the letter of R. Eybeschuetz in isolation, it would have misrepresented his integration of and selective deference to medical knowledge. Below is a provisional list of the guidelines for his incorporation of medical information into the halakhic process extracted from the sources presented.

1) Medical information may be accepted as long as it does not conflict with the tradition of Ḥazal (the heartless chicken, the nursing widow, bathhouse insemination [rabbinic tradition precludes acceptance of medical information]).

2) Medical information may be integrated to render a strict halakhic opinion, but not to render a lenient one (the nursing widow).

3) The reliability of physician testimony is restricted to visible, external medical conditions (laws of *nidda*).

4) While physician testimony is accepted in certain circumstances, if the information they provide is verifiable through testable means, such testing should be performed (laws of *nidda*).

5) In cases of *pikuaḥ nefesh*, we can accept the opinion of physicians, even if only to create enough doubt about the possibility of danger, to allow the violation of Shabbat (the nursing widow).

A complete picture of the unique position of R. Eybeschuetz to the integration of medical information will be revealed only through analysis of all his medical citations coupled with a proper comparison of his approach to those of other rabbinic authorities. This humble contribution will hopefully further this objective.

Glossary

Aḥaronim – leading rabbinic authorities during the period from roughly the sixteenth century through contemporary times.

al kiddush Hashem – to sanctify God's name.

Ammoraim – rabbinic scholars during the period 200 CE to 500 CE.

androgenus (**androgynous**) – hermaphrodite.

arayot – prohibition of illicit sexual relations.

asur behana'a – prohibited to derive benefit.

Bamidbar – Book of Numbers, the fourth book of the Five Books of Moses.

Bavli – Babylonian Talmud.

Beit HaMikdash – The Holy Temple in Jerusalem.

beitza/beitzim – egg, testicle, or ovary.

bekhor – first born male child.

Glossary

ben – son or son of.

Bereshit – Book of Genesis, the first book of the Five Books of Moses.

bi'ah – sexual intercourse.

bikur holim – (society for) visiting the sick.

brit – circumcision.

Devarim – Book of Deuteronomy, the fifth book of the Five Books of Moses.

egla arufa – calf that is required to be killed in a ritual which is held upon the finding of a victim murdered by an unknown perpetrator.

ever/evarim – organ or organs (can refer to the male reproductive organ specifically).

Eretz Yisrael – the Land of Israel.

erva – literally, nakedness, but often refers to prohibition of illicit sexual relations.

even – stone.

Gemara – collection of Jewish oral traditions which constitute a segment of the Oral Torah, redacted by Rav Ashi approximately 500 CE.

Geonim – heads of the rabbinic academies in Babylonia from roughly the seventh to the eleventh centuries.

ger – convert to Judaism.

gidim – vessels (veins, nerves, arteries).

gosses – one whose death is imminent.

haftara – passage from the prophets recited after the Torah reading on the Sabbath and holidays.

halakha/halakhic – either a specific provision of Jewish law or the entire corpus of Jewish law.

hana'at hamet – prohibition of deriving benefit from a corpse.

hashhatat zera – prohibition of wasting reproductive seed.

havala – wounding, causing bodily harm.

havhana – requisite period of waiting (three months) before remarrying.

Ḥazal – rabbinic sages of earlier generations.

ḥeder – room or uterus.

ḥidush – a novel idea.

ḥiyut – life or life force.

Ḥol HaMo'ed – intermediate days of the Jewish festivals of Passover and Sukkot.

ḥoleh lefaneinu – literally "an ill person before us," referring the requirement of direct and immediate life-saving benefit in order to allow violation of Torah prohibitions.

hotza'at zera levatala – wasteful emission of reproductive seed.

Kaddish – mourner's prayer.

kasher – kosher.

Glossary

kerut shafkha – see *petzua daka*.

ketoret – incense used in the Temple.

kiddush – prayer over wine recited on the Sabbath and holidays.

kiddushin – betrothal.

kis/bekis – bladder.

Kohen/Kohanim – member(s) of the priestly tribe.

Kohen Gadol – High Priest.

mamzer – bastard.

Masekhet – tractate of the Talmud.

mazik – wound or damage.

mazra'at – gives forth seed.

meineket – a nursing woman.

melaveh malka – meal customarily held on Saturday night after the conclusion of the Sabbath.

mesora – tradition.

metzitza – oral suction of the wound, part of the circumcision ceremony.

mezuza – a parchment inscribed with specific biblical verses, customarily placed on the doorpost of a home.

Mi Shebeirakh – prayer for the sick.

Midrash/*midrashim* – collection of early Jewish commentary on biblical text.

mikva – ritual bath.

mila – circumcision.

Minḥa – afternoon prayer.

minyan/minyanim – requisite quorum of ten men for certain prayers.

Mishkan – Tabernacle.

mishloaḥ manot – food items customarily given to one's neighbor or friend on the holiday of Purim.

Mishna – collection of Jewish oral traditions which constitute a segment of the Oral Torah, redacted by Rabbi Yehuda HaNasi approximately 200 CE.

mitzva – commandment.

mohel – ritual circumciser.

motza'ei Shabbat – Saturday night, after the conclusion of the Sabbath.

nefel – nonviable child.

nefesh – soul.

neshama – soul.

neshima – breath.

nidda – name for any woman during menstruation, or a woman who has menstruated and not yet completed the associated requirement of immersion in a *mikva* (ritual bath).

nishtaneh hateva – literally, nature has changed. A rabbinic expression, of varying interpretations, referring to areas of rabbinic literature where the understanding of science and medicine has evolved.

nivul – desecration.

nivul hamet – desecration of the dead.

orla – 1) foreskin; 2) fruit of a tree grown in Israel which is prohibited to be eaten for the first three years of the tree's growth.

parasha/parashat – weekly portion of the Torah read in the synagogue.

peru urevu – the obligation to be fruitful and multiply.

pesak – rabbinic decision.

petzua daka – damage or injury to male reproductive organs with halakhic ramifications.

pidyon haben – redemption of the first born.

pikuaḥ nefesh – for the sake of saving a life.

Pitum HaKetoret – account of the incense offering brought in the ancient Temple.

piyyut – liturgical poem.

posek/poskim – rabbinic decisor(s).

prozdor – literally, passageway/antechamber, metaphor for part of female reproductive anatomy.

Rashi – acronym for Rabbi Shlomo Yitzḥaki, prominent medieval commentator on the Bible and Talmud who lived in the eleventh century.

Rishonim – leading rabbinic authorities during the period from roughly the eleventh through the fifteenth centuries.

ruaḥ – spirit.

safek – doubt.

sakana – danger.

sefer/seforim – book(s).

sefira – period of counting the 49 days between Passover and Shavuot, during which period a form of communal mourning is observed in commemoration of the occurrence of historical tragic events for the Jewish people.

selaim – coins.

sevara – logical deduction.

Shabbat/Shabbos – the Jewish Sabbath.

sheḥita – ritual slaughter.

Shemot – Book of Exodus, the second book of the Five Books of Moses.

Shevatim – tribes.

shiva – seven-day period of mourning observed after the death of specific close family members.

Shlomo HaMelekh – King Solomon.

Shulḥan Arukh – authoritative code of Jewish law written in the sixteenth century.

sirus – sterilization.

Talmud – central text and primary source of Jewish law consisting of the Mishna and Gemara, compiled around 500 CE.

Tanakh – canonical collection of Hebrew scriptures, including the Torah (Five Books of Moses).

Tannaim – rabbinic sages whose opinions are recorded in the Mishna from approximately 10 CE – 200 CE.

Tazria – name of a specific Torah weekly portion.

tefillin – set of phylacteries, leather boxes containing sections of biblical text worn by Jewish men for morning prayers (except on the Sabbath and holidays).

tefillin shel rosh – phylacteries worn on the head.

tefillin shel yad – phylacteries worn on the arm.

teḥiyat hametim – resurrection of the dead.

Tosafot – medieval commentaries on the Talmud.

treifa/treifot – a member of a kosher species of mammal or bird, disqualified from being considered kosher due to pre-existing mortal injuries or physical defects.

tum'ah – ritual impurity or defilement.

tumtum – ambiguous genitalia.

tzara'at – biblical disease often identified (erroneously) with leprosy.

tzitzit – specially knotted ritual fringes worn on four-cornered garments.

Vayikra – Book of Leviticus, the third book of the Five Books of Moses.

Yerushalmi – Jerusalem Talmud.

yibum – levirate marriage.

zera – seed/reproductive seed.

Index

248 limbs, 38, 199–208, 232–244, 245, 249, 252, 515

A

abortion, xxvii, 9, 65, 73, 291–295, 322, 394–395, 401–402, 507

Abraham, Dr. Abraham S., 75, 107, 130, 147, 158, 202, 217, 368, 432, 449, 461, 466

Abudraham, 53, 242

Adam, xxi, 9, 140, 146, 250–251, 258, 273, 292

Adler, Rabbi Herman, 379–380

agriculture, 5

AIDS, 386, 391, 400, 404

Akiva, Rabbi 141, 179, 534

Albadaran, 260–261, 266

Aldabi, Meir Ibn, 13–14, 19, 53–54, 458

Alderotti, Taddeo, 5, 448

Alei Terufa, 376

Algazi, Rabbi Yom Tov, 52, 81–82

Anatoli, Jacob 43

anatomical dissection, xxvi, 5, 36, 38, 41, 199–200, 205, 208–210, 213–226, 229, 234–235, 239, 260–261, 345, 446–448, 455, 496, 512–513

animalculist, 9, 16, 20

anti-vaxxer, 374, 378, 380, 384

aorta, 439–440, 446, 448

Applebaum, Rabbi Dr. David, 161–162, 382

Aquinas, 32, 62

Arik, Rabbi Meir, 139, 142, 361–364, 366–369

Aristotle, 6–8, 10, 12–13, 15, 19, 41–42, 65, 71, 75, 140, 299–300, 304, 309, 435–439, 446–447, 450, 453–456, 459

arteries, 6, 66, 299–300, 436–438, 441, 444

artificial heart transplantation, 469

artificial insemination, xxviii, 4, 22–32, 35, 86, 103, 132, 154, 186–188, 193–194, 323

Arukh HaShulḥan, 19, 21, 251

Asaph, 434, 440, 489

Ashkenazi, Rabbi Eliezer, 331–332, 334

Ashkenazi, Rabbi Tzvi (Ḥakham Tzvi) 302–303, 525–526, 532

Ashmedai, 283

Assad, Rabbi Yehuda, 313, 316–317

Assia, 22, 24, 39, 73, 75, 84, 103, 108, 157, 216, 242, 250, 252, 275, 291, 348–349, 365, 370, 383, 386, 400, 443, 495, 505

Auerbach, Rabbi Shlomo Zalman, xiv, 217, 369, 382–383, 489, 504–506

autopsy, xxvi, 162, 209, 216–218, 226, 235, 272, 345, 348–350, 383, 513

Avers, Rabbi Rafael, 187, 202, 235–237

Avicenna, xxiv–xxv, 31–32, 34, 36, 199, 211, 285, 325–326, 330

Index

Azulai, Rabbi Ḥayyim Yosef David, 11, 25, 30, 46, 76, 78–82, 105, 136, 202, 273, 416, 455, 463, 467, 473

B

Baer, Karl Ernst von, 8, 114
balcony *minyan*, 416
Barkai, Ron, xiv, 5, 10, 24, 44, 47, 75, 403
barnacle goose, 139
Bartholin, Thomas, 512, 519
bathhouse insemination, 16, 18, 22–24, 26–33, 132, 134, 537–538, 542
Bauhinus, Caspar, 265, 267–268
Beit El, 246–247
bekhor, 121, 123–125, 131, 133, 140, 143, 169–171, 183
Ben Sira, 23–27, 86, 132–133
Benayahu, Meir, 214
Bentham, Jeremy, 226–228
Berlin, Rabbi Isaiah 10, 498
Betuel HaRamai, 251
Bick, Rabbi Ezra, 103, 109, 150, 167
Biesbrouck, Maurits, 210
bikur ḥolim, 388–389, 421–422
Billitzer, Rabbi Ephraim, 82
bitumen, 323–326, 329–331, 336–338, 342
Black Death, 374, 403–404, 411
bladder stone, 216-217, 345-349
Bleich, Rabbi J. David, xiv, 30, 73, 104, 106, 109, 112, 125, 133, 149–152, 156–159, 162–164, 167–168, 171, 183, 195, 230, 273, 283, 291, 346, 349, 361, 375, 381, 386, 400–401, 432, 469–470, 486, 503, 532
blood, 6–10, 12–13, 15, 17, 65–66, 129, 183, 219, 298, 300, 314–315, 323, 355, 370–371, 385, 392, 435, 437–439, 447, 456, 458, 469, 505–506, 523, 527, 535, 539
Blumenfeld, Rabbi Mayer, 282
body snatchers, 219, 221, 223–224, 327
Bondeson, Jan, 272, 274, 284, 287–289, 495

Bos, Gerrit, xiv, 32, 47, 330, 403, 454
Boss, Jeffrey, 461, 482–484
Brach, Rabbi Shaul 254
brain, 8–9, 18–19, 129, 161, 288, 394, 396–397, 431–432, 434–438, 450–456, 459–460, 462–463, 467–468, 496, 504–508, 531–532
Brandsdorfer, Rabbi Meir, 93, 100, 109
BRCA, 158–159
Breisch, Rabbi Yaakov, 256
Breitowitz, Rabbi Yitzḥak, 167, 375
Brim, Charles, 433, 516
Brown, Dr. Jeremy, xxix, 404, 524
Broyde, Rabbi Michael, 150, 167
Buchbinder, Dr. Shalom, 382
burial, 158, 161, 209, 218, 222–225, 227–228, 254–256, 328, 330, 388, 390, 422–424, 468, 478, 494–499, 501, 507–508, 524
Butler, Menachem xix, 7, 203, 219, 225
Butler, Samuel, 268–269
Buxtorf, Johannes, 268
Bynum, W. F., 301

C

Caesar, 478
caesarean section, 133, 162, 170–171, 276, 459–463, 477–508
Cantarini, Rabbi Dr. Isaac, 218
cardio-pulmonary resuscitation, 464, 467, 469–470
Carlbach, Rabbi Mordechai, 96, 101
Carmell, Rabbi Arye, xxix, 7
Carmoly, Eliakim, 448, 513
Carpi, Berengario de, 43
Castro, Jacob, 338–339
Catalano, Abraham, 407, 410–411, 413, 417
Catalano, Moshe, 407
Chagiz, Rabbi Yaakov, 284–285, 289, 317
Chapman, Israel, 221
cheese analogy, 309

chevra kadisha, 388, 414, 422–423

chloroform, 352–353, 358–360

cholera, 387–388, 404, 407, 409, 412, 414, 417–425

circulation, 7, 300, 323, 371, 438, 455–456, 458, 506

coccyx, 249–250, 260, 269

Cohn, Dr. Tobias (see *Ma'aseh Tuvia*), 14–15, 27, 434

contraception, 73, 322, 395, 398–400

corneal transplant- 147, 161–162, 470–473

coronary bypass, 469

coronavirus (see Covid-19), 403–405, 413, 422

Covid-19 (see coronavirus), x, 383, 388, 403, 420, 426

cowpox, 378–379

cremation, 253–256, 390, 422

D

Da Vinci, Leonardo, 36, 41, 43, 447

de Graaf, Renier, 7–8

Dead Sea, 324–326, 329, 434

death, vii, x, xxvii, 11, 50, 61, 74, 79–81, 99, 133, 161, 170, 179, 185–186, 200, 215–216, 218–219, 221, 229, 234–235, 239, 247, 251–256, 259, 283–285, 289–290, 294, 300, 303, 306, 312, 322–323, 364, 374, 383, 387–388, 390, 394, 403–404, 411–413, 423–426, 429, 431–463, 465–470, 472, 474, 476–508, 524, 526, 531–532, 534–535, 537

decapitation, 452, 454–455, 460, 499, 502, 505

Dessler, Rabbi Eliyahu, xxix, 7

Deutch, Rabbi Eliezer, 121–125, 127–129, 131, 133, 148, 168–171, 485

Dinah, 62, 67, 85–110

Dinerman, Rabbi Mordechai, xix, 538

Dioscorides, 325–326

Dipoce, Dr. James, 382

DNA, ix, 3, 71–72, 84, 114, 129, 175, 177, 183, 187–188, 191–195, 270, 384, 523

Duran, Rabbi Shimon ben Tzemaḥ, 13, 26, 34, 36, 77

E

Ebola, xxvii, 385–387, 389–393, 395, 397, 399, 401, 404

Ebstein, Wilhelm, 513–515, 521

Edelstein, Ludwig, 5, 128, 210, 448

egg, 3, 7–9, 14–17, 21, 64, 67–68, 78, 86, 93, 100, 103, 107–109, 114, 139, 142, 145, 147–149, 151, 164, 167, 176, 191–192, 194, 323, 401

Eiger, Rabbi Akiva, 56, 145–146, 286–287, 322, 418–419, 425–426, 500, 534

Einbinder, Professor Susan, 404, 407, 413

Elisha, 218, 306–308, 464–467, 470–471, 474, 476, 518

Eliyahu Hanavi, 271, 281

Elmagar, 327, 330–331, 336–337

Elyashiv, Rabbi Yosef Shalom, xiv, 188, 369, 372, 383–384, 505

embryology, 4–9, 11, 14–15, 37, 53, 59–61, 114, 309, 439, 442, 445, 449–450

Emden, Rabbi Yaakov, xxv, 16–17, 30, 171, 209, 215, 237, 251–252, 346, 348–350, 459, 512, 523–524, 530

encephalo-myelogenic doctrine, 8, 18–20

epigenesis, 8, 14, 20

Epstein, Rabbi Yaakov, 19, 21, 49, 259, 282, 295, 536–537

erva, 122, 127, 132–136, 138, 140, 142–143, 145–146, 152, 168–169, 171

Ettlinger, Rabbi Yaakov, 162, 228–229, 485–486

Etziony, Mordechai, 211, 232, 261

eugenics, 5, 60, 63, 439

Index

evarim, ix, 112, 158, 199–208, 232, 234, 236–241, 244, 370, 515

Eve (see Ḥavva), 9, 364

Eybeschuetz, Rabbi Yonatan, 30, 82–83, 229, 458–459, 522–542

F

fainting, 303–305, 310

Feinstein, Rabbi Moshe, xiv, 35, 125–126, 159–161, 163–164, 187, 194, 240, 290–291, 295, 303, 369, 390–391, 394–395, 401, 432, 463, 474

Feldman, Rabbi Daniel, xx, 96

Feldman, Rabbi David xiv, 9, 65–66, 73–74, 77

Feldman, Professor Louis, 31, 245, 262, 266

Feldman, William M., 5, 46, 60, 63, 273, 439

female seed, 6, 9–18, 21, 65–66, 68, 140, 186

fetus, xxii, 4, 6–8, 12, 14, 16–17, 40, 45, 53, 60, 62–66, 68–70, 73–76, 78, 87–94, 96, 123–125, 129, 131, 133–135, 137, 139–141, 145–146, 148, 152, 169–170, 178, 180, 228–229, 287, 290–294, 309, 354, 394–396, 398, 400–401, 439, 442, 450, 460, 462–463, 478–479, 486–493, 495, 498–508

fever, 299–301, 308, 311, 386, 394, 403–404

Fischer, Rabbi Yisrael, 491, 494–495

Fisher, Rabbi Amram, 359

Fisher, Rabbi Shlomo, 91–92, 94, 96–98, 102

Fleckeles, Rabbi Eliezer 91, 377, 383

fleeing (in times of plague), 400, 406–408

Fleischer, Rabbi Binyamin, 277–279

forty days, 61–64, 76–77, 89–90, 94, 178, 411

four elements, 435

Franklin, Benjamin, 377

Friedenwald, Dr. Harry, xiv, 26, 55, 210, 215, 415, 512–513, 520–521

Friedling, Rabbi Tzvi Hirsch, 105

Friedman, Rabbi Eliezer, 96–97, 100

Frigeis, Lazarus de, 211–212, 261

Frimer, Rabbi Dov, 39, 84, 443

Frizzi, Dr. Benzion (Benedetto), 215, 513

G

Galen, xxiv–xxv, 6, 10–13, 36, 41, 66, 199, 261, 298–300, 305, 309, 316, 325, 331, 433–441, 446–447, 450, 453–459, 512

gallstones, 216, 347–348

Garrison, Fielding H., 119, 250, 257, 260–261, 265–266, 268, 436, 438

gidim, 9, 252

Gintzburger, Benjamin Wolff, 171, 215, 512–514, 521

Goldhaber, Rabbi Yehiel, 495, 497–498

Goliath, ix, 175–177, 182, 189, 192, 194

Gordon, Rabbi Yaakov, 104–105, 121, 127, 130, 133, 154, 174

Goren, Rabbi Shlomo, 348

gosses, 218, 284–285, 289, 506–507

grave robbing, 213, 220, 223–225

Grazi, Dr. Richard, 475

Greek, xxiv, 5–6, 8, 10, 12, 31, 40–42, 65, 75, 211, 245, 298, 309, 324, 408, 433–437, 458, 515

Green, Monica, 6, 40–41

Greenblatt, Rabbi Ephraim, 278–279, 282

Grossberg, Rabbi Menashe, 104, 106

Grossnass, Rabbi Aryeh Leib, 226–227

Gutal, Rabbi Neriya, 24, 39, 75, 84, 142, 181, 252, 297, 311, 443

H

Habe'er, 105, 122, 132, 142, 144, 156, 162, 173

Hakalir, Rabbi Eliezer, 91, 105

Ḥakham Tzvi (see Ashenazi, Rabbi Tzvi)

Halakha Urefua, 107, 125–126, 159–161, 163, 382, 470, 472

Halevi, Rabbi Mordechai, 78–79, 81

Index

Halevi, Rabbi Avraham, 93, 106–107, 338–341
Halle, University of 459, 526, 528–531, 541
Haller, Albrecht, 21, 33
Halperin, Rabbi Dr. Mordechai, xiv, 13, 38–39, 84, 112, 130, 149, 157, 291, 383, 443, 449, 505
Halperin, Rabbi Levi Yitzhak, 292–294, 470, 476, 532
Harvey, William, 5, 7, 14–15, 20, 37, 41–42, 71, 210, 213, 300, 438, 448, 455–456, 506
hashhatat zera (prohibition of wasting male seed), 29, 146
Hatam Sofer, 35, 99, 142, 252–253, 276, 306, 313, 366, 387, 412, 414, 420, 423–425, 449, 466, 468
Havva (see Eve), 140, 273, 292, 368
Hazon Ish, 35, 75, 216–217, 348–349, 423, 432, 443, 483
heart, 161, 165, 204, 208, 260, 282, 290–295, 298–299, 302–304, 307, 310, 314, 323, 355, 384–385, 394, 421, 435–439, 441, 443–448, 450–451, 453–459, 469–470, 525–528, 532, 535
hematogenic doctrine, 8, 19
herd immunity, 381–382
hermaphrodite, 45–46, 49, 54, 56, 60
Herophilus, 128, 437, 439
Hershler, Rabbi Moshe 107, 125–126, 159–161, 163, 472
Herzog, Rabbi Yitzhak Isaac HaLevi, xxix, 235, 473
Heynick, Frank, xiv
Hippocrates, xxiv–xxv, 5–6, 8, 19, 36, 40–41, 45, 62, 66, 71, 129, 199, 265, 299, 435–436, 438–439, 444
Hizkuni, 48, 87, 95
Holocaust, 255, 398, 502
homunculus, 9, 17

Horowitz, Rabbi Avraham Yaakov, 93, 106, 142
Horowitz, Rabbi Pinchas Halevi, 30, 358–361
Hunter, John, 22, 29
Hurwitz, Pinchas Eliyahu, 17, 20, 375, 378
Hyrtl, Joseph, 205, 257
hysterectomy, 125–126, 153, 158–162, 173

I

Ibn Ezra, 46–52, 57, 87, 98, 232, 302–303, 409, 458, 540
Iggerot Moshe, 158–159, 161, 187, 240, 291, 369, 388, 390, 423, 463, 474, 532
Ilowy, Rabbi Bernard, 481
inheritance, 19, 118, 141, 184, 186
inheritance of conjoined twins, 283–285, 288, 291, 295
innate heat, x, xxv, 296, 298–303, 305–317, 436–438, 458, 465–466, 526
inoculation, 375–379, 381, 383
intubation, 243, 466, 518
Isaacs, Dr. Haskell, xxv, 34, 327, 357, 433
Isaacs, Rabbi Schachne, 223–225
Israels, Dr. Abraham Hartog, 481–482, 484, 514
Isserles, Rabbi Moshe, 388, 391, 406, 414, 461, 463

J

Jacquart, Danielle, 42
Jakobovits, Rabbi Lord Immanuel, xviii–xix, 22–23, 73, 76, 235, 353, 486
Jenner, Edward, 375, 378, 380, 382
Jeremiah, 23–25, 132, 303
Job, 309
Josephus, vii, 306, 324, 481

K

Kaddish, 416, 425–426
Kagen, Solomon, 516

Kahana, Maoz, xiv, 456, 523, 525

Kamelhar, Rabbi Yekutiel, 120, 126, 137–144, 147–151, 481

Kamenetsky, Rabbi Natan, 388

Kaplan, Rabbi Arye, 270

Karo, Rabbi Yosef, 11, 80, 139, 209, 243, 312, 314, 415, 492, 494, 525

Kasher, Rabbi Menachem, 46, 87, 92, 463

Katzburg, Rabbi David Tzvi, 129–131, 148, 170

Rabbi Yerachmiel Katzburg, 133

Katzenellenbogen, Rabbi Meir (*Maharam Padua*), 214, 414, 425

Katznelson, Dr. Yehuda Leib, 203, 205–208, 242, 433, 448, 514–515

ketoret, 412–414

kidney, 11, 157, 165, 231, 322, 346, 348, 475

Kimhi, Rabbi David, 303, 305, 307, 449

King David, 56, 305–306, 540–541

Klein, Rabbi Yisrael, 81–82

Klein, Rabbi Menashe, 106, 187–188, 190, 280–281, 294

Klein, Rabbi Shalom, 467, 473

Kluger, Rabbi Shlomo, 240

kohen, 23, 158, 182–184, 187–189, 192–193, 195, 218, 228–229, 256, 274, 276, 306, 338, 410, 459, 473–474, 489, 513, 523, 533

Koop, Dr. C. Everett, 290–291

Koren, Sharon, 44, 65

Koroth, xviii–xix, xxv, 10–11, 16, 27, 39, 45–46, 55, 66, 78, 130, 171, 208, 210–212, 214–216, 234, 324, 357, 415, 433, 437–439, 448–449, 466, 480, 512–513, 516–519, 524

Kottek, Dr. Samuel, xiv, xix, 5, 10, 60–62, 65, 73, 181, 211, 250, 304, 439, 495, 517–518

L

labor, 35, 77, 290, 364–365, 460–461, 479–480, 488

Lampronti, Rabbi Dr. Yitzhak, xxix, 7, 27, 77–78, 448

Landau, Rabbi Yehezkel, xxvi, 82–83, 128, 161, 166, 185–186, 209, 216–217, 314–315, 345–349, 420, 541

Lau, Rabbi Yisrael Meir, 108, 419, 473–474

Leah, xvii, 62–63, 86–99, 101–103, 105–108, 134–136

Leeuwenhoek, Antony von, 8–9, 14, 19

Leibowitz, Dr. Joshua, xiv, xix, xxv, 211, 438, 484, 517

Leiman, Dr. Shnayer, 8, 24, 39, 84, 137, 297, 443, 524, 526, 530

Lesky, Erna, 6

Levi, Dr. Yaakov, 66, 349, 503

Levi, Dr. Yehuda, xxix, 7, 39, 84, 297, 400, 443

levirate, 184–186, 189, 193

Levush Mordechai, 80, 361

Lieber, Elinor, xxiv, 433–434, 438, 440

Liebes, Rabbi Yitzhak Isaac, 112

Lifschutz, Rabbi Israel, 377–378

liver, 165, 315–316, 323, 435, 439, 446–450, 453

Loike, Dr. John, 157, 194

Lusitanus, 26, 28, 32

luz bone, x, xviii, 212, 241–242, 245, 247–257, 259–261, 263–265, 267–271

Luzzatto, Shmuel David, 48–50, 203

Luzzi, Mondino de, 42

M

Ma'aseh Tuvia, 14, 273, 285, 480

Macht, Dr. David, 5, 60, 413–414, 439, 516

Magen Avraham, 460, 495

Maggi, Girolmo, 262–268

Maharal, 52, 67, 181

Maimonides (Rambam), xiv, xx, 12–13, 28, 30, 38, 45, 47, 81, 122–125, 134, 168–169, 205, 209, 214, 237, 239, 276, 304–306,

313–314, 322, 330–332, 336, 340, 365, 386, 389, 396, 433–435, 449–450, 452–455, 483–484, 488, 494–495, 523, 525, 537

male seed, 5–6, 8, 12, 14, 17–19, 21, 65–66, 68, 75, 138–140, 147, 178

mamzer, 25–27, 81–82, 183–185, 193–194, 294

Margalit, Dr. David, xiv, 16, 27, 46, 77–78, 91, 93, 208, 234, 375, 438–439, 448, 512, 517

Margulies, Rabbi Reuven, 530

Markel, Nisan, 207–208, 242

masks, 408, 417

maternal impression, 179–181

measles, 374, 380–382, 384, 387, 389, 394, 422

Medical Leaves, 5, 60, 63, 214, 242, 327, 433, 439, 454, 516

Meiselman, Rabbi Moshe, xxix, 7, 39, 84, 297, 443

melaveh malka, 250–251, 271

Mendelsohn, Everett, 434, 436

menstrual blood, 7, 10, 12–13, 15, 17, 65–66, 129, 314, 535, 539

Meshekh Hokhma, 98, 102, 135–136

metzitza, 29, 366, 370, 391, 459, 523

Metzudat David, 306, 317

Meyerhof, Max, 327, 438, 454

mezuza, 419–420

microscope, 8, 15, 17, 20–21, 298

mila (circumcision), 29–30, 285, 352, 358–373

Minhat Elazar (see Spira, Rabbi Hayyim Elazar)

mitochondrial DNA, ix, 3, 175, 191–192, 194–195

Modena, Rabbi Yehuda Arye, 27, 213–214, 259, 421, 448–452

Montefiore, Moses, 412

Montpellier, xxiv, 11, 322

Morgagni, Giovanni Battista, 27, 213

Morris, Dr. Robert Tuttle, 7, 105, 114–121, 137–138, 141–142, 148, 151, 154

mourning, 79–81, 99, 255, 384, 424–425

Muenster, Sebastian, 257–259, 264, 267–268

mumia, x, xxvi, 111, 172, 230, 321, 323–343

mumps, 381, 387

Mundinus, 5, 209, 448

Muntner, Suessman, xiv, 45, 305, 330, 434, 513, 517, 521

Mussaphia, Benjamin, 512

N

Nadav and Avihu, 255–256

Nahmanides (see also Ramban), 11–12, 16–18, 44, 64–66, 81, 236, 303–305, 310, 322, 386, 454

Nansich, Abraham, 376

Nathanson, Rabbi Yosef Shaul, 31, 286–287, 467

navel, 60, 439–442, 444–445, 450

Needham, Joseph, 5–6, 8, 21, 61, 114, 309, 439, 441

Neuburger, Max, 436

nidda, xxii, xxvi, 9, 12–13, 16–18, 20, 25, 30, 38–39, 61–62, 65–67, 74, 77, 81, 90, 98, 128–132, 135, 142, 172–173, 286, 311, 314–315, 442, 449, 461, 467, 470–472, 474–475, 535, 538–539, 542

Nishmat Avraham (by Dr. Abraham S. Abraham), 38, 75, 107, 130, 147, 158, 202, 217, 273, 276, 368–369, 432, 449, 461, 505

nishtaneh hateva, xiii, 29, 36, 84

niskoy, 251–252

nivul hamet, 161, 485–486, 502, 507

nostrils, 231, 302–303, 440–442, 444–445, 450–451, 466

nursing mother, 536

Nutton, Vivian, 301

Index

O

obstetric anesthesia, 353, 365

Ofir Shemesh, Abraham, xiv, 216, 329, 340, 348

Olam Hafukh (by Abraham Catalano), 407, 410

Oppenheim, Rabbi Avraham Ḥayyim, 500–501

Or Zarua, 280

orla, 126, 138, 148, 166, 370

Oshry, Rabbi Ephraim, 364, 488, 502

ovaries, 12–16, 65, 114–119, 126, 131, 141–144, 151–152, 154, 159, 164, 166, 173, 401

ovist, 9

ovum, 7–8, 103, 109, 118, 150–151, 160, 167

P

Padua, University of, 14–15, 27, 37, 77, 202, 212–215, 218, 267, 407–408, 410–411, 413, 417, 425, 448, 451, 480, 531

Palimo, 274, 278, 280–283

pandemic, xxvii, 375, 383–384, 396, 404–406, 408–412, 414, 416–421, 423–426

pangenesis, 8, 19, 130

Pardes Yosef, 87, 91, 95, 97, 135, 202, 241, 273, 286

Park, Katherine, 479, 493

Pasteur, Louis, 7

Patai, Raphael, 329, 331, 333, 336, 338

paternity, ix, xxvii, 71, 77, 103, 150, 167, 175–196, 288

Pearlman, Moshe, 515

peru urevu, 81–82, 164, 202, 395–396, 398, 537

pidyon haben, 124, 151, 171, 189, 192–193, 274, 276–277, 291

Pines, Rabbi Michel, 203, 211–212, 220

Pliny, 71, 263, 266, 325, 478

pneuma, 436–438, 441–442, 450

Porjes, Meir Asher Zelig, 204–205

Portaleone, Dr. Abraham, 413–414

Posek, Rabbi Eliyahu, 105, 143–145, 147, 156, 162, 274, 494

Posek, Rabbi Hillel, 398

posthumous insemination, 476

Prager, Dr. Kenneth, 232, 243

Praxagoras of Cos, 439

preformation, 8–9, 14, 16–17, 20–21

premature burial, 468, 497

Preuss, Dr. Julius, xiv–xv, xviii, 5–6, 23, 26, 31–33, 36–37, 39, 45–46, 58, 60, 62, 66, 72–74, 76, 130–131, 141, 181, 203, 206–207, 242, 249, 357, 433, 439–440, 447, 449, 461, 482–484, 486, 513–515, 521

Puah, 466

pulse, 439–441, 457

Q

quarantine, 391, 396, 404, 411–412

R

Rabbenu Gershon, 285, 312, 454–455

Radak (see also Kimḥi, Rabbi David), 87, 182, 303, 306–308

Radbaz (Rabbi David ben Zimra), 230, 336–342, 360, 467, 473, 491–492, 498

Ralbag (Rabbi Levi ben Gershon), 285, 308–309, 315–317, 454

Rambam (see also Maimonides), xviii, xxvi, 183, 305, 330

Ramban (see also Naḥmanides), 11, 65, 217, 305, 381, 466

Rashbatz (see also, Duran, Rabbi Shimon ben Tzemaḥ), 80

Rashi, 5, 18, 33, 38–39, 52, 67, 73–77, 79, 96–97, 99–102, 131, 133, 135, 144, 156, 177–178, 181, 183, 187, 190, 194, 275–276, 279–280, 303, 308, 360, 445–449, 452,

457, 460, 483, 488–490, 499, 501–502, 505, 516

Rebbe (Rabbi Yehuda Hanasi), 274, 278, 280–283, 295

Recanati, Rabbi Menachem, 259

Redi, Francesco, xxix, 7

Regensberg, Rabbi Ḥayyim, 125–126, 159–161, 163, 470, 472–473

Reischer, Rabbi Yaakov, 30, 273, 276, 279, 284, 286–288, 388, 423, 463, 488, 491, 494, 496, 498–500, 502–503, 536

resurrectionists, 219, 221, 223

resuscitation, x, xxvii–xxviii, 147, 196, 306–307, 429, 432, 434, 436, 438, 440, 442, 444, 446, 448, 450, 452, 454, 456, 458, 460, 462, 464–476, 478, 480, 482, 484, 486, 488, 490, 492, 494, 496, 498, 500, 502, 504, 506, 508, 518

rete mirabile, 437

Rhazes, 325–326

right-left theory, 41, 44–45, 49, 52, 54

Riolan, Jean, 254

Rosanes, Rabbi Yehuda, 28–31, 171, 331, 340–342

Rosen, Rabbi Moshe, 277–279

Rosenfeld, Rabbi Dr. Azriel, 112, 149–150, 466, 470

Rosner, Dr. Fred, xiv, xviii–xx, 22, 39, 45–46, 58, 66, 71, 73, 84, 112, 130, 181, 191, 193, 203, 207, 235, 249, 297, 307, 331, 345–346, 354, 357, 375, 389, 391, 394–396, 399, 432–433, 443, 450, 454, 465, 473, 475, 482, 513–514, 518

Roth, Cecil, 14, 36, 46, 53, 137, 212–213, 218–219, 222–223, 247, 257, 261, 264, 267–268, 332, 334, 407–408, 410, 417

Roth, Rabbi Moshe Yosef, 101, 106, 134–136, 148, 150

Roth, Rabbi Pinchas, 449

Rousset, Francois, 478–479, 484

rubella, x, xxvii, 381, 393–397, 399, 401–402

Ruderman, David, xiv, xxix, 7, 14, 17, 27, 55, 77, 213, 375, 413, 480

Ryzman, Tzvi, 93, 152, 155

S

Salanter, Rabbi Israel 388

samma deshinta, 357, 363

Savitz, Dr. Harry, 27, 55, 78, 415, 514

Schachter, Rabbi Hershel, 405, 416, 423–424, 432, 435

Schachter, Rabbi Shay, 240

Schacter, Rabbi Dr. J. J. 524, 530

Schick, Barukh, 15–16, 20–21

Schick, Rabbi Moshe, 28

Schmelkes, Rabbi Yitzḥak, 182–186, 189, 193, 277, 284, 287–288

Schwadron, Rabbi Shalom Mordechai, 31, 227

Schwartz, Rabbi Yitzḥak Maier, 101–102

Schwartz, Rabbi Yosef, 121, 125, 156, 358

Scot, Michael, 42–43, 47, 50–51, 57

Sefer Habrit, 17–18, 20–21, 30, 67, 375, 378

Sefer Hagan, 46, 48, 51

Sefer Ḥasidim, 44, 77, 238

Sefer Toldot, 46–48, 50–51, 57

selling organs, 475

semen, 6, 12, 36–37, 65–66, 74, 300–301, 309, 313, 316

Sergei, Dr. Menachem Mendel, 447

sesamoid bone, 250

sex determination, 40–42, 45, 53, 66

Shafran, Rabbi Betzalel, 105, 136–137, 143–144, 369

Shafran, Rabbi Yigal, xiv, 186, 375, 460–461, 463, 504–506

Shakh, 312

Sharshevsky, Dr. Binyamin, 203, 205

Shatzmiller, Joseph, xiv, 11, 322, 434

Shaul ben Hakena'anit, 100, 106, 109, 134

Shema prayer, 201–202, 235–240

Shevilei Emuna (see Aldabi, Rabbi Meir), 13–14, 19, 53, 458

Shifra, 466

Shimon, 100, 106, 108–109, 134–135

shiva, 424–425

Shlomo Hamelekh (King Solomon), 277, 282–284, 288, 292

shoteh, 359, 362

Sherman, Silber, 151

Silverstein, Yeshaya, 127–131, 148, 166–167, 172–173

Singer, Charles, 5, 42, 210, 324, 437, 438, 446, 448, 455

Siraisi, Nancy, xxiv, 448

Slifkin, Natan, xxix, 7, 39, 84, 139, 155, 273, 297, 443

smallpox, xxvii, 111, 322, 375–380, 383–384, 389, 396, 404, 407, 422

social distancing, 416–418

Sofer, Rabbi Moses (see Ḥatam Sofer)

Sola, Abraham, de, 353

soul, 10, 20, 106, 231, 241, 260, 270, 299, 302, 304, 306, 310, 435, 445, 452, 457, 471, 514

Spanish flu, 404

Spektor, Rabbi Elḥanan, 225–227

sperm, 3, 8–9, 14, 18, 21–23, 25, 29, 32–33, 36–37, 115, 175, 193, 399, 401, 476

spinal cord, 8, 18–19, 129, 244, 436, 438

Spira, Rabbi Ḥayyim Elazar (Minḥat Elazar), 202, 219, 237, 239, 279, 283, 503

Spivak, Dr. Charles (Ḥayyim David), 232–235

spontaneous generation, 7

Sprecher, Dr Stanley (Shlomo), 38–39, 48, 84, 297, 443

Steinberg, Rabbi Dr. Avraham, ix, xii, xiv, xviii–xx, 22, 39, 73, 84, 107, 154,
160–161, 191, 193, 235, 250, 275, 291, 297, 345, 361, 364, 366, 369, 372, 383, 386, 394–395, 399, 405, 421, 432, 443, 460, 466, 473, 505, 523, 532, 538

sterilization, 125, 143–144, 152, 156–161, 173

Stern, Rabbi Gershon, 359–361

Stern, Menachem, 324–325, 433

Stern, Rabbi Moshe, 218

Sternbuch, Rabbi Moshe, 108, 157, 291, 422

Sternfeld, Rabbi Benzion, 223–225

superfecundation, 71–72, 78, 83, 541

superfetation, ix, 70–79, 81–84, 178, 540–541

T

tahara, 422

Targum Yonatan, 90–91, 93, 95, 97, 105, 135–136, 143, 306

Taub, Dr. Ira, 388

Taz (Turei Zahav), 80

tefillin, 250, 390

tefillin, for conjoined twins, 274, 276–282, 291, 295

Teitelbaum, Rabbi Moshe, 194, 499

Tel Talpiyot, 96, 100–101, 106, 127, 142, 146, 150–151, 166, 170, 358–361, 369

Tendler, Rabbi Moshe, xiv, xviii, 73, 157, 187, 194, 291, 303, 365, 368, 372, 432, 450, 452

testicles, 12, 15, 19, 34, 36, 65

Thorndyke, Lynn, 42–43, 139, 334, 340

Tiferet Adam, 16, 21

Tiferet Yisrael, 145–146, 377, 452

Toldot Yeshu, 484–485

Tosafot, 23, 29, 38, 46, 51, 74–75, 100, 124, 138, 170, 177, 194, 280, 283, 446, 449, 452, 478, 481, 483, 488–490, 492, 495, 499, 501–502, 505, 537

trachea, 313, 437, 446–448

Trachtenberg, Joshua, 44–45

Tradition Journal, xix, xxix, 48, 62, 103–104, 109, 112, 150, 159, 162, 167,

183, 195, 230, 361, 375, 385, 400, 404, 466, 475, 486, 532

Trammer, Rabbi Tzvi, 358–359

Trani, Rabbi Yosef, 315–316

treifa, 122, 127–128, 166–169, 275, 280–282, 286–287, 293–294, 312–314, 439, 455–456, 459, 525–526

tum'ah, 61, 128, 147, 172, 182, 218, 226–228, 252–256, 314, 338–339, 341, 467, 469, 471–474

tumtum, 45–46, 52, 56, 60

Turei Zahav (see Taz), 125, 143, 146

twins, x, 70–76, 78–80, 82–84, 87, 97–99, 272–276, 279–280, 283–295, 540–541

tzara'at, 307–309, 311, 315–316, 370, 408–410, 515, 519

Tzitz Eliezer (see Waldenberg, Rabbi Eliezer), xxiv, 21, 24–25, 35, 112, 147, 158, 257, 271, 287, 316, 368, 392, 421, 470, 474–475, 494, 506

tzitzit, 247, 278

Tzur Yaakov, 93, 106, 142

U

umbilical cord, 439

Unterman, Rabbi Yehuda, 147, 471–474

uterus, ix, xxv–xxvii, 5–6, 14, 31, 38–45, 47–49, 51–55, 57, 59–60, 66, 68, 106, 115–116, 121, 123–125, 127–134, 136, 147–148, 151, 153–155, 157–162, 165–173, 242–243, 309, 314–315, 415

V

vaccination, x, xxvii, 111, 322, 374–375, 377–384, 387, 395–396, 402, 404

Valmadonna Trust, 213, 267

Van der Horst, Pieter, Willem, 8, 24, 60, 65, 75

Vayelaket Yosef (journal), 81–82, 91, 94, 97, 101–102, 104–105, 121, 123, 127, 142–144, 146, 148, 154, 156, 164, 166, 168–169, 171

veins, 6, 66, 300, 438

Vesalius, Andreas, 5, 36–37, 43, 55, 209–214, 222, 259–264, 266, 437, 446, 448, 455, 484, 496

Vilna Gaon, 16, 488–489

von Baer, Ernst, 8, 114

Vozner, Rabbi Shmuel, 368, 394, 503–504

W

Waldenberg, Rabbi Eliezer (see Tzitz Eliezer), xiv, 21, 25, 112, 147–149, 271, 287, 316, 368, 382, 392, 394, 401, 474–475, 506

Weidenfeld, Rabbi Dov Ber, 219, 227

Weinreb, Rabbi Ḥayyim Zev, 122, 125, 132, 144–147, 156, 159, 163–164, 173

Weiss, Rav Asher, xiv, 194–195, 383, 388, 405, 416, 421,

Weiss, Rabbi Binyamin Arye, 125–127, 138, 142–144, 147–149, 156, 166

Weiss, David, xxix

Weiss, David Yoel (author *Megadim Hadashim*), 250, 252–253, 255, 269

Weiss, Rabbi Sheftel, 124–125, 150–151, 156, 164, 170–171

Weiss, Rabbi Yitzḥak Yaakov (*Minḥat Yitzḥak*), 133, 303, 317, 494

Well, Rabbi Don, 472

Winkler, Rabbi Mordechai Leib, 361, 369

Wolowelsky, Joel, 112, 475

Wunderbar, Reuben, 513–514, 521

Y

Yisraeli, Rabbi Shaul, 143, 163

Yosef, 87, 89–108, 134–136, 150, 398, 466

yotzei dofen, 479–481, 483

Z

Zachter, Jay, 234, 259, 485

Zahalon, Rabbi Dr. Yaakov (Jacob), 55, 415

Zika, x, xxvii, 393, 395–402

Zilberstein, Rabbi Yitzḥak, xiv, 188–190, 193, 389, 395–396

Zimmels, Rabbi H. J., xiv–xv, xviii, 5, 22, 44, 46, 60, 139, 273, 322, 329, 375, 404, 435, 439, 455, 463, 486, 492–493, 523, 529, 535–536, 540

Zohar, 251, 270, 283, 368